Posttraumatic Stress in Physical Illness

Posttraumatic Stress in Physical Illness

Man Cheung Chung

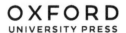

OXFORD
UNIVERSITY PRESS

OXFORD
UNIVERSITY PRESS

Great Clarendon Street, Oxford, OX2 6DP,
United Kingdom

Oxford University Press is a department of the University of Oxford.
It furthers the University's objective of excellence in research, scholarship,
and education by publishing worldwide. Oxford is a registered trade mark of
Oxford University Press in the UK and in certain other countries

Published in the United States of America by Oxford University Press
198 Madison Avenue, New York, NY 10016, United States of America

British Library Cataloguing in Publication Data

Data available

Library of Congress Control Number: 2023942746

ISBN 978-0-19-872732-3

DOI: 10.1093/oso/9780198727323.001.0001

Printed in the UK by
Ashford Colour Press Ltd, Gosport, Hampshire

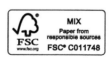

To my beloved Lia and Ethan, thank you for your love and for being who you are.

Contents

List of Abbreviations

ACS	acute coronary syndrome
aOR	adjusted odds ratio
ARDS	acute respiratory distress syndrome
ASD	acute stress disorder
ASD	acute stress syndrome
AWARE	Asian women's action for resilience and empowerment
BMT	bone marrow transplantation
CBSM	cognitive behavioural stress management
CBT	cognitive behavioural therapy
COPD	chronic obstructive pulmonary disease
Covid-19	coronavirus disease 2019
DSM	Diagnostic and statistical manual of mental disorders
EMDR	eye movement desensitisation and reprocessing
ES	epileptic seizures
FoP	fear of cancer progression
GDP	guided disclosure protocol
HIV/AIDS	human immunodeficiency virus
HPA axis	hypothalamic–pituitary–adrenal axis
HRV	heart rate variability
ICD	implantable cardioverter defibrillator
IPV	intimate partner violence
MDD	major depressive disorder
MI	myocardial infarction
MRI	magnetic resonance imaging
MSM	men who have sex with men
NES	non-epileptic seizures
NICE	National Institute for Health and Care Excellence
OR	odds ratio
PNES	psychogenic non-epileptic seizures
PTG	posttraumatic growth
PTSD	posttraumatic stress disorder
PTSS	posttraumatic stress symptoms
SAFE-IPV	safe alternatives for empowered sex for intimate partner violence
SAH	subarachnoid haemorrhage
SARS	severe acute respiratory syndrome
SES	socioeconomic status
TIA	transient ischaemic attack

1

Debates on posttraumatic stress disorder in physical illnesses

In 2013, the fifth edition of the *Diagnostic and statistical manual of mental disorders* (DSM-5) was published (American Psychiatric Association, 2013). Let us remind ourselves of some of the key differences between this version and DSM-IV (American Psychiatric Association, 1994). First, PTSD is no longer part of the classification of anxiety disorders. Instead, it has been placed in a new classification of traumatic and stressor-related disorders. Second, the DSM-5 makes explicit what constitutes a traumatic event, which includes sexual assault in particular. Third, intense fear, helplessness, or horror are no longer the terms used to describe the person's reactions to the traumatic event. Fourth, the DSM-5 describes PTSD reactions in terms of four symptom clusters: re-experiencing, avoidance, negative cognitions, and mood and arousal. These symptoms must last longer than one month; the DSM-5 no longer distinguishes between acute and chronic PTSD. It also specifies dissociative symptoms, namely depersonalisation and derealisation (see Table 1.1).

Despite these differences, the equivalence of psychometric properties between the two versions has been demonstrated (Moodliar et al., 2020). One study even claimed that the DSM-IV symptoms of PTSD can be used to approximate the DSM-5 diagnoses of PTSD. In other words, symptom-level data from previous studies using the DSM-IV criteria can be recoded to make inferences about DSM-5 PTSD (Rosellini et al., 2015). Furthermore, one component remains constant and has been recognised by the trauma research community, namely that PTSD is a chronic, debilitating psychological disorder that people can develop after being exposed to a traumatic life event. This is arguably the most consistent criterion for the diagnosis of PTSD across all the different versions of the DSM (Weathers et al., 2014).

However, the concordance between the two versions outlined above cannot hide the fact that trauma researchers have expressed their concerns and engaged in debates about this modified diagnostic tool both before and after the release of the DSM-5. The emergence of these concerns is not surprising given that psychiatric diagnostic criteria, including those for PTSD, have always been controversial

Posttraumatic Stress in Physical Illness. Man Cheung Chung, Oxford University Press. © Oxford University Press 2024.
DOI: 10.1093/oso/9780198727323.003.0001

Table 1.1 The comparison between DSM-IV and DSM-5 criteria for PTSD

DSM-IV diagnostic criteria for PTSD	DSM-5 diagnostic criteria for PTSD
A. The person has been exposed to a traumatic event in which both of the following were present: (1) the person experienced, witnessed, or was confronted with an event or events that involved actual or threatened death or serious injury, or a threat to the physical integrity of self or others (2) the person's response involved intense fear, helplessness, or horror. Note: In children, this may be expressed instead by disorganized or agitated behaviour	A. Exposure to actual or threatened death, serious injury, or sexual violence in one (or more) of the following ways: 1. Directly experiencing the traumatic event(s). 2. Witnessing, in person, the event(s) as it occurred to others. 3. Learning that the traumatic event(s) occurred to a close family member or close friend. In cases of actual or threatened death of a family member or friend, the event(s) must have been violent or accidental. 4. Experiencing repeated or extreme exposure to aversive details of the traumatic event(s) (e.g. first responders collecting human remains: police officers repeatedly exposed to details of child abuse). Note: Criterion A4 does not apply to exposure through electronic media, television, movies, or pictures, unless this exposure is work related.
B. The traumatic event is persistently reexperienced in one (or more) of the following ways: (1) recurrent and intrusive distressing recollections of the event, including images, thoughts, or perceptions. Note: In young children, repetitive play may occur in which themes or aspects of the trauma are expressed. (2) recurrent distressing dreams of the event. Note: In children, there may be frightening dreams without recognizable content. (3) acting or feeling as if the traumatic event were recurring (includes a sense of reliving the experience, illusions, hallucinations, and dissociative flashback episodes, including those that occur on awakening or when intoxicated). **Note:** In young children, trauma-specific reenactment may occur. (4) intense psychological distress at exposure to internal or external cues that symbolize or resemble an aspect of the traumatic event	B. Presence of one (or more) of the following intrusion symptoms associated with the traumatic event(s), beginning after the traumatic event(s) occurred: 1. Recurrent, involuntary, and intrusive distressing memories of the traumatic event(s). Note: In children older than 6 years, repetitive play may occur in which themes or aspects of the traumatic event(s) are expressed. 2. Recurrent distressing dreams in which the content and/or affect of the dream are related to the traumatic event(s). Note: In children, there may be frightening dreams without recognizable content. 3. Dissociative reactions (e.g. flashbacks) in which the individual feels or acts as if the traumatic event(s) were recurring. (Such reactions may occur on a continuum, with the most extreme expression being a complete loss of awareness of present surroundings.) Note: In children, trauma-specific reenactment may occur in play. 4. Intense or prolonged psychological distress at exposure to internal or external cues that symbolize or resemble an aspect of the traumatic event(s).

Table 1.1 Continued

DSM-IV diagnostic criteria for PTSD	DSM-5 diagnostic criteria for PTSD
(5) physiological reactivity on exposure to internal or external cues that symbolize or resemble an aspect of the traumatic event	5. Marked physiological reactions to internal or external cues that symbolize or resemble an aspect of the traumatic event(s).
C. Persistent avoidance of stimuli associated with the trauma and numbing of general responsiveness (not present before the trauma), as indicated by three (or more) of the following: (1) efforts to avoid thoughts, feelings, or conversations associated with the trauma (2) efforts to avoid activities, places, or people that arouse recollections of the trauma (3) inability to recall an important aspect of the trauma (4) markedly diminished interest or participation in significant activities (5) feeling of detachment or estrangement from others (6) restricted range of affect (e.g. unable to have loving feelings) (7) sense of a foreshortened future (e.g. does not expect to have a career, marriage, children, or a normal life span)	C. Persistent avoidance of stimuli associated with the traumatic event(s), beginning after the traumatic event(s) occurred, as evidenced by one or both of the following: 1. Avoidance of or efforts to avoid distressing memories, thoughts, or feelings about or closely associated with the traumatic event(s). 2. Avoidance of or efforts to avoid external reminders (people, places, conversations, activities, objects, situations) that arouse distressing memories, thoughts, or feelings about or closely associated with the traumatic event(s).
D. Persistent symptoms of increased arousal (not present before the trauma), as indicated by two (or more) of the following: (1) difficulty falling or staying asleep (2) irritability or outbursts of anger (3) difficulty concentrating (4) hypervigilance (5) exaggerated startle response	D. Negative alterations in cognitions and mood associated with the traumatic event(s), beginning or worsening after the traumatic event(s) occurred, as evidenced by two (or more) of the following: 1. Inability to remember an important aspect of the traumatic event(s) (typically due to dissociative amnesia and not to other factors such as head injury, alcohol, or drugs). 2. Persistent and exaggerated negative beliefs or expectations about oneself, others, or the world (e.g. 'I am bad', 'No one can be trusted', 'The world is completely dangerous', 'My whole nervous system is permanently ruined'). 3. Persistent, distorted cognitions about the cause or consequences of the traumatic event(s) that lead the individual to blame himself/herself or others. 4. Persistent negative emotional state (e.g. fear, horror, anger, guilt, or shame).

(continued)

Table 1.1 Continued

DSM-IV diagnostic criteria for PTSD	DSM-5 diagnostic criteria for PTSD
	5. Markedly diminished interest or participation in significant activities.
	6. Feelings of detachment or estrangement from others.
	7. Persistent inability to experience positive emotions (e.g. inability to experience happiness, satisfaction, or loving feelings).
E. Duration of the disturbance (symptoms in Criteria B, C, and D) is more than 1 month.	E. Marked alterations in arousal and reactivity associated with the traumatic event(s), beginning or worsening after the traumatic event(s) occurred, as evidenced by two (or more) of the following: 1. Irritable behaviour and angry outbursts (with little or no provocation) typically expressed as verbal or physical aggression toward people or objects. 2. Reckless or self-destructive behaviour. 3. Hypervigilance. 4. Exaggerated startle response. 5. Problems with concentration. 6. Sleep disturbance (e.g. difficulty falling or staying asleep or restless sleep).
F. The disturbance causes clinically significant distress or impairment in social, occupational, or other important areas of functioning.	F. Duration of the disturbance (criteria B, C, D, and E) is more than 1 month. G. The disturbance causes clinically significant distress or impairment in social, occupational, or other important areas of functioning. H. The disturbance is not attributable to the physiological effects of a substance (e.g., medication, alcohol) or another medical condition.
Specify if: Acute: if duration of symptoms is less than 3 months Chronic: if duration of symptoms is 3 months or more Specify if: With delayed onset: if onset of symptoms is at least 6 months after the stressor	*Specify* whether: With dissociative symptoms: The individual's symptoms meet the criteria for posttraumatic stress disorder, and in addition, in response to the stressor, the individual experiences persistent or recurrent symptoms of either of the following: 1. Depersonalization: Persistent or recurrent experiences of feeling detached from, and as if one were an outside observer of, one's mental processes or body (e.g. feeling as though one were in a dream; feeling a sense of unreality of self or body or of time moving slowly).

Table 1.1 Continued

DSM-IV diagnostic criteria for PTSD	DSM-5 diagnostic criteria for PTSD
	2. Derealization: Persistent or recurrent experiences of unreality of surroundings (e.g. the world around the individual is experienced as unreal, dreamlike, distant, or distorted).
	Note: To use this subtype, the dissociative symptoms must not be attributable to the physiological effects of a substance (e.g. blackouts, behaviour during alcohol intoxication) or another medical condition (e.g. complex partial seizures).
	Specify if:
	With delayed expression: If the full diagnostic criteria are not met until at least 6 months after the event (although the onset and expression of some symptoms may be immediate).

(North et al., 2009). The aim of this chapter is to capture some of these concerns. Before doing so, it is worth noting that, of all the responses to the diagnostic criteria for PTSD, the issue of PTSD as a label used to pathologise normal stress (McHugh & Treisman, 2007; Summerfield, 2001) does not seem to take precedence over other issues we will explore in this chapter. Despite this 'anti-pathologising' stance, trauma researchers seem increasingly sympathetic to the idea that PTSD can cause psychological difficulties that require psychological or medical attention. It is not a type of 'normal' stress that naturally resolves or self-corrects without having lasting detrimental psychological effects on the individuals affected. It impairs people's ability to adapt (e.g. Brewin, 2003; Shalev, 2003) and leads to long-term psychological difficulties (e.g. Morgan et al., 2003; Norris & Slone, 2007) and serious medical problems (Schnurr & Green, 2004). There is also evidence that there are biological patterns that are uniquely associated with PTSD compared with social anxiety disorder, specific phobia, and depression (Etkin & Wager, 2007; Kemp et al., 2007; Lanius et al., 2007; Whalley et al., 2009; Yehuda et al., 2004).

Criterion A

Concerns have been raised about the usefulness of criterion A for PTSD. It has been argued that this criterion, at least for DSM-IV, is too subjective; therefore, it needs to be defined more explicitly or objectively for the DSM-5

(Bensimon, Solomon, & Horesh, 2013). This narrower or tighter definition along with stringent symptom criteria would eliminate misconceptions about PTSD (Spitzer et al., 2007). In addition, a narrow definition is preferred, as a broad definition could lead to PTSD being associated with other disorders such as depression, generalised anxiety disorder, panic disorder, and substance abuse (Brewin et al., 2009; Friedman, 2013; Weathers & Keane, 2007).

Defining trauma, however, is by no means an easy task, and in fact has been a struggle in the last few versions of the DSMs (Weathers & Keane, 2007). Some researchers have therefore questioned why we should spend so much energy on tightening it up. After all, the change in Criterion A of the DSM-5 has not had a significant impact on our understanding of the phenomenology of PTSD (Roberts et al., 2012). Furthermore, the DSM-5 definition of trauma does not seem to be a good predictor of who would develop PTSD symptoms (Larsen & Berenbaum, 2017).

Criterion A events represent ambiguous, vaguely defined stressors that can cause different psychiatric comorbid symptoms in people. They are neither necessary nor sufficient to trigger PTSD (Rosen et al., 2008). Furthermore, it is not clear whether multiple criterion A events can be included in the assessment of PTSD symptoms (Kilpatrick et al., 2009, 2013). Criterion A is only useful in describing the usual context of PTSD, but not in contributing to diagnostic precision itself (i.e. the predictive value of criterion A for PTSD criteria B–D according to DSM-IV is low). Removing criterion A and focusing on the core PTSD symptoms does not affect the accuracy, selectivity, or validity of the PTSD diagnosis; therefore, focusing on the diagnosis of PTSD based on the predictive values of the PTSD symptoms is the way forward. Moreover, it is more useful to study the interaction between genetic and environmental factors than to specify triggering events (Brewin et al., 2009). All these controversies have led some researchers to conclude that the definition of trauma should be abolished altogether (Brewin et al., 2009; Karam et al., 2010).

However, this radical idea was not adopted in the DSM-5. In fact, the definition of trauma has become even narrower or more specific than in the previous version. In the DSM-5, events classified as traumatic must involve 'actual or threatened death, serious injury, or sexual violence' in one or more of the following ways: (1) directly experienced, (2) personally witnessed, (3) experienced as having happened to a close family member or friend (in the case of actual or threatened death of a family member or friend, the event must have been violent or accidental), or (4) experienced through repeated or extreme exposure to aversive details of the event.

The change in criterion A has led to debates about its impact on the prevalence rate of PTSD. One study shows that with the changes in traumatic stressors, estimates of current PTSD prevalence for the DSM-5 diagnostic algorithm were 0.4–1.8% points higher than for the DSM-IV (Elhai et al., 2012). This is at odds with other literature suggesting that the DSM-5 prevalence rate is somewhat lower than that of DSM-IV. For example, a study based on the criteria of DSM-IV showed that 98% met a criterion A1 event, but 89% met DSM-5 criterion A (Calhoun et al., 2012). Another study showed that (based on DSM-5 criterion) lifetime PTSD, PTSD in the last 12 and 6 months were 8.3%, 4.7%, and 3.8% respectively. They were slightly lower than the scores on DSM-IV (9.8%, 6.3%, 4.7%). The main reason for meeting the DSM-IV PTSD criteria but not the DSM-5 criteria is the exclusion of sudden unexpected death due to non-violence as a criterion A event in the DSM-5 (Kilpatrick et al., 2013). In other words, using the more restrictive definition of trauma in criterion A for DSM-5, where events involving indirect exposure to the death of a loved one are due to violent or accidental causes, the number of individuals eligible for a PTSD diagnosis decreased by 23% in one sample and 15% in another (Domino et al., 2021). This suggests that there are differences in the development of symptoms depending on the type of death. Those who experienced a sudden violent death tended to screen significantly more positive for possible PTSD than those who experienced the unexpected, non-violent death of a loved one. In other words, while a sudden violent death might be associated with increased PTSD symptoms, the unexpectedness or non-violent nature of the death was not (Kloep et al., 2014).

Life-threatening physical illness as a traumatic event

The DSM-IV has raised awareness of the importance of considering physical illness as a traumatic event for both patients and their families. For DSM-IV, a sudden, unexpected, potentially life-threatening illness (e.g. a heart attack) or diagnosis of a life-threatening illness (e.g. cancer) could broaden and enrich the study of PTSD (Buckley et al., 2004; Mundy & Baum, 2004; Tedstone & Tarrier, 2003). Learning that one's child has been diagnosed with a life-threatening illness, or learning of the sudden, unexpected death (e.g. heart attack) of a loved one, could also be considered traumatic events. It was claimed that PTSD was uniquely associated with cardiovascular disease, respiratory disease, chronic pain conditions, gastrointestinal disease, and cancer. This association persisted even after adjustment for sociodemographic factors and other mental disorders (Sareen et al., 2007). The enduring somatic threat model of PTSD may reflect this robust relationship, claiming that people experience PTSD life symptoms after a life-threatening illness because they are sensitised to the cues of persistent threat in the body (Edmondson et al., 2018). Early identification and treatment of PTSD associated with physical illness is warranted (Sareen et al., 2007).

On the contrary, the DSM-5 states, 'A life-threatening illness or debilitating medical condition is not necessarily considered a traumatic event. Medical incidents that qualify as traumatic events involve sudden, catastrophic events (e.g. waking during surgery, anaphylactic shock)' (DSM-5, p. 274). These events are thought to include heart attack, life-threatening asthma attack, severe acute respiratory syndrome (SARS), diabetic shock hypoglycaemia, stroke, and haemorrhage. However, it is debatable whether a diagnosis of cancer or HIV/AIDS could also constitute trauma, as such a diagnosis is a sudden and catastrophic medical event and the information received can be very stressful for the patient and their relatives (Kangas, 2013).

The DSM-5 also states that a traumatic event may be witnessing an unnatural death or medical catastrophe in a child (e.g. a life-threatening haemorrhage). Seemingly, witnessing their loved ones experiencing or dying from life-threatening heart attack, asthma attack, diabetic shock hypoglycaemia, stroke, or haemorrhage could constitute traumatic events. However, it is debatable whether witnessing or learning that a loved one has been diagnosed with cancer or HIV/AIDS can also be a traumatic event, even if such an event is sudden and catastrophic.

Criterion A2

With regard to criterion A2 of DSM-IV (i.e. the intense fear, helplessness, or horror one may experience in response to trauma), some trauma researchers have defended the importance of maintaining and redefining this criterion (Boals & Schuettler, 2009; Osei-Bonsu et al., 2012), for example by replacing the word 'or' with 'and' in the definition (Kubany et al., 2010). On the other hand, critics have argued that this criterion does not contribute to the accuracy of PTSD diagnoses (Adler et al., 2008; Breslau & Kessler, 2001; Schnurr et al., 2002). Some trauma victims may indeed experience intense peritraumatic emotional responses other than fear, helplessness, or horror. Instead, they may exhibit amnesia as part of their peritraumatic emotional experiences

(O'Donnell et al., 2010). In other words, not all traumatic events are fear-based (Schnurr, 2013).

Some trauma researchers have even argued that criterion A2 should be removed because it is mainly relevant for single traumatic events and not for chronic national traumatic events (e.g. ongoing political or terrorist conflicts) (Bensimon, Solomon, & Horesh, 2013). It should also be removed due to its redundancy, that is individuals who met criterion A2 tended to report higher severity of PTSD symptoms, even when trauma exposure was controlled for (Boals & Schuettler, 2009; Osei-Bonsu et al., 2012; Schnurr et al., 2002). Criterion A2 has been shown to have a high negative predictive value, that is the absence of A2 was a good indicator of the possible absence of PTSD (Osei-Bonsu et al., 2012). In other words, this criterion has no added value and its removal would simplify the diagnostic system and make it more efficient. The close relationship between this criterion and the severity of PTSD symptoms could mean that this criterion is a clinically significant factor that should be considered for indicating significant posttraumatic stress symptoms (Resick & Miller, 2009). The DSM-5 working group acknowledged the inherent problem with criterion A2, noting that for many trauma victims—for example soldiers and firefighters—fear, helplessness, or horror were simply irrelevant during their trauma exposure, partly because of their professional training (Friedman, Resick, Bryant, & Brewin, 2011). This criterion was later removed from the DSM-5 (Friedman, 2013).

Symptom clusters for PTSD (criteria B–E) and the prevalence rate of PTSD

As mentioned earlier, the change in criterion A could have an impact on the prevalence rate of PTSD. The clustering of PTSD symptoms (criteria B–E) in the DSM-5 could also have this impact. Some critics have argued that symptom clustering is controversial because it would only lead to a narrow definition of PTSD, which is problematic and should be avoided. Symptom clustering should be defined more broadly, that is including other non-specific symptoms following trauma (van der Kolk et al., 2005). A broader construct of PTSD would therefore include clinically important and relevant symptoms and thus improve the reliability of PTSD diagnosis (Kilpatrick, 2013). However, the inclusion of non-specific symptoms means an overlap of symptoms of other disorders, which is a major problem in understanding PTSD as a distinct clinical syndrome.

Over the years, various models of PTSD symptom clusters have emerged. Which model is best suited to represent PTSD as a clinical entity is not yet clear. Agreement on the exact number and type of PTSD factors has yet to be reached (Armour et al., 2016). It has been argued that the latent three-factor structure of PTSD symptoms from DSM-IV is not satisfactory, which was made clear using confirmatory factor analysis (Friedman, 2013). For example, it was problematic to group avoidance and emotional numbing together as one symptom cluster in criterion C of DSM-IV. Avoidance and numbing differ in their relationship to psychological outcomes (Malta et al., 2009; Taylor et al., 2003) and are distinct groups of PTSD symptoms that inherently imply different causal mechanisms. Pooling them would have missed important information that would help us understand the aetiology of PTSD (Asmundson & Taylor, 2009). To this end, it has been postulated that it would be best for the DSM-5 to reformulate the symptom clusters into re-experiencing, active avoidance, emotional numbing, and hyperarousal (Bensimon, Levine, et al., 2013). The DSM-5 has adopted a four-factor model but has not endorsed the symptom clusters mentioned above.

The idea of dividing PTSD symptoms into four factors rather than three was advocated some time ago. A four-factor model of numbing advocated grouping the factors of intrusion, avoidance, numbing, and hyperarousal (King et al., 1998). Subsequently, the four-factor model of dysphoria was developed (Simms et al., 2002). This is quite similar to the numbing model, except that the three hyperarousal symptoms of sleep problems, irritability, and concentration difficulties have been combined with the numbing symptoms to form a dysphoria factor. This model is thus composed of intrusion, avoidance, dysphoria, and two items of the hyperarousal factor (Carragher et al., 2010; Williams et al., 2011). There is evidence to support both the numbing (Armour et al., 2011; Asmundson et al., 2000; Elhai et al., 2009; Hoyt & Yeater, 2010; Kassam-Adams et al., 2010; Mansfield et al., 2010; Naifeh et al., 2008; Saul et al., 2008) and dysphoria models (Armour & Shevlin, 2010; Boelen et al., 2008; Carragher et al., 2010; Elklit et al., 2010; Hetzel-Riggin, 2009; Miller et al., 2013; Naifeh et al., 2010; Olff et al., 2009; Yufik & Simms, 2010). Using primary care patients exposed to trauma, confirmatory factor analyses confirmed good agreement with the DSM-5 PTSD dysphoria model as well as the DSM-5 numbing model (Contractor et al., 2014).

However, it has been noted that dysphoria is associated with negative affectivity (Charak et al., 2014), which also occurs in mood and anxiety disorders. Dysphoria is also more strongly associated with depression and generalised anxiety than with PTSD symptoms (Grant et al., 2008; Gros et al.,

2010; Palmieri et al., 2007; Simms et al., 2002). In other words, dysphoria is a non-specific component of PTSD, as opposed to intrusion, avoidance, and hyperarousal; therefore, to improve the diagnosis of PTSD, dysphoria should be de-emphasised. To understand the phenomenology of PTSD, one should focus only on the specific symptoms (Brewin et al., 2009; Simms et al., 2002; Watson, 2009), which calls into question the usefulness of dysphoria. Despite this problem, the dysphoria factor was retained in a five-factor model, with the hyperarousal factor separated off, into the dysphoric arousal and anxious arousal factors (Elhai et al., 2011). There is evidence that this five-factor model was significantly better than the two four-factor models mentioned above (Armour et al., 2013; Elhai et al., 2011; Wang et al., 2011). To extend the factor further, a hybrid seven-factor model encompassing re-experiencing, avoidance, negative affect, anhedonia, externalising behaviours, anxious arousal, and dysphoric arousal has been proposed and appears to have received some empirical support for its validity (Armour et al., 2015).

It is clear that these models have an influence on the emergence of the DSM-5 for PTSD (Charak et al., 2014). The DSM-5 model is also a four-factor model, defined by the criteria (B) re-experiencing, (C) avoidance, (D) negative cognitions and mood, and (E) arousal. Re-experiencing symptoms are characterised by spontaneous memories of the traumatic event, recurrent dreams related to the event, flashbacks or other intense or persistent psychological distress. Avoidance behaviour is characterised by the avoidance of distressing memories, thoughts, feelings, or external reminders of the event. Negative cognitions and moods are characterised by persistent and distorted feelings of self- or other-blame, alienation from others, markedly diminished interest in activities, and difficulty remembering important aspects of the event. Finally, arousal refers to aggressive, risky or reckless or self-destructive behaviour, sleep disturbances, and hypervigilance. It is worth noting that, to address the ambiguity of 'irritability or angry outbursts' in DSM-IV, angry feelings have been included with the other negative cognitions in criterion D of the DSM-5, and irritable behaviour or angry outbursts have been included in criterion E. These changes are attempts to distinguish between angry mood and angry behaviour (Friedman, 2013) and are consistent with the literature that argues for the importance of examining the specificity of anger in PTSD (Koffel et al., 2012; Orth & Wieland, 2006). This DSM-5 PTSD model has been shown to be a better fit than the dysphoria model (Biehn et al., 2013). While the current DSM-5 PTSD model has been considered an improvement over DSM-IV and a good representation of the latent structure of PTSD (Armour et al., 2016), the DSM-5 model may still not represent the true factor structure underlying PTSD (Gentes et al., 2014).

Some researchers have argued that the change in symptom clusters in the DSM-5 has led to a significant reduction in PTSD cases and a significantly lower rate of comorbid PTSD, especially among people with depression (Forbes et al., 2011). One study showed that, based on DSM-5 criteria, 49.3% of participants met criteria for PTSD, while 60.4% reported having PTSD using DSM-IV criteria (Schnyder et al., 2015). This means that the DSM-IV may have led to an overdiagnosis of PTSD (Forbes et al., 2011). However, one study showed that 50% met criteria for PTSD based on DSM-IV criteria, while 52% met DSM-5 criteria (Calhoun et al., 2012). Although the difference was not large, the DSM-5 showed a substantially higher prevalence than DSM-IV, when the actual DSM-IV prevalence ranged from 5% to 11% (Calhoun et al., 2012). Similarly, another study found a higher PTSD rate of 50% based on DSM-5 symptom criteria than that of 44% using DSM-IV criteria (Schaal et al., 2015). Regardless, there was a lower prevalence of PTSD compared to DSM-IV when the symptom requirements were one, one, three and three symptoms from criteria B, C, D, and E, respectively. However, when D (negative alternations in cognitions and mood) and E (marked alternations in arousal and reactivity) were changed to two symptoms each, as stated in the DSM-5, the prevalence estimates became more compatible (Miller et al., 2013).

Despite these differences between DSM-IV and DSM-5 in PTSD prevalence rates, some researchers have argued that with the changes in DSM-5 symptom criteria from DSM-IV, a large impact on PTSD prevalence rates is quite unlikely (Frueh et al., 2010). This claim has been supported by a review paper (Zoellner et al., 2013), an online study (Kilpatrick et al., 2013) and a study that found the same PTSD prevalence rate of 56% using DSM-IV and DSM-5 (Kuester et al., 2017). Nevertheless, this claim has been disputed elsewhere (Calhoun et al., 2012).

Criterion D in the DSM-5

A few words must be said about criterion D in the DSM-5. The DSM-5 focuses on a range of dysregulations of emotional states, including fear, anger, guilt, and shame. Unlike DSM-IV, fear is one of the emotional states rather than a dominant state. One reason for considering the role of emotional dysregulation is that PTSD is an affect systems disorder (Stone, 1992) that can be conceptualised in two pathways. One is referred to as the fear conditioning/stress sensitisation/kindling pathway. Following a traumatic event, people experience fear and symptoms of re-experiencing, which then trigger a sensitisation/

kindling process—a complex process involving the interplay of psychological distress, psychophysiological reactivity, and neurological responses, leading to the emergence of general emotional dysregulation including anger, grief, numbing, and dissociation. Kindling is the process by which generalised epileptic seizures are triggered by repeated electrophysiological stimulation in the brain, particularly in the amygdala. People involved in this pathway have usually not experienced childhood trauma, that is they are not predisposed to distorted neurodevelopment of emotion regulation systems resulting from childhood trauma.

The second pathway is called early life vulnerabilities with the stress diathesis model as the important starting point. An impoverished childhood environment resulting from problematic attachment styles, childhood abuse or trauma leads to the development of distorted emotion and arousal regulation systems and associated emotional dysregulation. People are then unable to regulate physiological arousal in fear, anger, guilt and shame. When they experience a traumatic event later in life, there is an exacerbation of emotional dysregulation, including PTSD symptoms associated with that event (Lanius et al., 2010).

Although the validity of these previous models remains to be empirically tested, there is evidence that difficulties in emotion regulation are associated with PTSD symptom severity. Increased difficulties in accepting one's emotions were associated with increased avoidance and hyperarousal symptoms. Similarly, greater difficulty accepting one's emotions and using effective emotion regulation strategies to cope with stress were associated with distorted cognitions and a cluster of mood symptoms (criterion D in DSM-5) (O'Bryan et al., 2015). This new criterion D has been shown to have relatively high sensitivity (0.76–0.91), specificity (0.70–0.75), positive predictive power (0.75–0.76), and negative predictive power (0.75–0.89). It is useful for clinicians to determine the likelihood of meeting criteria for PTSD (Schnyder et al., 2015).

Dissociation in the DSM-5

In addition to the changes in the definition of trauma (criterion A) and symptom clusters (Criteria B-E), the role of dissociative symptoms characterised by depersonalisation or derealisation has also been highlighted in the DSM-5 (Friedman, 2013). This is not surprising, as the link between dissociation and PTSD is widely recognised (Dalenberg et al., 2012; Frewen et al., 2015; van der Kolk et al., 1996; Waelde et al., 2005; Wolf et al., 2012). This dissociative subtype of PTSD involves chronic dissociative experiences that can be triggered by stressful or traumatic events. They are chronic and can persist for decades after exposure to a traumatic event (Chu et al., 1999; Dalenberg et al., 2012; van der Kolk et al., 1996; Wolf et al., 2012). The DSM-5 PTSD symptom clusters are closely related to this dissociative subtype of PTSD (Carlson et al., 2012; Ginzburg et al., 2009; Spiegel, 2012; Steuwe et al., 2012). Dissociation has been associated with hyperarousal (Bryant & Panasetis, 2005; Ginzburg et al., 2006; Krystal et al., 1995; Sterlini & Bryant, 2002), dysfunctional avoidance strategies aimed at coping with PTSD (Briere et al., 2010; Waelde et al., 2009), and emotional numbing (Frewen et al., 2008; Lanius et al., 2010). This leads to changes in arousal and reactivity with specific underlying mechanisms (Armour et al., 2014). Individuals with depersonalisation/derealisation symptoms respond differently to cognitive behavioural therapy for PTSD than individuals with PTSD only (Lanius et al., 2012; Spiegel, 2012).

This strong link between PTSD symptoms and dissociation has led some researchers to conclude that PTSD should be considered a dissociative disorder, that is PTSD symptoms are expressed through dissociative processes (e.g. Twaite & Rodriguez-Srednicki, 2004). However, this conclusion is controversial because for some researchers dissociation and PTSD are two separate clinical entities, although they often coexist (Marshall et al., 1999; Simeon et al., 2008). Dissociative symptoms do not occur in all patients, but they are much more likely to occur if they also have PTSD (Carlson et al., 2012). Nevertheless, people with PTSD who have dissociative symptoms are qualitatively different from those who do not. There are also differences in psychiatric symptoms between well-adjusted trauma individuals, individuals with PTSD only, and those with PTSD/dissociation. The group with PTSD/dissociation had higher scores on all PTSD symptoms than the well-adjusted group. They also scored higher than the other two groups on all depersonalisation/derealisation symptoms, somatic conversion symptoms, borderline traits, and some schizophrenic symptoms (Blevins et al., 2014). Individuals with a dissociative subtype of PTSD also had a higher number of comorbid Axis I disorders and a significant history of childhood abuse and neglect (Steuwe et al., 2012).

People with a dissociative subtype of PTSD also differ in terms of neurobiological mechanisms (Griffin et al., 1997; Lanius et al., 2010; Putnam et al., 1996). In relation to the emotional dysregulation mentioned earlier, people with this subtype appear to have functional and structural brain changes and to overcontrol their emotional states. Such over-modulation is mediated by prefrontal inhibition of the limbic regions. This is different from PTSD re-experiencing or hyperarousal symptoms, a form of emotion dysregulation in which individuals tend to undercontrol their emotional states. This under-modulation is mediated by a problem of prefrontal inhibition of activity in limbic regions (Friedman, Resick, Bryant, Strain, et al., 2011). However, more research is needed, especially to understand the neurobiological mechanisms underlying dissociative subtypes of PTSD and their treatment (Lanius et al., 2012; Steuwe et al., 2012).

Impairment of functional capacity

While it is important to focus on what has changed, it is also intriguing to point out what has not changed. Criteria F and G (impairment in social, occupational, or other important areas of functioning) for DSM-IV and DSM-5, respectively, are virtually identical. The reason that no changes have been made to these criteria could be that trauma researchers are largely in agreement with the status of these criteria. However, another reason could be that they tend to focus mainly on subjectively reported symptoms rather than objective indicators of impairment of functioning. Nevertheless, the importance of revising and clarifying this criterion has been pointed out. Some researchers have even argued that, after meeting the criteria for trauma, criterion F/G is probably the next important factor to be examined (Gaughwin, 2009). It points to a level of clinical significance by which victims can be distinguished as suffering from posttraumatic stress or posttraumatic stress 'disorder' (Friedman et al., 2016; Garcia & Mullen, 2008; McNally, 2009).

Should PTSD be part of an anxiety disorder?

Having discussed issues about the diagnostic criteria for PTSD, let us now turn to the debate over the fact that PTSD is no longer part of the classification of anxiety disorders in the DSM-5. For some trauma researchers, considering PTSD as a clinical syndrome distinct from anxiety disorder is a dubious and highly problematic proposition, as well as an alarming change. There is simply no evidence to justify such a change. The main symptoms of PTSD are so intertwined with the symptoms of anxiety or mood disorders that they should not be separated (Brown et al., 2001; Kessler et al., 2005). For example, PTSD is characterised by 'alarms' associated with anxious apprehension (e.g. intrusion and nightmares) (Jones & Barlow, 1990). PTSD avoidance overlaps with phobic and anxious avoidance. Intrusive thoughts also occur in people who have generalised anxiety disorder, obsessive-compulsive disorder, panic disorder, and social phobia (Bryant et al., 2011; Friedman, Resick, Bryant, Strain, et al., 2011; Hackmann et al., 2000; Salkovskis, 1985). Hyperarousal is a symptom that overlaps with symptoms of anxiety disorders such as insomnia, irritability, difficulty concentrating, and startle responses (Zoellner et al., 2011). Social phobia is considered one of the most common comorbid emotional disorders in individuals who meet criteria for PTSD (Gallagher & Brown, 2015). People with anxiety disorders tend to report elevated fear when responding to stimuli that signal a threat. They also experience heightened anxiety in situations where they anticipate aversive stimuli and are confronted with non-specific stressors or stressors that have personal meaning to them. These features bear strong similarities to PTSD reactions, suggesting that PTSD should be conceptualised as an anxiety disorder (Craske et al., 2009).

But just because the symptoms of PTSD and anxiety disorders overlap, does this mean that PTSD should be classified as an anxiety disorder? This is similar to saying that Chinese people should be classified as Korean just because they share physical similarities with Koreans. This is absurd, one could argue. Chinese are 'uniquely' or 'distinctly' different from Koreans. Indeed, one could argue that the problem of symptom overlap, that is lack of specificity, is precisely the argument for distinguishing between PTSD and anxiety disorder (Brewin, 2003; Brewin et al., 2009; McHugh & Treisman, 2007; Spitzer et al., 2007). Otherwise, a diagnosis of PTSD raises the question of whether the patient is really suffering from PTSD and not from an anxiety disorder. As an aside, this uncertainty in diagnosis would have implications for lawyers who might rely on clearly differentiated diagnoses and an identified link between symptoms and behaviour to defend their clients (Zoellner et al., 2013).

The question arises as to how PTSD can be distinguished from anxiety disorder when there is considerable overlap between the two. In fact, the symptoms of anxiety disorder are only some of the symptoms that are comorbid with the symptoms of PTSD. For example, major depressive disorder is another common comorbid emotional disorder in individuals who meet criteria for PTSD (Gallagher & Brown, 2015). There is evidence of specificity between PTSD factors and depression types. Somatic and non-somatic depression factors were more strongly associated with PTSD-related dysphoria and mood/cognition factors than with re-experiencing and avoidance factors (Biehn et al., 2013; Contractor et al., 2014). Similarly, network analysis revealed bridging symptoms between PTSD and depression by finding the highest edge-weights for sleep disturbance, irritability and difficulty concentrating in both disorders, supporting the role of dysphoria-related symptoms in PTSD/MDD comorbidity (Afzali et al., 2017). People who meet symptom criteria for

PTSD and major depressive disorder have about three-fifths of the symptoms in common (Olbert et al., 2014). The two disorders are not independent of each other, but are determined in part by genetic susceptibility to experiencing stressful life events (Horwitz & Wakefield, 2007). In addition to major depression and anxiety disorders, chronic pain, neurocognitive disorders resulting from traumatic brain injury, substance use disorders, and personality disorders are also considered common comorbidities of PTSD (Young et al., 2014).

In other words, how can PTSD be conceptualised as a distinct clinical syndrome when it overlaps with extensive comorbidities that have their own underlying biopsychosocial vulnerabilities (Lockwood & Forbes, 2014)? Would the comorbidity of PTSD make this validity unattainable (Barglow, 2012), given the need to establish clear boundaries to ensure the validity of a diagnosis? The diagnostic criteria for PTSD are becoming increasingly non-specific. Distinguishing between PTSD and other disorders is becoming increasingly difficult (Brewin et al., 2009; Rosen et al., 2010; Simms et al., 2002; Watson, 2009), although it is claimed that the differential diagnosis of PTSD can be improved by emphasising symptoms specific to PTSD and attenuating symptoms common to many mental disorders (Rosen et al., 2008). It has been concluded that PTSD symptoms are unlikely to help improve differential diagnosis (Koffel et al., 2012). The diagnostic reliability of PTSD is therefore questioned (Resick et al., 2012).

One might succumb to the fact that overlapping symptoms will always be an obstacle to differentiating PTSD from other disorders. This is partly because the DSM-5 retains the descriptive phenomenological approach. Such an approach is based on surface features with limited reference to underlying pathophysiology or psychotherapeutics. As a result, it lacks explanatory power and construct validity. Insistence on such an approach would only lead to overlapping syndromes and blurring of boundaries between diagnostic entities, resulting in overdiagnosis of 'comorbidities' (Eppel, 2013). Alternative ways of conceptualising PTSD are therefore needed.

Alternative conceptualisation of PTSD symptoms

It has been recommended that symptoms of different disorders be prioritised according to primary (e.g. unique markers), secondary (core and essential symptoms), and tertiary levels (common and cross-diagnosis symptoms). In this way, clinicians and other professionals (e.g. lawyers) can find these different levels of symptoms useful for their own purposes (Young et al., 2014).

However, one could argue that the above proposal is simply another form of symptom classification. It does not really solve the problem of the overlap of PTSD with other mental health symptoms. Therefore, it does not help to distinguish PTSD from other disorders.

An alternative way advocates not losing sight of the fact that PTSD results from adverse life events, the impact of which can affect people's predispositional vulnerability (diathesis–stress model) to psychological difficulties. The causal mechanisms underlying this diathesis–stress interaction are different for different individuals in terms of the expression of PTSD symptoms. Anxiety is only one of the symptoms resulting from this diathesis–stress interaction. Other symptoms include those grouped under the terms acute stress disorder, adjustment disorder, complex PTSD and traumatic grief. These symptoms are qualitatively different from other disorders. One consequence is that one should focus on a spectrum of PTSD (Resick & Miller, 2009).

One must not undermine the need for trauma to precede the onset of PTSD symptoms (Blanchard et al., 1995; Mayou et al., 2001; O'Donnell et al., 2004; Shalev et al., 1998). A distinction must be made between disorders that are directly dependent on a traumatic event or stressor and those that may be exacerbated by such an event (Friedman, Resick, Bryant, Strain, et al., 2011). The onset of PTSD symptoms is necessarily triggered by a specific traumatic event or stressor, although the trauma itself is not sufficient for all individuals to develop PTSD. This is different from mood and anxiety disorders, where many symptoms are gradual rather than suddenly triggered by trauma. Depression is also not necessarily triggered by a stressful event (Friedman, Resick, Bryant, Strain, et al., 2011). In other words, the exclusivity of trauma must be defended. It is therefore important to define what is meant by trauma (see the debates already mentioned).

Staying with the theme of the diathesis–stress model, there is also the view that people show different clinical responses such as fear-based anxiety, dysphoria, anhedonia, aggression, substance abuse, guilt, shame, dissociation, and the like due to different individual diatheses following trauma. Some people may even experience more than one of the above reactions. As a result, one must accept this inevitable fact of overlapping symptoms and consider PTSD as a separate category of trauma-related disorders alongside, for example, anxiety disorders or other disorders (Resick & Miller, 2009). If you cannot beat them, join them, so to speak! This collaboration could also be seen as people 'expressing' their PTSD symptoms through other psychological responses. Externalisers are those who tend to manifest their PTSD symptoms outwardly by having conflicts with others, interacting antagonistically with others, and having conflicts with social norms and values. They tend to suffer from psychological difficulties such as substance-related disorders. Internalisers, on the other hand, tend to manifest PTSD symptoms inwardly. They tend to have high negative emotionality, depression, anxiety, withdrawal, and indeed shame and guilt (Miller et al., 2004).

All of the aforementioned alternative approaches to conceptualising PTSD focus on how PTSD can be understood by clarifying the presentation, emergence, organisation, or expression of symptoms. There are alternative views that focus on underlying mechanisms rather than symptom presentation. One view is that the overlap of symptoms *per se* should not be emphasised so much. Instead, one should emphasise the maladaptive responses to stressors, that is how their affect regulation systems are impaired, leading to the occurrence of certain reactions (e.g. numbing, avoidance, dissociation, flashback, irritability, impulsivity, and aggression). These reactions are not just any reactions, but a pattern of psychological reactions characterised, for example, by under- or over-regulating one's distressing emotions, cognitive thoughts, and behaviours (Friedman, Resick, Bryant, Strain, et al., 2011).

PTSD can be conceptualised in terms of the affective neuroscience attachment framework. This framework aims to integrate the biological and psychotherapeutic developmental perspectives. It can be applied to various psychiatric disorders, not only to PTSD. This framework describes the neuroanatomy and neurochemistry involved in our affect systems that regulate our emotions. The attachment component focuses on our developmental and interpersonal experiences in our lives. Psychological problems, including PTSD, should be viewed in terms of the interaction between these two aspects or specifically the disruption of this interaction process (Eppel, 2013). This approach is based on the tenet that mental health problems are closely related to the interaction between brain pathophysiology, the environment, or psychosocial contributing factors (e.g. the effects of stress) (Andrews et al., 2009).

PTSD can also be conceptualised in terms of endophenotypes that stand between genetics and disease. It can be understood in terms of the pathways between different brain regions, neural networks and stress systems (e.g. the hypothalamic–pituitary–adrenal (HPA) axis) and their genetic and neurogenetic bases. Understanding these pathways would give us more information about individual differences in response to trauma than using symptom criteria (DSM-5) for PTSD (Young, 2014). Understanding specific epigenetic changes in risk for PTSD is also another avenue, although the evidence for this is still somewhat limited (Yehuda & Bierer, 2009). Although the researchers proposing the above alternative biopsychosocial approaches would argue that they seek a balance between nature and nurture, they arguably lean more towards the side of nature than nurture, which basically contradicts the spirit of the title 'trauma and stress-related disorders' (Kilpatrick, 2013).

To what extent these alternative conceptualisations of PTSD stand up to scientific scrutiny and pave the way for a better understanding of PTSD remains to be seen. However, from what has been said so far, one thing is clear: DSM-5 PTSD is far from being a clear, satisfactory, or ideal nosology for many PTSD experts (Frueh et al., 2010). Indeed, these diagnostic criteria may be an obstacle to truly understanding traumatic reactions (McHugh & Treisman, 2007). It is hardly surprising, then, that for some critics the entire DSM-5 represents a bundle of scientific difficulties. The revised definition of PTSD in the DSM-5 has not improved clinical utility, differentiated, but rather has excluded many individuals who met the previous criteria (Hoge et al., 2016).

The reason why the term DSM-5 is used as opposed to DSM-V is because the DSM committee wants to pave the way for further improvements, that is DSM-5.2 or -5.4 and the like (Friedman, 2013). However, some critics believe that further 'improvements' will still be problematic because DSM-5 is simply a product that came out of a flawed process. It will not make clinical diagnosis clearer, but will continue to cause confusion and turmoil. The expansion of DSM-5 in terms of psychological disorders makes it difficult to distinguish between a psychological disorder and a normal distress. However, one thing that the DSM-5 has achieved is that it has raised many questions that scientists, psychologists, and medical practitioners will have to deal with in the future (Wakefield, 2013). Attempting to resolve the conceptual confusion surrounding the DSM-5, questioning the expansion and changes in PTSD diagnosis, and ultimately limiting the misuse of the diagnosis, is essential but a difficult challenge to overcome (Rosen et al., 2008).

Despite the above sceptical views of the DSM-5 or the DSM in general, it will continue to evolve over many years (Rosen et al., 2008). The DSM-5 will continue to be used for practical and legal purposes, although it should be used with caution (Brewin et al., 2009; Young, 2014). This is similar to what the prisoner does in Plato's cave (*The Republic*, Plato, 2007). In this story, a group of prisoners were chained to the wall of a cave and therefore faced a blank wall for their entire lives. Behind them a fire was burning, so they could see the shadows of things passing in front of them on the wall. It was these shadows that represented reality for these prisoners. The story goes on to say that one of the prisoners is freed and forced to turn around and look at the fire and finally see the 'truth' or the 'light', the new knowledge or reality that he is experiencing. He does not want to return to ignorance, but continues to see the 'truth' and wants his fellow prisoners to experience the same.

Of course, the philosophical meaning behind this story is complex and has led to many philosophical debates. It is not our intention to engage in these longstanding debates. One could argue that some of the PTSD experts are like the prisoners trying to make sense of the shadows (the DSM-5 or the DSM in general). Unlike the prisoners in Plato's cave, however, they are free to turn around and observe the clinical phenomena that pass by their clinics every day. Then they can turn back to the shadow and see to what extent the clinical phenomena and the shadows correspond. The prisoners (PTSD experts) can even exchange information with each other about the extent to which the shadows and the clinical phenomena match. In other words, they work with two 'realities'.

The problem is that both realities are not necessarily the truths or lights they can see. When they look at the shadow (DSM-5), on what basis do they make sense of it? The clinical phenomena, perhaps—which is why they turn to the symptoms of their patients who pass through their psychiatric outpatient clinics or psychotherapeutic rehabilitation centres. However, given what we have outlined in this chapter, the clinical phenomena are not clear either, which is why the prisoners (the PTSD experts) want to turn to the problematic reality of the shadow in the hope that it might help them to structure and make sense of the confusing clinical phenomena. So the prisoners or the PTSD professionals shuttle back and forth between the shadows and what is happening in their clinics, looking for a way to make sense of both blurred realities. Interestingly, different prisoners come up with different versions of the blurred realities. This will go on for a long time, but it is useful to keep working on this blurring because it allows them to stay out of the cave and stare at the wall.

PTSD affecting or resulting from a life-threatening illness

As mentioned above, on DSM-IV a life-threatening physical illness has been considered a traumatic event that can cause symptoms of PTSD. Whether this should always be the case has been questioned in the DSM-5. This new version of the DSM does not exclude a life-threatening illness as trauma. Rather, it emphasises the importance of exercising caution in distinguishing whether or not the illness meets the trauma criteria. Therefore, studies that consider an illness as trauma are found throughout this book. In terms of intervention for patients suffering from PTSD induced by physical illness, one systematic review examined patients with PTSD triggered by events related to cardiovascular problems, cancer, HIV, multiple sclerosis and stem cell transplantation, finding that exposure-based cognitive behavioural therapy (CBT) reduced PTSD symptoms (Hedges's $g = -0.47$). It was also found that imaginal exposure-based therapy was able to reduce PTSD symptoms. Eye movement desensitisation and reprocessing (EMDR) was more effective than imaginal exposure, conventional CBT, and relaxation therapy. It appears that both CBT and EMDR were effective interventions for reducing PTSD symptoms resulting from events related to physical illness (Haerizadeh et al., 2020).

Notwithstanding this, there appear to be more studies looking at how PTSD due to past trauma can affect the development or severity of a physical illness. This is not surprising, as past trauma can alter our physical state or increase physiological arousal, a marker of increased PTSD (Nugent et al., 2006). Such arousal could in turn increase the likelihood of developing physical illness (Boscarino, 1997; Fetzner et al., 2012; McFarlane et al., 1994). A graded relationship between trauma exposure, PTSD, and chronic physical illness has been suggested (Norman et al., 2006; Pengpid & Peltzer, 2020). People with full PTSD have the highest risk of various diseases, whereas people without PTSD (i.e. they have experienced the trauma but do not meet the criteria for PTSD) have the lowest risk. This association between PTSD and physical illness may also be influenced by the number of lifetime traumas, whether single, repeated, or chronic (D'Andrea et al., 2011). Multiple traumas can have a cumulative effect on physical health (Sledjeski et al., 2008). A dose–response phenomenon has also been observed, where an increased number of these traumatic events was associated with an increased likelihood of all physical illnesses (Atwoli et al., 2016; Husarewycz et al., 2014).

These physical illnesses have a wide spectrum (Boscarino, 1997; D'Andrea et al., 2011; Fetzner et al., 2012; Ouimette et al., 2006; Pengpid & Peltzer, 2020) and affect people from different backgrounds and experiences (Sareen et al., 2007; Spitzer et al., 2009). One population study found that trauma or PTSD can increase the likelihood of musculoskeletal, neurological, cardiovascular, gastrointestinal, hepatobiliary, endocrine/metabolic, respiratory, cancer, sleep disorders, and anaemia. At the symptom level, re-experiencing symptoms were associated with cardiovascular and endocrine/metabolic-related illnesses, while negative changes in mood and cognitive symptoms were correlated with sleep disturbances. These findings persisted after controlling for demographic variables and comorbid psychiatric symptoms (Sommer et al., 2019; Sommer et al., 2021). Another population study also found that injury and witnessing trauma were correlated with a variety of physical illnesses (e.g. cardiovascular and gastrointestinal diseases, diabetes, arthritis), while natural disasters or terrorism were associated with cardiovascular, gastrointestinal illnesses, and arthritis (Husarewycz et al., 2014).

In addition, PTSD was associated with the above physical health conditions in people of different ages (b range: 0.62–1.29: young, middle-aged, young–old, and older adults). Across these age categories, PTSD was associated with increased odds of cardiovascular and musculoskeletal disease (adjusted odds ratio (aOR) range: 1.54–2.34), gastrointestinal, hepatobiliary, endocrine/metabolic, respiratory and neurological disease, cancer, sleep disorders, and anaemia (aOR range: 1.70–3.31). For these physical illnesses, the largest effect sizes were found in younger adults and middle-aged adults. In other words, whereas PTSD is associated with the above physical health conditions at different ages, it is especially pronounced in younger and middle-aged adults (Sommer et al., 2021).

Evidence is also accumulating on the impact PTSD may have on hyperreactive immune responses, autoimmune diseases (e.g. rheumatoid arthritis, psoriasis, insulin-dependent diabetes, thyroid disease) (Norman et al., 2006) and inflammation (Hori & Kim, 2019). The link between PTSD and an increased likelihood of a whole range of inflammation-related conditions has been established. These include hypercholesterolaemia, insulin resistance, angina, myocardial infarction, and emphysema, with the greatest likelihood of myocardial infarction (OR: 3.94) and emphysema (OR: 4.06) (Tsai & Shen, 2017). Chronic inflammation is a condition associated with cardiovascular disease risk (Dennis et al., 2016). PTSD is also associated with increased circulating T-cell lymphocytes (von Kanel et al., 2010) and lower cortisol levels (von Kanel et al., 2010). Lower cortisol levels are correlated with the severity of PTSD symptoms, especially hyperarousal symptoms, even after controlling for depression (von Känel et al., 2010). Other conditions include endocrine disorders, pulmonary disease, renal disease, liver disease, peripheral arterial disease, neurohormonal as well as psychosomatic conditions such as fibromyalgia, chronic fatigue syndrome, and back pain (Boscarino, 2004; D'Andrea et al., 2011; Eglinton & Chung, 2011; Glaesmer et al., 2011; Ouimette et al., 2006; Spitzer et al., 2009).

To further explore the broad understanding that the previous studies have given us regarding the relationship between PTSD and physical illness, one can focus on the different types of victims in the literature. Veterans with full PTSD were more likely to develop musculoskeletal disorders, neurological disorders, and gastrointestinal disorders, for example, than those without PTSD. Veterans with subsyndromal PTSD were more likely to develop the same disorders with respiratory illness as an additional disorder than veterans without PTSD (Fetzner et al., 2012). In another study, Vietnam veterans were also found to have disorders of the circulatory system, digestive system, endocrine–nutritional–metabolic, nervous system, and non-sexually transmitted infectious diseases (Boscarino, 1997). Even 15 years after the war, veterans in Croatia suffered from musculoskeletal, pulmonary, and metabolic diseases significantly more often than those who had not been exposed to combat. They also suffered more frequently from cardiovascular and dermatological illnesses (Britvic et al., 2015).

A dose–response phenomenon appeared to occur, as prolonged combat exposure was associated with cardiac arrhythmias in veterans with PTSD along with other psychiatric comorbidities (Britvic et al., 2015). Female veterans with PTSD and comorbid mental health problems also had increases in cardiovascular disease as well as diabetes, gastrointestinal disorders, hypertension, obesity, pain, and urinary problems (Creech et al., 2021). Among active military personnel, increased deployment was positively correlated with PTSD and comorbid psychiatric disorders (e.g. depression, generalised anxiety disorder). In particular, those with PTSD and depression tended to be at increased risk for medical conditions, including cardiovascular disease (Lazar, 2014).

Police officers with high levels of PTSD severity were about three times more likely to meet criteria for metabolic syndrome than those with lower levels of PTSD severity (Violanti et al., 2006). This finding is consistent with research showing that PTSD alters metabolism (de Vries et al., 2015) and leads to metabolic abnormalities, which in turn can affect cardiovascular health and central nervous system function. Metabolic syndrome is characterised by a combination of health parameters, including obesity, increased blood pressure, decreased high-density lipoprotein cholesterol, increased triglycerides, and abnormal glucose levels (Violanti et al., 2006). Interestingly, PTSD has been associated with increased cardiometabolic risk, characterised by metabolic syndrome and insulin resistance (Blessing et al., 2017).

Former prisoners of war with PTSD reported still suffering from musculoskeletal, cardiovascular, and gastrointestinal conditions twenty-five years after their captivity (Jukić et al., 2019). Torture victims tended to report musculoskeletal disorders and respiratory problems (Shrestha et al., 1998). Among Holocaust survivors, there was an increase in chronic degenerative diseases, myocardial infarction, and cancer (Sperling et al., 2012). After a fire rescue, firefighters reported frequent musculoskeletal symptoms, neurological symptoms (e.g. headaches), and respiratory symptoms (McFarlane et al., 1994). Survivors of child abuse tended to have cardiovascular, metabolic and autoimmune disorders, as well as an increased likelihood of depression, PTSD, substance abuse, and obesity (Moog et al., 2021).

It is also worth noting that, whereas past trauma and PTSD were used interchangeably in the above studies, they are two distinct psychological constructs that interact to affect physical health. One of these interactions is the postulate that trauma exposure can impact physical health via PTSD. That is, PTSD can be seen as a mediator. One study concluded that PTSD symptoms mediated the impact of war exposure on the severity of post-deployment physical illnesses (cardiovascular, dermatological, gastrointestinal, genitourinary, musculoskeletal, neurological, and pulmonary) with a reasonably high percentage of mediation ranging from 44% to 75% for both genders (Wachen et al., 2013). Similarly, trauma in childhood is associated with an increased likelihood of physical illnesses such as cardiovascular, metabolic, endocrine, and respiratory diseases in adulthood. Although such trauma is also associated with increased health-risk behaviours such as smoking and alcohol abuse, these behaviours alone cannot account for these physical illnesses. On the other hand, PTSD has been shown to be a consistent factor influencing the association between trauma exposure and poor physical health (Schnurr, 2015).

The persistent mediating role of PTSD does not mean that it is the only mediating factor. On the contrary, in addition to respiratory sinus arrhythmia, smoking and alcohol dependence have been shown to mediate the effects of PTSD due to past trauma on inflammation (Dennis et al., 2016). In young adults, increased PTSD and depressive symptoms were associated with decreased high-density lipoprotein cholesterol and increased triglyceride levels. Smoking and poor sleep quality mediated these associations. Specifically, poor sleep quality explained 83% and 9% of the effects of PTSD and depression on high-density lipoprotein and triglyceride levels, respectively. Thus, the influence that health behaviours may have on the association between PTSD and cardiovascular risk cannot be ignored (Dennis et al., 2014).

Summary

This chapter has articulated the background against which this book should be read. While researchers or clinicians may take comfort in the fact that the DSM-5 represents an advanced understanding of PTSD resulting from thousands of clinical observations, systematic assessments, treatments, or reports of subjective experiences of trauma victims, in reality this understanding raises new questions and debates and exposes itself to new critiques and challenges. This chapter describes what some trauma researchers find difficult and challenging about the conceptualisation or classification of PTSD in the DSM-5. Debates include the usefulness of the definition of trauma, the volatility of life-threatening physical illness as a traumatic event, whether the terms fear, helplessness, or horror should be modified or removed, how PTSD symptoms should be composed in different models, whether these models would affect prevalence rates of PTSD, and whether PTSD should be considered a dissociative disorder or treated as a clinical entity separate from dissociation. Another controversy is whether PTSD should be included in anxiety disorders, as the symptoms of both disorders overlap. At the same time, there is the question of how to delineate PTSD as a distinct clinical syndrome when it overlaps not only with anxiety disorder symptoms but also with other comorbidities that have their own underlying biopsychosocial vulnerabilities. For some researchers, these issues may not be resolvable at all. Therefore, an alternative conceptualisation of PTSD is needed, some candidates for which have been presented in this chapter.

Although the above issues and debates might be considered purely academic, they may significantly alter the findings, interpretations, and conclusions about PTSD in physical illness. Nevertheless, most of the studies presented in the following chapters do not address or resolve these issues in their investigation. One could realistically say that it would be unreasonable to do so. In other words, most researchers would take a biased approach, for example, by using a particular assessment instrument that reflects a particular classification and conceptualisation of PTSD. They would examine psychological comorbidities without considering whether they should be grouped together as one clinical entity with PTSD or as separate clinical responses. In other words, one must accept the fact that the studies presented in the following chapters are only 'versions' of scientific accounts waiting to be further debated, challenged, revised, or extended.

References

Adler, A. B., Wright, K. M., Bliese, P. D., Eckford, R., & Hoge, C. W. (2008). A2 diagnostic criterion for combat-related posttraumatic stress disorder. *Journal of Traumatic Stress, 21*(3), 301–308. https://doi.org/10.1002/jts.20336

Afzali, M. H., Sunderland, M., Teesson, M., Carragher, N., Mills, K., & Slade, T. (2017). A network approach to the comorbidity between posttraumatic stress disorder and major depressive disorder: The role of overlapping symptoms. *Journal of Affective Disorders, 208*, 490–496.

American Psychiatric Association. (1994). *Diagnostic and statistical manual of mental disorders* (4th ed.).

American Psychiatric Association. (2013). *Diagnostic and statistical manual of mental disorders* (5th ed.). https://doi.org/10.1176/appi.books.9780890425596

Andrews, G., Charney, D., Sirovatka, P., & Regier, D. A. (2009). *Stress-induced and fear circuitry disorders: Refining the research agenda for DSM-V.* American Psychiatric Publishing, Inc.

Armour, C., & Shevlin, M. (2010). Testing the dimensionality of PTSD and the specificity of the dysphoria factor. *Journal of Loss and Trauma, 15,* 11–27. https://doi.org/10.1080/153250 20903373110

Armour, C., Contractor, A. A., Palmieri, P. A., & Elhai, J. D. (2014). Assessing latent level associations between PTSD and dissociative factors: Is depersonalization and derealization related to PTSD factors more so than alternative dissociative factors? *Psychological Injury and Law, 7,* 131–142. https://doi.org/10.1007/s12207-014-9196-9

Armour, C., Layne, C. M., Naifeh, J. A., Shevlin, M., Duraković-Belko, E., Djapo, N., Pynoos, R. S., & Elhai, J. D. (2011). Assessing the factor structure of posttraumatic stress disorder symptoms in war-exposed youths with and without criterion A2 endorsement. *Journal of Anxiety Disorders, 25*(1), 80–87. https://doi.org/10.1016/j.janxdis.2010.08.006

Armour, C., Müllerová, J., & Elhai, J. D. (2016). A systematic literature review of PTSD's latent structure in the Diagnostic and Statistical Manual of Mental Disorders: DSM-IV to DSM-5. *Clinical Psychology Review, 44,* 60–74. https://doi.org/10.1016/j.cpr.2015.12.003

Armour, C., Raudzah Ghazali, S., & Elklit, A. (2013). PTSD's latent structure in Malaysian tsunami victims: Assessing the newly proposed Dysphoric Arousal model. *Psychiatry Research, 206*(1), 26–32. https://doi.org/https://doi.org/10.1016/j.psychres.2012.09.012

Armour, C., Tsai, J., Durham, T. A., Charak, R., Biehn, T. L., Elhai, J. D., & Pietrzak, R. H. (2015). Dimensional structure of DSM-5 posttraumatic stress symptoms: Support for a hybrid Anhedonia and Externalizing Behaviors model. *Journal of Psychiatric Research, 61,* 106–113.

Asmundson, G. J., & Taylor, S. (2009). PTSD diagnostic criteria: understanding etiology and treatment. *American Journal of Psychiatry, 166*(6), 726; author reply 727. https://doi.org/ 10.1176/appi.ajp.2009.08121799

Asmundson, G. J., Frombach, I., McQuaid, J., Pedrelli, P., Lenox, R., & Stein, M. B. (2000). Dimensionality of posttraumatic stress symptoms: A confirmatory factor analysis of DSM-IV symptom clusters and other symptom models. *Behavioral Research and Therapy, 38*(2), 203–214. https://doi.org/10.1016/s0005-7967(99)00061-3

Atwoli, L., Platt, J. M., Basu, A., Williams, D. R., Stein, D. J., & Koenen, K. C. (2016). Associations between lifetime potentially traumatic events and chronic physical conditions in the South African Stress and Health Survey: A cross-sectional study. *BMC Psychiatry Vol 16 2016, ArtID 214, 16.*

Barglow, P. (2012). We can't treat soldiers' PTSD without a better diagnosis. *Skeptical Inquirer, 36*(3).

Bensimon, M., Levine, S. Z., Zerach, G., Stein, E., Svetlicky, V., & Solomon, Z. (2013). Elaboration on posttraumatic stress disorder diagnostic criteria: a factor analytic study of PTSD exposure to war or terror. *Israeli Journal of Psychiatry and Related Sciences, 50*(2), 84–90.

Bensimon, M., Solomon, Z., & Horesh, D. (2013). The utility of Criterion A under chronic national terror. *Israeli Journal of Psychiatry and Related Sciences, 50*(2), 81–83.

Biehn, T. L., Elhai, J. D., Seligman, L. D., Tamburrino, M., Armour, C., & Forbes, D. (2013). Underlying dimensions of DSM-5 posttraumatic stress disorder and major depressive disorder symptoms. *Psychological Injury and Law, 6,* 290–298. https://doi.org/10.1007/s12 207-013-9177-4

Blanchard, E. B., Hickling, E. J., Taylor, A. E., & Loos, W. (1995). Psychiatric morbidity associated with motor vehicle accidents. *Journal of Nervous and Mental Diseases, 183*(8), 495–504. https://doi.org/10.1097/00005053-199508000-00001

Blessing, E. M., Reus, V., Mellon, S. H., Wolkowitz, O. M., Flory, J. D., Bierer, L., Lindqvist, D., Dhabhar, F., Li, M., Qian, M., Abu-Amara, D., Galatzer-Levy, I., Yehuda, R., & Marmar, C. R.

(2017). Biological predictors of insulin resistance associated with posttraumatic stress disorder in young military veterans. *Psychoneuroendocrinology, 82,* 91–97.

Blevins, C. A., Weathers, F. W., & Witte, T. K. (2014). Dissociation and posttraumatic stress disorder: a latent profile analysis. *Journal of Traumatic Stress, 27*(4), 388–396. https://doi.org/10.1002/jts.21933

Boals, A., & Schuettler, D. (2009). PTSD symptoms in response to traumatic and non-traumatic events: The role of respondent perception and A2 criterion. *Journal of Anxiety Disorders, 23*(4), 458–462. https://doi.org/10.1016/j.janxdis.2008.09.003

Boelen, P. A., van den Hout, M. A., & van den Bout, J. (2008). The factor structure of posttraumatic stress disorder symptoms among bereaved individuals: A confirmatory factor analysis study. *Journal of Anxiety Disorders, 22,* 1377–1383. https://doi.org/10.1016/j.janxdis.2008.01.018

Boscarino, J. A. (1997). Diseases among men 20 years after exposure to severe stress: implications for clinical research and medical care. *Psychosomatic Medicine, 59*(6), 605–614. https://doi.org/10.1097/00006842-199711000-00008

Boscarino, J. A. (2004). Posttraumatic stress disorder and physical illness: results from clinical and epidemiologic studies. In R. Yehuda, & B. McEwen (Eds.), *Biobehavioral stress response: Protective and damaging effects* (pp. 141–153). New York Academy of Sciences.

Breslau, N., & Kessler, R. C. (2001). The stressor criterion in DSM-IV posttraumatic stress disorder: an empirical investigation. *Biological Psychiatry, 50*(9), 699–704. https://doi.org/10.1016/s0006-3223(01)01167-2

Brewin, C. R. (2003). *Posttraumatic stress disorder: Malady or myth?* Yale University Press.

Brewin, C. R., Lanius, R. A., Novac, A., Schnyder, U., & Galea, S. (2009). Reformulating PTSD for DSM-V: life after Criterion A. *Journal of Traumatic Stress, 22*(5), 366–373. https://doi.org/10.1002/jts.20443

Briere, J., Hodges, M., & Godbout, N. (2010). Traumatic stress, affect dysregulation, and dysfunctional avoidance: a structural equation model. *Journal of Traumatic Stress, 23*(6), 767–774. https://doi.org/10.1002/jts.20578

Britvic, D., Anticevic, V., Kaliterna, M., Lusic, L., Beg, A., Brajevic-Gizdic, I., Kudric, M., Stupalo, Z., Krolo, V., & Pivac, N. (2015). Comorbidities with posttraumatic stress disorder (PTSD) among combat veterans: 15 years postwar analysis. *International Journal of Clinical and Health Psychology, 15*(2), 81–92.

Brown, T. A., Campbell, L. A., Lehman, C. L., Grisham, J. R., & Mancill, R. B. (2001). Current and lifetime comorbidity of the DSM-IV anxiety and mood disorders in a large clinical sample. *Journal of Abnormal Psychology, 110*(4), 585–599. https://doi.org/10.1037//0021-843x.110.4.585

Bryant, R. A., & Panasetis, P. (2005). The role of panic in acute dissociative reactions following trauma. *British Journal of Clinical Psychology, 44*(Pt 4), 489–494. https://doi.org/10.1348/014466505x28766

Bryant, R. A., O'Donnell, M. L., Creamer, M., McFarlane, A. C., & Silove, D. (2011). Posttraumatic intrusive symptoms across psychiatric disorders. *Journal of Psychiatric Research, 45*(6), 842–847. https://doi.org/10.1016/j.jpsychires.2010.11.012

Buckley, T. C., Green, B. L., & Schnurr, P. P. (2004). Trauma, PTSD, and physical health: clinical issues. In J. P. Wilson & T. M. Keane (Eds.), *Assessing psychological trauma and PTSD* (pp. 441–465). The Guilford Press.

Calhoun, P. S., Hertzberg, J. S., Kirby, A. C., Dennis, M. F., Hair, L. P., Dedert, E. A., & Beckham, J. C. (2012). The effect of draft DSM-V criteria on posttraumatic stress disorder prevalence. *Depression and Anxiety, 29,* 1032–1042.

Carlson, E. B., Dalenberg, C., & McDade-Montez, E. (2012). Dissociation in posttraumatic stress disorder part I: Definitions and review of research. *Psychological Trauma: Theory, Research, Practice, and Policy, 4,* 479–489. https://doi.org/10.1037/a0027748

Carragher, N., Mills, K., Slade, T., Teesson, M., & Silove, D. (2010). Factor structure of post-traumatic stress disorder symptoms in the Australian general population. *Journal of Anxiety Disorders, 24*(5), 520–527. https://doi.org/10.1016/j.janxdis.2010.03.009

Charak, R., Armour, C., Elklit, A., Koot, H. M., & Elhai, J. D. (2014). Assessing the latent factor association between the dysphoria model of PTSD and positive and negative affect in trauma victims from India. *Psychological Injury and Law, 7,* 122–130.

Chu, J. A., Frey, L. M., Ganzel, B. L., & Matthews, J. A. (1999). Memories of childhood abuse: dissociation, amnesia, and corroboration. *American Journal of Psychiatry, 156*(5), 749–755. https://doi.org/10.1176/ajp.156.5.749

Contractor, A. A., Durham, T. A., Brennan, J. A., Armour, C., Wutrick, H. R., Christopher Frueh, B., & Elhai, J. D. (2014). DSM-5 PTSD's symptom dimensions and relations with major depression's symptom dimensions in a primary care sample. *Psychiatry Research, 215*(1), 146–153. https://doi.org/https://doi.org/10.1016/j.psychres.2013.10.015

Craske, M. G., Rauch, S. L., Ursano, R., Prenoveau, J., Pine, D. S., & Zinbarg, R. E. (2009). What is an anxiety disorder? *Depress Anxiety, 26*(12), 1066–1085. https://doi.org/10.1002/da.20633

Creech, S. K., Pulverman, C. S., Crawford, J. N., Holliday, R., Monteith, L. L., Lehavot, K., Olson-Madden, J., & Kelly, U. A. (2021). Clinical complexity in women veterans: A systematic review of the recent evidence on mental health and physical health comorbidities. *Behavioral Medicine, 47*(1), 69–87. https://doi.org/10.1080/08964289.2019.1644283

D'Andrea, W., Sharma, R., Zelechoski, A. D., & Spinazzola, J. (2011). Physical health problems after single trauma exposure: When stress takes root in the body. *Journal of the American Psychiatric Nurses Association, 17*(6), 378–392.

Dalenberg, C. J., Brand, B. L., Gleaves, D. H., Dorahy, M. J., Loewenstein, R. J., Cardeña, E., Frewen, P. A., Carlson, E. B., & Spiegel, D. (2012). Evaluation of the evidence for the trauma and fantasy models of dissociation. *Psychological Bulletin, 138*(3), 550–588. https://doi.org/10.1037/a0027447

de Vries, G.-J., Lok, A., Mocking, R., Assies, J., Schene, A., & Olff, M. (2015). Altered one-carbon metabolism in posttraumatic stress disorder. *Journal of Affective Disorders, 184,* 277–285.

Dennis, P. A., Ulmer, C. S., Calhoun, P. S., Sherwood, A., Watkins, L. L., Dennis, M. F., & Beckham, J. C. (2014). Behavioral health mediators of the link between posttraumatic stress disorder and dyslipidemia. *Journal of Psychosomatic Research, 77*(1), 45–50.

Dennis, P. A., Weinberg, J., Calhoun, P. S., Watkins, L. L., Sherwood, A., Dennis, M. F., & Beckham, J. C. (2016). An investigation of vago-regulatory and health-behavior accounts for increased inflammation in posttraumatic stress disorder. *Journal of Psychosomatic Research, 83,* 33–39.

Domino, J. L., Whiteman, S. E., Davis, M. T., Witte, T. K., & Weathers, F. W. (2021). Sudden unexpected death as a traumatic stressor: The impact of the DSM-5 revision of Criterion A for posttraumatic stress disorder. *Traumatology, 27,* 168–176. https://doi.org/10.1037/trm0000272

Edmondson, D., Birk, J. L., Ho, V. T., Meli, L., Abdalla, M., & Kronish, I. M. (2018). A challenge for psychocardiology: Addressing the causes and consequences of patients' perceptions of enduring somatic threat. *American Psychologist, 73,* 1160–1171. https://doi.org/10.1037/amp0000418

Eglinton, R., & Chung, M. C. (2011). The relationship between posttraumatic stress disorder, illness cognitions, defence styles, fatigue severity and psychological well-being in chronic fatigue syndrome. *Psychiatry Research, 188*(2), 245–252.

Elhai, J. D., Biehn, T. L., Armour, C., Klopper, J. J., Frueh, B. C., & Palmieri, P. A. (2011). Evidence for a unique PTSD construct represented by PTSD's D1–D3 symptoms. *Journal of Anxiety Disorders, 25*(3), 340–345. https://doi.org/10.1016/j.janxdis.2010.10.007

Elhai, J. D., Engdahl, R. M., Palmieri, P. A., Naifeh, J. A., Schweinle, A., & Jacobs, G. A. (2009). Assessing posttraumatic stress disorder with or without reference to a single, worst traumatic event: Examining differences in factor structure. *Psychological Assessment, 21,* 629–634. https://doi.org/10.1037/a0016677

Elhai, J. D., Miller, M. E., Ford, J. D., Biehn, T. L., Palmieri, P. A., & Frueh, B. (2012). Posttraumatic stress disorder in DSM-5: Estimates of prevalence and symptom structure in a nonclinical sample of college students. *Journal of Anxiety Disorders, 26*(1), 58–64.

Elklit, A., Armour, C., & Shevlin, M. (2010). Testing alternative factor models of PTSD and the robustness of the dysphoria factor. *Journal of Anxiety Disorders, 24*(1), 147–154. https://doi.org/10.1016/j.janxdis.2009.10.002

Eppel, A. B. (2013). Paradigms lost and the structure of psychiatric revolutions. *Australian & New Zealand Journal of Psychiatry, 47*(11), 992–994. https://doi.org/10.1177/0004867413492222

Etkin, A., & Wager, T. D. (2007). Functional neuroimaging of anxiety: a meta-analysis of emotional processing in PTSD, social anxiety disorder, and specific phobia. *American Journal of Psychiatry, 164*(10), 1476–1488. https://doi.org/10.1176/appi.ajp.2007.07030504

Fetzner, M. G., McMillan, K. A., & Asmundson, G. J. (2012). Similarities in specific physical health disorder prevalence among formerly deployed Canadian forces veterans with full and subsyndromal PTSD. *Depression and Anxiety, 29*(11), 958–965. https://doi.org/10.1002/da.21976

Forbes, D., Fletcher, S., Lockwood, E., O'Donnell, M., Creamer, M., Bryant, R. A., McFarlane, A., & Silove, D. (2011). Requiring both avoidance and emotional numbing in DSM-V PTSD: Will it help? *Journal of Affective Disorders, 130,* 483–486. https://doi.org/10.1016/j.jad.2010.10.032

Frewen, P. A., Brown, M. F. D., Steuwe, C., & Lanius, R. A. (2015). Latent profile analysis and principal axis factoring of the DSM-5 dissociative subtype. *European Journal of Psychotraumatology, 6,* 26406.

Frewen, P. A., Lanius, R. A., Dozois, D. J., Neufeld, R. W., Pain, C., Hopper, J. W., Densmore, M., & Stevens, T. K. (2008). Clinical and neural correlates of alexithymia in posttraumatic stress disorder. *Journal of Abnormal Psychology, 117*(1), 171–181.

Friedman, M. J. (2013). Finalizing PTSD in DSM-5: getting here from there and where to go next. *Journal of Traumatic Stress, 26*(5), 548–556. https://doi.org/10.1002/jts.21840

Friedman, M. J., Kilpatrick, D. G., & Schnurr, P. P. (2016). Changes to the definition of posttraumatic stress disorder in the DSM-5-Reply. *JAMA Psychiatry, 73*(11), 1203. https://doi.org/10.1001/jamapsychiatry.2016.2401

Friedman, M. J., Resick, P. A., Bryant, R. A., & Brewin, C. R. (2011). Considering PTSD for DSM-5. *Depress Anxiety, 28*(9), 750–769. https://doi.org/10.1002/da.20767

Friedman, M. J., Resick, P. A., Bryant, R. A., Strain, J., Horowitz, M., & Spiegel, D. (2011). Classification of trauma and stressor-related disorders in DSM-5. *Depress Anxiety, 28*(9), 737–749. https://doi.org/10.1002/da.20845

Frueh, B. C., Elhai, J. D., & Acierno, R. (2010). The future of posttraumatic stress disorder in the DSM. *Psychological Injury and Law, 3,* 260–270. https://doi.org/10.1007/s12207-010-9088-6

Gallagher, M. W., & Brown, T. A. (2015). Bayesian analysis of current and lifetime comorbidity rates of mood and anxiety disorders in individuals with posttraumatic stress disorder. *Journal of Psychopathology and Behavioral Assessment, 37*(1), 60–66. https://doi.org/10.1007/s10862-014-9436-z

Garcia, J. I., & Mullen, R. (2008). Follow up of post-traumatic stress disorder symptoms in Australian servicemen hospitalized in 1942–1952. *Australia and New Zealand Journal of Psychiatry, 42*(6), 547. https://doi.org/10.1080/00048670802050629

Gaughwin, P. (2009). The PTSD supremacy: Criterion F in three Voyager cases. *Australasian Psychiatry, 17*(2), 97–104. https://doi.org/10.1080/10398560802582868

Gentes, E. L., Dennis, P. A., Kimbrel, N. A., Rissling, M. B., Beckham, J. C., & Calhoun, P. S. (2014). DSM-5 posttraumatic stress disorder: Factor structure and rates of diagnosis. *Journal of Psychiatric Research, 59*, 60–67. https://doi.org/10.1016/j.jpsychires.2014.08.014

Ginzburg, K., Butler, L. D., Saltzman, K., & Koopman, C. (2009). Dissociative reactions in PTSD. In P. F. Dell, & J. A. O'Neil (Eds.), *Dissociation and the dissociative disorders: DSM-V and beyond* (pp. 457–469). Routledge/Taylor & Francis Group.

Ginzburg, K., Koopman, C., Butler, L. D., Palesh, O., Kraemer, H. C., Classen, C. C., & Spiegel, D. (2006). Evidence for a dissociative subtype of post-traumatic stress disorder among help-seeking childhood sexual abuse survivors. *Journal of Trauma Dissociation, 7*(2), 7–27. https://doi.org/10.1300/J229v07n02_02

Glaesmer, H., Brahler, E., Gundel, H., & Riedel-Heller, S. G. (2011). The association of traumatic experiences and posttraumatic stress disorder with physical morbidity in old age: A German population-based study. *Psychosomatic Medicine, 73*, 401–406.

Grant, D. M., Beck, J. G., Marques, L., Palyo, S. A., & Clapp, J. D. (2008). The structure of distress following trauma: Posttraumatic stress disorder, major depressive disorder, and generalized anxiety disorder. *Journal of Abnormal Psychology, 117*(3), 662–672. https://doi.org/10.1037/a0012591

Griffin, M. G., Resick, P. A., & Mechanic, M. B. (1997). Objective assessment of peritraumatic dissociation: psychophysiological indicators. *American Journal of Psychiatry, 154*(8), 1081–1088. https://doi.org/10.1176/ajp.154.8.1081

Gros, D. F., Simms, L. J., & Acierno, R. (2010). Specificity of posttraumatic stress disorder symptoms: an investigation of comorbidity between posttraumatic stress disorder symptoms and depression in treatment-seeking veterans. *Journal of Nervous and Mental Disease, 198*(12), 885–890. https://doi.org/10.1097/NMD.0b013e3181fe7410

Hackmann, A., Clark, D. M., & McManus, F. (2000). Recurrent images and early memories in social phobia. *Behavioral Research and Therapy, 38*(6), 601–610. https://doi.org/10.1016/s0005-7967(99)00161-8

Haerizadeh, M., Sumner, J. A., Birk, J. L., Gonzalez, C., Heyman-Kantor, R., Falzon, L., Gershengoren, L., Shapiro, P., & Kronish, I. M. (2020). Interventions for posttraumatic stress disorder symptoms induced by medical events: A systematic review. *Journal of Psychosomatic Research, 129*, 109908. https://doi.org/10.1016/j.jpsychores.2019.109908

Hetzel-Riggin, M. D. (2009). A test of structural invariance of posttraumatic stress symptoms in female survivors of sexual and/or physical abuse or assault. *Traumatology, 15*, 46–59. https://doi.org/10.1177/1534765608331294

Hoge, C. W., Yehuda, R., Castro, C. A., McFarlane, A. C., Vermetten, E., Jetly, R., Koenen, K. C., Greenberg, N., Shalev, A. Y., Rauch, S. A. M., Marmar, C. R., & Rothbaum, B. O. (2016). Unintended consequences of changing the definition of posttraumatic stress disorder in DSM-5: Critique and call for action. *JAMA Psychiatry, 73*, 750–752. https://doi.org/10.1001/jamapsychiatry.2016.0647

Hori, H., & Kim, Y. (2019). Inflammation and post-traumatic stress disorder. *Psychiatry and Clinical Neurosciences, 73*(4), 143–153. https://doi.org/https://doi.org/10.1111/pcn.12820

Horwitz, A. V., & Wakefield, J. C. (2007). *The loss of sadness: How psychiatry transformed normal sorrow into depressive disorder*. Oxford University Press.

Hoyt, T., & Yeater, E. A. (2010). Comparison of posttraumatic stress disorder symptom struc-ture models in Hispanic and White college students. *Psychological Trauma: Theory, Research, Practice, and Policy, 2*(1), 19–30.

Husarewycz, M., El-Gabalawy, R., Logsetty, S., & Sareen, J. (2014). The association between number and type of traumatic life experiences and physical conditions in a nationally repre-sentative sample. *General Hospital Psychiatry, 36*(1), 26–32.

Jones, J. C., & Barlow, D. H. (1990). The etiology of posttraumatic stress disorder. *Clinical Psychology Review, 10*, 299–328.

Jukić, M., Filaković, P., Požgain, I., & Glavina, T. (2019). Health-related quality of life of ex-prisoners of war affected by posttraumatic stress disorder 25 years after captivity. *Psychiatria Danubina, 31*(2), 189–200. https://doi.org/10.24869/psyd.2019.189

Kangas, M. (2013). DSM-5 trauma and stress-related disorders: Implications for screening for cancer-related stress. *Frontiers in Psychiatry, 4*, 122. https://doi.org/10.3389/fpsyt.2013.00122

Karam, E. G., Andrews, G., Bromet, E., Petukhova, M., Ruscio, A. M., Salamoun, M., Sampson, N., Stein, D. J., Alonso, J., Andrade, L. H., Angermeyer, M., Demyttenaere, K., de Girolamo, G., de Graaf, R., Florescu, S., Gureje, O., Kaminer, D., Kotov, R., Lee, S., et al. (2010). The role of criterion A2 in the DSM-IV diagnosis of posttraumatic stress disorder. *Biological Psychiatry, 68*(5), 465–473. https://doi.org/10.1016/j.biopsych.2010.04.032

Kassam-Adams, N., Marsac, M. L., & Cirilli, C. (2010). Posttraumatic stress disorder symptom structure in injured children: Functional impairment and depression symptoms in a confirmatory factor analysis. *Journal of the American Academy of Child and Adolescent Psychiatry, 49*(6), 616–625.

Kemp, A. H., Felmingham, K., Das, P., Hughes, G., Peduto, A. S., Bryant, R. A., & Williams, L. M. (2007). Influence of comorbid depression on fear in posttraumatic stress dis-order: An fMRI study. *Psychiatry Research, 155*(3), 265–269. https://doi.org/10.1016/j.pscychresns.2007.01.010

Kessler, R. C., Chiu, W. T., Demler, O., Merikangas, K. R., & Walters, E. E. (2005). Prevalence, severity, and comorbidity of 12-month DSM-IV disorders in the National Comorbidity Survey Replication. *Archives of General Psychiatry, 62*(6), 617–627. https://doi.org/10.1001/archpsyc.62.6.617

Kilpatrick, D. G. (2013). The DSM-5 Got PTSD right: Comment on Friedman (2013). *Journal of Traumatic Stress, 26*(5), 563–566. https://doi.org/10.1002/jts.21844

Kilpatrick, D. G., Resnick, H. S., & Acierno, R. (2009). Should PTSD Criterion A be retained? *Journal of Traumatic Stress, 22*(5), 374–383. https://doi.org/10.1002/jts.20436

Kilpatrick, D. G., Resnick, H. S., Milanak, M. E., Miller, M. W., Keyes, K. M., & Friedman, M. J. (2013). National estimates of exposure to traumatic events and PTSD prevalence using DSM-IV and DSM-5 criteria. *Journal of Traumatic Stress, 26*(5), 537–547. https://doi.org/10.1002/jts.21848

King, D. W., Leskin, G. A., King, L. A., & Weathers, F. W. (1998). Confirmatory factor anal-ysis of the clinician-administered PTSD Scale: Evidence for the dimensionality of post-traumatic stress disorder. *Psychological Assessment, 10*, 90–96. https://doi.org/10.1037/1040-3590.10.2.90

Kloep, M. L., Lancaster, S. L., & Rodriguez, B. F. (2014). Sudden unexpected versus violent death and PTSD symptom development. *Journal of Aggression, Maltreatment & Trauma, 23*, 286–300. https://doi.org/10.1080/10926771.2014.882464

Koffel, E., Polusny, M. A., Arbisi, P. A., & Erbes, C. R. (2012). A preliminary investigation of the new and revised symptoms of posttraumatic stress disorder in DSM-5. *Depression and Anxiety, 29*(8), 731–738.

Krystal, J. H., Bennett, A. L., Bremner, J. D., Southwick, S. M., & Charney, D. S. (1995). Toward a cognitive neuroscience of dissociation and altered memory functions in post-traumatic stress disorder. In M. J. Friedman, D. S. Charney, & A. Y. Deutch (Eds.), *Neurobiological and clinical consequences of stress: From normal adaptation to post-traumatic stress disorder* (pp. 239–269). Lippincott–Raven.

Kubany, E. S., Ralston, T. C., & Hill, E. E. (2010). Intense fear, helplessness, "and" horror? An empirical investigation of DSM-IV PTSD Criterion A2. *Psychological Trauma: Theory, Research, Practice, and Policy, 2*(2), 77–82. https://doi.org/10.1037/a0019185

Kuester, A., Köhler, K., Ehring, T., Knaevelsrud, C., Kober, L., Krüger-Gottschalk, A., Schäfer, I., Schellong, J., Wesemann, U., & Rau, H. (2017). Comparison of DSM-5 and proposed ICD-11 criteria for PTSD with DSM-IV and ICD-10: changes in PTSD prevalence in military personnel. *European Journal of Psychotraumatology, 8*(1), 1386988. https://doi.org/10.1080/20008198.2017.1386988

Lanius, R. A., Brand, B., Vermetten, E., Frewen, P. A., & Spiegel, D. (2012). The dissociative subtype of posttraumatic stress disorder: Rationale, clinical and neurobiological evidence, and implications. *Depression and Anxiety, 29*(8), 701–708. https://doi.org/10.1002/da.21889

Lanius, R. A., Frewen, P. A., Girotti, M., Neufeld, R. W., Stevens, T. K., & Densmore, M. (2007). Neural correlates of trauma script-imagery in posttraumatic stress disorder with and without comorbid major depression: a functional MRI investigation. *Psychiatry Research, 155*(1), 45–56. https://doi.org/10.1016/j.pscychresns.2006.11.006

Lanius, R. A., Frewen, P. A., Vermetten, E., & Yehuda, R. (2010). Fear conditioning and early life vulnerabilities: Two distinct pathways of emotional dysregulation and brain dysfunction in PTSD. *European Journal of Psychotraumatology, 1*, 5467. https:10.3402/ejpt.v1i0.5467.

Lanius, R. A., Vermetten, E., Loewenstein, R. J., Brand, B., Schmahl, C., Bremner, J. D., & Spiegel, D. (2010). Emotion modulation in PTSD: Clinical and neurobiological evidence for a dissociative subtype. *American Journal of Psychiatry, 167*(6), 640–647. https://doi.org/10.1176/appi.ajp.2009.09081168

Larsen, S. E., & Berenbaum, H. (2017). Did the DSM-5 improve the traumatic stressor criterion?: Association of DSM-IV and DSM-5 Criterion A with posttraumatic stress disorder symptoms. *Psychopathology, 50*(6), 373–378. https://doi.org/10.1159/000481950

Lazar, S. G. (2014). The mental health needs of military service members and veterans. *Psychodynamic Psychiatry, 42*(3), 459–478.

Lockwood, E., & Forbes, D. (2014). Posttraumatic stress disorder and comorbidity: Untangling the Gordian knot. *Psychological Injury and Law, 7*, 108–121. https://doi.org/10.1007/s12207-014-9189-8

Malta, L. S., Wyka, K. E., Giosan, C., Jayasinghe, N., & Difede, J. (2009). Numbing symptoms as predictors of unremitting posttraumatic stress disorder. *Journal of Anxiety Disorders, 23*(2), 223–229. https://doi.org/10.1016/j.janxdis.2008.07.004

Mansfield, A. J., Williams, J., Hourani, L. L., & Babeu, L. A. (2010). Measurement invariance of posttraumatic stress disorder symptoms among U.S. military personnel. *Journal of Traumatic Stress, 23*(1), 91–99. https://doi.org/10.1002/jts.20492

Marshall, R. D., Spitzer, R., & Liebowitz, M. R. (1999). Review and critique of the new DSM-IV diagnosis of acute stress disorder. *American Journal of Psychiatry, 156*(11), 1677–1685. https://doi.org/10.1176/ajp.156.11.1677

Mayou, R., Bryant, B., & Ehlers, A. (2001). Prediction of psychological outcomes one year after a motor vehicle accident. *American Journal of Psychiatry, 158*(8), 1231–1238. https://doi.org/10.1176/appi.ajp.158.8.1231

McFarlane, A. C., Atchison, M., Rafalowicz, E., & Papay, P. (1994). Physical symptoms in posttraumatic stress disorder. *Journal of Psychosomatic Research, 38*(7), 715–726. https://doi.org/10.1016/0022-3999(94)90024-8

McHugh, P. R., & Treisman, G. (2007). PTSD: a problematic diagnostic category. *Journal of Anxiety Disord, 21*(2), 211–222. https://doi.org/10.1016/j.janxdis.2006.09.003

McNally, R. J. (2009). Can we fix PTSD in DSM-V? *Depression and Anxiety, 26*(7), 597–600. https://doi.org/https://doi.org/10.1002/da.20586

Miller, M. W., Kaloupek, D. G., Dillon, A. L., & Keane, T. M. (2004). Externalizing and internalizing subtypes of combat related PTSD: A replication and extension using the PSY-5 scales. *Journal of Abnormal Psychology, 112*, 636–645.

Miller, M. W., Wolf, E. J., Kilpatrick, D., Resnick, H., Marx, B. P., Holowka, D. W., Keane, T. M., Rosen, R. C., & Friedman, M. J. (2013). The prevalence and latent structure of proposed DSM-5 posttraumatic stress disorder symptoms in U.S. national and veteran samples. *Psychological Trauma: Theory, Research, Practice, and Policy, 5*, 501–512. https://doi.org/10.1037/a0029730

Moodliar, R., Russo, J., Bedard-Gilligan, M., Moloney, K., Johnson, P., Seo, S., Vaziri, N., & Zatzick, D. (2020). A pragmatic approach to psychometric comparisons between the DSM-IV and DSM-5 posttraumatic stress disorder (PTSD) checklists in acutely injured trauma patients. *Psychiatry, 83*(4), 390–401. https://doi.org/10.1080/00332747.2020.1762396

Moog, N. K., Wadhwa, P. D., Entringer, S., Heim, C. M., Gillen, D. L., & Buss, C. (2021). The challenge of ascertainment of exposure to childhood maltreatment: Issues and considerations. *Psychoneuroendocrinology, 125*, 105102. https://doi.org/10.1016/j.psyneuen.2020.105102

Morgan, L., Scourfield, J., Williams, D., Jasper, A., & Lewis, G. (2003). The Aberfan disaster: 33-year follow-up of survivors. *British Journal of Psychiatry, 182*, 532–536. https://doi.org/10.1192/bjp.182.6.532

Mundy, E., & Baum, A. (2004). Medical disorders as a cause of psychological trauma and posttraumatic stress disorder. *Current Opinion in Psychiatry, 17*, 123–127. https://doi.org/10.1097/00001504-200403000-00009

Naifeh, J. A., Elhai, J. D., Kashdan, T. B., & Grubaugh, A. L. (2008). The PTSD Symptom Scale's latent structure: An examination of trauma-exposed medical patients. *Journal of Anxiety Disorders, 22*, 1355–1368. https://doi.org/10.1016/j.janxdis.2008.01.016

Naifeh, J. A., Richardson, J. D., Del Ben, K. S., & Elhai, J. D. (2010). Heterogeneity in the latent structure of PTSD symptoms among Canadian veterans. *Psychological Assessment, 22*, 666–674. https://doi.org/10.1037/a0019783

Norman, S. B., Means-Christensen, A. J., Craske, M. G., Sherbourne, C. D., Roy-Byrne, P. P., & Stein, M. B. (2006). Associations between psychological trauma and physical illness in primary care. *Journal of Traumatic Stress, 19*(4), 461–470. https://doi.org/10.1002/jts.20129

Norris, F. H., & Slone, L. B. (2007). The epidemiology of trauma and PTSD. In M. J. Friedman, T. M. Keane, & P. A. Resick (Eds.), *Handbook of PTSD* (pp. 78–98.). The Guilford Press.

North, C. S., Suris, A. M., Davis, M., & Smith, R. P. (2009). Toward validation of the diagnosis of posttraumatic stress disorder. *American Journal of Psychiatry, 166*(1), 34–41. https://doi.org/10.1176/appi.ajp.2008.08050644

Nugent, N. R., Christopher, N. C., & Delahanty, D. L. (2006). Emergency medical service and in-hospital vital signs as predictors of subsequent PTSD symptom severity in pediatric injury patients. *Journal of Child Psychology and Psychiatry, 47*(9), 919–926.

O'Bryan, E. M., McLeish, A. C., Kraemer, K. M., & Fleming, J. B. (2015). Emotion regulation difficulties and posttraumatic stress disorder symptom cluster severity among trauma-exposed college students. *Psychological Trauma: Theory, Research, Practice, and Policy, 7*, 131–137. https://doi.org/10.1037/a0037764

O'Donnell, M. L., Creamer, M., McFarlane, A. C., Silove, D., & Bryant, R. A. (2010). Should A2 be a diagnostic requirement for posttraumatic stress disorder in DSM-V? *Psychiatry Research, 176*(2–3), 257–260. https://doi.org/10.1016/j.psychres.2009.05.012

O'Donnell, M. L., Creamer, M., Pattison, P., & Atkin, C. (2004). Psychiatric morbidity following injury. *American Journal of Psychiatry, 161*(3), 507–514. https://doi.org/10.1176/appi.ajp.161.3.507

Olbert, C. M., Gala, G. J., & Tupler, L. A. (2014). Quantifying heterogeneity attributable to polythetic diagnostic criteria: Theoretical framework and empirical application. *Journal of Abnormal Psychology, 123*(2), 452–462. https://doi.org/10.1037/a0036068

Olff, M., Sijbrandij, M., Opmeer, B. C., Carlier, I. V., & Gersons, B. P. (2009). The structure of acute posttraumatic stress symptoms: 'reexperiencing', 'active avoidance', 'dysphoria', and 'hyperarousal'. *Journal of Anxiety Disorders, 23*(5), 656–659. https://doi.org/10.1016/j.janxdis.2009.02.003

Orth, U., & Wieland, E. (2006). Anger, hostility, and posttraumatic stress disorder in trauma-exposed adults: a meta-analysis. *Journal of Consulting and Clinical Psychology, 74*(4), 698–706. https://doi.org/10.1037/0022-006x.74.4.698

Osei-Bonsu, P. E., Spiro, A., III, Schultz, M. R., Ryabchenko, K. A., Smith, E., Herz, L., & Eisen, S. V. (2012). Is DSM-IV criterion A2 associated with PTSD diagnosis and symptom severity? *Journal of Traumatic Stress, 25*(4), 368–375. https://doi.org/10.1002/jts.21720

Ouimette, P., Goodwin, E., & Brown, P. J. (2006). Health and well being of substance use disorder patients with and without posttraumatic stress disorder. *Addictive Behaviors, 31*(8), 1415–1423.

Palmieri, P. A., Weathers, F. W., Difede, J., & King, D. W. (2007). Confirmatory factor analysis of the PTSD Checklist and the Clinician-Administered PTSD Scale in disaster workers exposed to the World Trade Center Ground Zero. *Journal of Abnormal Psychology, 116*, 329–341. https://doi.org/10.1037/0021-843X.116.2.329

Pengpid, S., & Peltzer, K. (2020). Mental morbidity and its associations with socio-behavioural factors and chronic conditions in rural middle- and older-aged adults in South Africa. *Journal of Psychology in Africa, 30*(3), 257–263. https://doi.org/10.1080/14330237.2020.1767956

Plato. (2007). *The Republic* (D. Lee, Trans.; 2nd ed.). Penguin.

Putnam, F. W., Carlson, E. B., Ross, C. A., Anderson, G., Clark, P., Torem, M., Bowman, E. S., Coons, P., Chu, J. A., Dill, D. L., Loewenstein, R. J., & Braun, B. G. (1996). Patterns of dissociation in clinical and nonclinical samples. *Journal of Nervous and Mental Disease, 184*(11), 673–679. https://doi.org/10.1097/00005053-199611000-00004

Resick, P. A., & Miller, M. W. (2009). Posttraumatic stress disorder: Anxiety or traumatic stress disorder? *Journal of Traumatic Stress, 22*(5), 384–390. https://doi.org/10.1002/jts.20437

Resick, P. A., Bovin, M. J., Calloway, A. L., Dick, A. M., King, M. W., Mitchell, K. S., Suvak, M. K., Wells, S. Y., Stirman, S. W., & Wolf, E. J. (2012). A critical evaluation of the complex PTSD literature: implications for DSM-5. *Journal of Traumatic Stress, 25*(3), 241–251. https://doi.org/10.1002/jts.21699

Roberts, A. L., Dohrenwend, B. P., Aiello, A. E., Wright, R. J., Maercker, A., Galea, S., & Koenen, K. C. (2012). The stressor criterion for posttraumatic stress disorder: Does it matter? *Journal of Clinical Psychiatry, 73*(2), e264–e270. https://doi.org/10.4088/JCP.11m07054

Rosellini, A. J., Stein, M. B., Colpe, L. J., Heeringa, S. G., Petukhova, M. V., Sampson, N. A., Schoenbaum, M., Ursano, R. J., Kessler, R. C., on behalf of the Army STARRS Collaborators (2015). Approximating a DSM-5 diagnosis of PTSD using DSM-IV criteria. *Depression and Anxiety, 32*(7), 493–501. https://doi.org/https://doi.org/10.1002/da.22364

Rosen, G. M., Lilienfeld, S. O., Frueh, B. C., McHugh, P. R., & Spitzer, R. L. (2010). Reflections on PTSD's future in DSM-V. *British Journal of Psychiatry, 197*(5), 343–344. https://doi.org/10.1192/bjp.bp.110.079699

Rosen, G. M., Spitzer, R. L., & McHugh, P. R. (2008). Problems with the post-traumatic stress disorder diagnosis and its future in DSM V. *British Journal of Psychiatry, 192*(1), 3–4. https://doi.org/10.1192/bjp.bp.107.043083

Salkovskis, P. M. (1985). Obsessional-compulsive problems: A cognitive-behavioural analysis. *Behaviour Research and Therapy, 23*(5), 571–583. https://doi.org/https://doi.org/10.1016/0005-7967(85)90105-6

Sareen, J., Cox, B. J., Stein, M. B., Afifi, T. O., Fleet, C., & Asmundson, G. J. (2007). Physical and mental comorbidity, disability, and suicidal behavior associated with posttraumatic stress disorder in a large community sample. *Psychosomatic Medicine, 69*(3), 242–248.

Saul, A. L., Grant, K. E., & Carter, J. S. (2008). Post-traumatic reactions in adolescents: how well do the DSM-IV PTSD criteria fit the real life experience of trauma exposed youth? *Journal of Abnormal Child Psychology, 36*(6), 915–925. https://doi.org/10.1007/s10802-008-9222-z

Schaal, S., Koebach, A., Hinkel, H., & Elbert, T. (2015). Posttraumatic stress disorder according to DSM-5 and DSM-IV diagnostic criteria: a comparison in a sample of Congolese ex-combatants. *European Journal of Psychotraumatology, 6*, 24981. https://doi.org/10.3402/ejpt.v6.24981

Schnurr, P. P. (2013). The Changed Face of PTSD Diagnosis [Article]. *Journal of Traumatic Stress, 26*(5), 535–536. https://doi.org/10.1002/jts.21851

Schnurr, P. P. (2015). Understanding pathways from traumatic exposure to physical health. In U. Schnyder, & M. Cloitre (Eds.), *Evidence based treatments for trauma-related psychological disorders: A practical guide for clinicians* (pp. 87–103). Springer.

Schnurr, P. P., & Green, B. L. (2004). Understanding relationships among trauma, posttraumatic stress disorder and health outcomes. In P. P. Schnurr & B. L. Green (Eds.), *Trauma and health: Physical health consequences of exposure to extreme stress* (pp. 247–275). American Psychological Association.

Schnurr, P. P., Spiro Iii, A., Vielhauer, M. J., Findler, M. N., & Hamblen, J. L. (2002). Trauma in the lives of older men: Findings from the Normative Aging Study. *Journal of Clinical Geropsychology, 8*(3), 175–187. https://doi.org/10.1023/A:1015992110544

Schnyder, U., Muller, J., Morina, N., Schick, M., Bryant, R. A., & Nickerson, A. (2015). A comparison of DSM-5 and DSM-IV diagnostic criteria for posttraumatic stress disorder in traumatized refugees. *Journal of Traumatic Stress, 28*(4), 267–274.

Shalev, A. Y. (2003). The interdisciplinary study of posttraumatic stress disorder. *CNS Spectrums, 8*(9), 640. https://doi.org/10.1017/S1092852900008828

Shalev, A. Y., Freedman, S., Peri, T., Brandes, D., Sahar, T., Orr, S. P., & Pitman, R. K. (1998). Prospective study of posttraumatic stress disorder and depression following trauma. *American Journal of Psychiatry, 155*(5), 630–637. https://doi.org/10.1176/ajp.155.5.630

Shrestha, N. M., Sharma, B., Van Ommeren, M., Regmi, S., Makaju, R., Komproe, I., Shrestha, G. B., & de Jong, J. T. (1998). Impact of torture on refugees displaced within the developing world: Symptomatology among Bhutanese refugees in Nepal. *JAMA, 280*(5), 443–448. https://doi.org/10.1001/jama.280.5.443

Simeon, D., Yehuda, R., Knutelska, M., & Schmeidler, J. (2008). Dissociation versus posttraumatic stress: cortisol and physiological correlates in adults highly exposed to the World Trade Center attack on 9/11. *Psychiatry Research, 161*(3), 325–329. https://doi.org/10.1016/j.psychres.2008.04.021

Simms, L. J., Watson, D., & Doebbeling, B. N. (2002). Confirmatory factor analyses of posttraumatic stress symptoms in deployed and nondeployed veterans of the Gulf War. *Journal of Abnormal Psychology, 111*(4), 637–647. https://doi.org/10.1037//0021-843x.111.4.637

Sledjeski, E. M., Speisman, B., & Dierker, L. C. (2008). Does number of lifetime traumas explain the relationship between PTSD and chronic medical conditions? Answers from the National Comorbidity Survey-Replication (NCS-R). *Journal of Behavioral Medicine, 31*(4), 341–349.

Sommer, J. L., El-Gabalawy, R., & Mota, N. (2019). Understanding the association between posttraumatic stress disorder characteristics and physical health conditions: A population-based study. *Journal of Psychosomatic Research, 126*, 109776. https://doi.org/10.1016/j.jpsychores.2019.109776

Sommer, J. L., Reynolds, K., El-Gabalawy, R., Pietrzak, R. H., Mackenzie, C. S., Ceccarelli, L., Mota, N., & Sareen, J. (2021). Associations between physical health conditions and posttraumatic stress disorder according to age. *Aging & Mental Health, 25*(2), 234–242. https://doi.org/10.1080/13607863.2019.1693969

Sperling, W., Kreil, S., & Biermann, T. (2012). Somatic diseases in child survivors of the Holocaust with posttraumatic stress disorder: A comparative study. *Journal of Nervous and Mental Disease, 200*(5), 423–428.

Spiegel, D. (2012). Divided consciousness: Dissociation in DSM-5. *Depression and Anxiety, 29*(8), 667–670. https://doi.org/https://doi.org/10.1002/da.21984

Spitzer, C., Barnow, S., Volzke, H., John, U., Freyberger, H. J., & Grabe, H. J. (2009). Trauma, posttraumatic stress disorder, and physical illness: Findings from the general population. *Psychosomatic Medicine, 71*(9), 1012–1017.

Spitzer, R. L., First, M. B., & Wakefield, J. C. (2007). Saving PTSD from itself in DSM-V. *Journal of Anxiety Disorder, 21*(2), 233–241. https://doi.org/10.1016/j.janxdis.2006.09.006

Sterlini, G. L., & Bryant, R. A. (2002). Hyperarousal and dissociation: A study of novice skydivers. *Behaviour Research and Therapy, 40*, 431–437. https://doi.org/10.1016/S0005-7967(01)00021-3

Steuwe, C., Lanius, R. A., & Frewen, P. A. (2012). Evidence for a dissociative subtype of PTSD by latent profile and confirmatory factor analyses in a civilian sample. *Depress Anxiety, 29*(8), 689–700. https://doi.org/10.1002/da.21944

Stone, A. M. (1992). The role of shame in post-traumatic stress disorder. *American Journal of Orthopsychiatry, 62*(1), 131–136. https://doi.org/10.1037/h0079308

Summerfield, D. (2001). The invention of post-traumatic stress disorder and the social usefulness of a psychiatric category. *BMJ, 322*(7278), 95–98. https://doi.org/10.1136/bmj.322.7278.95

Taylor, S., Thordarson, D. S., Maxfield, L., Fedoroff, I. C., Lovell, K., & Ogrodniczuk, J. (2003). Comparative efficacy, speed, and adverse effects of three PTSD treatments: exposure therapy, EMDR, and relaxation training. *Journal of Consulting and Clinical Psychology, 71*(2), 330–338. https://doi.org/10.1037/0022-006x.71.2.330

Tedstone, J. E., & Tarrier, N. (2003). Posttraumatic stress disorder following medical illness and treatment. *Clinical Psychology Review, 23*(3), 409–448. https://doi.org/10.1016/S0272-7358(03)00031-X

Tsai, J., & Shen, J. (2017). Exploring the link between posttraumatic stress disorder and inflammation-related medical conditions: An epidemiological examination. *Psychiatric Quarterly, 88*(4), 909–916. https://doi.org/10.1007/s11126-017-9508-9

Twaite, J. A., & Rodriguez-Srednicki, O. (2004). Childhood sexual and physical abuse and adult vulnerability to PTSD: the mediating effects of attachment and dissociation. *Journal of Child Sexual Abuse, 13*(1), 17–38. https://doi.org/10.1300/J070v13n01_02

van der Kolk, B. A., Pelcovitz, D., Roth, S., Mandel, F. S., McFarlane, A., & Herman, J. L. (1996). Dissociation, somatization, and affect dysregulation: the complexity of adaptation of trauma. *American Journal of Psychiatry, 153*(7 Suppl), 83–93. https://doi.org/10.1176/ajp.153.7.83

van der Kolk, B. A., Roth, S., Pelcovitz, D., Sunday, S., & Spinazzola, J. (2005). Disorders of extreme stress: The empirical foundation of a complex adaptation to trauma. *Journal of Traumatic Stress, 18*(5), 389–399. https://doi.org/10.1002/jts.20047

Violanti, J. M., Fekedulegn, D., Hartley, T. A., Andrew, M. E., Charles, L. E., Mnatsakanova, A., & Burchfiel, C. M. (2006). Police trauma and cardiovascular disease: Association between PTSD symptoms and metabolic syndrome. *International Journal of Emergency Mental Health, 8*(4), 227–238.

von Känel, R., Abbas, C. C., Begré, S., Saner, H., Gander, M.-L., & Schmid, J.-P. (2010). Posttraumatic stress disorder and soluble cellular adhesion molecules at rest and in response to a trauma-specific interview in patients after myocardial infarction. *Psychiatry Research, 179*(3), 312–317. https://doi.org/10.1016/j.psychres.2009.06.005

Wachen, J. S., Shipherd, J. C., Suvak, M., Vogt, D., King, L. A., & King, D. W. (2013). Posttraumatic stress symptomatology as a mediator of the relationship between warzone exposure and physical health symptoms in men and women. *Journal of Traumatic Stress*, 26(3), 319–328.

Waelde, L. C., Silvern, L., Carlson, E., Fairbank, J. A., & Kletter, H. (2009). Dissociation in PTSD. In P. F. Dell, J. A. & O'Neil (Eds.), *Dissociation and the dissociative disorders: DSM-V and beyond* (pp. 447–456). Routledge/Taylor & Francis Group.

Waelde, L. C., Silvern, L., & Fairbank, J. A. (2005). A taxometric investigation of dissociation in Vietnam veterans. *Journal of Traumatic Stress*, 18, 359–369. https://doi.org/10.1002/jts.20034

Wakefield, J. C. (2013). *DSM-5: An overview of changes and controversies. Clinical Social Work Journal* 41(2), 139–154.

Wang, L., Zhang, J., Shi, Z., Zhou, M., Li, Z., Zhang, K., Liu, Z., & Elhai, J. D. (2011). Comparing alternative factor models of PTSD symptoms across earthquake victims and violent riot witnesses in China: Evidence for a five-factor model proposed by Elhai et al. (2011). *Journal of Anxiety Disorders*, 25(6), 771–776. https://doi.org/10.1016/j.janxdis.2011.03.011

Watson, D. (2009). Differentiating the mood and anxiety disorders: a quadripartite model. *Annual Review of Clinical Psychology*, 5, 221–247. https://doi.org/10.1146/annurev.clin psy.032408.153510

Weathers, F. W., & Keane, T. M. (2007). The Criterion A problem revisited: controversies and challenges in defining and measuring psychological trauma. *Journal of Traumatic Stress*, 20(2), 107–121. https://doi.org/10.1002/jts.20210

Weathers, F. W., Marx, B. P., Friedman, M. J., & Schnurr, P. P. (2014). Posttraumatic stress disorder in DSM-5: New criteria, new measures, and implications for assessment. *Psychological Injury and Law*, 7, 93–107. https://doi.org/10.1007/s12207-014-9191-1

Whalley, M. G., Rugg, M. D., Smith, A. P. R., Dolan, R. J., & Brewin, C. R. (2009). Incidental retrieval of emotional contexts in post-traumatic stress disorder and depression: An fMRI study. *Brain and Cognition*, 69, 98–107. https://doi.org/10.1016/j.bandc.2008.05.008

Williams, J. L., Monahan, C. J., & McDevitt-Murphy, M. E. (2011). Factor structure of the PTSD Checklist in a sample of OEF/OIF veterans presenting to primary care: Specific and nonspecific aspects of dysphoria. *Journal of Psychopathology and Behavioral Assessment*, 33(4), 514–522. https://doi.org/10.1007/s10862-011-9248-3

Wolf, E. J., Miller, M. W., Reardon, A. F., Ryabchenko, K. A., Castillo, D., & Freund, R. (2012). A latent class analysis of dissociation and posttraumatic stress disorder: Evidence for a dissociative subtype. *Archives of General Psychiatry*, 69(7), 698–705. https://doi.org/10.1001/archge npsychiatry.2011.1574

Yehuda, R., & Bierer, L. M. (2009). The relevance of epigenetics to PTSD: implications for the DSM-V. *Journal of Traumatic Stress*, 22(5), 427–434. https://doi.org/10.1002/jts.20448

Yehuda, R., Halligan, S. L., Golier, J. A., Grossman, R., & Bierer, L. M. (2004). Effects of trauma exposure on the cortisol response to dexamethasone administration in PTSD and major depressive disorder. *Psychoneuroendocrinology*, 29(3), 389–404. https://doi.org/10.1016/s0306-4530(03)00052-0

Young, G. (2014). PTSD, Endophenotypes, the RDoC, and the DSM-5. *Psychological Injury and Law*, 7(1), 75–91. https://doi.org/10.1007/s12207-014-9187-x

Young, G., Lareau, C., & Pierre, B. (2014). One quintillion ways to have PTSD comorbidity: Recommendations for the disordered DSM-5. *Psychological Injury and Law*, 7, 61–74. https://doi.org/10.1007/s12207-014-9186-y

Yufik, T., & Simms, L. J. (2010). A meta-analytic investigation of the structure of posttraumatic stress disorder symptoms. *Journal of Abnormal Psychology*, 119, 764–776. https://doi.org/10.1037/a0020981

Zoellner, L. A., Bedard-Gilligan, M. A., Jun, J. J., Marks, L. H., & Garcia, N. M. (2013). The evolving construct of posttraumatic stress disorder (PTSD): DSM-5 criteria changes and legal implications. *Psychological Injury and Law*, 6(4), 277–289. https://doi.org/10.1007/s12 207-013-9175-6

Zoellner, L. A., Rothbaum, B. O., & Feeny, N. C. (2011). PTSD not an anxiety disorder? DSM committee proposal turns back the hands of time. *Depression and Anxiety*, 28(10), 853–856. https://doi.org/10.1002/da.20899

2

Posttraumatic stress disorder and cardiovascular disease

Preamble

Before we begin the subsequent chapters on the relationship between post-traumatic stress disorder (PTSD) and different types of physical illness, it is important to point out some features of those chapters. First, it was indicated in Chapter 1 that the list of illnesses covered in this book is potentially very long. Of course, it would be beyond the scope to list all possible illnesses here. Instead, the focus is mainly on potentially life-threatening or debilitating physical illnesses that may be interpreted differently by different researchers. Therefore, some readers may or may not agree with the types of illnesses listed here. Some may feel that other relevant illnesses have been neglected. Second, the terms PTSD and PTSS (posttraumatic stress symptoms) are used depending on the studies selected for the book. This may reflect an ambivalent attitude of the researchers towards PTSD, the reasons for which were outlined in Chapter 1. In using the term PTSD, some may have adhered strictly to the diagnostic criteria of DSM-IV (American Psychiatric Association, 1994) or DSM-5 (American Psychiatric Association, 2013). On the other hand, some might have preferred to avoid the debate about whether the index event, e.g. the illness itself, should be treated as trauma, or not to be constrained by the strict diagnostic criteria, which would mean dividing their samples into those with PTSD or without PTSD. Instead, they would prefer to focus on the severity of symptoms. Third, although this book is mainly concerned with PTSD or PTSS in physical illness, it also 'draws attention' to posttraumatic growth (PTG). In other words, PTG is not a major focus of the book, but in reviewing the literature it became clear that PTG is an important area that cannot be ignored. However, to explore it meaningfully in people with life-threatening physical illnesses, a separate project is needed.

Posttraumatic Stress in Physical Illness. Man Cheung Chung, Oxford University Press. © Oxford University Press 2024.
DOI: 10.1093/oso/9780198727323.003.0002

Trauma and cardiovascular disease

According to the World Health Organization (2021), cardiovascular disease is the leading cause of death worldwide. In 2019, an estimated 17.9 million people died from these diseases, 85% of which were due to heart attacks and strokes. This estimate represented 32% of all deaths worldwide. Cardiovascular diseases can affect people of all ages, genders, ethnicities, and socioeconomic status (Sheikh & Marotta, 2008). Stress-related disorders are associated with a whole range of cardiovascular diseases such as ischaemic heart disease, cerebrovascular disease, embolism or thrombosis, hypertension, heart failure, and cardiac arrhythmias. These associations persist even after controlling for factors such as family history, previous somatic disease, and past and current psychiatric problems (Song et al., 2019).

Cumulative trauma exposure is also associated with increased risk of recurrent cardiovascular disease, increased mortality from heart disease (Boscarino, 2008a; Hendrickson et al., 2013) and early death (Cohen, Marmar, Neylan, et al., 2009) after accounting for psychiatric comorbidities and health risk behaviours such as smoking, physical inactivity, and substance abuse. This association between trauma and cardiovascular disease is not a new phenomenon, but has been observed and discussed in soldiers in the American Civil War as early as the nineteenth century. As a result of the war, they showed the so-called 'soldier's heart syndrome', which is comparable to some of today's PTSD reactions and is associated with exaggerated cardiovascular reactivity (Bremner et al., 2020).

The type of trauma also appears to play a role in cardiovascular disease. For example, women who had experienced physical and sexual abuse in childhood reported more cardiovascular symptoms than those who had not experienced such trauma (Farley & Patsalides, 2001). This is consistent with the literature that advocates dividing traumatic events into interpersonal or non-interpersonal trauma. The former is intentionally or deliberately brought about by the perpetrator. This includes physical or sexual abuse/assault and domestic violence. The latter occurs naturally or unintentionally, meaning that the occurrence of the trauma is beyond one's control. Trauma includes natural disasters (e.g. earthquakes, floods, hurricanes) and man-made disasters (e.g. train or plane accidents). Interpersonal trauma tends to be associated with higher severity of PTSD and psychiatric comorbidities than non-interpersonal trauma (Breslau et al., 1999; Creamer et al., 2001;

Kilpatrick et al., 1997). The reason for this may be that interpersonal trauma triggers a strong sense of betrayal (Freyd, 1994) and can violate victims' core beliefs and basic assumptions about the trustworthiness and benevolence of others (Janoff-Bulman, 1992). It appears that this type of betrayal trauma, or trauma characterised by a severe assault of the self, can have major effects on the cardiovascular system.

The risk factors for PTSD and cardiovascular risks

PTSD has been associated with cardiovascular disease in various popula-tions (Boscarino, 2004), with an odds ratio (OR) of 2.10 in one study (Vidal et al., 2018). These diseases include angina, coronary artery disease, conges-tive heart failure, peripheral vascular disease (Falger et al., 1992; Ford, 2004; Glaesmer et al., 2011; Kibler, 2009; Spitzer et al., 2009; Taylor-Clift et al., 2016; Wilson et al., 2019; Zen et al., 2012), ischaemic heart disease, throm-boembolic stroke (Vaccarino & Bremner, 2017), myocardial ischaemia (Turner et al., 2013), and circulatory diseases such as hypertension and dyslipidaemia that may contribute to coronary heart disease (Dyball et al., 2019; Taylor-Clift et al., 2016).

Certain PTSD symptoms have been shown to be associated with spe-cific cardiovascular disease or risk factors. For example, high levels of in-trusion symptoms have been associated with hospitalisation for myocardial infarction, unstable angina or emergency coronary revascularisation pro-cedures. Avoidance and hyperarousal symptoms, on the other hand, have not. Intrusive memory may also have a persistent deleterious effect on the cardiovascular system (Vaccarino & Bremner, 2017) and act as a strong and unique predictor of increased risk for serious adverse cardiac events and mortality (Edmondson et al., 2011). In other words, not having control over distressing images intruding into one's consciousness may increase the risk of cardiovascular disease in a way that conscious (implying an element of control) avoidant coping behaviours and the resulting physiological arousal do not.

Whereas the link between PTSD and cardiovascular disease has been estab-lished, PTSD alone is not the only factor contributing to such disease. Studies have been conducted to explore specific variables that influence this associ-ation between PTSD and cardiovascular risk (Dedert et al., 2010), some of which are listed below.

Gender differences

The presentation, pathophysiology, and clinical course of cardiovascular disease may differ between genders. For example, compared to men, these diseases tend to manifest later in life in women and have similar or worse morbidity and mortality rates (Vaccarino & Bremner, 2017). Women are also more prone to microvascular coronary disease (a problem for small coronary arteries to dilate under stress) and endothelial dysfunction (an imbalance between vasodilating and vasoconstricting substances that regulate the endothelium) than men (Bugiardini & Bairey Merz, 2005). As women are more likely than men to suffer from psychological disorders such as depression, PTSD, and early trauma, they may be at higher long-term risk for stress-related cardiometabolic diseases, especially coronary heart disease. Young women are particularly vulnerable to the negative effects of stress, which increases the risk of developing cardiovascular disease and worsens prognosis (Vaccarino & Bremner, 2017).

A systematic review also concluded that indigenous women overall were more vulnerable to cardiovascular disease risk factors than men. Women tended to have higher levels of anxiety, perceived stress, feelings of cultural loss, racism, and discrimination than men. Women's mental health problems, particularly depression, anxiety, PTSD, and substance abuse were associated with cardiovascular disease. They were also more prone to elevated levels of C-reactive protein, a marker of cardiovascular disease, higher levels of high-density lipoprotein, and a higher prevalence of diabetes. Men exercised more than women to protect themselves from cardiovascular disease. Women, on the other hand, exercised less because of their high family responsibilities. Poor diet and obesity, diabetes, hypertension, and cholesterol were behavioural or physical factors related to their cardiovascular risks (Burnette et al., 2020).

Whereas one study has shown that women (12%) have less cardiovascular disease associated with PTSD, diabetes, and comorbid PTSD-diabetes than men (22%) (Gibson et al., 2018), other studies examining gender-specific cardiovascular stress responses have contradicted the findings overall. In addition, female military personnel showed greater psychological effects of stress exposure than males. During stress exposure, women had lower systolic blood pressure than men. During the recovery period, women reported greater residual systolic blood pressure and lower diastolic blood pressure than men (Taylor et al., 2014). Although both genders have experienced long-term war-related health effects, women have higher cardiovascular risk associated with war exposure than men with similar levels of exposure (Korinek et al., 2020). The above studies appear to have supported the 'feminine vulnerability hypothesis', which states that women have poorer health outcomes than men following a traumatic event (in this case, cardiovascular disease) (Breslau et al., 1999).

If we focus only on women, women who experienced trauma but did not receive a PTSD diagnosis (OR: 1.30) and women who experienced six or seven trauma symptoms (OR: 1.69) may be at higher risk for cardiovascular disease than women who were not exposed to trauma. Compared to women without trauma, every five additional years of PTSD symptoms among those exposed to trauma was associated with a 9% increase in the incidence of cardiovascular disease (Gilsanz et al., 2017).

Age

After Hurricane Katrina, among older adults with hypertension and PTSD symptoms, 8.6% reported PTSD symptoms and 11.6% had a cardiovascular event during follow-up (PTSD was assessed between 12 and 24 months after the disaster). PTSD symptoms were associated with cardiovascular events with an adjusted hazard ratio of 1.70 (Lenane et al., 2019). Other studies focused on older victims exposed to war-related trauma. A prospective study showed that in older men, most of whom were veterans living in the community, elevated PTSD symptoms increased the risk of coronary heart disease. After excluding pre-existing coronary heart disease and controlling depressive symptoms, for every standard deviation increase in PTSD symptoms in men, there was a relative risk of 1.26 for non-fatal myocardial infarction and fatal coronary heart disease combined, and 1.21 for these conditions combined with angina (Kubzansky et al., 2007). A large-scale study focusing on Vietnamese older adults who had been exposed to war in their young adulthood showed that a large proportion of them suffered from cardiovascular diseases. The participants reported one of these conditions: hypertension and dyslipidaemia (primary risk factors for cardiovascular disease), as well as heart attack and stroke, which are major causes of mortality and disability worldwide. Specifically, nearly 60% reported hypertension; 21%, 23%, and 7.5% reported high cholesterol, heart disease, and stroke, respectively (Korinek et al., 2020).

The impact of PTSD on increased incidence of cardiovascular disease in older veterans may be long-lasting. After controlling for demographics, medical and psychiatric comorbidities, and substance abuse, those with late-life PTSD (i.e. a continual suffering from PTSD after service and into late life) were at a 49%, 45%, 35%, and 26% increased risk of myocardial infarction, cardiovascular disease, peripheral vascular disease, or congestive heart failure, respectively, compared to individuals without late-life PTSD (Beristianos et al., 2016). Similarly, exposure to combat and violence and adverse living conditions (e.g. war-related displacement, lack of clean water and food shortage, sleep problems due to an inhospitable environment) during the Vietnam War were positively correlated with hypertension, dyslipidaemia, heart disease, and stroke in older adults. The severity of recent PTSD symptoms mediated these associations. In other words, the trauma of war and resulting PTSD could impact cardiovascular disease later in life (Korinek et al., 2020).

Ethnic differences

An epidemiological study has shown that Latino people have a higher risk of a number of diseases than non-Latino whites. These diseases were cardiovascular disease (OR: 3.23 (Latino) vs 1.28 (non-Latino white)), hypertension (OR: 1.61 (Latino) vs 0.98 (non-Latino white)), and diabetes (OR: 2.18 (Latino) vs 0.81 (non-Latino white)) (Valentine et al., 2017). Non-Latino whites and non-Latino blacks reported the highest rates of trauma (84% and 82%, respectively) and cardiovascular disease (29% and 35%, respectively). The co-occurrence of trauma and cardiovascular disease was highest among non-Latino blacks (30%) and lowest among Asians (15%) (Vidal et al., 2018). PTSD symptoms were also associated with cardiovascular disease (adjusted hazard ratio: 1.7) among Hurricane Katrina survivors of different ethnicities. PTSD was associated with an increased risk of incident cardiovascular disease in black older adults with hypertension (adjusted hazard ratio: 3.3), but not in whites (adjusted hazard ratio: 0.9) (Lenane et al., 2019).

Comorbid psychological factors

The relationship between PTSD and cardiovascular disease may be influenced by a complex interaction with comorbid psychological factors. While cardiovascular risk may increase with PTSD, the risk increases more in patients with comorbid PTSD-diabetes (Gibson et al., 2018). Similarly, patients suffering from comorbid cardiovascular disease and diabetes were found to have high rates of PTSD in addition to depression and suicidal thoughts. This was particularly the case in men (Annunziato et al., 2015).

Veterans who have been diagnosed with a psychological disorder tend to have a higher prevalence of cardiovascular risk factors than those who have not been diagnosed. Specifically, those who had PTSD with or without other mental health diagnoses reported an adjusted rate (adjusted for age, race, component type (active duty vs National Guard/Reserve), rank, branch of service, and multiple deployments) of 3.63 for smoking, 2.88 for hypertension, 2.70 for dyslipidaemia, and 2.35 for obesity, compared with the corresponding ORs of 3.04, 2.42, 2.33, and 2.05 for those with mental health diagnoses without PTSD (Cohen, Marmar, Ren, et al., 2009). In other words, PTSD does not exclusively increase the prevalence of cardiovascular risk factors. Mental health conditions such as anxiety and substance abuse may act as confounders that need to be controlled for when examining the association between PTSD and cardiovascular risk factors (Burnette et al., 2020).

After controlling for sociodemographic variables and substance abuse, it was found that veterans with PTSD and comorbid major depressive disorder (MDD) were more likely to have heart disease, migraine, fibromyalgia, and rheumatoid arthritis compared to those with MDD alone. They were also more likely to be diagnosed with hypertension and hypercholesterolaemia than those with PTSD alone. Veterans with both PTSD and MDD tended to have poorer physical functioning and were three times more likely to be affected by disability than those with MDD alone (Nichter et al., 2019).

It is not surprising for researchers to examine the combined effects of PTSD and MDD, as traumatised individuals tend to suffer from depression more often compared to the general population (Eberly & Engdahl, 1991). PTSD cannot be studied independently of depression as it is an important confounding factor (von Känel, Schmid, et al., 2010). There are indeed common underlying mechanisms of aetiology between these two psychological conditions. To understand the heightened sensitisation of people with multiple traumatic experiences is to understand these common mechanisms. The neural circuits in these conditions include the amygdala, medial prefrontal cortex, and anterior cingulate. The common aetiological mechanisms would have implications for the treatment of both depression and PTSD (McFarlane, 2010).

Conversely, cardiovascular risk may exacerbate the effects of mental health risk factors such as anxiety sensitivity and stress tolerance, which in turn could impact on PTSD and depression. High levels of anxiety sensitivity and low stress tolerance have been associated with increased PTSD and depression symptoms in firefighters. Among those who were at high cardiovascular risk, increased anxiety sensitivity was more strongly associated with increased PTSD symptoms than among those who were at low cardiovascular risk (Ranney et al., 2020).

Lifestyle and health risk behaviours

Patients with PTSD are more likely than those without PTSD to lead unhealthy lifestyles that increase their cardiovascular risk factors such as obesity, diabetes, and hypertension (Vaccarino & Bremner, 2017). People with PTSD also tend to have increased symptom burden, physical limitations, high rates of physical inactivity in terms of total exercise (OR: 1.6) and light exercise (OR: 1.7), a long smoking history, and poor quality of life in general. These results occurred even after controlling for factors such as cardiovascular risk factors, depression, and income level (Cohen, Marmar, Neylan, et al., 2009; Zen et al., 2012). These findings were also confirmed by another study in which PTSD symptoms were associated with a sharp decline in physical activity over time in women (Winning et al., 2017).

A systematic review and meta-analysis also confirmed that compared to people without PTSD, people with PTSD are 5% and 9% less likely to eat a healthy diet and exercise regularly, respectively, but 31% and 22% more likely to be obese and smoke, respectively. These behaviours would in turn contribute to an increased risk of cardiometabolic diseases such as cardiovascular disease and diabetes (van den Berk-Clark et al., 2018). Increased tobacco use and obesity may also influence the association between PTSD and circulatory diseases, including hypertension, which then contributes to the development of cardiovascular disease (Dyball et al., 2019).

Relational issues

Attachment is a natural human phenomenon where we develop strong emotional bonds with some significant person or 'attachment figure' in our lives. The experience with these figures helps us regulate our emotions when faced with stress or danger (Ainsworth & Bell, 1970; Bowlby, 1969, 2005). When our attachment experience is 'secure', that is, we are able to seek emotional support and comfort from an attachment figure in stressful situations, we feel reassured, secure, and less anxious, and therefore perceive others or the outside world as safe and trustworthy. However, some of us may have developed an 'insecure' attachment where we worry that our attachment figures will not be available or supportive when we need them or want reassurance. As a result, we distrust our attachment figures and avoid seeking emotional support or closeness from them (avoidant attachment). This insecure experience often makes us feel distressed, vulnerable, and anxious rather than calm or secure (anxious attachment), which then motivates us to reassure ourselves by maintaining emotional distance.

It has been argued that insecure attachment experiences can contribute to the development of chronic illness (McWilliams & Bailey, 2010; Pietromonaco & Collins, 2017; Pietromonaco et al., 2013). Attachment anxiety, a form of insecure attachment, has been shown to increase PTSD distress, which in turn can impact cardiovascular disease. Increased attachment anxiety was associated with fasting blood glucose and glycated haemoglobin (HbA1c), as well as with poor physical and mental health (anxiety, depression), via increased severity of PTSD symptoms in patients participating in a cardiac rehabilitation programme. In other words, patients' anxiety about the lack of support from key attachment figures may exacerbate some trauma symptoms, which in turn may affect not only physical and mental health, but also cardiovascular disease risk factors. Surprisingly, attachment avoidance, another form of insecure attachment, did not predict poor physical and mental health outcomes, although it was correlated with increased fasting blood glucose levels (Heenan et al., 2020). It appears that different types of insecure attachment may influence health outcomes and cardiovascular disease risk factors in different ways. Similarly, one might wonder whether or how different types of secure attachment might mitigate the aforementioned outcomes differently. Further research is clearly needed to address this question.

It is tempting to speculate that one reason for the association between insecure attachment and poor health outcomes is lack of social support, particularly emotional support or closeness. The implication is that the lack of opportunities for patients to talk about and share their feelings and emotions with someone they trust may have a negative impact on their health. However, this observation is not what some researchers have found. They have argued that, even when cardiovascular disease patients feel that they have someone available to talk to about their problems or emotional issues, this is not enough to protect them from PTSD, which in turn contributes to health issues, although these patients may develop adaptive coping strategies. If instead they perceive the availability of material help (e.g. having someone to help them with practical things like moving house) or the availability of people to do things with (e.g. going to the cinema), this may reduce patients' perceptions of threat and increase active coping, feelings of self-efficacy, and control. Thus, they may be less likely to develop future PTSD (Dinenberg et al., 2014).

To look at the relationship between PTSD and cardiovascular disease from a different relationship perspective, male veterans with PTSD reported greater couple conflict, less warmth, increased anger, and raised systolic blood pressure in response to stress. Their partners' responses were similar. In other words, anger and physiological responses to relationship conflict may contribute to cardiovascular risk (Caska et al., 2014). Similarly, PTSD may also increase cardiac sympathetic activity in both veterans and partners through mutual blame or criticism during marital conflict. The physiological reactivity in PTSD couples may be due to hostility or attempts to control each other during marital disagreements (Smith et al., 2021).

PTSD and cardiovascular risks: heart rate variability and blood pressure

PTSD, a history of victimisation, and cumulative trauma (dose effect) can affect the autonomic nervous system, increasing hyperarousal, immune dysfunction, and physiological reactivity to trauma-related stimuli, thereby increasing cardiovascular activity (Blanchard, 1990; Hamner, 1994; Kibler, 2009; Newton et al., 2005; Rabe et al., 2006; Tedstone & Tarrier, 2003). Because intrusive images can remind victims of their traumas, victims are likely to regularly repeat episodes of sustained over-reactivity that impair emotional regulation. Such repetition may make it more difficult for them to recover from this heightened physiological reactivity or arousal (Norte et al., 2013), which in turn would contribute to the risk of cardiovascular disease (Forneris et al., 2004).

For instance, fear following trauma may increase autonomic nervous system dysregulation and increase cardiovascular risk for traumatised individuals (Sumner et al., 2020). Autonomic imbalance, characterised by increased sympathetic activation and parasympathetic withdrawal, is thought to play a role in the development of PTSD (Arditte Hall et al., 2018). Stronger parasympathetic responses appeared to be related to greater depersonalisation or derealisation during trauma recall (Chou et al., 2018). In men with moderate to high combat exposure, PTSD sufferers tend to exhibit decreased diurnal differences and blunted tonic parasympathetic activity, suggesting central neuroautonomic dysregulation that may indicate increased cardiovascular disease (Agorastos et al., 2013). Dysregulation of the autonomic system could lead to immune system dysfunction, which could also influence the relationship between PTSD and cardiovascular disease (Pope & Wood, 2019).

Autonomic nervous system dysregulation could include increased heart rate, heart rate variability (variations from beat to beat produced by fluctuations in autonomic nervous system activity at the sinus node), or increased blood pressure, which may cause people with PTSD to develop cardiovascular disease (Arditte Hall et al., 2018). Veterans with PTSD, for example, tend to report higher heart rates over a 24 h cycle than people without PTSD (T. C. Buckley et al., 2004; Buckley & Kaloupek, 2001). Similarly, PTSD survivors of motor vehicle accidents showed increased baseline heart rate and increased heart rate reactivity during exposure to the trauma-related image (Rabe et al., 2006). Heart rate scores shortly after trauma were related to both short-term (e.g. 6 weeks) and long-term (e.g. 6 months) severity of PTSD symptoms, even when depressive symptoms were taken into account (Nugent et al., 2006). To gain a better understanding of PTSD and increased heart rate, it has been suggested that autonomic arousal associated with momentary negative affect should be considered. This type of autonomic arousal associated with negative affect is thought to be a major factor influencing cardiovascular risk in PTSD (Dennis et al., 2017). There are studies that show decreased heart rate in trauma victims. Whether heart rate increases or decreases in trauma victims may be related to different trauma symptoms. An overall decrease during trauma recall has been associated with increased fear and perceived threat, whereas an increase has been related to flashbacks (Chou et al., 2018), symptoms of re-experiencing (Norte et al., 2013), and threat appraisal (Lee et al., 2020).

Memory of trauma and severity of PTSD symptoms may influence heart rate variability (HRV) (Bedi & Arora, 2007; Cohen et al., 1999; Dyball et al., 2019; Hopper et al., 2006; Keary et al., 2009; Newton et al., 2005; Norte et al., 2013; Scheeringa et al., 2004) and respiratory sinus arrhythmia (Jovanovic et al., 2009; Sack et al., 2004) with gender differences (women are more at risk) (Kleim et al., 2010). Changes in HRV may indicate autonomic nervous system dysregulation or cardiac autonomic dysfunction, which is a risk factor for developing cardiovascular disease. For example, low HRV is associated with a 32–45% increased risk of a first cardiovascular event in people who have no history of cardiovascular disease (Hillebrand et al., 2013).

People with PTSD tend to show higher levels of ambulatory distress and heart rate, but lower levels of ambulatory LF (low frequency) HRV and HF (high frequency) HRV (Dennis et al., 2016). The association between PTSD symptom severity and decreased LF HRV was also found in traumatised young adults after controlling for age and activity level (Green et al., 2016). Katrina disaster survivors with high levels of PTSD and depression symptoms have shown higher resting heart rate, lower baseline parasympathetic (high frequency normalised unit) HRV activity and lower reactivity to trauma cues, but higher baseline sympathovagal activity (low frequency:HF ratio) than controls (Tucker et al., 2012).

Heart rate during sleep has been found to be higher in veterans with PTSD than those without PTSD (Bedi & Arora, 2007; Blanchard, 1990; Muraoka et al., 1998). A later study showed that individuals with high PTSD symptom severity tended to have lower HF-HRV during sleep than those with low PTSD symptom severity. In other words, individuals with elevated PTSD symptoms may have decreased parasympathetic control during sleep (Rissling et al., 2016). One study focused on sleep type and compared non-rapid eye movement (NREM) sleep with rapid eye movement (REM) sleep in veterans. Those with PTSD had lower HF-HRV in the first and fourth NREM cycles and in total NREM sleep than those without PTSD. The two groups did not appear to differ in terms of total HF-HRV during REM sleep. These results essentially suggest that the veterans may have experienced impaired parasympathetic modulation during NREM sleep. This impaired parasympathetic nervous system function could be a mechanism by which cardiovascular risks may increase (Ulmer et al., 2018).

Taken together, some researchers conclude that people with PTSD respond differently to heart rate variability than patients with other types of psychological disorders (e.g. panic disorder) (Cohen et al., 2000). The findings on the relationship between heart rate variability and increased risk of cardiovascular disease or death need to be further explored in light of health risk behaviours, especially smoking and alcohol abuse, as well as sleep disturbances. These behavioural factors could mediate the effects of PTSD on HRV-based indices of autonomic nervous system dysregulation (Dennis et al., 2014).

When people with PTSD respond to stress, they may have problems not only with heart rate variability but also with blood pressure, another parameter associated with cardiovascular disease risk (Lee et al., 2020). For example, the increase of heart rate during stress and the decrease of blood pressure after stress was lower in people with PTSD, which may indicate a dysregulation of the cardiovascular system as it reacts to stress (Diener et al., 2012). Lifetime victimisation and PTSD symptoms, especially intrusive symptoms, have been jointly associated with ambulatory blood pressure (Kibler et al., 2008; Newton et al., 2005). Compared to non-PTSD individuals, PTSD individuals showed higher blood pressure reactivity when reminded of the stressor (T. C. Buckley et al., 2004), although the effect size for the association between PTSD and elevated blood pressure tended to be smaller in magnitude than that for HRV (Buckley & Kaloupek, 2001).

Specifically, veterans with PTSD had higher systolic blood pressure, diastolic blood pressure and heart rate. Trauma-exposed patients without PTSD also had higher blood pressure than those who had not been exposed to war. The prevalence of hypertension was 34.1% of PTSD patients (Paulus et al., 2013). Although age, education level, body mass index, smoking, and diabetes were associated with hypertension status, only PTSD was associated with the occurrence of incident hypertension (hazard ratio: 1.94), which was defined as the first occurrence at follow-up of (1) systolic blood pressure (≥140 mmHg) or diastolic blood pressure (≥90 mmHg), (2) patients taking antihypertensive medication, or (3) a new diagnosis of hypertension (Mendlowicz et al., 2021).

The association between PTSD and elevated systolic blood pressure may be partly due to anxiety during the day (Edmondson, Sumner, et al., 2018). Threat appraisal may mediate the impact of PTSD on the increase in systolic PTSD response (Lee et al., 2020). Young women (premenopausal, aged 19–49 years) with PTSD tend to have higher systolic and diastolic blood pressure and other cardiovascular disease risk factors, as well as lower high-density lipoprotein levels and higher triglycerides. In other words, PTSD could increase cardiovascular risks early in life (Kibler et al., 2018; Kibler et al., 2013). The association between PTSD and blood pressure is found to be independent of other psychological problems such as depression (Kibler et al., 2008; Newton et al., 2005). This finding was also confirmed in a later study in which PTSD was associated with increased blood pressure (brachial and central systolic and diastolic pressures) in veterans; this association was also independent of depression and other risk factors (Moazen-Zadeh et al., 2016).

There seems to be evidence that PTSD, blood pressure, and heart rate are associated with strong emotions such as anger. Veterans with PTSD felt angry much faster than those without PTSD. During their anger, they also responded with higher diastolic blood pressure and mean heart rate than those without PTSD. This anger has been associated with hostility (Beckham et al., 2004; Beckham et al., 2002), which in turn was associated with greater increases in heart rate and poorer cardiovascular outcomes (Beckham et al., 2009). Women with PTSD reported greater anxiety, greater hostility, and higher resting heart rate during anger than women without PTSD. Similar to previous studies, hostility was associated with higher diastolic blood pressure and heart rate during re-experienced anger and recovery from anger in women with PTSD, but not in the group without PTSD (Vrana et al., 2009).

However, previous findings on the relationship between PTSD, heart rate variability, and blood pressure are not always consistent. One study found no significant differences between female veterans with and without PTSD in terms of blood pressure levels (Forneris et al., 2004). Another study also found no significant differences in mean ambulatory heart rate, systolic blood pressure, or diastolic blood pressure between veterans with and without PTSD (Beckham et al., 2000). Similarly, no significant associations were found between levels of heart rate and blood pressure in victims of car crashes with acute PTSD. These contradictory findings have even led to questioning the usefulness of these cardiovascular parameters as predictors of acute PTSD (B. Buckley et al., 2004), although one cannot deny the abundance of evidence demonstrating the association between heart rate variability, blood pressure, and PTSD.

PTSD and cardiovascular risks: other clinical parameters

In addition to heart rate, heart rate variability, or blood pressure, trauma may also be related to other clinical parameters. Childhood abuse, for example, can have unique effects on neurobiology and cognition, leading to a whole range of physical and mental health problems. Trauma in childhood can affect brain areas such as the hippocampus, amygdala, and medial prefrontal cortex, all of which are involved with memory and emotion. These brain areas could in turn affect the peripheral sympathetic and hormonal systems that activate the cardiovascular response to stress (Bremner & Vaccarino, 2015). It has also been postulated that childhood trauma is specifically related to altered function of catecholaminergic systems in the brain stem, which may result in abnormal patterns of catecholamine activity. This would then affect central nervous system function, including a dysregulated brain stem, which in turn may influence cardiovascular regulation as well as anxiety, startle responses, and sleep disturbances (Perry, 1994).

PTSD has also been linked to increased cardiovascular risk through alterations in the hypothalamic–pituitary–adrenal (HPA) axis and the sympathetic nervous system, although this claim has not been consistently verified in various studies (Wingenfeld et al., 2015; Zaba et al., 2015). Anxiety-related disorders, including PTSD, can increase autonomic arousal via the HPA axis to increase circulating catecholamines (Player & Peterson, 2011). This increased arousal has been linked to an increased risk of hypertension and a pro-inflammatory state, and consequently to the development of coronary heart disease (Player & Peterson, 2011). Overall, these findings are consistent with the hypothesis that stress-related diseases may be expressed through a number of biological pathways, including the HPA axis and the sympathetic–adrenal–medullary stress axes (Boscarino, 2004).

Regarding the sympathetic nervous system, some studies have found higher levels of plasma norepinephrine and 24 h urinary norepinephrine in veterans with PTSD than in veterans without PTSD. PTSD is associated with hyper-function of the central noradrenergic system (Bedi & Arora, 2007). These biological pathways may also involve the amygdala and hippocampus, which interpret what is stressful and regulate emotional responses. The amygdala may become hyperactive in people with PTSD and depression (Bedi & Arora, 2007; McEwen, 2003). Another study suggests that PTSD is associated with decreased parasympathetic nervous system (PNS) function, particularly in women with PTSD. Such reduced PNS activity may predispose them to poor cardiovascular health (Hughes et al., 2006).

Persistently elevated levels of inflammation appear to be associated with the development of PTSD symptoms 3 months after an acute coronary syndrome (Bielas et al., 2018). Myocardial infarction patients with PTSD have been shown to release increased levels of interleukin-6 in response to stress, which may indicate a mechanistic link between PTSD and adverse cardiovascular outcomes as well as other diseases associated with inflammation (Lima et al., 2019). Another study shows that people with severe PTSD symptoms tend to have higher levels of inflammation, greater impairment of arterial baroreflex sensitivity—which can be seen as a trend towards higher resting heart rate—and exaggerated withdrawal of the parasympathetic nervous system, possibly contributing to cardiovascular risks (Fonkoue et al., 2020).

Other clinical parameters are as follows: 66.7% of patients with PTSD after their war experiences have electrocardiogram (ECG) abnormalities, which may contribute to the risk of cardiovascular disease (Khazaie et al., 2013). PTSD is also associated with impaired coronary distensibility, which reflects the endothelial-dependent process associated with vulnerable plaque composition. These two factors may independently contribute and simultaneously interact to increase the risk of severe cardiovascular events later in life (Ahmadi et al., 2018). PTSD may increase cardiovascular risk through hyper-coagulability of the blood (Von Kanel et al., 2006; von Känel, Kraemer, et al., 2010). Police officers with high levels of PTSD symptoms also had a nearly twofold reduction in brachial artery (flow-mediated dilation), a biomarker of subclinical cardiovascular disease, compared to those with low levels of PTSD (Violanti et al., 2006). PTSD is also associated with increased risk of cardiometabolic health problems, with preclinical and clinical studies providing evidence of behavioural (e.g. poor sleep, cigarette use, poor diet, and insufficient exercise) and biological (e.g. autonomic reactivity, inflammation) mediators for these associations. These behavioural and biological mechanisms could lead to accelerated cellular ageing, which may contribute to premature deterioration in cardiometabolic health (Wolf & Schnurr, 2016).

From what has been said, a few observations are worth mentioning. First, trauma or PTSD interacts with biological factors to affect cardiovascular disease. This observation is consistent with the psychobiological model of the allostatic load hypothesis (McEwen & Stellar, 1993), which can be considered as a way to explain the relationship between PTSD and cardiovascular disease. This allostatic load is not only evident in PTSD, but also in major depressive disorder. This hypothesis states that chronic stress can prolong allostasis, which then leads, for example, to long-term increased neuroendocrine responses that have a negative impact on the body. Fluctuation of the neuroendocrine system can increase immune function and cause overactive platelet function, which leads to the development of atherosclerosis, a risk factor for cardiovascular disease. A long-term response to trauma can increase allostatic load by activating the HPA axis and sympathetic nervous system, resulting in long-term lower and higher levels of norepinephrine and cortisol, respectively. This dysfunctional regulation of the HPA axis and nervous system could increase blood pressure and lipid levels (Bedi & Arora, 2007; Boscarino, 2008b; Coughlin, 2011; Kendall-Tackett, 2009; McEwen, 2003; Wentworth et al., 2013).

Second, PTSD and cardiovascular disease can increase hospital admissions, lengthen hospital stays, and increase the use of resources, particularly health services (Boscarino, 2004; Wilson et al., 2019). Patients with PTSD resulting from trauma such as domestic violence or childhood abuse frequently accessed medical or primary care services in the 12 months prior to diagnosis. When using these services, patients mainly focused on treating physical symptoms (cardiovascular symptoms) and in other words were not aware that they needed psychological treatment for PTSD symptoms. Whereas primary care doctors are able to recognise depression or anxiety symptoms, they do not necessarily recognise PTSD. This could be due to overlapping symptoms as well as their lack of experience in recognising this condition (Samson et al., 1999) in coronary patients. Instead, doctors tend to see PTSD as a reaction to external stressful events such as accidents (Doerfler et al., 1994). Therefore, PTSD is likely to be under-diagnosed and therefore not treated in patients with cardiovascular disease who seek help from primary care (Cohen, Marmar, Neylan, et al., 2009). In other words, if the literature argues that PTSD patients or patients with anxiety and a comorbid condition such as acute myocardial infarction incur the highest medical costs and therefore have the greatest need for primary care interventions, then some of these medical costs should be set aside to treat this hidden clinical condition, namely cardiovascular-related PTSD (Marciniak et al., 2005; Player & Peterson, 2011). The ability of these patients to improve their daily functioning and quality of life would be severely compromised (Cohen, Marmar, Neylan, et al., 2009).

PTSD after acute coronary syndrome or myocardial infarction

Rather than focusing on the impact of past trauma or PTSD on the development of physical illness later in life, some studies have focused on how PTSD may result from acute life-threatening illness (e.g. heart attack, stroke, and cancer), which has been confirmed in 12–25% of patients (Edmondson, 2014). Some studies have specifically looked at PTSD following acute coronary syndrome (post-ACS PTSD) or myocardial infarction (post-MI PTSD). That is, the acute coronary event and MI are treated as the index trauma. The psychological consequences of PTSD related to cardiovascular disease can have a significant impact on recovery, quality of life, recurrent cardiovascular events, medication adherence, and mortality (Kronenberg et al., 2017).

After the acute coronary event, studies showed that about 15% of patients developed PTSD (Edmondson, Richardson, et al., 2012; Edmondson et al., 2011; Gander & von Känel, 2006), while an aggregate prevalence estimate of 12% was also reported. A meta-analysis estimated a wider range of prevalence rates between 0% and 32%. Compared to patients without PTSD, ACS patients with clinically significant PTSD symptoms had twice the risk of recurrent cardiac events or death (Edmondson, Richardson, et al., 2012). Patients tend to experience enduring somatic threat, where they are sensitised to the signs of persistent threat in their bodies, which in turn perpetuates PTSD symptoms (Edmondson, Birk, et al., 2018). Post-ACS PTSD is also associated with sleep disturbance, which in turn may increase the risk of cardiovascular risk (Shaffer et al., 2013). Looking at the course of post-ACS PTSD, one year after an ACS, 12.2% of patients met criteria for PTSD; 36 months later, 12.8% of patients met criteria, indicating the persistent nature of this psychological syndrome. PTSD at 36 months was predicated by PTSD at 12 months and depressed mood at admission. In other words, early emotional reactions are related to longer-term PTSD reactions (Wikman et al., 2008).

Anxiety sensitivity and depressive symptoms, but not experiential avoidance, have been shown to contribute to post-ACS PTSD. Depressive and PTSD symptoms have been associated with perceived health, but not anxiety sensitivity or experiential avoidance. Posttraumatic symptoms of acute coronary syndrome significantly mediated the association between depressive symptoms and perceived health. In other words, increased depressive symptomatology was significantly associated with higher levels of posttraumatic symptoms, which in turn predicted lower levels of perceived health (García-Encinas et al., 2020). A notable observation from the above study is that fear of anxiety-related symptoms—due to the belief that these symptoms cause oneself physical, social, or cognitive harm (Reiss, 1991)—could heighten sensitization to trauma and the possibility of eliciting posttraumatic reactions following trauma exposure. Alternatively, a traumatic event could elicit this fear of anxiety-related symptoms and posttraumatic stress, while anxiety sensitivity could in turn exacerbate negative reactions (Marshall et al., 2010). Meanwhile, it was somewhat surprising that efforts to escape and avoid distressing emotions, thoughts, and memories did not contribute to post-ACS PTSD. This avoidance strategy is often used by trauma victims and is associated with PTSD symptoms (Orcutt et al., 2020).

It has been suggested that PTSD can also result from myocardial infarction (MI). PTSD is associated with reduced quality of life and increased risk of recurrent adverse cardiovascular events and mortality (Jacquet-Smailovic et al., 2021). One of the first studies to focus on MI as an index trauma drew attention to this syndrome of post-MI PTSD by examining the case studies of four adult MI patients (Kutz et al., 1988). A later study found 16% and 9% for chronic and acute PTSD, respectively, in MI patients (Kutz et al., 1994). Another study claimed that one in eight patients with MI or other acute heart condition in the USA would develop PTSD each year (Voelker, 2012). One review study concluded that the prevalence rate for post-MI PTSD is between 0% and 38%. The rate for the best-powered studies is 15% (Spindler & Pedersen, 2005). Post-MI patients reported more PTSD symptoms than the control group of colonoscopy patients (Neumann, 1991).

It is worth noting that prevalence rates for post-MI PTSD or rates of other life-threatening physical illnesses (e.g. HIV and cancer) tend to be lower than those of combat or sexual assault (Tedstone & Tarrier, 2003), although their traumatic symptoms overlap with others (Doerfler & Paraskos, 2011). In addition, there are patients who have not developed full PTSD but have developed subsyndromal or partial PTSD (van Driel & Op den Velde, 1995), for which a prevalence rate of 16% has been identified (Rocha et al., 2008). This is important because PTSD occurs along a continuum from normal to abnormal stress responses. Even if people do not meet the full diagnostic criteria for PTSD, they may still experience severe impairments in their functioning and require the same level of care as people with a full diagnosis of PTSD. Therefore, it is considered important to classify PTSD reactions at different levels (Blank, 1993; Carlier & Gersons, 1995; Joseph et al., 1997).

There are studies that suggest that post-MI PTSD is a persistent condition. Patients retained the PTSD diagnosis over time (Abbas et al., 2009; Wikman et al., 2008), which affects their health-related quality of life (Ginzburg et al., 2003). The risk of recurrent MI or recurrent cardiovascular events and mortality should not be underestimated (Edmondson, Richardson, et al., 2012; Pedersen, 2001). One study showed that just over 2 years later, about two-thirds of patients still met the diagnostic criteria for PTSD (Abbas et al., 2009). Specifically, avoidance and hyperarousal symptoms did not appear to decrease longitudinally (Abbas et al., 2009). However, the persistent nature of post-MI PTSD is not without controversy. There are studies claiming that the severity of post-MI PTSD gradually decreases over time (e.g. on average 2 years later), especially in terms of re-experiencing and avoidance symptoms (Abbas et al., 2009; Doerfler et al., 1994). In one study, most coronary patients were found to have only mild symptoms 6–22 months later, although a small minority continued to meet criteria for PTSD along with psychiatric comorbid symptoms such as anxiety, depression, and anger (Doerfler et al., 1994).

To shed light further on the course of post-MI PTSD, the diagnosis of acute stress syndrome (ASD) was considered. According to a longitudinal study, over a 7-month period, 6% of MI patients had both ASD and PTSD, 10% had no ASD but PTSD, and 12% had ASD but no PTSD (Ginzburg et al., 2003). Over an 8-year period after MI, among resilient patients (i.e. those who recovered from MI), the rate of ASD changed from 12.4% at time 1 (1 week after MI) to 6.1% of PTSD at time 3 (8 years later). Among chronic patients, the rate of PTSD was 85.3% at time 1 and decreased to 75.7% at time 3. They also reported lower quality of life than the resilient individuals at time 3 (Ginzburg & Ein-Dor, 2011). From the preceding complex or inconclusive results, one could at best conclude that there are individual differences in the expression, maintenance, or recovery of ASD and PTSD symptoms after MI over time.

The explanation for the above complexity is difficult to fathom. It could be related to methodological issues. For example, while some studies have relied on self-report measures such as the Posttraumatic Stress Diagnostic Scale to assess PTSD symptoms, others have used structured interviews. When using self-report, people tend to report a higher prevalence. For this reason, some studies have attempted to use self-report as a screening tool, followed by a structured interview. It is understandable that such studies are labour intensive. In addition, several studies have used DSM-III-revised and DSM-VI, which could have an impact on prevalence. The arguments in this regard have already been discussed in Chapter 1. It has been pointed out that a prospective design with multiple assessments and an adequate sample size is needed for future research (Spindler & Pedersen, 2005).

Alternatively, the complexity described above may reflect the sceptical view that cardiac-induced PTSD may not be a unique subtype of PTSD (Tully & Cosh, 2019). However, this claim has yet to be verified. Also, cardiac-induced PTSD does not necessarily have a higher level of medical comorbidities and psychiatric vulnerabilities than non-cardiac-related PTSD. For example, the latter have been shown to have more substance abuse and depression problems than the former (Tully & Cosh, 2019). Despite these inconclusive findings and complexities, it has been argued that the consequences of under-recognition, under-diagnosis, and under-treatment of this psychological condition can be devastating (Sareen et al., 2007; Voelker, 2012).

Post-MI PTSD and psychiatric comorbidity

In addition to post-MI PTSD symptoms, patients may also have other psychiatric comorbidities such as anxiety, social dysfunction, depression, and somatic complaints that affect their health-related quality of life (Ginzburg et al., 2003). In MI patients with full-PTSD, these comorbid symptoms were more pronounced than in patients without and with partial-PTSD or in the healthy control group (e.g. Chung et al., 2007; Ginzburg, 2006; Ginzburg et al., 2003), even after controlling for age, bypass surgery, previous mental health problems, and angioplasty (Chung et al., 2007). Regarding depression, one study showed that 7 months after MI, 8% had comorbid PTSD and depression, while 14% had high levels of depression without full-PTSD. Both PTSD and depression were associated with higher levels of adjustment difficulties (Ginzburg, 2006). Another study found that post-MI PTSD was associated with increased dissociation. Seemingly, patients could develop two comorbid disorders (depression or dissociation) or a dissociative subtype of PTSD (Ginzburg et al., 2006).

In other words, post-MI PTSD is not a separate and discrete psychological syndrome, but is related to or expressed through other psychological disorders. This observation can be conceptualised using the distinction between externalisers and internalisers (Keane et al., 2007; Miller et al., 2004), mentioned in Chapter 1. As a reminder, externalisers are those who tend to manifest PTSD symptoms externally by having conflicts with others, interacting antagonistically with others, and having conflicts with social norms and values. Internalisers, on the other hand, tend to manifest PTSD symptoms internally. They tend to have high negative emotionality, depression, anxiety, withdrawal, shame, and guilt. Both types had a higher mortality rate and were more likely to die from cardiovascular causes than people without PTSD (Flood et al., 2010).

The coexisting relationship between PTSD and other psychiatric symptoms reflects the idea that other mental health problems may act as covariates that need to be controlled for when examining the impact of PTSD on health outcomes in cardiovascular patients or patients with other life-threatening illnesses. Adjusting for these comorbidities is likely to significantly affect estimates of the burden of disease (Gadermann et al., 2012) for these patients.

The risk factors for post-MI PTSD

The prevalence rate of post-MI PTSD implies that not all MI patients will later develop PTSD. This is consistent with the general PTSD literature. Even in a large-scale disaster, less than 50% would develop PTSD (McFarlane, 1990). Similarly, large-scale epidemiological studies of PTSD have shown that while 40–90% of the general population will experience a traumatic event at some point in their lives, less than 10% will develop PTSD (Breslau et al., 1991, 1998; Davidson et al., 1991; Helzer et al., 1987; Kessler et al., 1995; Norris, 1992). In other words, exposure to a traumatic experience, in this case MI, is not sufficient to explain the aetiology of PTSD. There are other factors at play. So what are some of the factors involved in the development of post-MI PTSD? Broadly speaking, they can be divided into three groups: patient demographic characteristics, subjective appraisal, and personality and coping strategies.

Demographic characteristics

Myocardial infarction may affect short-term rather than long-term PTSD symptoms in women (Hari et al, 2010). In addition, PTSD symptoms have been associated with younger age, ethnicity (e.g. Asian or African) (Bennett & Brooke, 1999; Kutz et al., 1994; Rocha et al., 2008), social disadvantage (Kutz et al., 1994; Wikman et al., 2008), a history of cardiac hospitalisation (Kutz et al., 1994) or recurrence of cardiac symptoms (Wikman et al., 2008).

In addition, previous mental health problems (e.g. depression) may influence PTSD symptoms (Wikman et al., 2008). Other factors include work and social dysfunction (Kutz et al., 1994).

Subjective appraisal

It has been postulated that the emotional state of patients at the time of MI and their subjective response to it are important factors in the development of PTSD symptoms (Rocha et al., 2008). For example, anxiety at the time of MI and depressed mood during hospitalisation have been associated with post-MI PTSD (Rocha et al., 2008; Wikman et al., 2008). Awareness of having MI was also strongly associated with PTSD symptoms, even when controlling for negative affect (Bennett & Brooke, 1999). Because patients were aware that they had MI, the way they perceived the severity of the condition was associated with the trajectory of PTSD (Ginzburg et al., 2003). Experiencing pain and feeling helpless predicted more severe PTSD at baseline. Increased PTSD over time was also predicted by increased PTSD at baseline and higher perception of pain during MI. In contrast, lower PTSD over time was found in patients with lower pain experience during MI. One implication is that short-term PTSD may perpetuate long-term PTSD. Another implication is that the intense emotional experience of pain may influence long-term PTSD and its recovery (Hari et al., 2010). This was confirmed in another study after controlling for sociodemographic, clinical, and psychological factors (age, gender, ethnicity, social disadvantage, severity of acute coronary syndrome, negative affectivity, and recurrence of cardiac symptoms) (Wikman et al., 2012).

During MI, some patients need to be resuscitated. Such emergency procedure may be associated with PTSD symptoms. One study has shown that patients who have survived cardiac arrest may exhibit PTSD symptoms and have problems regulating their affects and social functioning (Ladwig et al., 1999). To prevent the development of PTSD, studies have shown that the administration of morphine during resuscitation and early trauma care can usually be protective (Bryant et al., 2009; Saxe et al., 2001). The rationale for this intervention is based on the idea that physical injuries with severe pain caused by trauma are a risk factor for the later development of PTSD. Therefore, the earlier the pain is relieved, the lower the risk of PTSD.

Three months after acute myocardial infarction, subjective perceptions of illness, higher illness concerns, and higher emotional impairment were associated with PTSD symptoms. Beliefs about harmful consequences after an acute MI were associated with PTSD symptoms after controlling for demographic factors, cognitive depressive symptoms, and fear of dying during MI (Princip et al., 2018). These findings also reflect previous findings that MI increases the risk of developing not only acute stress disorder but also PTSD. Consequences after illness and worry about illness, as well as identity (patients' perception of symptoms as part of their illness) predicted the development of both disorders (Oflaz et al., 2014).

As MI is an unpredictable and uncontrollable negative event, patients may have shattered their sense of invulnerability but adopted their negative assumptions about the world. Patients with post-MI PTSD tend to perceive themselves as less worthy immediately after MI and to view the world as more random (e.g. that our lives are largely determined by chance) than the group without PTSD or without trauma. The patients with post-MI PTSD also had a decrease in their sense of luck (they felt they were not lucky individuals). On the other hand, the other groups without PTSD remained stable in terms of their perception of luck (Ginzburg, 2004). The above studies have led to the argument that the importance of looking at subjective appraisal cannot be underestimated. Some have even concluded that these subjective factors influence mental health more than objective measures of cardiac function (e.g. left ventricular ejection fraction, treadmill exercise capacity, and inducible ischaemia on stress echocardiography) (Cohen, Marmar, Neylan, et al., 2009).

Personality and coping

Based on the Big Five general personality traits, patients with full-PTSD were significantly more neurotic than patients without PTSD and with partial-PTSD. This is not surprising given that neuroticism is a risk factor for poor mental and physical health problems (Khan et al., 2005; Lahey, 2009; Smith & MacKenzie, 2006), including cardiovascular disease (Suls & Bunde, 2005), eczema (Buske-Kirschbaum et al., 2001), asthma (Huovinen et al., 2001), and irritable bowel syndrome (Spiller et al., 2007). Neuroticism predicted distress outcomes and health complaint outcomes after controlling for demographic and clinical variables (Pedersen et al., 2002). A meta-analysis based on 33 population-based samples showed that neuroticism was associated with mood disorders, anxiety disorders, somatoform disorders, alcohol and drug disorders, schizophrenia, and eating disorders, with effect sizes ranging from 0.54 to 1.54 (Cohen's d) (Malouff et al., 2005). Neuroticism may also influence comorbidity between these psychological disorders (Khan et al., 2005; Middeldorp et al., 2006; Weinstock & Whisman, 2006). For example, it can explain 20–45% of comorbidity in people with depression and anxiety and 19–88% of comorbidity in people with substance dependence (Khan et al., 2005).

Another distress-prone personality is Type D, which is associated with coronary artery disease (Denollet, 1998). Type D describes a personality trait characterised by an interaction between negative affectivity (the tendency to feel negative emotions) and social inhibition (the tendency to deliberately suppress the expression of these emotions in social interaction in order to avoid the disapproval of others), which influences health outcomes. The argument is that the likelihood of cardiac events occurring is higher in individuals who exhibit high levels of negative affectivity and social inhibition. Type D personality predicted PTSD symptoms over and above other factors (gender, age, MI, neuroticism and extroversion) (Pedersen & Denollet, 2004). People with Type D personality trait tend to have higher scores for MI-PTSD symptoms (especially arousal and avoidance), depression, and anxiety than people without Type D. This trait is used as a marker for general emotional distress (Pedersen & Denollet, 2004).

As mentioned earlier, social inhibition, one of the personality domains of Type D, refers to a person's tendency to inhibit the expression of emotions. Some researchers have focused specifically on this aspect of personality, arguing that alexithymia is also a risk factor for post-MI PTSD. Put simply, alexithymia is characterised by (1) difficulty identifying and distinguishing emotions from bodily sensations and differentiating between cognition and emotions, (2) difficulty expressing and describing feelings to others, and (3) a literal, utilitarian, and externally oriented cognitive style (Nemiah & Sifneos, 1970; Taylor et al., 1997). Thus, people with high levels of alexithymia tend to have problems recognising, processing, regulating, or expressing emotions using appropriate emotional regulation strategies (Fink et al., 2010; Shishido et al., 2013). Alexithymia has been shown to be predictive of post-MI PTSD. In particular, difficulty identifying feelings was positively correlated with PTSD symptoms (Bennett & Brooke, 1999). Extending this study, further research showed that in addition to difficulty identifying feelings, difficulty describing feelings was significantly correlated with PTSD after MI (Gao et al., 2015).

In addition to the personality traits mentioned above, some researchers have also examined the role of attachment and found that a greater increase in attachment anxiety was associated with an increase in PTSD symptoms in these MI patients (Gao et al., 2015). Hostility was also a factor (Wikman et al., 2008), which may reflect why patients with full-PTSD were less agreeable (i.e. antagonistic) than patients without PTSD (Chung et al., 2007).

Research has also examined the role of coping. Overall, research suggests that social support is an adaptive coping strategy. Patients who received little social support reported an increased risk of post-MI PTSD and depression. Patients who were dissatisfied with the type of social support they received also had an increased risk of PTSD along with depression, anxiety, and health complaints (Pedersen et al., 2002). This type of coping had a unique effect on PTSD symptoms after controlling for negative affect (Bennett & Brooke, 1999) and neuroticism (Pedersen et al., 2002). Repression is another adaptive or protective coping strategy in both the immediate (e.g. 1 week) and long-term (7 months) aftermath of MI. Patients who used this coping strategy showed fewer symptoms of acute stress disorder (ASD) and post-MI PTSD than those who did not repress (Ginzburg et al., 2002). These results may be surprising to some, as repression means preventing the processing and integration of trauma memories, which in turn should maintain PTSD (Brewin et al., 1996; Horowitz, 1976). Another adaptive form of coping is the trait resilience, which has been shown to buffer against PTSD, although one study has shown that in patients with acute MI, the trait resilience does not buffer the perception of the acute MI as stressful *per se*. Nevertheless, it may contribute to better coping with the traumatic experience in the long term. This in turn would prevent the development of MI-associated PTSD. Resilience could thus play an important role in coping with PTSD symptoms triggered by acute MI (Meister et al., 2016).

Unfortunately, the traumatogenic potential of sudden and unexpected chronic illnesses (e.g. MI) and the traumatogenic changes in life circumstances can lead to maladaptive coping with illness. This type of coping develops throughout life (Alonzo, 2000; Alonzo & Reynolds, 1998). Some patients use avoidance-focused coping, detaching mentally and behaviourally from the traumatic effects of MI. After controlling for age, bypass surgery, psychological problems prior to MI, and angioplasty, patients who applied avoidance-focused and emotion-focused coping tended to report more comorbid symptoms than PTSD symptoms. In other words, the way in which MI patients' coping strategies relate to health outcomes appears to be symptom-specific (Chung, Berger, & Rudd, 2008). Furthermore, there seems to be an age effect in coping, as older patients with full-PTSD tend to use both maladaptive and problem-focused coping strategies. In these older patients, coping was a partial mediator between the different levels of post-MI PTSD and comorbidity (Chung, Berger, Jones, & Rudd, 2008).

For some MI patients, the consequences of using maladaptive avoidance coping can be severe and even life-threatening. Due to the cumulative stress of the condition, individuals may experience a 'spectrum of posttraumatic disturbances' ranging from anxiety to PTSD. These disturbances could put patients at greater risk for acute myocardial infarction (AMI) and sudden cardiac death (Alonzo, 2000; Alonzo & Reynolds, 1998). The reason for this is that they want to avoid being reminded of MI in the context of their PTSD symptoms. This also means that they may not take medication (e.g. aspirin) because taking it would be a reminder of MI. A meta-analysis based on a very large sample ($n = 376,162$) of MI patients showed that only 66% adhered to their cardiac medication for a median of 2 years (Naderi et al., 2012). Thus, medication non-adherence was associated with severe PTSD symptoms, which in turn perpetuated non-adherence. No other psychological symptoms independently predicted non-adherence (Shemesh et al., 2001). Not surprisingly, non-adherence to medication increases poor disease control and the risk of subsequent cardiovascular readmissions, clinical adverse events and mortality (Shemesh et al., 2001, 2004; Spindler & Pedersen, 2005; Zen et al., 2012). As a result, people with PTSD are more prone to increased likelihood of medication non-adherence, including forgetting or skipping medication (Zen et al., 2012) and leaving medication at home (Cornelius et al., 2018). Some also have reasons related to emotional processes, such as wondering if the medication would help or not having answers about the medication (Cornelius et al., 2018). These individuals are therefore likely to experience recurrent attack and require repeated emergency medical treatment (Kutz et al., 1994).

This problem of poor medication adherence affects not only MI patients, but also patients suffering from acute coronary syndrome. Patients with elevated PTSD symptoms triggered by an acute coronary syndrome were more likely to have aversive cognitions towards cardiovascular medications after controlling for age, gender, race, ethnicity, education, depression and acute coronary syndrome status. Elevated PTSD scores were associated with lack of medication to avoid traumatic memories not only of heart disease, but also fears and thoughts of ongoing and future risks (Husain et al., 2018).

Furthermore, patients with acute coronary syndrome diagnosed with current PTSD showed significantly greater optimistic bias than patients without a PTSD diagnosis, after adjustment for demographics, ACS severity, medical comorbidities, depression, and self-confidence in their ability to control their heart disease. In other words, PTSD might be associated with poor adherence to medical advice due to an overly optimistic perception of the risk of recurrence. They might tend to believe that they themselves are less likely to experience a negative event. This belief could be conceptualised as a form of avoidance or numbing response as part of their PTSD symptoms that minimises risk perception in relation to the future MI threat (Edmondson, Shaffer, et al., 2012).

It is worth noting that patients who have high levels of anxiety sensitivity, that is, fear of the negative consequences of anxiety-related sensations, also tend to avoid taking medication. Compared to patients with low anxiety sensitivity, patients with high anxiety sensitivity are more inclined to make catastrophic interpretations of arousal-related sensations of anxiety (e.g. believing that palpitations can lead to cardiac arrest or heart attack), which in turn would exacerbate anxiety. As a result, they want to avoid occasions when they might experience anxiety-provoking triggers, situations or contexts. Presumably, taking medication could be considered one of these triggers. One study showed that patients with high levels of anxiety sensitivity (65%) were more likely to not take their blood pressure medication (BP) compared to patients with low anxiety sensitivity (37%) (adjusted relative risk: 1.76). Such non-adherence would naturally increase cardiovascular risk (Alcantara et al., 2014).

Intervention: Cognitive behavioural therapy

Since MI patients may not take medication (e.g. aspirin) which, as mentioned earlier, is part of their posttraumatic avoidance coping, intervention studies have been conducted to improve PTSD symptoms, which in turn may improve treatment adherence and ultimately cardiovascular risk (Shemesh et al., 2006, 2001). The benefits of various forms of cognitive behavioural therapy (CBT) have been demonstrated in several studies. These studies examined patients with PTSD triggered not only by cardiac events but also by cancer, HIV, multiple sclerosis and stem cell transplantation. They compared exposure-based CBT with an assessment-only control and found that the former was effective in reducing PTSD symptoms. Imaginal exposure, another form of exposure-based CBT, was also compared to an attentional control. The results also showed a trend towards a reduction in PTSD symptoms (Haerizadeh et al., 2020). Trauma-focused cognitive-behavioural therapy, which involves imaginal exposure in 3 to 5 sessions, is also a treatment that has been proposed as a safe and effective treatment for improving PTSD, depression and cardiovascular risk factors (Shemesh et al., 2006, 2011).

However, Eye Movement Desensitisation and Reprocessing (EMDR) is claimed to be more effective than imaginal exposure in reducing not only PTSD symptoms but also depressive and anxiety symptoms in patients with life-threatening cardiac events (Arabia et al., 2011). Studies have compared EMDR with imaginal exposure, conventional CBT and relaxation therapy and found EMDR to be more effective. From the above, it has been inferred that patients suffering from medical events, including cardiovascular events, may benefit from both CBT and EMDR (Haerizadeh et al., 2020). It is therefore not surprising that CBT and EMDR have been recommended by the National Institute for Health and Care Excellence (2018) as appropriate treatment approaches for PTSD.

It is worth noting that CBT alone is not the most effective method to help these patients. In addition to CBT, a non-specific educational programme explaining to patients the importance of adhering to medical recommendations post-MI has been shown to be helpful in improving adherence to the aspirin regimen. Therefore, it has been recommended that this non-specific intervention, which focuses on adherence, be used as a first line of treatment, especially for patients who are unwilling or unable to undergo CBT treatment (Shemesh et al., 2006).

Cognitive behavioural therapy has also been used to normalise physiological responses and reduce heart rate reactivity. Patients who have received this therapy have had a significantly greater reduction in heart rate reactivity than those who have not (Rabe et al., 2006). Similarly, prolonged exposure and virtual reality exposure therapies may reduce cardiovascular risk associated with PTSD by reducing heart rate reactivity and resting heart rate in soldiers with PTSD from baseline to post-treatment. This reduction would in turn lead to improved cardiovascular function (Bourassa et al., 2020). Despite this evidence, whether PTSD treatments improve health by improving tonic (i.e. resting) cardiovascular function and cardiovascular reactivity is inconclusive, although the evidence that PTSD treatments, for example cognitive–behavioural interventions, reduce cardiovascular reactivity to traumatic events was stronger (Bourassa et al., 2021).

The above studies demonstrating the effectiveness of therapies for PTSD symptoms in patients with cardiovascular disease may be encouraging overall; however, one study examined the effectiveness of trauma-focused counselling on the incidence of posttraumatic stress symptoms triggered by acute coronary syndrome. The results showed no differences between trauma-focused counselling and stress counselling in terms of PTSD symptoms, depressive symptoms, global psychological distress and risk of cardiovascular-related hospitalisation/general mortality. On the contrary, in patients who had received trauma-focused counselling, symptom burden increased significantly more over time than in patients who had received stress counselling. Trauma-focused early treatment should be avoided (von Känel et al., 2018).

One must also be careful about placing emphasis on the effective or immediate results of treating psychological disorders such as PTSD and heart problems. Such emphasis can have an opposite effect, that is, harmful medical treatment. It is important that health professionals accept the fact that effective treatments often take time (Theorell, 1997). The timing of therapy for patients also needs to be carefully considered. A single psychological debriefing aimed at alleviating traumatic reactions within a few hours or days of trauma exposure has been discouraged. It neither reduces psychological distress nor prevents the onset of PTSD. It may even cause harm and increase the risk of PTSD, as emotional catharsis can be performed in the acute phase without a good understanding of the patient's distress (Bryant, 2015; Witteveen et al., 2012).

Other interventions

Limited evidence shows that physical fitness is associated with greater reductions in avoidance and hyperarousal symptoms, as well as physical and social symptoms of anxiety sensitivity. It may also provide a buffer against cardiovascular risk and associated mortality (Vancampfort et al., 2017). However, more research is needed in this area. Other interventions that could potentially help people with PTSD include autogenic training. It is considered effective in improving PTSD symptoms along with disrupting cardiac autonomic nerve activity (Mitani et al., 2006). Simply put, autogenic training aims to teach the body to respond to verbal commands. These commands direct the body to relax and control breathing, blood pressure, heart rate, and body temperature using visual imagery and verbal cues. This is to enable patients to reduce stress and achieve deep relaxation (Schultz & Luthe, 1959). Mindfulness-informed approaches are also increasingly being used with patients suffering from myocardial ischaemia, hypertension, and a whole range of other physical conditions such as respiratory diseases (e.g. asthma, chronic obstructive pulmonary disease) and psychosomatic conditions (e.g. fibromyalgia, irritable bowel syndrome) (McCown & Reibel, 2010).

In addition, some researchers focus on reducing traumatic memories through physical treatments such as administering glucocorticoids (stress doses of hydrocortisone) to patients. The idea behind this is that PTSD patients often have inadequate endogenous glucocorticoid signalling, that is, critical illness-related corticosteroid insufficiency. Stress doses of hydrocortisone can remedy this, which in turn leads to down-regulation of the stress response, inhibition of the retrieval of traumatic memories, facilitation of the extinction of aversive information, and ultimately PTSD symptoms (Schelling et al., 2006). Similarly, stress doses of hydrocortisone may also reduce the intensity of chronic stress and PTSD symptoms over time in patients who have undergone cardiac surgery (Schelling et al., 2004). Another study examined the association between active treatment with blood pressure medications (i.e. angiotensin-converting enzyme inhibitors (ACE) and angiotensin receptor blockers (ARBs)) and PTSD. A significant association was found between the presence of an ACE inhibitor/ARB drug and reduced PTSD symptoms. Interestingly, other blood pressure medications, including beta-blockers, calcium channel blockers, and diuretics, did not appear to reduce PTSD symptoms (Khoury et al., 2012).

Posttraumatic growth and cardiovascular problems

The foregoing implies that patients suffer from some pathologies that can be treated with a whole range of psychological or physical interventions. However, positive psychologists advocate not emphasising pathology so much (Sheikh & Marotta, 2008). In the context of supporting MI patients, it has been argued that counsellors should be used in cardiac rehabilitation to promote posttraumatic growth (PTG). There are potential benefits that may arise from this traumatic condition MI (Sheikh & Marotta, 2008). Posttraumatic growth also appears to be beneficial for other groups of patients. For example, there are no group differences between MI and brain injury patients in terms of posttraumatic growth overall or all five growth domains except for 'relationship with others', which was higher in the brain injury group (Karagiorgou & Cullen, 2016).

Posttraumatic growth is a psychological phenomenon in which people can experience positive psychological changes in self-perception, relationships with others and views of life after coping with a very stressful or challenging life circumstance, in this case MI (Tedeschi et al., 1998). According to the organismic valuing theory of growth, adversity can enhance an intrinsic motivation to grow. Adversity can lead to the emergence of cognitive–emotional processing after trauma, characterised by intrusion and avoidance. Assimilation, negative accommodation, and positive accommodation can be the result of this processing. Some people experience positive changes in their psychological well-being after trauma by accommodating the new trauma-related information. This positive accommodation is possible if the environment can support this positive process (Joseph & Linley, 2005).

Using a large ($n = 2636$) cohort of MI patients, one study showed that a larger PTG was associated with a higher predicted risk of recurrent events, but not with the actual frequency of events. In other words, patient reflection on the risk of cardiac events may lead to the emergence of PTG. In addition, greater PTG has been associated with proactive measures to prevent the recurrence of cardiac events, including increased doctor visits, participation in rehabilitation programmes, and seeking non-urgent medical care (Leung et al., 2012), that is, a type of proactive coping with one's illness and thus preventing a recurrence of a cardiac event. This illustrates the close relationship between patients' perceived risk of a cardiac event → PTG → coping. In other words, PTG can be seen as a mediator. However, it can also be seen as an outcome. One study has shown that patients perceive social support → coping → PTG. More research is needed to find out the dynamic interaction between these factors, which might affect the way people cope with their illness (Senol-Durak & Ayvasik, 2010).

In the passage above, it was suggested that the reason posttraumatic growth is beneficial for MI patients is because posttraumatic growth facilitates proactive or adaptive coping strategies. Evidence suggests that PTG is actually associated with a whole range of positive, adaptive, or resilient human characteristics that are helpful for MI patients. For example, PTG may help build personal resilience. Patients with coronary heart disease who have high levels of personal resilience (e.g. perceived control) tend to have better quality of life, lower cholesterol levels, and more physical activity than patients with low levels of personal resilience (Chan et al., 2006). Similarly, patients with increasing levels of personal resilience are more likely to experience PTG, which in turn is associated with positive health outcomes (Senol-Durak & Ayvasik, 2010).

After an MI incident, PTG was positively correlated with extraversion, agreeableness, conscientiousness and openness to experience, but negatively correlated with neuroticism. In other words, PTG may counteract neuroticism while being correlated with the increase of other traits. PTG was also positively correlated with perceived social support and problem-focused and active emotional coping, but negatively correlated with avoidant emotional coping. It seems that individuals with these growth traits are the ones who deal with the problems at hand and actively engage with social support. This active engagement may reflect the negative relationship between growth and avoidant emotional coping (Javed & Dawood, 2016). In addition, PTG in general and specific domains of posttraumatic growth (changes in self, relationships or life affirmation) was related to cognitive coping strategies measured in terms of refocusing on planning, positive refocusing, positive reappraisal, and putting events into perspective (Łosiak & Nikiel, 2014).

However, research on PTG in cardiovascular patients is not without controversy. First of all, the sustained effect of PTG in MI patients has been questioned. One study showed that 74.4% of MI patients reported PTG in the first 5 days to 2 weeks and 23.3% reported PTG after 8 weeks (Zhao et al., 2015). The aforementioned cognitive coping was also not related to spiritual changes, another feature of posttraumatic growth. Surprisingly, spiritual change correlated more strongly with the severity of the life threat posed by the MI (Łosiak & Nikiel, 2014). Indeed, spiritual change seems to be controversial in the patient population of MI. Looking at the change in spiritual well-being from preoperative to one year after surgery in non-emergency cardiovascular disease patients, 48.4% of patients reported some increase in spiritual well-being associated with PTG characterised by relating to others, finding new possibilities and accepting one's circumstances. However, for 40.8%, spiritual well-being decreased overall. In addition, 10.9% reported no change (Kearns et al., 2020).

Furthermore, positive changes following trauma were not necessarily related to overall life satisfaction. However, when looking at specific satisfaction dimensions, satisfaction with leisure time was positively correlated with changes in relationships with others, appreciation of life, and spiritual changes (Ogińska-Bulik, 2014). Although most patients have developed growth during hospitalisation, the degree to which patients have developed growth may vary depending on early life experiences. Those who had high levels of attachment avoidance were more likely to have PTG (OR: 1.01–1.07) during hospitalisation (Zhao et al., 2015). However, this increase was smaller in patients who had experienced emotional neglect in childhood (OR: 0.76–0.96) (Zhao et al., 2015).

Controversial results associated with PTG are not uncommon, as it could be argued that this construct is inherently controversial due to its paradoxical and double-edged phenomenon. PTG often occurs in patients who have concurrent levels of posttraumatic growth and distress. One study showed that whereas PTSD symptoms were associated with increased psychological distress and decreased well-being and health-related quality of life in MI and survivors of acute bypass surgery, they were also associated with increased PTG. However, growth may moderate the negative impact of PTSD symptoms on stress outcomes (Bluvstein et al., 2013).

Best practice recommendations have been made for counsellors helping people with traumatic heart disease. One of these recommendations is that patients' appraisals of life-threatening cardiovascular disease can influence psychological and physical recovery, as well as social support. They must therefore be empowered to re-evaluate their value systems, avoid blame, but allow for posttraumatic growth. This in turn would reduce recurrence and complications not only for the patient but also for others affected, including family members. In addition, facilitating growth would enable patients to facilitate their own health care and take charge of their condition, including following the treatment recommendations of their medical consultants. Ultimately, PTG is a form of problem-focused coping that creates a sense of control and hope, which is important and useful for MI patients.

The assumption is that patients who are able to perceive benefits in their struggles tend to have a better prognosis than those who maintain a negative evaluation of their current situation. Counsellors can empower their patients to see the importance of meaning-making and change from the negative view that there is no recovery to the recognition of recovery, the possibility of future improvement, and the improvement of depressive symptoms. Counsellors can also empower their patients to move from blaming themselves and others to minimising helplessness and anger, which are risk factors for MI. In this way, patients would increase their acceptance and motivation and take planned action. Finding meaning in their traumatic illness would enable them to reconstruct their basic assumptions about themselves, others, control, and predictability in life (Sheikh & Marotta, 2008). Put simply, facilitating posttraumatic growth means minimising maladaptive coping with posttraumatic avoidance. Otherwise, the risk of cardiovascular readmission, recurrent cardiac events, and mortality would only increase.

Passing remarks on PTSD in relation to medical procedures

To close this chapter, it is worth briefly mentioning existing research that addresses PTSD symptoms that may occur in patients following invasive physical treatments or medical procedures to treat cardiovascular events. It has been claimed that patients who have undergone medical procedures or interventions such as bypass surgery and angioplasty report PTSD symptoms. In other words, medical procedures or interventions to treat MI may play an important role in the maintenance of PTSD symptoms in patients with MI (Chung, Berger, & Rudd, 2008). Similarly, the literature has previously demonstrated the development of PTSD following heart transplantation (Stukas et al., 1999), cardiopulmonary bypass (Rothenhäusler et al., 2005) and surgery for congenital cyanotic heart disease (Toren & Horesh, 2007). In addition to PTSD, patients may also develop postoperative delirium, adjustment disorders, depression, and cognitive deficits (Favaro et al., 2011; Rothenhäusler et al., 2005).

One study examined the 1-year mortality risk associated with preoperative mental health problems in patients who had undergone non-ambulatory cardiac or vascular surgery. It was found that 14% of patients with PTSD died, 16% suffered from bipolar disorder, 18% from major depression, 24% from schizophrenia, but 20% had no mental health problems. Mental health problems were associated with increased mortality after heart surgery only in patients with bipolar disorder. Bipolar disorder and PTSD were associated with lower mortality after vascular surgery. The study concluded that the impact of mental health problems before surgery on mortality after surgery is unclear. In other words, whether patients with mental health problems should receive needed surgery in a timely manner remains unclear, although it is an important factor to consider before surgical referral (Copeland et al., 2014). On the other hand, some studies have investigated whether patients can develop adjustment disorder with depressive and PTSD symptoms and cognitive deficits after cardiac surgery. One year later, the severity of these symptoms, especially depression and anxiety, improved and returned to pre-surgery levels. Quality of life improved over time. However, impaired cognitive functions were associated with a lower quality of life 1 year later (Rothenhäusler et al., 2005).

Some studies specifically look at the impact of living with an implantable cardioverter defibrillator (ICD). Although there are fewer studies looking at PTSD after implantation of an ICD than those looking at the post-MI PTSD, the negative impact of PTSD on the long-term mortality risk of patients living with an ICD cannot be underestimated. Living with an ICD can be a stressful experience for many patients. To prevent sudden cardiac death, the ICD is a standard therapy (DiMarco, 2003). An ICD monitors cardiac arrhythmias and can deliver an electric shock to the heart for cardioversion or defibrillation if ventricular tachycardia or fibrillation occurs. Although this shock can potentially save lives and reduce the risk of death, it can be uncomfortable or frightening for patients. Patients may have fears of recurrent arrhythmias, sudden death, proper functioning of the device and loss of control of the ICD discharge (Fricchione et al., 1989). These fears can be traumatic and constantly remind patients of their potentially fatal cardiovascular disease (Hamner et al., 1999).

In addition to anxiety and depression symptoms, which ranged from 24 to 87% in different studies (Sears & Conti, 2002), patients living with an ICD also report PTSD (Habibović et al., 2012; Hamner et al., 1999; Ladwig et al., 2008; von Känel et al., 2011; Yuan Ng & Mela, 2016), although one study showed no significant differences compared to non-PTSD patients in terms of disease severity (left ventricular ejection fraction status) or extent of ICD discharges (Ladwig et al., 2008). In a follow-up study, 12% met the cut-off for PTSD and about two years later 18% met this cut-off. Some of these were consistent in that 19% met the cut-off for both assessments (von Känel et al., 2011). However, a much lower prevalence rate of 7.6% was found 18 months after implantation (Habibović et al., 2012). Patients with ICD who met the criteria for PTSD had a higher mortality risk than those without PTSD (Ladwig et al., 2008).

In terms of risk factors, among patients living with an ICD, more women than men reported PTSD at baseline (von Känel et al., 2011) and poor quality of life (Irvine et al., 2011). The relative risk of developing PTSD was 13.4 times higher in women than in men. People with a low level of education tended to maintain PTSD in the long term (about 24 months later) (von Känel et al., 2011). Patients' feelings of helplessness were related to both immediate and long-term PTSD (von Känel et al., 2011). The severity of PTSD at baseline and the presence of alexithymia predicted more severe long-term PTSD. Other factors were the extent of patients' peritraumatic dissociation and depression (von Känel et al., 2011).

Personality traits may also play a role in influencing PTSD after ICD implantation. In one study, Type D personality (OR: 3.5) (a personality trait with high levels of negative affectivity and social inhibition (Denollet, 2005)) and baseline anxiety (OR: 4.3) were found to predict PTSD 18 months after implantation. This association was independent of shocks and other clinical and demographic covariates. Shocks were not significantly associated with PTSD, which contradicts another study in which the impact of a shock (e.g. >5) by ICD was associated with greater long-term PTSD (von Känel et al., 2011). It seems important to identify patients with Type D personality and anxiety at the time of implantation to prevent the development of PTSD in ICD patients (Habibović et al., 2012).

Studies have been conducted to investigate whether psychological interventions can reduce PTSD symptoms, which in turn could improve survival rates. This is consistent with the rationale behind psychosocial interventions in cardiac rehabilitation programmes, particularly for people who have experienced traumatic cardiac illness (Sheikh & Marotta, 2008). A study using eight sessions of cognitive behavioural therapy (CBT) for ICD patients showed that PTSD symptoms, especially avoidance symptoms in both genders, as well as depressive symptoms and quality of life in women improved under CBT than under usual cardiac care. However, no significant differences between treatment conditions were found at follow-up. In other words, CBT as a potential psychological intervention improved psychological functioning or adjustment in the first year but not in the long term (Irvine et al., 2011). However, the results changed when the severity of PTSD symptoms was taken into account. ICD patients in the CBT group who had high levels of PTSD symptoms reported significantly greater symptom reduction from baseline to 12 months than those in the usual cardiac care group. In contrast, patients with low levels of PTSD symptoms reported little reduction in symptoms regardless of group membership (Ford et al., 2016). These results suggest the importance of a multidisciplinary approach with input from cardiologists and mental health professionals, in line with the interventions already mentioned to support patients with cardiovascular disease (Yuan Ng & Mela, 2016).

Summary

There is ample evidence that PTSD due to past trauma is associated with cardiovascular risk. Several risk factors are implicated in influencing this relationship, including female gender, older age and ethnicity. This relationship may also be influenced by a complex interaction with comorbid psychological factors. Patients with PTSD tend to have unhealthy lifestyles that would exacerbate cardiovascular risk factors such as obesity, diabetes, and hypertension. Another risk factor is relationships, including insecure attachment and attachment anxiety, both of which can increase the distress of PTSD. This in turn can affect physical and mental health as well as cardiovascular disease risk factors. Trauma can increase dysregulation of the autonomic nervous system and increase cardiovascular risk. Autonomic nervous system dysregulation includes increased heart rate, heart rate variability and increased blood pressure, which can cause people with PTSD to develop cardiovascular disease.

In addition to examining the relationship between PTSD due to past trauma and cardiovascular disease, previous research has also looked at PTSD following acute coronary syndrome (post-ACS PTSD) or myocardial infarction (post-MI PTSD). Anxiety sensitivity and depressive symptoms may contribute to the former. For the latter, risk factors include demographic variables, subjective appraisal, feeling anxious during the onset of MI and feeling depressed during hospitalisation, experiencing pain, and feeling helpless. Other risk factors for post-MI PTSD include the perception of a higher level of harmful consequences after the disease, worry about the disease, and emotional impairment of patients.

Personality traits and coping strategies are also considered risk factors for post-MI PTSD including neuroticism, Type D, and alexithymia. Coping strategies include low levels of social support, and avoidance- and emotion-focused coping strategies. Avoidance coping especially can have serious and life-threatening consequences, as patients can avoid being reminded of MI by not adhering to medication. On the other hand, repression and resilience are adaptive coping strategies. To improve PTSD symptoms, which in turn could improve medication adherence and ultimately cardiovascular risk, different types of cognitive behavioural therapy (exposure-based, imaginal exposure, trauma-focused) and eye movement desensitisation and reprocessing have been shown effective.

Although the benefits of PTG in cardiovascular patients can be controversial, it is broadly considered to be something that can facilitate proactive, positive, and adaptive coping strategies that patients can use to manage their illness and prevent recurrence of cardiac events. PTG can also promote resilient human qualities that are helpful for MI patients. It may buffer neuroticism, increase social support, promote problem-focused and active emotional coping, and decrease avoidant emotional coping.

References

Abbas, C. C., Schmid, J.-P., Guler, E., Wiedemar, L., Begre, S., Saner, H., Schnyder, U., & von Kanel, R. (2009). Trajectory of posttraumatic stress disorder caused by myocardial infarction: A two-year follow-up study. *International Journal of Psychiatry in Medicine, 39*(4), 359–379.

Agorastos, A., Boel, J. A., Heppner, P. S., Hager, T., Moeller-Bertram, T., Haji, U., Motazedi, A., Yanagi, M. A., Baker, D. G., & Stiedl, O. (2013). Diminished vagal activity and blunted diurnal variation of heart rate dynamics in posttraumatic stress disorder. *Stress, 16*(3), 300–310. https://doi.org/10.3109/10253890.2012.751369

Ahmadi, N., Hajsadeghi, F., Nabavi, V., Olango, G., Molla, M., Budoff, M., Vaidya, N., Quintana, J., Pynoos, R., Hauser, P., & Yehuda, R. (2018). The long-term clinical outcome of posttraumatic stress disorder with impaired coronary distensibility. *Psychosomatic Medicine, 80*(3), 294–300. https://doi.org/10.1097/psy.0000000000000565

Ainsworth, M. D., & Bell, S. M. (1970). Attachment, exploration, and separation: Illustrated by the behavior of one-year-olds in a strange situation. *Child Development, 41*, 49–67. https://doi.org/10.2307/1127388

Alcantara, C., Edmondson, D., Moise, N., Oyola, D., Hiti, D., & Kronish, I. M. (2014). Anxiety sensitivity and medication nonadherence in patients with uncontrolled hypertension. *Journal of Psychosomatic Research, 77*(4), 283–286.

Alonzo, A. A. (2000). The experience of chronic illness and posttraumatic stress disorder: the consequences of cumulative adversity. *Social Science and Medicine, 50*, 1475–1484.

Alonzo, A., & Reynolds, N. (1998). The structure of emotions during acute myocardial infarction: a model of coping. *Social Science & Medicine, 46*, 1099–1110.

American Psychiatric Association. (1994). *Diagnostic and statistical manual of mental disorders* (4th ed.).

American Psychiatric Association. (2013). *Diagnostic and statistical manual of mental disorders* (5th ed.).https://doi.org/10.1176/appi.books.9780890425596

Annunziato, R. A., Kim, S.-K., Fussner, M., Ahmad, T., Jerson, B., & Rubinstein, D. (2015). Utilizing correspondence analysis to characterize the mental health of cardiac patients with diabetes. *Journal of Health Psychology, 20*(10), 1275–1284.

Arabia, E., Manca, M. L., & Solomon, R. M. (2011). EMDR for survivors of life-threatening cardiac events: Results of a pilot study. *Journal of EMDR Practice and Research, 5*, 2–13.

Arditte Hall, K. A., Osterberg, T., Orr, S. P., & Pineles, S. L. (2018). The cardiovascular consequences of autonomic nervous system dysregulation in PTSD. In G. Pinna & T. Izumi (Eds.), *Facilitating resilience after PTSD: A translational approach* (pp. 127–156). Nova Biomedical Books.

Beckham, J. C., Feldman, M. E., Barefoot, J. C., Fairbank, J. A., Helms, M. J., Haney, T. L., Hertzberg, M. A., Moore, S. D., & Davidson, J. R. (2000). Ambulatory cardiovascular activity in Vietnam combat veterans with and without posttraumatic stress disorder. *Journal of Consulting and Clinical Psychology, 68*(2), 269–276.

Beckham, J. C., Flood, A. M., Dennis, M. F., & Calhoun, P. S. (2009). Ambulatory cardiovascular activity and hostility ratings in women with chronic posttraumatic stress disorder. *Biological Psychiatry, 65*(3), 268–272.

Beckham, J. C., Gehrman, P. R., McClernon, F., Collie, C. F., & Feldman, M. E. (2004). Cigarette smoking, ambulatory cardiovascular monitoring, and mood in Vietnam veterans with and without chronic posttraumatic stress disorder. *Addictive Behaviors, 29*(8), 1579–1593.

Beckham, J. C., Vrana, S. R., Barefoot, J. C., Feldman, M. E., Fairbank, J., & Moore, S. D. (2002). Magnitude and duration of cardiovascular response to anger in Vietnam veterans with and without posttraumatic stress disorder. *Journal of Consulting and Clinical Psychology, 70*(1), 228–234.

Bedi, U. S., & Arora, R. (2007). Cardiovascular manifestations of posttraumatic stress disorder. *Journal of the National Medical Association, 99*(6), 642–649.

Bennett, P., & Brooke, S. (1999). Intrusive memories, post-traumatic stress disorder and myocardial infarction. *British Journal of Clinical Psychology, 38*(4), 411–416. https://doi.org/10.1348/014466599163015

Beristianos, M. H., Yaffe, K., Cohen, B., & Byers, A. L. (2016). PTSD and risk of incident cardiovascular disease in aging veterans. *American Journal of Geriatric Psychiatry, 24*(3), 192–200. https://doi.org/10.1016/j.jagp.2014.12.003

Bielas, H., Meister-Langraf, R. E., Schmid, J.-P., Barth, J., Znoj, H., Schnyder, U., Princip, M., & von Kanel, R. (2018). C-reactive protein as a predictor of posttraumatic stress induced by acute myocardial infarction. *General Hospital Psychiatry, 53*, 125–130. https://doi.org/10.1016/j.genhosppsych.2018.03.008

Blanchard, E. B. (1990). Elevated basal level of cardiovascular responses in Vietnam veterans with PTSD: A health problem in the making? *Journal of Anxiety Disorders, 4*(3), 233–237.

Blank, A. (1993). The longitudinal course of posttraumatic stress disorder. In J. R. T. Davidson & E. B. Foa (Eds.), *Posttraumatic stress disorder: DSM-IV and beyond* (pp. 3–22). American Psychiatric Press.

Bluvstein, I., Moravchick, L., Sheps, D., Schreiber, S., & Bloch, M. (2013). Posttraumatic growth, posttraumatic stress symptoms and mental health among coronary heart disease survivors. *Journal of Clinical Psychology in Medical Settings, 20*(2), 164–172. https://doi.org/10.1007/s10880-012-9318-z

Boscarino, J. A. (2004). Posttraumatic stress disorder and physical illness: results from clinical and epidemiologic studies. In R. Yehuda & B. McEwen (Eds.), *Biobehavioral stress response: Protective and damaging effects* (pp. 141–153). New York Academy of Sciences.

Boscarino, J. A. (2008a). A prospective study of PTSD and early-age heart disease mortality among Vietnam veterans: Implications for surveillance and prevention. *Psychosomatic Medicine, 70*(6), 668–676.

Boscarino, J. A. (2008b). Psychobiologic predictors of disease mortality after psychological trauma: Implications for research and clinical surveillance. *Journal of Nervous and Mental Disease, 196*(2), 100–107.

Bourassa, K. J., Hendrickson, R. C., Reger, G. M., & Norr, A. M. (2021). Posttraumatic stress disorder treatment effects on cardiovascular physiology: a systematic review and agenda for future research. *Journal of Traumatic Stress, 34*(2), 384–393. https://doi.org/https://doi.org/10.1002/jts.22637

Bourassa, K. J., Stevens, E. S., Katz, A. C., Rothbaum, B. O., Reger, G. M., & Norr, A. M. (2020). The impact of exposure therapy on resting heart rate and heart rate reactivity among active-duty soldiers with posttraumatic stress disorder. *Psychosomatic Medicine, 82*(1), 108–114. https://doi.org/10.1097/psy.0000000000000758

Bowlby, J. (1969). *Attachment and loss*. Basic Books.

Bowlby, J. (2005). *A secure base*. Routledge.

Bremner, J., & Vaccarino, V. (2015). Neurobiology of early life stress in women. In K. Orth-Gomer, N. Schneiderman, V. Vaccarino, & H.-C. Deter (Eds.), *Psychosocial stress and cardiovascular disease in women: Concepts, findings, future perspectives* (pp. 161–178). Springer.

Bremner, J. D., Wittbrodt, M. T., Shah, A. J., Pearce, B. D., Gurel, N. Z., Inan, O. T., Raggi, P., Lewis, T. T., Quyyumi, A. A., & Vaccarino, V. (2020). Confederates in the attic: Posttraumatic stress disorder, cardiovascular disease, and the return of soldier's heart. *Journal of Nervous and Mental Disease, 208*, 171–180. https://doi.org/10.1097/NMD.0000000000001100

Breslau, N., Chilcoat, H. D., Kessler, R. C., Peterson, E. L., & Lucia, V. C. (1999). Vulnerability to assaultive violence: Further speculation of the sex difference in post-traumatic stress disorder. *Psychological Medicine, 29*, 813–821.

Breslau, N., Davis, G. C., Andreski, P., & Peterson, E. (1991). Traumatic events and post-traumatic stress disorder in an urban population of young adults. *Archives of General Psychiatry, 48*(3), 216–222. https://doi.org/10.1001/archpsyc.1991.01810270028003

Breslau, N., Kessler, R., Chilcoat, H., Schultz, L., Davis, G., & Andreski, P. (1998). Trauma and posttraumatic stress disorder in the community: the 1996 Detroit Area Survey of Trauma. *Archives of General Psychiatry, 55*(7), 626–632.

Brewin, C. R., Dalgleish, T., & Joseph, S. (1996). A dual representation theory of posttraumatic stress disorder. *Psychological Review, 103*(4), 670–686.

Bryant, R. A. (2015). Early intervention after trauma. In *Evidence based treatments for trauma-related psychological disorders: A practical guide for clinicians.* (pp. 125–142). Springer International Publishing/Springer Nature. https://doi.org/10.1007/978-3-319-07109-1_7

Bryant, R. A., Creamer, M., O'Donnell, M., Silove, D., & McFarlane, A. C. (2009). A study of the protective function of acute morphine administration on subsequent posttraumatic stress disorder. *Biological Psychiatry, 65*(5), 438–440. https://doi.org/10.1016/j.biopsych.2008.10.032

Buckley, B., Nugent, N., Sledjeski, E., Raimonde, A., Spoonster, E., Bogart, L. M., & Delahanty, D. L. (2004). Evaluation of initial posttrauma cardiovascular levels in association with acute PTSD symptoms following a serious motor vehicle accident. *Journal of Traumatic Stress, 17*(4), 317–324.

Buckley, T. C., Holohan, D., Greif, J. L., Bedard, M., & Suvak, M. (2004). Twenty-four-hour ambulatory assessment of heart rate and blood pressure in chronic PTSD and non-PTSD veterans. *Journal of Traumatic Stress, 17*(2), 163–171.

Buckley, T. C., & Kaloupek, D. G. (2001). A meta-analytic examination of basal cardiovascular activity in posttraumatic stress disorder. *Psychosomatic Medicine, 63*(4), 585–594.

Bugiardini, R., & Bairey Merz, C. N. (2005). Angina with "normal" coronary arteries: a changing philosophy. *JAMA, 293*(4), 477–484. https://doi.org/10.1001/jama.293.4.477

Burnette, C. E., Ka'apu, K., Scarnato, J. M., & Liddell, J. (2020). Cardiovascular health among U.S. indigenous peoples: a holistic and sex-specific systematic review. *Journal of Evidence Based Social Work (2019), 17*(1), 24–48. https://doi.org/10.1080/26408066.2019.1617817

Buske-Kirschbaum, A., Geiben, A., & Hellhammer, D. (2001). Psychobiological aspects of atopic dermatitis: an overview. *Psychotherapy and Psychosomatics, 70*(1), 6–16. https://doi.org/10.1159/000056219

Carlier, I. V. E., & Gersons, B. P. R. (1995). Partial posttraumatic stress disorder (PTSD): The issue of psychological scars and the occurrence of PTSD symptoms. *Journal of Nervous and Mental Disease, 183*, 107–109.

Caska, C. M., Smith, T. W., Renshaw, K. D., Allen, S. N., Uchino, B. N., Birmingham, W., & Carlisle, M. (2014). Posttraumatic stress disorder and responses to couple conflict: Implications for cardiovascular risk. *Health Psychology, 33*(11), 1273–1280.

Chan, I. W. S., Lai, J. C. L., & Wong, K. W. N. (2006). Resilience is associated with better recovery in Chinese people diagnosed with coronary heart disease. *Psychology & Health, 21*, 335–349. https://doi.org/10.1080/14768320500215137

Chou, C. Y., La Marca, R., Steptoe, A., & Brewin, C. R. (2018). Cardiovascular and psychological responses to voluntary recall of trauma in posttraumatic stress disorder. *European Journal of Psychotraumatology, 9*(1), 1472988. https://doi.org/10.1080/20008198.2018.1472988

Chung, M. C., Berger, Z., Jones, R., & Rudd, H. (2008). Posttraumatic stress and co-morbidity following myocardial infarction among older patients: The role of coping. *Ageing and Mental Health, 12*, 124–133.

Chung, M. C., Berger, Z., & Rudd, H. (2007). Comorbidity and personality traits in patients with different levels of posttraumatic stress disorder following myocardial infarction. *Psychiatry Research, 152*(2–3), 243–252.

Chung, M. C., Berger, Z., & Rudd, H. (2008). Coping with posttraumatic stress disorder and comorbidity after myocardial infarction. *Comprehensive Psychiatry, 49*, 55–64.

Cohen, B. E., Marmar, C., Ren, L., Bertenthal, D., & Seal, K. H. (2009). Association of cardiovascular risk factors with mental health diagnoses in Iraq and Afghanistan war veterans using VA health care. *JAMA, 302*(5), 489–492.

Cohen, B. E., Marmar, C. R., Neylan, T. C., Schiller, N. B., Ali, S., & Whooley, M. A. (2009). Posttraumatic stress disorder and health-related quality of life in patients with coronary heart disease: Findings from the heart and soul study. *Archives of General Psychiatry, 66*(11), 1214–1220.

Cohen, H., Benjamin, J., Geva, A. B., Matar, M. A., Kaplan, Z., & Kotler, M. (2000). Autonomic dysregulation in panic disorder and in post-traumatic stress disorder: Application of power spectrum analysis of heart rate variability at rest and in response to recollection of trauma or panic attacks. *Psychiatry Research, 96*(1), 1–13.

Cohen, H., Matar, M. A., Kaplan, Z., & Kotler, M. (1999). Power spectral analysis of heart rate variability in psychiatry. *Psychotherapy and Psychosomatics, 68*(2), 59–66.

Copeland, L. A., Sako, E. Y., Zeber, J. E., Pugh, M. J., Wang, C.-P., MacCarthy, A. A., Restrepo, M. I., Mortensen, E. M., & Lawrence, V. A. (2014). Mortality after cardiac or vascular operations by preexisting serious mental illness status in the Veterans Health Administration. *General Hospital Psychiatry, 36*(5), 502–508. https://doi.org/10.1016/j.genhosppsych.2014.04.003

Cornelius, T., Voils, C. I., Birk, J. L., Romero, E. K., Edmondson, D. E., & Kronish, I. M. (2018). Identifying targets for cardiovascular medication adherence interventions through latent class analysis. *Health Psychology, 37*(11), 1006–1014. https://doi.org/10.1037/hea0000661

Coughlin, S. S. (2011). Post-traumatic stress disorder and cardiovascular disease. *Open Cardiovascular Medicine Journal, 5,* 164–170. https://doi.org/10.2174/18741924011005010164

Creamer, M., Burgess, P., & McFarlane, A. C. (2001). Post-traumatic stress disorder: findings from the Australian National Survey of Mental Health and Well-being. *Psychological Medicine, 31*(7), 1237–1247. https://doi.org/10.1017/s0033291701004287

Davidson, J. R., Hughes, D., Blazer, D. G., & George, L. K. (1991). Post-traumatic stress disorder in the community: An epidemiological study. *Psychological Medicine, 21*(3), 713–721.

Dedert, E. A., Calhoun, P. S., Watkins, L. L., Sherwood, A., & Beckham, J. C. (2010). Posttraumatic stress disorder, cardiovascular, and metabolic disease: A review of the evidence. *Annals of Behavioral Medicine, 39*(1), 61–78.

Dennis, P. A., Dedert, E. A., Van Voorhees, E. E., Watkins, L. L., Hayano, J., Calhoun, P. S., Sherwood, A., Dennis, M. F., & Beckham, J. C. (2016). Examining the crux of autonomic dysfunction in posttraumatic stress disorder: Whether chronic or situational distress underlies elevated heart rate and attenuated heart rate variability. *Psychosomatic Medicine, 78*(7), 805–809.

Dennis, P. A., Kimbrel, N. A., Sherwood, A., Calhoun, P. S., Watkins, L. L., Dennis, M. F., & Beckham, J. C. (2017). Trauma and autonomic dysregulation: episodic- versus systemic-negative affect underlying cardiovascular risk in posttraumatic stress disorder. *Psychosomatic Medicine, 79*(5), 496–505.

Dennis, P. A., Watkins, L. L., Calhoun, P. S., Oddone, A., Sherwood, A., Dennis, M. F., Rissling, M. B., & Beckham, J. C. (2014). Posttraumatic stress, heart rate variability, and the mediating role of behavioral health risks. *Psychosomatic Medicine, 76*(8), 629–637.

Denollet, J. (1998). Personality and coronary heart disease: the type-D scale-16 (DS16). *Annals of Behavioral Medicine, 20*(3), 209–215. https://doi.org/10.1007/bf02884962

Denollet, J. (2005). DS14: standard assessment of negative affectivity, social inhibition, and Type D personality. *Psychosomatic Medicine, 67*(1), 89–97. https://doi.org/10.1097/01.psy.0000149256.81953.49

Diener, S. J., Wessa, M., Ridder, S., Lang, S., Diers, M., Steil, R., & Flor, H. (2012). Enhanced stress analgesia to a cognitively demanding task in patients with posttraumatic stress disorder. *Journal of Affective Disorders, 136*(3), 1247–1251.

DiMarco, J. P. (2003). Implantable cardioverter-defibrillators. *New England Journal of Medicine, 349*(19), 1836–1847. https://doi.org/10.1056/NEJMra035432

Dinenberg, R. E., McCaslin, S. E., Bates, M. N., & Cohen, B. E. (2014). Social support may protect against development of posttraumatic stress disorder: Findings from the Heart and Soul Study. *American Journal of Health Promotion, 28*(5), 294–297.

Doerfler, L. A., & Paraskos, J. A. (2011). Posttraumatic stress disorder following myocardial infarction or cardiac surgery. In *Heart and mind: The practice of cardiac psychology* (2nd ed., pp. 249–268). American Psychological Association. https://doi.org/10.1037/13086-010

Doerfler, L. A., Pbert, L., & DeCosimo, D. (1994). Symptoms of posttraumatic stress disorder following myocardial infarction and coronary artery bypass surgery. *General Hospital Psychiatry, 16,* 193–199.

Dyball, D., Evans, S., Boos, C. J., Stevelink, S. A. M., & Fear, N. T. (2019). The association between PTSD and cardiovascular disease and its risk factors in male veterans of the Iraq/Afghanistan conflicts: a systematic review. *International Review of Psychiatry, 31*(1), 34–48. https://doi.org/10.1080/09540261.2019.1580686

Eberly, R. E., & Engdahl, B. E. (1991). Prevalence of somatic and psychiatric disorders among former prisoners of war. *Hospital & Community Psychiatry, 42*(8), 807–813.

Edmondson, D. (2014). An enduring somatic threat model of posttraumatic stress disorder due to acute life-threatening medical events. *Social and Personality Psychology Compass*, 8(3), 118–134. https://doi.org/10.1111/spc3.12089

Edmondson, D., Birk, J. L., Ho, V. T., Meli, L., Abdalla, M., & Kronish, I. M. (2018). A challenge for psychocardiology: Addressing the causes and consequences of patients' perceptions of enduring somatic threat. *American Psychologist*, 73, 1160–1171. https://doi.org/10.1037/amp0000418

Edmondson, D., Richardson, S., Falzon, L., Davidson, K. W., Mills, M. A., & Neria, Y. (2012). Posttraumatic stress disorder prevalence and risk of recurrence in acute coronary syndrome patients: A meta-analytic review. *PLoS ONE*, 7(6). https://doi.org/10.1371/journal.pone.0038915

Edmondson, D., Rieckmann, N., Shaffer, J. A., Schwartz, J. E., Burg, M. M., Davidson, K. W., Clemow, L., Shimbo, D., & Kronish, I. M. (2011). Posttraumatic stress due to an acute coronary syndrome increases risk of 42-month major adverse cardiac events and all-cause mortality. *Journal of Psychiatric Research*, 45(12), 1621–1626. https://doi.org/10.1016/j.jpsychires.2011.07.004

Edmondson, D., Shaffer, J. A., Denton, E.-G., Shimbo, D., & Clemow, L. (2012). Posttraumatic stress and myocardial infarction risk perceptions in hospitalized acute coronary syndrome patients. *Frontiers in Psychology*, 3, 144. https://doi.org/10.3389/fpsyg.2012.00144

Edmondson, D., Sumner, J. A., Kronish, I. M., Burg, M. M., Oyesiku, L., & Schwartz, J. E. (2018). The association of posttraumatic stress disorder with clinic and ambulatory blood pressure in healthy adults. *Psychosomatic Medicine*, 80(1), 55–61. https://doi.org/10.1097/psy.0000000000000523

Falger, P. R., Op den Velde, W., Hovens, J. E., Schouten, E. G., De Groen, J. H., & Van Duijn, H. (1992). Current posttraumatic stress disorder and cardiovascular disease risk factors in Dutch Resistance veterans from World War II. *Psychotherapy and Psychosomatics*, 57(4), 164–171.

Farley, M., & Patsalides, B. M. (2001). Physical symptoms, posttraumatic stress disorder, and healthcare utilization of women with and without childhood physical and sexual abuse. *Psychological Reports*, 89(3), 595–606.

Favaro, A., Gerosa, G., Caforio, A. L., Volpe, B., Rupolo, G., Zarneri, D., Boscolo, S., Pavan, C., Tenconi, E., d'Agostino, C., Moz, M., Torregrossa, G., Feltrin, G., Gambino, A., & Santonastaso, P. (2011). Posttraumatic stress disorder and depression in heart transplantation recipients: the relationship with outcome and adherence to medical treatment. *General Hospital Psychiatry*, 33(1), 1–7. https://doi.org/10.1016/j.genhosppsych.2010.10.001

Fink, E. L., Anestis, M. D., Selby, E. A., & Joiner, T. E. (2010). Negative urgency fully mediates the relationship between alexithymia and dysregulated behaviours. *Personality and Mental Health*, 4(4), 284–293. https://doi.org/10.1002/pmh.138

Flood, A. M., Boyle, S. H., Calhoun, P. S., Dennis, M. F., Barefoot, J. C., Moore, S. D., & Beckham, J. C. (2010). Prospective study of externalizing and internalizing subtypes of posttraumatic stress disorder and their relationship to mortality among Vietnam veterans. *Comprehensive Psychiatry*, 51(3), 236–242.

Fonkoue, I. T., Marvar, P. J., Norrholm, S., Li, Y., Kankam, M. L., Jones, T. N., Vemulapalli, M., Rothbaum, B., Bremner, J. D., Le, N. A., & Park, J. (2020). Symptom severity impacts sympathetic dysregulation and inflammation in post-traumatic stress disorder (PTSD). *Brain, Behavior, and Immunity*, 83, 260–269. https://doi.org/10.1016/j.bbi.2019.10.021

Ford, D. E. (2004). Depression, trauma, and cardiovascular health. In P. P. Schnurr, & B. L. Green (Eds.), *Trauma and health: Physical health consequences of exposure to extreme stress* (pp. 73–97). American Psychological Association.

Ford, J., Rosman, L., Wuensch, K., Irvine, J., & Sears, S. F. (2016). Cognitive–behavioral treatment of posttraumatic stress in patients with implantable cardioverter defibrillators: Results from a randomized controlled trial. *Journal of Traumatic Stress*, *29*(4), 388–392. https://doi.org/10.1002/jts.22111

Forneris, C. A., Butterfield, M. I., & Bosworth, H. B. (2004). Physiological arousal among women veterans with and without posttraumatic stress disorder. *Military Medicine*, *169*(4), 307–312.

Freyd, J. (1994). Betrayal trauma: Traumatic amnesia as an adaptive response to childhood abuse. *Ethics & Behavior*, *4*, 307–329. https://doi.org/10.1207/s15327019eb0404_1

Fricchione, G. L., Olson, L. C., & Vlay, S. C. (1989). Psychiatric syndromes in patients with the automatic internal cardioverter defibrillator: Anxiety, psychological dependence, abuse, and withdrawal. *American Heart Journal*, *117*(6), 1411–1414. https://doi.org/10.1016/0002-8703(89)90457-2

Gadermann, A. M., Alonso, J., Vilagut, G., Zaslavsky, A. M., & Kessler, R. C. (2012). Comorbidity and disease burden in the National Comorbidity Survey Replication (NCS-R). *Depression and Anxiety*, *29*(9), 797–806.

Gander, M. L., & von Känel, R. (2006). Myocardial infarction and post-traumatic stress disorder: frequency, outcome, and atherosclerotic mechanisms. *European Journal of Cardiovascular Prevention and Rehabilitation*, *13*(2), 165–172. https://doi.org/10.1097/01.hjr.0000214606.60995.46

Gao, W., Zhao, J., Li, Y., & Cao, F. L. (2015). Post-traumatic stress disorder symptoms in first-time myocardial infarction patients: Roles of attachment and alexithymia. *Journal of Advanced Nursing*, *71*(11), 2575–2584. https://doi.org/10.1111/jan.12726

García-Encinas, A., Ramírez-Maestre, C., Esteve, R., & López-Martínez, A. E. (2020). Predictors of posttraumatic stress symptoms and perceived health after an acute coronary syndrome: The role of experiential avoidance, anxiety sensitivity, and depressive symptoms. *Psychology and Health*, *35*(12), 1497–1515. https://doi.org/10.1080/08870446.2020.1761974

Gibson, C. J., Li, Y., Inslicht, S. S., Seal, K. H., & Byers, A. L. (2018). Gender differences in cardiovascular risk related to diabetes and posttraumatic stress disorder. *Am Journal of Geriatr Psychiatry*, *26*(12), 1268–1272. https://doi.org/10.1016/j.jagp.2018.09.012

Gilsanz, P., Winning, A., Koenen, K. C., Roberts, A. L., Sumner, J. A., Chen, Q., Glymour, M. M., Rimm, E. B., & Kubzansky, L. D. (2017). Post-traumatic stress disorder symptom duration and remission in relation to cardiovascular disease risk among a large cohort of women. *Psychological Medicine*, *47*(8), 1370–1378. https://doi.org/10.1017/s0033291716003378

Ginzburg, K. (2004). PTSD and world assumptions following myocardial infarction: a longitudinal study. *American Journal of Orthopsychiatry*, *74*(3), 286–292. https://doi.org/10.1037/0002-9432.74.3.286

Ginzburg, K. (2006). Comorbidity of PTSD and depression following myocardial infarction. *Journal of Affective Disorders*, *94*, 135–143.

Ginzburg, K., & Ein-Dor, T. (2011). Posttraumatic stress syndromes and health-related quality of life following myocardial infarction: 8-year follow-up. *General Hospital Psychiatry*, *33*(6), 565–571. https://doi.org/10.1016/j.genhosppsych.2011.08.015

Ginzburg, K., Solomon, Z., & Bleich, A. (2002). Repressive coping mechanism, acute stress disorder and posttraumatic stress disorder after myocardial infarction. *Psychosomatic Medicine*, *64*, 748–757.

Ginzburg, K., Solomon, Z., Dekel, R., & Bleich, A. (2006). Longitudinal study of acute stress disorder, posttraumatic stress disorder and dissociation following myocardial infarction. *Journal of Nervous and Mental Disease*, *194*, 945–950. https://doi.org/10.1097/01.nmd.0000249061.65454.54

Ginzburg, K., Solomon, Z., Koifman, B., Keren, G., Roth, A., Kriwisky, M., Kutz, I., David, D., & Bleich, A. (2003). Trajectories of posttraumatic stress disorder following myocardial infarction: a prospective study. *Journal of Clinical Psychiatry, 64*(10), 1217–1223.

Glaesmer, H., Brahler, E., Gundel, H., & Riedel-Heller, S. G. (2011). The association of traumatic experiences and posttraumatic stress disorder with physical morbidity in old age: A German population-based study. *Psychosomatic Medicine, 73*(5), 401–406.

Green, K. T., Dennis, P. A., Neal, L. C., Hobkirk, A. L., Hicks, T. A., Watkins, L. L., Hayano, J., Sherwood, A., Calhoun, P. S., & Beckham, J. C. (2016). Exploring the relationship between posttraumatic stress disorder symptoms and momentary heart rate variability. *Journal of Psychosomatic Research, 82*, 31–34.

Habibović, M., van den Broek, K. C., Alings, M., Van der Voort, P. H., & Denollet, J. (2012). Posttraumatic stress 18 months following cardioverter defibrillator implantation: Shocks, anxiety, and personality. *Health Psychology, 31*(2), 186–193. https://doi.org/10.1037/a0024701

Haerizadeh, M., Sumner, J. A., Birk, J. L., Gonzalez, C., Heyman-Kantor, R., Falzon, L., Gershengoren, L., Shapiro, P., & Kronish, I. M. (2020). Interventions for posttraumatic stress disorder symptoms induced by medical events: A systematic review. *Journal of Psychosomatic Research, 129*, 109908. https://doi.org/10.1016/j.jpsychores.2019.109908

Hamner, M., Hunt, N., Gee, J., Garrell, R., & Monroe, R. (1999). PTSD and automatic implantable cardioverter defibrillators. *Psychosomatics, 40*(1), 82–85. https://doi.org/10.1016/s0033-3182(99)71277-6

Hamner, M. B. (1994). Exacerbation of posttraumatic stress disorder symptoms with medical illness. *General Hospital Psychiatry, 16*(2), 135–137. https://doi.org/10.1016/0163-8343(94)90058-2

Hari, R., Begré, S., Schmid, J.-P., Saner, H., Gander, M.-L., & von Känel, R. (2010). Change over time in posttraumatic stress caused by myocardial infarction and predicting variables. *Journal of Psychosomatic Research, 69*(2), 143–150. https://doi.org/10.1016/j.jpsychores.2010.04.011

Heenan, A., Greenman, P. S., Tassé, V., Zachariades, F., & Tulloch, H. (2020). Traumatic stress, attachment style, and health outcomes in cardiac rehabilitation patients. *Frontiers in Psychology, 11*, 75. https://doi.org/10.3389/fpsyg.2020.00075

Helzer, J. E., Robins, L. N., & McEvoy, L. (1987). Post-traumatic stress disorder in the general population. Findings of the epidemiologic catchment area survey. *New England Journal of Medicine, 317*(26), 1630–1634. https://doi.org/10.1056/nejm198712243172604

Hendrickson, C. M., Neylan, T. C., Na, B., Regan, M., Zhang, Q., & Cohen, B. E. (2013). Lifetime trauma exposure and prospective cardiovascular events and all-cause mortality: Findings from the Heart and Soul Study. *Psychosomatic Medicine, 75*(9), 849–855.

Hillebrand, S., Gast, K. B., de Mutsert, R., Swenne, C. A., Jukema, J. W., Middeldorp, S., Rosendaal, F. R., & Dekkers, O. M. (2013). Heart rate variability and first cardiovascular event in populations without known cardiovascular disease: meta-analysis and dose-response meta-regression. *Europace, 15*(5), 742–749. https://doi.org/10.1093/europace/eus341

Hopper, J. W., Spinazzola, J., Simpson, W. B., & van der Kolk, B. A. (2006). Preliminary evidence of parasympathetic influence on basal heart rate in posttraumatic stress disorder. *Journal of Psychosomatic Research, 60*(1), 83–90.

Horowitz, M. J. (1976). *Stress response syndromes.* Aronson.

Hughes, J. W., Feldman, M. E., & Beckham, J. C. (2006). Posttraumatic stress disorder is associated with attenuated baroreceptor sensitivity among female, but not male, smokers. *Biological Psychology, 71*(3), 296–302.

Huovinen, E., Kaprio, J., & Koskenvuo, M. (2001). Asthma in relation to personality traits, life satisfaction, and stress: A prospective study among 11,000 adults. *Allergy, 56*(10), 971–977. https://doi.org/10.1034/j.1398-9995.2001.00112.x

Husain, S. A., Edmondson, D., Kautz, M., Umland, R., & Kronish, I. M. (2018). Posttraumatic stress disorder due to acute cardiac events and aversive cognitions towards cardiovascular medications. *Journal of Behavioral Medicine, 41*(2), 261–268. https://doi.org/10.1007/s10 865-017-9906-3

Irvine, J., Firestone, J., Ong, L., Cribbie, R., Dorian, P., Harris, L., Ritvo, P., Katz, J., Newman, D., Cameron, D., Johnson, S., Bilanovic, A., Hill, A., O'Donnell, S., & Sears, S., Jr. (2011). A randomized controlled trial of cognitive behavior therapy tailored to psychological adaptation to an implantable cardioverter defibrillator. *Psychosomatic Medicine, 73*(3), 226–233. https://doi.org/10.1097/PSY.0b013e31820afc63

Jacquet-Smailovic, M., Tarquinio, C., Alla, F., Denis, I., Kirche, A., Tarquinio, C., & Brennstuhl, M. J. (2021). Posttraumatic stress disorder following myocardial infarction: A systematic review. *Journal of Traumatic Stress, 34*(1), 190–199. https://doi.org/10.1002/jts.22591

Janoff-Bulman, R. (1992). *Shattered assumptions: Towards a new psychology of trauma.* Free Press.

Javed, A., & Dawood, S. (2016). Psychosocial predictors of post-traumatic growth in patients after myocardial infarction. *Pakistan Journal of Psychological Research, 31*(2), 365–381.

Joseph, S., Williams, R., & Yule, W. (1997). *Understanding posttraumatic stress: A psychosocial perspective on PTSD and treatment.* John Wiley & Sons.

Joseph, S., & Linley, P. A. (2005). Positive adjustment to threatening events: an organismic valuing theory of growth through adversity. *Review of General Psychology, 9*(3), 262–280. https://doi.org/10.1037/1089-2680.9.3.262

Jovanovic, T., Norrholm, S. D., Sakoman, A. J., Esterajher, S., & Kozarić-Kovačić, D. (2009). Altered resting psychophysiology and startle response in Croatian combat veterans with PTSD. *International Journal of Psychophysiology, 71*(3), 264–268. https://doi.org/10.1016/j.ijpsycho.2008.10.007

Karagiorgou, O., & Cullen, B. (2016). A comparison of posttraumatic growth after acquired brain injury or myocardial infarction. *Journal of Loss and Trauma, 21*(6), 589–600. https://doi.org/10.1080/15325024.2016.1161427

Keane, T. M., Brief, D. J., Pratt, E. M., & Miller, M. W. (2007). Assessment of PTSD and its comorbidities in adults. In M. J. Friedman., T. M. Keane., & P. A. Resick (Eds.), *Handbook of PTSD* (pp. 279–305). The Guilford Press.

Kearns, N. T., Becker, J., McMinn, K., Bennett, M. M., Powers, M. B., Warren, A. M., & Edgerton, J. (2020). Increased spiritual well-being following cardiovascular surgery influences one-year perceived posttraumatic growth. *Psychology of Religion and Spirituality, 12*, 288–293. https://doi.org/10.1037/rel0000291

Keary, T. A., Hughes, J. W., & Palmieri, P. A. (2009). Women with posttraumatic stress disorder have larger decreases in heart rate variability during stress tasks. *International Journal of Psychophysiology, 73*, 257–264. https://doi.org/10.1016/j.ijpsycho.2009.04.003

Kendall-Tackett, K. (2009). Psychological trauma and physical health: A psychoneuroimmunology approach to etiology of negative health effects and possible interventions. *Psychological Trauma: Theory, Research, Practice, and Policy, 1*, 35–48. https://doi.org/10.1037/a0015128

Kessler, R., Sonnega, A., Bromet, E., Hughes, M., & Nelson, C. (1995). Posttraumatic stress disorder in the National Comorbidity Survey. *Archives of General Psychiatry, 52*(12), 1048–1060.

Khan, A. A., Jacobson, K. C., Gardner, C. O., Prescott, C. A., & Kendler, K. S. (2005). Personality and comorbidity of common psychiatric disorders. *British Journal of Psychiatry, 186*, 190–196. https://doi.org/10.1192/bjp.186.3.190

Khazaie, H., Saidi, M. R., Sepehry, A. A., Knight, D. C., Ahmadi, M., Najafi, F., Parvizi, A. A., Samadzadeh, S., & Tahmasian, M. (2013). Abnormal ECG patterns in chronic post-war PTSD patients: A pilot study. *International Journal of Behavioral Medicine, 20*(1), 1–6.

Khoury, N. M., Marvar, P. J., Gillespie, C. F., Wingo, A., Schwartz, A., Bradley, B., Kramer, M., & Ressler, K. J. (2012). The renin–angiotensin pathway in posttraumatic stress disorder: Angiotensin-converting enzyme inhibitors and angiotensin receptor blockers are associated with fewer traumatic stress symptoms. *Journal of Clinical Psychiatry, 73*(6), 849–855.

Kibler, J. l. (2009). Posttraumatic stress and cardiovascular disease risk. *Journal of Trauma & Dissociation, 10*(2), 135–150.

Kibler, J. L., Joshi, K., & Ma, M. (2008). Hypertension in relation to posttraumatic stress disorder and depression in the US National Comorbidity Survey. *Behavioral Medicine, 34*(4), 125–131.

Kibler, J. L., Ma, M., Tursich, M., Malcolm, L., Llabre, M. M., Greenbarg, R., Gold, S. N., & Beckham, J. C. (2018). Cardiovascular risks in relation to posttraumatic stress severity among young trauma-exposed women. *Journal of Affective Disorders, 241*, 147–153. https://doi.org/10.1016/j.jad.2018.08.007

Kibler, J. L., Malcolm, L. R., Lerner, R. S., Findon, K. R., & Ma, M. (2013). Women's cardiovascular health risks associated with posttraumatic stress. In J. Marich (Ed.), *The psychology of women: Diverse perspectives from the modern world* (pp. 173–201). Nova Science Publishers.

Kilpatrick, D. G., Acierno, R., Resnick, H. S., Saunders, B. E., & Best, C. L. (1997). A 2-year longitudinal analysis of the relationships between violent assault and substance use in women. *Journal of Consulting and Clinical Psychology, 65*(5), 834–847. https://doi.org/10.1037//0022-006x.65.5.834

Kleim, B., Wilhelm, F. H., Glucksman, E., & Ehlers, A. (2010). Sex differences in heart rate responses to script-driven imagery soon after trauma and risk of posttraumatic stress disorder. *Psychosomatic Medicine, 72*(9), 917–924. https://doi.org/10.1097/PSY.0b013e318 1f8894b

Korinek, K., Young, Y., Teerawichitchainan, B., Kim Chuc, N. T., Kovnick, M., & Zimmer, Z. (2020). Is war hard on the heart? Gender, wartime stress and late life cardiovascular conditions in a population of Vietnamese older adults. *Social Science & Medicine, 265*, 113380. https://doi.org/10.1016/j.socscimed.2020.113380

Kronenberg, G., Schoner, J., Nolte, C., Heinz, A., Endres, M., & Gertz, K. (2017). Charting the perfect storm: Emerging biological interfaces between stress and stroke. *European Archives of Psychiatry and Clinical Neuroscience, 267*(6), 487–494.

Kubzansky, L. D., Koenen, K. C., Spiro, A., Vokonas, P. S., & Sparrow, D. (2007). Prospective study of posttraumatic stress disorder symptoms and coronary heart disease in the Normative Aging study. *Archives of General Psychiatry, 64*, 109–116.

Kutz, I., Garb, R., & David, D. (1988). Post-traumatic stress disorder following myocardial infarction. *General Hospital Psychiatry, 10*(3), 169–176. https://doi.org/10.1016/0163-8343(88)90016-3

Kutz, I., Shabtai, H., Solomon, Z., Neumann, M., & David, D. (1994). Post-traumatic stress disorder in myocardial infarction patients: Prevalence study. *Israel Journal of Psychiatry and Related Sciences, 31*, 48–56.

Ladwig, K. H., Baumert, J., Marten-Mittag, B., Kolb, C., Zrenner, B., & Schmitt, C. (2008). Posttraumatic stress symptoms and predicted mortality in patients with implantable cardioverter-defibrillators: results from the prospective living with an implanted cardioverter-defibrillator study. *Archives of General Psychiatry, 65*(11), 1324–1330. https://doi.org/10.1001/archpsyc.65.11.1324

Ladwig, K. H., Schoefinius, A., Dammann, G., Danner, R., Gürtler, R., & Herrmann, R. (1999). Long-acting psychotraumatic properties of a cardiac arrest experience. *American Journal of Psychiatry, 156*(6), 912–919. https://doi.org/10.1176/ajp.156.6.912

Lahey, B. B. (2009). Public health significance of neuroticism. *American Psychologist, 64*, 241–256. https://doi.org/10.1037/a0015309

Lee, S. Y., Park, C. L., & Pescatello, L. S. (2020). How trauma influences cardiovascular responses to stress: Contributions of posttraumatic stress and cognitive appraisals. *Journal of Behavioral Medicine, 43*(1), 131–142. https://doi.org/10.1007/s10865-019-00067-8

Lenane, Z., Peacock, E., Joyce, C., Frohlich, E. D., Re, R. N., Muntner, P., & Krousel-Wood, M. (2019). Association of post-traumatic stress disorder symptoms following Hurricane Katrina with incident cardiovascular disease events among older adults with hypertension. *American Journal of Geriatric Psychiatry, 27*(3), 310–321. https://doi.org/10.1016/j.jagp.2018.11.006

Leung, Y. W., Alter, D. A., Prior, P. L., Stewart, D. E., Irvine, J., & Grace, S. L. (2012). Posttraumatic growth in coronary artery disease outpatients: Relationship to degree of trauma and health service use. *Journal of Psychosomatic Research, 72*(4), 293–299. https://doi.org/10.1016/j.jps ychores.2011.12.011

Lima, B. B., Hammadah, M., Wilmot, K., Pearce, B. D., Shah, A., Levantsevych, O., Kaseer, B., Obideen, M., Gafeer, M. M., Kim, J. H., Sullivan, S., Lewis, T. T., Weng, L., Elon, L., Li, L., Bremner, J. D., Raggi, P., Quyyumi, A., & Vaccarino, V. (2019). Posttraumatic stress disorder is associated with enhanced interleukin-6 response to mental stress in subjects with a recent myocardial infarction. *Brain, Behavior, and Immunity, 75*, 26–33. https://doi.org/10.1016/ j.bbi.2018.08.015

Łosiak, W., & Nikiel, J. (2014). Posttraumatic growth in patients after myocardial infarction: The role of cognitive coping and experience of life threat. *Health Psychology Report, 2*(4), 256–262. https://doi.org/10.5114/hpr.2014.45894

Malouff, J. M., Thorsteinsson, E. B., & Schutte, N. S. (2005). The relationship between the five-factor model of personality and symptoms of clinical disorders: a meta-analysis. *Journal of Psychopathology and Behavioral Assessment, 27*(2), 101–114. https://doi.org/10.1007/s10 862-005-5384-y

Marciniak, M. D., Lage, M. J., Dunayevich, E., Russell, J. M., Bowman, L., Landbloom, R. P., & Levine, L. R. (2005). The cost of treating anxiety: The medical and demographic correlates that impact total medical costs. *Depression and Anxiety, 21*(4), 178–184. https://doi.org/ 10.1002/da.20074

Marshall, G. N., Miles, J. N. V., & Stewart, S. H. (2010). Anxiety sensitivity and PTSD symptom severity are reciprocally related: Evidence from a longitudinal study of physical trauma survivors. *Journal of Abnormal Psychology, 119*, 143–150. https://doi.org/10.1037/a0018009

McCown, D., & Reibel, D. (2010). Mindfulness and mindfulness-based stress reduction. In D. A. Monti, & B. D. Beitman (Eds.), *Integrative psychiatry* (pp. 289–338). Oxford University Press. http://zulib.idm.oclc.org/login?url=https://search.ebscohost.com/login.aspx?direct= true&AuthType=ip&db=psyh&AN=2009-13409-013&site=ehost-live

McEwen, B. S. (2003). Mood disorders and medical illness: Mood disorders and allostatic load. *Biological Psychiatry, 54*(3), 200–207.

McEwen, B. S., & Stellar, E. (1993). Stress and the individual. Mechanisms leading to disease. *Archives of Internal Medicine, 153*(18), 2093–2101.

McFarlane, A. C. (1990). Vulnerability to posttraumatic stress disorder. In M. E. Wolf & A. D. Mosnaim (Eds.), *Posttraumatic stress disorder: Etiology, phenomenology and treatment* (pp. 3–20). American Psychiatric Association.

McFarlane, A. C. (2010). The delayed and cumulative consequences of traumatic stress: Challenges and issues in compensation settings. *Psychological Injury and Law, 3*(2), 100–110.

McWilliams, L. A., & Bailey, S. J. (2010). Associations between adult attachment ratings and health conditions: evidence from the National Comorbidity Survey Replication. *Health Psychology, 29*(4), 446–453. https://doi.org/10.1037/a0020061

Meister, R. E., Princip, M., Schnyder, U., Barth, J., Znoj, H., Schmid, J. P., Wittmann, L., & von Känel, R. (2016). Association of trait resilience with peritraumatic and posttraumatic stress in patients with myocardial infarction. *Psychosomatic Medicine, 78*(3), 327–334. https://doi.org/10.1097/psy.0000000000000278

Mendlowicz, V., Garcia-Rosa, M. L., Gekker, M., Wermelinger, L., Berger, W., Luz, M. P. d., Pires-Dias, P. R. T., Marques-Portela, C., Figueira, I., & Mendlowicz, M. V. (2021). Posttraumatic stress disorder as a predictor for incident hypertension: A 3-year retrospective cohort study. *Psychological Medicine, 53*(1), 132–139. https://doi.org/10.1017/S0033291721001227

Middeldorp, C. M., Cath, D. C., Berg, M. van den, Beem, A. L., Dyck, R. van, & Boomsma, D. I. (2006). The association of personality with anxious and depressive psychopathology. In T. Canli (Ed.), *Biology of personality and individual differences* (pp. 251–272). The Guilford Press.

Miller, M. W., Kaloupek, D. G., Dillon, A. L., & Keane, T. M. (2004). Externalizing and internalizing subtypes of combat related PTSD: A replication and extension using the PSY-5 scales. *Journal of Abnormal Psychology, 112*, 636–645.

Mitani, S., Fujita, M., Sakamoto, S., & Shirakawa, T. (2006). Effect of autogenic training on cardiac autonomic nervous activity in high-risk fire service workers for posttraumatic stress disorder. *Journal of Psychosomatic Research, 60*(5), 439–444. https://doi.org/https://doi.org/10.1016/j.jpsychores.2005.09.005

Moazen-Zadeh, E., Khoshdel, A., Avakh, F., & Rahmani, A. (2016). Increased blood pressures in veterans with post traumatic stress disorder: A case–control study. *International Journal of Psychiatry in Medicine, 51*(6), 576–586.

Muraoka, M. Y., Carlson, J. G., & Chemtob, C. M. (1998). Twenty-four-hour ambulatory blood pressure and heart rate monitoring in combat-related posttraumatic stress disorder. *Journal of Traumatic Stress, 11*(3), 473–484.

Naderi, S. H., Bestwick, J. P., & Wald, D. S. (2012). Adherence to drugs that prevent cardiovascular disease: meta-analysis on 376,162 patients. *American Journal of Medicine, 125*(9), 882–887.e881. https://doi.org/10.1016/j.amjmed.2011.12.013

Nemiah, J. C., & Sifneos, P. E. (1970). Psychosomatic illness: A problem in communication. *Psychotherapy and Psychosomatics, 18*, 154–160. https://doi.org/10.1159/000286074

Neumann, J. K. (1991). Psychological post-traumatic effects of MI: A comparison study. *Medical Psychotherapy, 4*, 105–110.

Newton, T. L., Parker, B. C., & Ho, I. K. (2005). Ambulatory cardiovascular functioning in healthy postmenopausal women with victimization histories. *Biological Psychology, 70*(2), 121–130.

National Institute for Health and Care Excellence. (2018). https://www.health-ni.gov.uk/articles/nice-endorsed-clinical-guidelines-20182019.

Nichter, B., Norman, S., Haller, M., & Pietrzak, R. H. (2019). Physical health burden of PTSD, depression, and their comorbidity in the US veteran population: Morbidity, functioning, and disability. *Journal of Psychosomatic Research, 124*, 109744. https://doi.org/10.1016/j.jpsychores.2019.109744

Norris, F. H. (1992). Epidemiology of trauma: Frequency and impact of different potentially traumatic events on different demographic groups. *Journal of Consulting and Clinical Psychology, 60*, 409–418. https://doi.org/10.1037/0022-006X.60.3.409

Norte, C. E., Souza, G. G. L., Vilete, L., Marques-Portella, C., Coutinho, E. S. F., Figueira, I., & Volchan, E. (2013). They know their trauma by heart: An assessment of psychophysiological failure to recover in PTSD. *Journal of Affective Disorders, 150*(1), 136–141. https://doi.org/10.1016/j.jad.2012.11.039

Nugent, N. R., Christopher, N. C., & Delahanty, D. L. (2006). Emergency medical service and in-hospital vital signs as predictors of subsequent PTSD symptom severity in pediatric injury patients. *Journal of Child Psychology & Psychiatry, 47*(9), 919–926.

Oflaz, S., Yüksel, Ş., Şen, F., Özdemİroğlu, F., Kurt, R., Oflaz, H., & Kaşikcioğlu, E. (2014). Does illness perception predict posttraumatic stress disorder in patients with myocardial infarction? *Nöropsikiyatri Arşivi, 51*(2), 103–109. https://doi.org/10.4274/npa.y6394

Ogińska-Bulik, N. (2014). Satisfaction with life and posttraumatic growth in persons after myocardial infarction. *Health Psychology Report, 2*(2), 105–114. https://doi.org/10.5114/hpr.2014.43917

Orcutt, H. K., Reffi, A. N., & Ellis, R. A. (2020). Experiential avoidance and PTSD. In M. T. Tull, & N. A. Kimbrel (Eds.), *Emotion in posttraumatic stress disorder: Etiology, assessment, neurobiology, and treatment* (pp. 409–436). Elsevier Academic Press.

Paulus, E. J., Argo, T. R., & Egge, J. A. (2013). The impact of posttraumatic stress disorder on blood pressure and heart rate in a veteran population. *Journal of Traumatic Stress, 26*(1), 169–172.

Pedersen, S. S. (2001). Posttraumatic stress disorder in patients with coronary artery disease: A review and evaluation of the risk. *Scandinavian Journal of Psychology, 42*, 445–451.

Pedersen, S. S., & Denollet, J. (2004). Validity of the Type D personality construct in Danish post-MI patients and healthy controls. *Journal of Psychosomatic Research, 57*(3), 265–272. https://doi.org/10.1016/S0022-3999(03)00614-7

Pedersen, S. S., Middel, B., & Larsen, M. L. (2002). The role of personality variables and social support in distress and perceived health in patients following myocardial infarction. *Journal of Psychosomatic Research, 53*, 1171–1175.

Perry, B. D. (1994). Neurobiological sequelae of childhood trauma: PTSD in children. In M. M. Murburg (Ed.), *Catecholamine function in posttraumatic stress disorder: Emerging concepts* (pp. 233–255). American Psychiatric Association.

Pietromonaco, P., & Collins, N. (2017). Interpersonal mechanisms linking close relationships to health. *American Psychologist, 72*, 531–542. https://doi.org/10.1037/amp0000129

Pietromonaco, P. R., Uchino, B., & Dunkel Schetter, C. (2013). Close relationship processes and health: Implications of attachment theory for health and disease. *Health Psychology, 32*, 499–513. https://doi.org/10.1037/a0029349

Player, M. S., & Peterson, L. E. (2011). Anxiety disorders, hypertension, and cardiovascular risk: A review. *International Journal of Psychiatry in Medicine, 41*(4), 365–377.

Pope, B. S., & Wood, S. K. (2019). Stress-induced inflammation as the "connexin" between posttraumatic stress disorder and cardiovascular disease. *Brain, Behavior, and Immunity, 82*, 3–5. https://doi.org/10.1016/j.bbi.2019.08.182

Princip, M., Gattlen, C., Meister-Langraf, R. E., Schnyder, U., Znoj, H., Barth, J., Schmid, J.-P., & von Känel, R. (2018). The role of illness perception and its association with posttraumatic stress at 3 months following acute myocardial infarction. *Frontiers in Psychology, 9.* https://doi.org/10.3389/fpsyg.2018.00941

Rabe, S., Dorfel, D., Zollner, T., Maercker, A., & Karl, A. (2006). Cardiovascular correlates of motor vehicle accident related posttraumatic stress disorder and its successful treatment. *Applied Psychophysiology and Biofeedback, 31*(4), 315–330.

Ranney, R. M., Bing-Canar, H., Paltell, K. C., Tran, J. K., Berenz, E. C., & Vujanovic, A. A. (2020). Cardiovascular risk as a moderator of associations among anxiety sensitivity, distress tolerance, PTSD and depression symptoms among trauma-exposed firefighters. *Journal of Psychosomatic Research, 139*, 110269. https://doi.org/10.1016/j.jpsychores.2020.110269

Reiss, S. (1991). Expectancy model of fear, anxiety, and panic. *Clinical Psychology Review, 11*, 141–153. https://doi.org/10.1016/0272-7358(91)90092-9

Rissling, M. B., Dennis, P. A., Watkins, L. L., Calhoun, P. S., Dennis, M. F., Beckham, J. C., Hayano, J., & Ulmer, C. S. (2016). Circadian contrasts in heart rate variability associated with posttraumatic stress disorder symptoms in a young adult cohort. *Journal of Traumatic Stress, 29*(5), 415–421.

Rocha, L. P., Peterson, J. C., Meyers, B., Boutin-Foster, C., Charlson, M. E., Jayasinghe, N., & Bruce, M. L. (2008). Incidence of posttraumatic stress disorder (PTSD) after myocardial infarction (MI) and predictors of PTSD symptoms post-MI: A brief report. *International Journal of Psychiatry in Medicine, 38*(3), 297–306. https://doi.org/10.2190/PM.38.3.f

Rothenhäusler, H. B., Grieser, B., Nollert, G., Reichart, B., Schelling, G., & Kapfhammer, H. P. (2005). Psychiatric and psychosocial outcome of cardiac surgery with cardiopulmonary bypass: a prospective 12-month follow-up study. *General Hospital Psychiatry, 27*(1), 18–28. https://doi.org/10.1016/j.genhosppsych.2004.09.001

Sack, M., Hopper, J. W., & Lamprecht, F. (2004). Low respiratory sinus arrhythmia and prolonged psychophysiological arousal in posttraumatic stress disorder: Heart rate dynamics and individual differences in arousal regulation. *Biological Psychiatry, 55*(3), 284–290. https://doi.org/10.1016/s0006-3223(03)00677-2

Samson, A. Y., Bensen, S., Beck, A., Price, D., & Nimmer, C. (1999). Posttraumatic stress disorder in primary care. *Journal of Family Practice, 48*(3), 222–227.

Sareen, J., Cox, B. J., Stein, M. B., Afifi, T. O., Fleet, C., & Asmundson, G. J. (2007). Physical and mental comorbidity, disability, and suicidal behavior associated with posttraumatic stress disorder in a large community sample. *Psychosomatic Medicine, 69*(3), 242–248.

Saxe, G., Stoddard, F., Courtney, D., Cunningham, K., Chawla, N., Sheridan, R., King, D., & King, L. (2001). Relationship between acute morphine and the course of PTSD in children with burns. *Journal of the American Academy of Child and Adolescent Psychiatry, 40*(8), 915–921. https://doi.org/10.1097/00004583-200108000-00013

Scheeringa, M. S., Zeanah, C. H., Myers, L., & Putnam, F. (2004). Heart period and variability findings in preschool children with posttraumatic stress symptoms. *Biological Psychiatry, 55*, 685–691. https://doi.org/10.1016/j.biopsych.2004.01.006

Schelling, G., Kilger, E., Roozendaal, B., de Quervain, D. J., Briegel, J., Dagge, A., Rothenhäusler, H. B., Krauseneck, T., Nollert, G., & Kapfhammer, H. P. (2004). Stress doses of hydrocortisone, traumatic memories, and symptoms of posttraumatic stress disorder in patients after cardiac surgery: a randomized study. *Biological Psychiatry, 55*(6), 627–633. https://doi.org/10.1016/j.biopsych.2003.09.014

Schelling, G., Roozendaal, B., Krauseneck, T., Schmoelz, M., Quervain, D. D E., & Briegel, J. (2006). Efficacy of hydrocortisone in preventing posttraumatic stress disorder following critical illness and major surgery. *Annals of the New York Academy of Science, 1071*, 46–53. https://doi.org/10.1196/annals.1364.005

Schultz, J. H., & Luthe, W. (1959). *Autogenic training: A psychophysiologic approach to psychotherapy.* Grune & Stratton.

Sears, S. F., Jr., & Conti, J. B. (2002). Quality of life and psychological functioning of ICD patients. *Heart, 87*(5), 488–493. https://doi.org/10.1136/heart.87.5.488

Senol-Durak, E., & Ayvasik, H. B. (2010). Factors associated with posttraumatic growth among myocardial infarction patients: Perceived social support, perception of the event and coping. *Journal of Clinical Psychology in Medical Settings, 17*(2), 150–158. https://doi.org/10.1007/s10880-010-9192-5

Shaffer, J. A., Kronish, I. M., Burg, M., Clemow, L., & Edmondson, D. (2013). Association of acute coronary syndrome-induced posttraumatic stress disorder symptoms with self-reported sleep. *Annals of Behavioral Medicine, 46*(3), 349–357.

Sheikh, A. I., & Marotta, S. A. (2008). Best practices for counseling in cardiac rehabilitation settings. *Journal of Counseling & Development, 86*(1), 111–119. https://doi.org/https://doi.org/10.1002/j.1556-6678.2008.tb00632.x

Shemesh, E., Annunziato, R. A., Weatherley, B. D., Cotter, G., Feaganes, J. R., Santra, M., Yehuda, R., & Rubinstein, D. (2011). A randomized controlled trial of the safety and promise of cognitive–behavioral therapy using imaginal exposure in patients with posttraumatic stress disorder resulting from cardiovascular illness. *Journal of Clinical Psychiatry, 72*(2), 168–174.

Shemesh, E., Koren-Michowitz, M., Yehuda, R., Milo-Cotter, O., Murdock, E., Vered, Z., Shneider, B. L., Gorman, J. M., & Cotter, G. (2006). Symptoms of posttraumatic stress disorder in patients who have had a myocardial infarction. *Psychosomatics: Journal of Consultation and Liaison Psychiatry, 47*(3), 231–239.

Shemesh, E., Rudnick, A., Kaluski, E., Milovanov, O., Salah, A., Alon, D., Dinur, I., Blatt, A., Metzkor, M., Golik, A., Verd, Z., & Cotter, G. (2001). A prospective study of posttraumatic stress symptoms and nonadherence in survivors of a myocardial infarction (MI). *General Hospital Psychiatry, 23*(4), 215–222. https://doi.org/10.1016/S0163-8343(01)00150-5

Shemesh, E., Yehuda, R., Milo, O., Dinur, I., Rudnick, A., Vered, Z., & Cotter, G. (2004). Posttraumatic stress, nonadherence, and adverse outcome in survivors of a myocardial infarction. *Psychosomatic Medicine, 66*(4), 521–526.

Shishido, H., Gaher, R. M., & Simons, J. S. (2013). I don't know how I feel, therefore I act: alexithymia, urgency, and alcohol problems. *Addictive Behaviors, 38*(4), 2014–2017. https://doi.org/10.1016/j.addbeh.2012.12.014

Smith, T. W., Baron, C. E., Caska-Wallace, C. M., Knobloch-Fedders, L. M., Renshaw, K. D., & Uchino, B. N. (2021). PTSD in veterans, couple behavior, and cardiovascular response during marital conflict. *Emotion, 21*, 478–488. https://doi.org/10.1037/emo0000727

Smith, T. W., & MacKenzie, J. (2006). Personality and risk of physical illness. *Annual Review of Clinical Psychology, 2*, 435–467. https://doi.org/10.1146/annurev.clinpsy.2.022305.095257

Song, H., Fang, F., Arnberg, F. K., Mataix-Cols, D., Fernández de la Cruz, L., Almqvist, C., Fall, K., Lichtenstein, P., Thorgeirsson, G., & Valdimarsdóttir, U. A. (2019). Stress related disorders and risk of cardiovascular disease: Population based, sibling controlled cohort study. *BMJ, 365*, l1255. https://doi.org/10.1136/bmj.l1255

Spiller, R., Aziz, Q., Creed, F., Emmanuel, A., Houghton, L., Hungin, P., Jones, R., Kumar, D., Rubin, G., Trudgill, N., & Whorwell, P. (2007). Guidelines on the irritable bowel syndrome: Mechanisms and practical management. *Gut, 56*(12), 1770–1798. https://doi.org/10.1136/gut.2007.119446

Spindler, H., & Pedersen, S. S. (2005). Posttraumatic stress disorder in the wake of heart disease: prevalence, risk factors and future research directions. *Psychosomatic Medicine, 67*, 715–723.

Spitzer, C., Barnow, S., Volzke, H., John, U., Freyberger, H. J., & Grabe, H. J. (2009). Trauma, posttraumatic stress disorder, and physical illness: Findings from the general population. *Psychosomatic Medicine, 71*(9), 1012–1017.

Stukas, A. A., Jr., Dew, M. A., Switzer, G. E., DiMartini, A., Kormos, R. L., & Griffith, B. P. (1999). PTSD in heart transplant recipients and their primary family caregivers. *Psychosomatics, 40*(3), 212–221. https://doi.org/10.1016/s0033-3182(99)71237-5

Suls, J., & Bunde, J. (2005). Anger, anxiety, and depression as risk factors for cardiovascular disease: the problems and implications of overlapping affective dispositions. *Psychological Bulletin, 131*(2), 260–300. https://doi.org/10.1037/0033-2909.131.2.260

Sumner, J. A., Kubzansky, L. D., Roberts, A. L., Chen, Q., Rimm, E. B., & Koenen, K. C. (2020). Not all posttraumatic stress disorder symptoms are equal: fear, dysphoria, and risk of developing hypertension in trauma-exposed women. *Psychological Medicine, 50*(1), 38–47. https://doi.org/10.1017/s0033291718003914

Taylor-Clift, A., Holmgreen, L., Hobfoll, S. E., Gerhart, J. I., Richardson, D., Calvin, J. E., & Powell, L. H. (2016). Traumatic stress and cardiopulmonary disease burden among low-income, urban heart failure patients. *Journal of Affective Disorders, 190,* 227–234. https://doi.org/10.1016/j.jad.2015.09.023

Taylor, G. J., Bagby, R. M., & Parker, J. D. A. (1997). *Disorders of affect regulation: Alexithymia in medical and psychiatric illness.* Cambridge University Press. https://doi.org/10.1017/CBO9780511526831

Taylor, M. K., Larson, G. E., Lauby, M. D., Padilla, G. A., Wilson, I. E., Schmied, E. A., Highfill-McRoy, R. M., & Morgan, C. A., III. (2014). Sex differences in cardiovascular and subjective stress reactions: Prospective evidence in a realistic military setting. *Stress, 17*(1), 70–78.

Tedeschi, R. G., Park, C. L., & Calhoun, L. G. (1998). *Posttraumatic growth: Positive transformations in the aftermath of crisis.* Lawrence Erlbaum Associates.

Tedstone, J. E., & Tarrier, N. (2003). Posttraumatic stress disorder following medical illness and treatment. *Clinical Psychology Review, 23*(3), 409–448. https://doi.org/10.1016/S0272-7358(03)00031-X

Theorell, T. (1997). Absurd emphasis on effectiveness and immediate results will harm medical treatment. *Psychotherapy and Psychosomatics, 66*(5), 227–228. https://doi.org/10.1159/000289139

Toren, P., & Horesh, N. (2007). Psychiatric morbidity in adolescents operated in childhood for congenital cyanotic heart disease. *Journal of Paediatrics and Child Health, 43*(10), 662–666. https://doi.org/10.1111/j.1440-1754.2007.01183.x

Tucker, P., Pfefferbaum, B., Jeon-Slaughter, H., Khan, Q., & Garton, T. (2012). Emotional stress and heart rate variability measures associated with cardiovascular risk in relocated Katrina survivors. *Psychosomatic Medicine, 74*(2), 160–168.

Tully, P., & Cosh, S. (2019). Post-traumatic stress disorder in heart failure patients: A test of the cardiac disease-induced PTSD hypothesis. *Current Psychiatry Research and Reviews, 15.* https://doi.org/10.2174/2666082215666191113121558

Turner, J. H., Neylan, T. C., Schiller, N. B., Li, Y., & Cohen, B. E. (2013). Objective evidence of myocardial ischemia in patients with posttraumatic stress disorder. *Biological Psychiatry, 74*(11), 861–866.

Ulmer, C. S., Hall, M. H., Dennis, P. A., Beckham, J. C., & Germain, A. (2018). Posttraumatic stress disorder diagnosis is associated with reduced parasympathetic activity during sleep in US veterans and military service members of the Iraq and Afghanistan wars. *Sleep, 41*(12). https://doi.org/10.1093/sleep/zsy174

Vaccarino, V., & Bremner, J. D. (2017). Behavioral, emotional and neurobiological determinants of coronary heart disease risk in women. *Neuroscience and Biobehavioral Reviews, 74*(Pt B), 297–309. https://doi.org/10.1016/j.neubiorev.2016.04.023

Valentine, S. E., Nobles, C. J., Gerber, M. W., Vaewsorn, A. S., Shtasel, D. L., & Marques, L. (2017). The association of posttraumatic stress disorder and chronic medical conditions by ethnicity. *Journal of Latina/o Psychology, 5*(3), 227–241.

van den Berk-Clark, C., Secrest, S., Walls, J., Hallberg, E., Lustman, P. J., Schneider, F., & Scherrer, J. F. (2018). Association between posttraumatic stress disorder and lack of exercise, poor diet, obesity, and co-occuring smoking: A systematic review and meta-analysis. *Health Psychology, 37*(5), 407–416.

van Driel, R. C., & Op den Velde, W. (1995). Myocardial infarction and post-traumatic stress disorder. *Journal of Traumatic Stress, 8*(1), 151–159. https://doi.org/10.1002/jts.2490080111

Vancampfort, D., Stubbs, B., Richards, J., Ward, P. B., Firth, J., Schuch, F. B., & Rosenbaum, S. (2017). Physical fitness in people with posttraumatic stress disorder: A systematic review. *Disability and Rehabilitation, 39*(24), 2461–2467.

Vidal, C., Polo, R., Alvarez, K., Falgas Bague, I., Wang, Y., Cook, B., & Alegria, M. (2018). Co-occurrence of posttraumatic stress disorder and cardiovascular disease among ethnic/racial groups in the United States. *Psychosomatic Medicine, 80*, 1. https://doi.org/10.1097/PSY.0000000000000601

Violanti, J. M., Andrew, M. E., Burchfiel, C. M., Dorn, J., Hartley, T., & Miller, D. B. (2006). Posttraumatic stress symptoms and subclinical cardiovascular disease in police officers. *International Journal of Stress Management, 13*(4), 541–554.

Voelker, R. (2012). Study: Acute coronary events linked with PTSD. *JAMA, 308*(2), 121. https://doi.org/10.1001/jama.2012.7948

von Känel, R., Barth, J., Princip, M., Meister-Langraf, R. E., Schmid, J. P., Znoj, H., Herbert, C., & Schnyder, U. (2018). Early psychological counseling for the prevention of posttraumatic stress induced by acute coronary syndrome: The MI-SPRINT Randomized Controlled Trial. *Psychotherapy and Psychosomatics, 87*(2), 75–84. https://doi.org/10.1159/000486099

von Känel, R., Baumert, J., Kolb, C., Cho, E.-Y. N., & Ladwig, K.-H. (2011). Chronic posttraumatic stress and its predictors in patients living with an implantable cardioverter defibrillator. *Journal of Affective Disorders, 131*(1–3), 344–352. https://doi.org/10.1016/j.jad.2010.12.002

Von Kanel, R., Hepp, U., Buddeberg, C., Keel, M., Mica, L., Aschbacher, K., & Schnyder, U. (2006). Altered blood coagulation in patients with posttraumatic stress disorder. *Psychosomatic Medicine, 68*(4), 598–604.

von Känel, R., Kraemer, B., Saner, H., Schmid, J.-P., Abbas, C. C., & Begré, S. (2010). Posttraumatic stress disorder and dyslipidemia: Previous research and novel findings from patients with PTSD caused by myocardial infarction. *World Journal of Biological Psychiatry, 11*(1–2), 141–147. https://doi.org/10.3109/15622970903449846

von Känel, R., Schmid, J.-P., Abbas, C. C., Gander, M.-L., Saner, H., & Begré, S. (2010). Stress hormones in patients with posttraumatic stress disorder caused by myocardial infarction and role of comorbid depression. *Journal of Affective Disorders, 121*(1–2), 73–79. https://doi.org/10.1016/j.jad.2009.05.016

Vrana, S. R., Hughes, J. W., Dennis, M. F., Calhoun, P. S., & Beckham, J. C. (2009). Effects of posttraumatic stress disorder status and covert hostility on cardiovascular responses to relived anger in women with and without PTSD. *Biological Psychology, 82*(3), 274–280.

Weinstock, L. M., & Whisman, M. A. (2006). Neuroticism as a common feature of the depressive and anxiety disorders: A test of the revised integrative hierarchical model in a national sample. *Journal of Abnormal Psychology, 115*, 68–74. https://doi.org/10.1037/0021-843X.115.1.68

Wentworth, B. A., Stein, M. B., Redwine, L. S., Xue, Y., Taub, P. R., Clopton, P., Nayak, K. R., & Maisel, A. S. (2013). Post-traumatic stress disorder: a fast track to premature cardiovascular disease? *Cardiology in Review, 21*(1), 16–22. https://doi.org/10.1097/crd.0b013e318265343b

World Health Organization. (2021). *Cardiovascular diseases (CVDs).* https://www.who.int/news-room/fact-sheets/detail/cardiovascular-diseases-(cvds)

Wikman, A., Bhattacharyya, M., Perkins-Porras, L., & Steptoe, A. (2008). Persistence of posttraumatic stress symptoms 12 and 36 months after acute coronary syndrome. *Psychosomatic Medicine, 70*(7), 764–772. https://doi.org/10.1097/PSY.0b013e3181835c07

Wikman, A., Messerli-Bürgy, N., Molloy, G. J., Randall, G., Perkins-Porras, L., & Steptoe, A. (2012). Symptom experience during acute coronary syndrome and the development of posttraumatic stress symptoms. *Journal of Behavioral Medicine, 35*(4), 420–430. https://doi.org/10.1007/s10865-011-9369-x

Wilson, M. A., Liberzon, I., Lindsey, M. L., Lokshina, Y., Risbrough, V. B., Sah, R., Wood, S. K., Williamson, J. B., & Spinale, F. G. (2019). Common pathways and communication between the brain and heart: connecting post-traumatic stress disorder and heart failure. *Stress*, *22*(5), 530–547. https://doi.org/10.1080/10253890.2019.1621283

Wingenfeld, K., Whooley, M. A., Neylan, T. C., Otte, C., & Cohen, B. E. (2015). Effect of current and lifetime posttraumatic stress disorder on 24-h urinary catecholamines and cortisol: Results from the Mind Your Heart Study. *Psychoneuroendocrinology*, *52*, 83–91.

Winning, A., Gilsanz, P., Koenen, K. C., Roberts, A. L., Chen, Q., Sumner, J. A., Rimm, E. B., Maria Glymour, M., & Kubzansky, L. D. (2017). Post-traumatic stress disorder and 20-year physical activity trends among women. *American Journal of Preventive Medicine*, *52*(6), 753–760. https://doi.org/10.1016/j.amepre.2017.01.040

Witteveen, A. B., Bisson, J. I., Ajdukovic, D., Arnberg, F. K., Bergh Johannesson, K., Bolding, H. B., Elklit, A., Jehel, L., Johansen, V. A., Lis-Turlejska, M., Nordanger, D. O., Orengo-García, F., Polak, A. R., Punamaki, R. L., Schnyder, U., Wittmann, L., & Olff, M. (2012). Post-disaster psychosocial services across Europe: the TENTS project. *Social Science & Medicine*, *75*(9), 1708–1714. https://doi.org/10.1016/j.socscimed.2012.06.017

Wolf, E. J., & Schnurr, P. P. (2016). Posttraumatic stress disorder-related cardiovascular disease and accelerated cellular aging. *Psychiatric Annals*, *46*(9), 527–532. https://doi.org/10.3928/00485713-20160729-01

Yuan Ng, C., & Mela, T. (2016). A primer on cardiac devices: Psychological and pharmacological considerations. *Psychiatric Annals*, *46*(12), 683–690. https://doi.org/10.3928/00485713-20161107-01

Zaba, M., Kirmeier, T., Ionescu, I. A., Wollweber, B., Buell, D. R., Gall-Kleebach, D. J., Schubert, C. F., Novak, B., Huber, C., Kohler, K., Holsboer, F., Putz, B., Muller-Myhsok, B., Hohne, N., Uhr, M., Ising, M., Herrmann, L., & Schmidt, U. (2015). Identification and characterization of HPA-axis reactivity endophenotypes in a cohort of female PTSD patients. *Psychoneuroendocrinology*, *55*, 102–115.

Zen, A. L., Whooley, M. A., Zhao, S., & Cohen, B. E. (2012). Post-traumatic stress disorder is associated with poor health behaviors: Findings from the Heart and Soul Study. *Health Psychology*, *31*(2), 194–201.

Zhao, J., Cao, F.-L., & Xu, Y.-H. (2015). Predictive factors of posttraumatic growth in patients with acute myocardial infarction. *Chinese Mental Health Journal*, *29*(2), 87–91.

3

Posttraumatic stress disorder associated with cancer experiences

The growth in research into PTSD in cancer patients results in part from the definition of trauma using the 'A' criteria of DSM-IV (American Psychiatric Association, 1994). Trauma is defined as reactions after experiencing, witnessing, or confronting an event (or events) involving actual or threatened violence or physical injury, or a threat to the physical integrity of oneself or others (criterion A1), causing intense fear, helplessness, and/or horror (criterion A2). Based on this definition, a life-threatening illness such as cancer and its treatment can therefore be viewed as a potentially traumatic event that may trigger PTSD responses (Andrykowski & Kangas, 2010). Research shows that the cancer experience is a traumatic stressor in 37–57% of patients. Between 50% and 60% of cancer survivors perceived the diagnosis and treatment of cancer as a threat to their life and physical integrity. They also reported fear, helplessness, or horror, with the former reactions apparently more common than the latter (Cordova et al., 2017).

Should cancer be conceptualised in terms of a trauma framework?

However, conceptualising cancer in terms of a trauma framework, that is cancer-related PTSD, is controversial. How useful is PTSD as a model for understanding cancer experiences? (Phipps et al., 2006). This kind of question, with a sceptical tone, is not surprising as many medical professionals tend to associate PTSD with soldiers returning from a battlefield or with abused victims rather than with a cancer diagnosis and subsequent treatment (Bush, 2009). Interestingly, paediatric cancer has been postulated as a form of childhood trauma because it is life-threatening and requires invasive treatments. This childhood trauma is similar to child abuse in that both types of trauma involve exposure to threats to life or physical integrity, which has been shown to affect neural development (Marusak et al., 2018; Marusak et al., 2015).

Posttraumatic Stress in Physical Illness. Man Cheung Chung, Oxford University Press. © Oxford University Press 2024.
DOI: 10.1093/oso/9780198727323.003.0003

Cancer-related stress occurs at some key transition points, such as finding an abnormality during self-examination, participating in a screening procedure or routine imaging or clinical examination, receiving a diagnosis that may be considered an acute life threat, undergoing invasive treatments or procedures, enduring side-effects or complications of the treatments or disease, receiving news of treatment results, disease recurrence, and a reduction in life expectancy. This distress can be characterised by shock, denial, fear, anxiety, depression, sleep disturbance, loss of appetite, and feelings of vulnerability, unpredictability, and uncontrollability (Bush, 2009; Cordova et al., 2017). Following cancer diagnosis and treatment, patients often face issues such as extreme and chronic fatigue, pain, gastrointestinal symptoms, skin irritation, hot flashes, sexual difficulties, fertility, neurological or cognitive impairment, disfigurement, and risk of secondary malignancies and recurrences, which in turn can impact daily functioning (e.g. education, work) and interpersonal relationships and increase anxiety, depression, and PTSD (Cordova et al., 2017; Vuotto et al., 2018). Such distress is a constant or repetitive threat. Cancer appears to correspond to the experience of type I (sudden and one-time traumatic event) and type II (repetitive and anticipated trauma) traumas, which can elicit different psychological responses (Stuber et al., 1998), including PTSD symptoms (Ingerski et al., 2010). A meta-analysis shows that cancer survivors are 1.66 times more likely to have PTSD after a cancer diagnosis compared to the general non-cancer population (based on the DSM-IV criteria) (Swartzman et al., 2017).

For some trauma researchers, then, the question is not whether it is appropriate or useful to view the cancer experience in a trauma framework. Rather, the question is how best to understand cancer-related PTSD. One study concludes that a four-symptom cluster model of re-experiencing, avoidance, numbing, and arousal is best model fit for understanding PTSD responses in cancer survivors. This model seems to be superior to the three-symptom cluster model of DSM-IV (re-experiencing, avoidance/numbing, and arousal) (DuHamel et al., 2004). On the contrary, a confirmatory factorial study has confirmed the symptom structure of PTSD in breast cancer survivors using the DSM-IV criteria (Cordova et al., 2000). Specifically, intrusion and avoidance appear to have a unique relationship with distress outcomes, as the former was a much stronger predictor of distress than the latter in breast cancer patients (Baider & Kaplan De-Nour, 1997).

Notwithstanding this, a study that focused on women with breast cancer did not support the DSM-IV three-symptom cluster model. Furthermore, it found that symptoms in the four-factor model had poor factor loadings.

Similarly, the three- or four-factor structure in those at high risk of melanoma due to an identified family-specific CDKN2A mutation was not confirmed. The two-factor structure of cancer-related PTSD (based on the Impact of Event Scale) in melanoma patients was also not confirmed by factor analysis. Instead, a unidimensional account of emotional distress corresponded to all items of the Impact of Event Scale, suggesting that a single dimension of emotional distress in response to melanoma risk appears to be more relevant for assessing psychological adjustment in these cancer survivors. In addition, the two-factor structure of anxiety and depression was found to fit the data well (Kasparian et al., 2012).

These conflicting findings have led to the conclusion that using the symptoms above to measure cancer survivors' experiences may be problematic. Whether the posttraumatic stress framework is best suited to conceptualise or measure the nature of melanoma or cancer-related distress remains controversial (Kasparian et al., 2012). The sceptics would also argue that although PTSD symptoms were present in some studies that focused on cancer survivors, this does not mean that they would all meet the diagnostic criteria for PTSD. A large-scale study of 2141 cancer patients with different types of cancer found that the prevalence rate of PTSD after the first four weeks was 2%, but only 9% of these four-week PTSD cases were cancer-related (Esser et al., 2019). Another large-scale study (n = 2969) also showed that 14.5% described cancer as a traumatic event. However, there were no significant differences in PTSD scores between those who described cancer as the most stressful event and those who described non-cancer events as most stressful. The study concluded that cancer cannot be directly linked to PTSD symptoms (Allen et al., 2018).

Similarly, whereas children undergoing cancer treatment may show PTSD symptoms, one year after a bone marrow transplant (BMT) (Pot-Mees & Zeitlin, 1987; Stuber et al., 1991) they did not meet a PTSD diagnosis (Brown et al., 2003; Stuber et al., 1998), although more than 36% had mild subthreshold symptomatology (Brown et al., 2003). Furthermore, a study of women who had ovarian cancer found that none developed full PTSD, although a small proportion (14%) of them had subsyndromal PTSD (Guglietti et al., 2010). Another study showed that no women who underwent autologous BMT met the diagnostic criteria for PTSD. Women with breast cancer who underwent mastectomy and received extensive and aggressive cytotoxic treatment were also not found to have PTSD. However, they were more likely to report 'PTSD-like symptoms' than women who received other treatment (Khalid & Gul, 2000).

One study showed that about 16% of female cancer survivors reported 'probable' PTSD, in addition to anxiety (29%) and depression (20%) (Urbaniec et al., 2011). Among older adults who were long-term cancer survivors, most were not found to have clinical levels of PTSD. However, more than 25% reached clinical levels of depression and other psychological distress symptoms related to the continuing effects of cancer and its treatment. Cancer-related symptoms were the strongest predictors of hyperarousal symptom, not PTSD diagnosis, and depression (Deimling et al., 2002). This echoes a study suggesting that 44.2% of cancer survivors predominantly experienced hyper-arousal symptoms as their main cancer-related traumatic response (Zhou et al., 2019). Although 41% of breast cancer patients met the A2 criterion of the DSM-IV PTSD diagnosis (i.e. the person's reaction to the event (in this case cancer) involves intense fear, helplessness, or horror), only a small minority (4%) met the full diagnostic criteria, while 38% had other significant psychological distress (Kangas, 2013).

According to a study of latent profiles, 37% and 12.2% of their cancer patients were classified as having moderate or severe co-occurring PTSD and depression symptom groups, respectively (Yang et al., 2020). Given the presence of comorbid psychiatric symptoms such as depression, one might wonder to what extent these comorbidities or pre-existing psychological disorders exacerbate the burden of post-cancer diagnosis or increase the prevalence rate of PTSD or other disorders (Kangas, 2013).

In short, these studies suggest that PTSD diagnosis may not be a useful indicator for capturing the psychological changes that result from the cancer experience (Kasparian et al., 2012). It has even been argued that using the PTSD diagnostic criteria, e.g. the A2 criterion from DSM-IV, is a poor indicator of cancer-related PTSD (Palmer et al., 2004). Furthermore, relying on diagnostic criteria can have serious consequences. For example, as mentioned in Chapter 1, a slight change in diagnostic criteria or a restructuring of symptom structure would affect the prevalence rate of PTSD and its relationship to other predictors. This could increase the risk of inflating the severity and diagnosis of PTSD (Shelby et al., 2005). For example, a study looking at young adult survivors of childhood cancer showed that the prevalence rates of PTSD changed from an odds ratio of 4.21 when PTSD was defined as a full symptom with functional impairment to an odds ratio of 1.42 when PTSD was defined as a partial symptom with functional impairment (Stuber et al., 2011).

The sceptics could further discuss the problem by saying that PTSD symptoms may have overlapped with symptoms resulting from the effects of cancer and that therefore these were amplified. For example, symptoms of re-experiencing may overlap with the cancer survivor's intrusions or fear of relapse. In addition, many patients cannot avoid thinking or talking about the cancer because of ongoing treatments or follow-up appointments. In addition, hyperarousal symptoms such as sleep disturbances, difficulty concentrating and irritability are often side-effects of cancer treatment (Bruce, 2006). These co-existing PTSD and cancer-related symptoms may make it difficult to clearly identify the phenomenology of cancer-related PTSD. This is a similar problem to that of concurrent PTSD and psychiatric comorbidity mentioned earlier.

Taken together, the sceptics have concluded that (1) cancer-related PTSD is indeed rare and (2) therefore the experience of most cancer patients cannot be properly understood (Palmer et al., 2004). To decipher these conclusions, it could be argued that the rarity of this condition is precisely the reason for future empirical research, without which an appropriate clinical guide for the management of PTSD in cancer patients cannot be produced (Kangas et al., 2002). The first conclusion could also mean that cancer-related PTSD is a real clinical syndrome, but rare. What follows is more of a puzzling conclusion. Just because this psychologically traumatic condition is rare, it is therefore inaccurate to understand the experiences of cancer patients in terms of the trauma framework. This is rather like a doctor diagnosing Sanfilippo, a rare but real genetic condition that causes fatal brain damage in children, saying that it is not accurate to understand the experiences of these children in the light of a genetic condition!

Proponents of cancer-related PTSD might argue that the sceptics may have been misled by cross-sectional studies that have found no significant association between PTSD and cancer experience (Kangas et al., 2005b) In fact, cancer diagnosis and treatment can precipitate PTSD (Black & White, 2005) and other psychological symptoms in cancer survivors (Gold et al., 2012). However, cancer-related PTSD takes time to develop; 22% of patients with acute stress disorder have changed diagnostic status to full PTSD 6 months after initial assessment (Kangas et al., 2005b). The way patients coped at the time of their cancer diagnosis appears to have an impact on the development of PTSD. For example, to cope with the traumatic impact of the diagnosis, patients may have developed peritraumatic dissociative symptoms that predict PTSD at the six-month follow-up. The repressed grief at baseline may have exacerbated the later severity of PTSD (Kangas et al., 2005a).

The above controversies about the nature of cancer-related PTSD have led to it being under-diagnosed and untreated. Access to mental health services for this condition is limited. This in turn has led to increased medical and psychiatric morbidity and a reduction in quality of life, while at the same time patient survival rates have improved due to advances in treatment. In other words, the proportion of cancer patients who spend their lives dealing with the traumatic effects of cancer may be increasing (Brunet et al., 2008; French-Rosas et al., 2011). It is understandable that awareness of this problem needs to be raised. Therefore, cancer-related PTSD cannot be ignored as a clinical syndrome in its own right (Kelly et al., 1995).

The prevalence of cancer-related PTSD

Prevalence rates for cancer-related PTSD vary from 4% to 45% depending on cancer type (gastric cancer, breast cancer, haematological cancer, paediatric sarcoma, head and neck or lung malignancy), sample size of >30 to 1000 patients, assessment tools (e.g. PTSD Checklist—Civilian version; the Impact of Event Scale—Revised; University of California at Los Angeles Post Traumatic Stress Disorder Index), and stressor criteria (e.g. the impact of experiencing cancer, the impact of receiving a life-threatening diagnosis, or the impact of undergoing treatment) (Alter et al., 1996; Andrykowski & Kangas, 2010; Black & White, 2005; Cordova et al., 1995; Gold et al., 2012; Hobbie et al., 2000; Kangas et al., 2005a; Li Liu et al., 2015; Mehnert & Koch, 2008; Mystakidou et al., 2012; Schwartz et al., 2012; Widows et al., 2000; Wiener et al., 2006).

Adult long-term cancer survivors in a large population survey ($n = 9282$) who had received a diagnosis for at least five years were one and a half times more likely to have an anxiety disorder, which included PTSD according to the criteria of DSM-IV (Greer et al., 2011). It was shown that 45% of these adult oncology patients met the diagnostic criteria for PTSD and partial PTSD. Compared to patients without PTSD, those with PTSD had significantly lower levels of social functioning, had recently received the cancer diagnosis, had higher levels of mood disturbance, and had lower levels of physical functioning and quality of life. Lower levels of social functioning and a diagnosis of bone metastases predicted an increased risk of PTSD (Gold et al., 2012). PTSD is accompanied by comorbid symptoms such as clinical anxiety, depressive symptoms and a lack of positive affectivity (e.g. Curda, 2011; Deimling et al., 2002; Mehnert & Koch, 2008; Naidich & Motta, 2000; Palgi et al., 2011; Salsman et al., 2009; Urbaniec et al., 2011; Wiener et al., 2006). Early detection and intervention can mediate the onset of psychological distress and better health outcomes (Gold et al., 2012). Ninety-four per cent of cancer patients in one study described their cancer as the most traumatic experience in their lives; 13% later developed PTSD (Petersen et al., 2005). A higher prevalence rate of 17% was found using the DSM-IV criteria in haematological cancer patients (Black & White, 2005). Looking at symptom severity, 13% of patients with various haematological malignancies had high levels of intrusive thoughts, 26% avoidance behaviours, 20.5% anxiety, and 16.8% depression. Patients with a recent diagnosis had higher levels of intrusive thoughts than patients with a previous diagnosis. Patients who received intravenous chemotherapy had higher levels of anxiety than patients who did not receive this therapy (Santos et al., 2006).

Among women with ovarian cancer, 9.25% reported PTSD, 5.6% reported depression, and 13.9% reported anxiety. Low levels of quality of life were associated with total PTSD symptoms, avoidance symptoms, and intrusive symptoms, while depression was associated with avoidance and intrusive symptoms. Anxiety was associated with total, avoidant, intrusive, and hyperarousal symptoms. Substance use/self-blame as coping strategies were associated with total, avoidant, and hyperarousal PTSD symptoms. It appears that poor quality of life, depression, anxiety, and maladaptive coping (avoidance, substance use, and self-blame) are related to increases in PTSD symptoms in women with ovarian cancer (Shand et al., 2015).

A study focusing on survivors of gynaecological cancers found a prevalence rate of 6.3% for posttraumatic stress symptoms (PTSS) in women who were at stage 1 to 3 of breast cancer. PTSS was also associated with anxiety (Vazquez et al., 2020). Between 12% and 19% met PTSD criteria in cancer survivors who had undergone autologous BMT for breast cancer. Increased PTSD symptoms were associated with low levels of physical and mental health, sleep quality, and health-related quality of life (Jacobsen et al., 1998). Another study found a higher incidence of PTSD following a diagnosis of breast cancer (29.4%) in women who had undergone BMT. Interestingly, these women did not differ from women who had not undergone BMT in the incidence of PTSD, severity of depression, and anxiety at baseline and at 3, 6, and 12 months (Mundy et al., 2000). This finding seems to indicate that the severity of psychological distress in breast cancer patients persisted over time whether or not they underwent invasive treatment such as BMT. The PTSD rate of 12% was also found in a large-scale study of >1000 long-term breast cancer survivors. Moderate to high levels of anxiety (38%) and depression (22%) were also found (Mehnert & Koch, 2008). Women who have a PTSD diagnosis within 6 months of receiving a breast cancer diagnosis tend to have significantly lower plasma cortisol levels (Luecken et al., 2004). These studies reflect the claim that there are distinct PTSD symptoms following gynaecological cancer, characterised by avoidance behaviour and intrusive thoughts in relation to breast cancer stimuli, as well as psychiatric comorbidity (Naidich & Motta, 2000).

In addition to the traumatic effects of invasive treatments or a traumatic diagnosis, one study focused on women who had received BRCA1/2 (genetic tests for cancer risk) results. About 8% reported threshold or subthreshold PTSD related to the genetic testing process. However, when rates were examined based on carrier status, 25% of BRCA1/2 carriers reported test-related threshold or subthreshold PTSD compared to 2.3% of non-carriers. In other words, rates of threshold and subthreshold PTSD associated with genetic testing appear to be less common, although carriers may be at higher risk for significant posttraumatic symptoms (Hamann et al., 2005).

The trajectory of PTSD symptoms appeared to decrease after surgery, particularly in individuals without premorbid health problems and negative life events (Tjemsland et al., 1996). However, this decrease in PTSD symptoms over time is not sustained in survivors of aggressive and life-threatening ovarian cancer who have received chemotherapy. In 36–45% of them, there appears to have been a steady increase in symptoms, although the increase was not statistically significant. In more than half (57%), symptoms occurred sporadically, while in some (13%) they persisted for a longer period of time (Gonçalves et al., 2011). A study examining breast cancer patients showed that although the total and subscale of PTSD symptoms were stable over a one-year period, there was evidence of a decrease in PTSD symptoms over time in women who had received higher levels of social support and who had experienced fewer traumatic stressors prior to their breast cancer diagnosis. On the other hand, women who had higher levels of PTSD at the initial screening were less likely to participate at follow-up. This unwillingness to participate could be interpreted as a form of avoidance of PTSD. After all, participation in the follow-up would represent a reminder of the trauma that those with high levels of PTSD would want to avoid (Andrykowski et al., 2000).

The incidence of PTSD in paediatric cancer survivors is consistent with epidemiological estimates for the general population (Butler et al., 1996). The effects of trauma symptoms can be long-lasting (Erickson & Steiner, 2000), interfering with the developmental process and leading to significant impairment in paediatric cancer survivors. Those who underwent BMT reported persistent PTSD symptoms for about 1 year (Stuber et al., 1991). A systematic review showed that rates of PTSD symptoms in childhood cancer survivors using the PTSD symptom scale ranged from 0 to 12.5%, while the use of a structured clinical interview revealed rates of current cancer-related PTSD ranging from 4.7% to 20.8%. Meanwhile, rates of lifetime cancer-related PTSD among childhood cancer survivors ranged from 20.5% to 35% (Bruce,

2006; Cordova et al., 2017). One study showed that 33% met lifetime criteria for PTSD (Pelcovitz, 1992). An even longer study found that, 5 years after completion of treatment, the majority (78%) still had at least partial PTSD symptoms. Somatisation also occurred and was positively correlated with PTSD and negatively correlated with general adjustment (Erickson & Steiner, 1999). On average, 17 years after the end of multi-model cancer therapy, 12% of paediatric sarcoma survivors still met diagnostic criteria for PTSD, and 77% met the clinical cut-off for global symptom severity. This severity was associated with intrusive thoughts and avoidance behaviours, as well as difficulties reintegrating into work or school and concerns about health (Wiener et al., 2006).

Reaching adulthood does not appear to increase resistance to the traumatic effects of childhood cancer. Survivors have been shown to be four times more likely to suffer from PTSD than their healthy peers. Those with PTSD reported more depression, negative affect, poor quality of life, and lower life satisfaction than those without PTSD (Schwartz & Drotar, 2006). Long-term adult survivors of childhood cancer typically report high levels of global distress, perceived stress, and cancer-related anxiety (Allen et al., 2018). They have not only psychosocial but also neurocognitive problems, characterised by increased impairment in psychological (relative risk (RR): 3.42) and physical (RR: 2.26) aspects of health-related quality of life. PTSD symptoms were also associated with increased impairment in emotion regulation (RR: 3.67), followed by task efficiency (RR: 3.09), working memory (RR: 2.55), and organisational skills (RR: 2.11). Compared to individuals without PTSD, individuals with PTSD were significantly more likely to use health services (cancer-specific health services (odds ratio (OR): 1.89) and primary care services (OR: 1.89)) (Crochet et al., 2019). Survivors of childhood cancer may suffer from Damocles syndrome, where they feel an overwhelming sense of fear about what might happen to them in the future. This fear is debilitating and affects them so much that they can no longer enjoy life and are unable to make important decisions in their lives, such as marriage or employment. This fear often relates to different organ systems, depending on the type of cancer and the treatment they have received (Cupit-Link et al., 2018).

From what has been articulated, a few observations are worth mentioning. First, cancer-related PTSD is not an uncommon psychological condition, but is rather a non-discrete clinical syndrome that is often associated with other psychiatric comorbid symptoms. In addition to PTSD symptoms, survivors tend to have high levels of depression, anxiety, antisocial behaviour, and adjustment disorders. This in turn affects quality of life, relationships with others, and the ability to succeed at work. Women tend to be more vulnerable to these problems than men. In gastric cancer patients, increased PTSD is associated with a fifteen-fold increased risk of depression (Palgi et al., 2011). This interwoven relationship between PTSD and psychiatric comorbidity has been mentioned in several places in earlier chapters. The impact of this interconnectedness cannot be underestimated (Gold et al., 2012; Jacobsen et al., 1998; Mystakidou et al., 2012). So treatment for cancer does not stop after treatment. Treatment for the physical and psychological symptoms associated with surviving cancer continues for the rest of life (Curda, 2011). While the sceptics echo the aforementioned concern that the presence of co-occurring symptoms may be a problem in inflating the prevalence rate of PTSD or making it difficult to distinguish the phenomenology of cancer-related PTSD from other disorders, the way in which these symptoms influence each other is bidirectional. The reverse could also be true. Attention can therefore be drawn not only to the PTSD symptoms, but also to the comorbid symptoms, both of which need to be addressed through psychological interventions (Kangas et al., 2005a; Palgi et al., 2011).

Second, there may be biological evidence that could serve as additional support for the use of PTSD as a framework to represent the cancer experience. Using three-dimensional magnetic resonance imaging (MRI), women who had breast cancer surgery more than 3 years ago, and who had a history of distressing cancer-related intrusion, had significantly smaller left hippocampal volume (5%) than women without this history. This finding persisted even after controlling for previous trauma and depression prior to cancer (Nakano et al., 2002). Similarly, another study showed that, based on volumetric MRI analyses, increased intrusion was associated with decreased hippocampal volume, although volumes were similar in individuals with cancer-related PTSD, without cancer-related PTSD, and compared to healthy individuals (Hara et al., 2008). Breast cancer survivors with a history of cancer-related intrusion also tended to have smaller amygdala volumes than those without intrusion, according to a volumetric analysis of MRI (Matsuoka et al., 2003).

Risk factors for cancer-related PTSD

In light of the research evidence outlined in the previous section, risk factors associated with the severity of PTSD are now discussed for patients with various types of cancer—breast, haematological, prostate, colorectal, paediatric, or ovarian cancer, and in patients who have received a BMT. Broadly speaking, risk factors can be categorised into demographic variables, past trauma, coping styles, and subjective appraisal, and some other clinical parameters.

Demographic variables

Cancer-related PTSD is more likely to occur in people who are financially poor (Cordova et al., 1995) and unemployed (Santos et al., 2006), although these findings are not consistent with a study showing that higher household income is associated with higher severity of PTSD (Zhou et al., 2019). Cancer-related PTSD has been found in people with low levels of education (Allen et al., 2018; Jacobsen et al., 1998; Mehnert & Koch, 2008; Vazquez et al., 2020). They also tend to be younger (Cordova et al., 1995; Gold et al., 2012; Gonçalves et al., 2011; Turner-Sack et al., 2012), although one study showed that younger adolescents between 2 and 10 years after cancer treatment appeared to have lower levels of psychological distress at the time of diagnosis (Turner-Sack et al., 2012). On the contrary, older women with breast cancer tend to experience less psychological distress characterised by anxiety, depression, and PTSD symptoms than younger women (Mosher & Danoff-Burg, 2005). However, the relationship between age and PTSD response 6 weeks after surgery has not been demonstrated (Tjemsland et al., 1996). Some would argue that younger and older patients simply channel their distress differently. Behavioural changes are more likely to occur in children and adolescents than in adults. Adults seem to experience more clearly defined emotional responses (Andrykowski & Kangas, 2010). In addition, age differences would imply differences in health status, treatment care, social support, coping strategies and other life circumstances that could explain differences in patient adjustment (Mosher & Danoff-Burg, 2005).

Both genders appear to report distress related to different aspects of the cancer experience. Men appear to be more vulnerable to distress than women (Wiener et al., 2006). These findings are contradicted by studies showing that women are more prone to increased PTSD symptoms (Allen et al., 2018; Liu et al., 2015; Zhou et al., 2019). They also reported significantly higher treatment intensity, greater number and type of treatments, and they had more problems with health professionals than did men. Interpersonal and relational aspects of their illness were perceived as most stressful, while men were more concerned with behavioural avoidance, work, and finances (Hampton & Frombach, 2000). Perceptions of doctors' interpersonal skills during the diagnostic interview (i.e. perceptions of being cared for through doctor–patient communication) influence subsequent psychological adjustment in more women than in men (Mager & Andrykowski, 2002). In other words, although doctor–patient interaction is thought to be important in the care of cancer patients (Mehnert et al., 2010), this issue may be more important for women than for men.

A psychiatric history also seems to be a risk factor, as women with ovarian cancer who suffered from depression before the cancer diagnosis also tended to have increased PTSD symptoms (Guglietti et al., 2010). This could be the reason why negative affect also correlates with the same outcomes (Kristensen et al., 2012). Somewhat surprisingly, previous consultations for anxiety problems had no influence on the response to PTSD after surgery (Tjemsland et al., 1996). However, this was contradicted by later studies which found that pre-cancer anxiety disorder was responsible for cancer-related PTSD in breast cancer patients 18 months after surgery (Shelby et al., 2008). Compared to patients without PTSD, cancer patients who met criteria for PTSD were four times more likely to report suicidal ideation (Spencer et al., 2012). To reduce suicidal ideation, feelings of self-efficacy, spirituality, and support need to be strengthened, while physical distress needs to be reduced through palliative care interventions (Spencer et al., 2012).

Clinical parameters associated with cancer

A longer time since cancer diagnosis was associated with fewer hyperarousal symptoms and less severe PTSS (Zhou et al., 2019). This finding is at odds with a previous study which found that time since diagnosis had no significant impact on psychological comorbidity and quality of life in cancer survivors (Mehnert & Koch, 2008). In other words, the vividness of the memory of the time of diagnosis has a limited impact on the psychological well-being of survivors. However, this seems to depend on how 'certain' the diagnosis is, the effects of which have been associated with increased severity of PTSD symptoms in women with ovarian cancer (Guglietti et al., 2010). On the other hand, a shorter waiting time for treatment probably increased the severity of PTSD symptoms. In other words, too early treatment could have a negative impact on patients (Guglietti et al., 2010). In children with cancer, PTSD is related to the preparation phase before BMT and the timing of treatment. It seems that children's anticipation of treatment can trigger PTSD symptoms. However, the cessation of anticipation and confrontation with 'reality' can also trigger PTSD. After completion of treatment, the incidence of PTSD was similar to the estimated incidence in the general population (Butler et al., 1996). These studies are at odds with previous research indicating that cancer-related PTSD is not related to the timing of cytotoxic treatment (Cordova et al., 1995) and that adjuvant cytostatic treatment also does not affect the PTSD response 6 weeks after surgery (Tjemsland et al., 1996).

In addition, treatment intensity and the number and type of treatments received could also be related to cancer-related PTSD (Hampton & Frombach, 2000). Hospitalisation could also be related to PTSD (Jacobsen et al., 1998). Those who had a longer hospital stay for autologous BMT for breast cancer tended to report more symptoms of PTSD (Jacobsen et al., 1998). For children and adolescents, hospital treatment means external changes such as hair or weight loss, which can be traumatic (Andrykowski & Kangas, 2010).

Somewhat controversial is the non-significant association between PTSD and stage of illness (Cordova et al., 1995). Perception of disease stage does not appear to influence PTSD response 6 weeks after surgery (Tjemsland et al., 1996), but this has not been confirmed by later studies (Andrykowski & Cordova, 1998; Cordova et al., 2017; Mehnert & Koch, 2008; Vazquez et al., 2020) on women with advanced disease who underwent autologous BMT for breast cancer (Jacobsen et al., 1998). The lack of a significant correlation may also contradict the claim that limited knowledge about the stage of cancer progression was associated with PTSD symptoms in women with breast cancer (Naidich & Motta, 2000).

Past trauma

Past traumatic life events or the number of low-magnitude stressors experienced in the past may influence the severity of cancer-related PTSD (Andrykowski & Cordova, 1998; Libov et al., 2002; Tjemsland et al., 1996). Cancer surviving children who have experienced more life stressors tend to have more severe cancer-related PTSD than those who have experienced fewer life stressors (Currier et al., 2009), even after controlling for demographic factors (age, gender, ethnicity, and socioeconomic status), cancer factors (treatment status, time since diagnosis, and cancer type), and the intensity of PTSS experienced by parents (Currier et al., 2009). Stressful events or life stressors include family problems, non-cancer-related illnesses, and bereavement (Tjemsland et al., 1996). About 11% of advanced cancer patients reported experiencing the death of a loved one. Bereavement is, next to cancer diagnosis, the most traumatic event for patients in advanced stages of cancer (Mystakidou et al., 2012). According to the mortality salience hypothesis

(Greenberg et al., 1990), after a trauma involving death or threat to life, awareness, anxiety, or sensitivity to death tends to be heightened, which then affects later life. Previous violent trauma is particularly associated with PTSD, low levels of functioning, and poor quality of life in patients (Shelby et al., 2008). The same is true for interpersonal trauma (physical or sexual), which indirectly affects cancer-related PTSD through the loss of interpersonal resources (Banou et al., 2009). On the other hand, the absence of prior trauma seems to provide a buffer against stress. In the study of breast cancer patients before and after surgery, it was found that PTSD decreased after surgery, especially in those who had no previous negative life events.

In a large cohort study of 214,649 men diagnosed with prostate cancer, 5.7% also had a previous diagnosis of PTSD. Compared to the men without PTSD, the men with PTSD used more health services and therefore had a lower risk of cancer at the time of diagnosis. However, they suffered more suicide deaths and fewer non-suicide deaths than their peers. PTSD predicted suicide risk (hazard ratio: 2.35), with depression, substance abuse, and prostate cancer treatments acting as partial mediators. In other words, patients with pre-existing PTSD had a higher risk of suicide but a lower risk of death by non-suicide. They were also more likely to attend a clinic and to be diagnosed early with a lower-risk cancer (Aboumrad et al., 2021).

While the above studies seem to suggest that prior trauma may influence the severity of cancer-related PTSD, there is evidence that pre-existing PTSD does not increase the risk of lung, breast, prostate, and colorectal cancer. This nested case–control study included over 19,000 to just over 31,000 cases of patients who had the above cancers. No association was found between PTSD and cancer risk for any of the cancers, with OR ranging from 0.73 to 1.24 (Cohn et al., 2018).

Subjective appraisal

It has been documented that subjective appraisal or perception of life threat from cancer is associated with more severe PTSD symptoms and psychiatric comorbidity and may complicate adjustment to cancer (Cordova et al., 2007; Mehnert et al., 2010). In patients who have undergone prostatectomy, it has a long-term impact on psychological distress and quality of life on average 27 months after surgery (Hampton & Frombach, 2000). There is evidence that subjective appraisal indirectly influences outcomes through PTSD symptoms (Barakat et al., 1997; Laubmeier & Zakowski, 2004).

The feeling of uncertainty about the impact of cancer can be seen as a form of appraisal that triggers stress (Mehnert et al., 2010). It contributed to the fear of cancer recurrence. This fear has in turn been associated with increased PTSD symptoms (Black & White, 2005; Libov et al., 2002; Mehnert et al., 2009; Mehnert et al., 2010; Zhou et al., 2019) and poor quality of life (Laubmeier & Zakowski, 2004). This is not surprising given that such fear can be perceived as a direct and immediate threat to life, a trauma definition not far removed from that advocated in the DSM-5 (American Psychiatric Association, 2013; Black & White, 2005). Fear of cancer progression (FoP) can also affect distress and is associated with cancer-related intrusive cognitions, avoidance behaviours, hyperarousal, PTSD diagnoses, perceived impairment, and physical and psychological quality of life. Moderate and high levels of FoP are associated with a depressive coping style and an active problem-focused coping style. For about 24% of women who have moderate to high levels of this fear, the main fear is that of attending a doctor's appointment or examination and being dependent on outside help to cope with daily life. This fear is particularly pronounced in younger women or those who have children and have received chemotherapy (Mehnert et al., 2009).

The subjective appraisal of cancer requires a cognitive process of observing and thinking about one's immediate situation. In this sense, rumination can be considered a form of subjective appraisal. It is a form of perception that focuses on negative contents of the past and the present, and therefore triggers emotional distress. According to response style theory (Nolen-Hoeksema, 1991), rumination is a way for some people to cope with stress (Ehring & Ehlers, 2014; Nolen-Hoeksema, 1991). It is a trait-like process in which they repeatedly and passively focus on depressive symptoms, their causes, meanings, effects, and consequences. Essentially, they use a cognitive avoidance strategy (Rosebrock et al., 2019) in which they do not solve problems or change circumstances associated with distress. Instead, they preoccupy themselves with the problems and distress without taking concrete action. This preoccupation would only lead to compulsive or excessive rumination, unproductive thoughts, 'Why me?' or 'What if?' questions, and negative evaluations of situations (Michael et al., 2007).

Ruminating on traumatic cancer experiences can trigger intrusive traumatic memories and impair cognitive reconstruction of traumatic events. This in turn impairs instrumental behaviours such as help-seeking and decreases problem-solving skills, which in turn exacerbates PTSD (Yu et al., 2008). As pain is a major problem for patients diagnosed with cancer, the phenomenon of pain rumination cannot be ignored, which could lead to the development of PTSD (Andrykowski et al., 2003). To underscore the harmful effect of rumination, one study has also shown that intrusive cancer-related rumination mediates the effects of difficulties in emotional processing and PTSD symptoms after cancer diagnosis (Ogińska-Bulik & Michalska, 2020).

Similarly, metacognition refers to beliefs about one's cognition and involves monitoring, controlling, and evaluating one's thoughts. It acts as an internal guide that directs people's attention to identifying their own thoughts and taking action. Research has shown that adolescent and young adult survivors of cancer have some metacognitive beliefs (particularly negative beliefs about worry and the need to control one's thoughts) that account for 50% and 41% of the variance in psychological distress (anxiety and depression) and PTSD symptoms, respectively. This finding was replicated after controlling for demographic information and physical health problems (Fisher et al., 2018).

Coping strategies

In terms of coping strategies, increased avoidant coping in BMT patients is associated with increased severity of PTSD and general distress in the long term (Fuemmeler et al., 2001; Jacobsen et al., 2002). Cognitive and behavioural avoidant coping strategies have been associated with PTSD in women with cancer (Hampton & Frombach, 2000). However, there are gender differences in this avoidant coping. Whereas cognitive avoidance coping predicted cancer-related PTSD in women, behavioural avoidance was the predictor in men (Hampton & Frombach, 2000). Endorsement of avoidant coping is a barrier to the development of self-efficacy, the lack of which has been linked to cancer-related PTSD (Spencer et al., 2012). Lower avoidant coping, on the other hand, predicts lower levels of psychological distress in adolescents who have completed cancer treatment (Turner-Sack et al., 2012).

Peritraumatic or increased dissociative symptoms at the time of receiving a cancer diagnosis can be considered another form of avoidant coping. Although dissociation can help protect oneself by emotionally distancing oneself from the stressor (e.g. a cancer diagnosis), it has been associated with the severity of PTSD in the long term (Kangas et al., 2005a). Although repression is also an attempt to protect oneself by not allowing the traumatic emotions of the stressor to overwhelm oneself, it is a different psychological process (i.e. low distress and high restraint). This appears to be an adaptive coping style for cancer patients. Adolescent cancer survivors who identified themselves as repressors reported lower levels of PTSD and psychosocial stress, with moderate or large differences in effect size, and they had better quality of life than non-repressors (Erickson & Steiner, 1999; Erickson & Steiner, 2000; Erickson et al., 2008). This coping strategy enables children with cancer to develop a sense of resilience. This is also true for parents of children with cancer (Phipps, 2007; Phipps et al., 2006). Repression seems to have a protective function and could be an important way to identify and treat trauma-related distress (Erickson & Steiner, 1999; Erickson et al., 2008; Erickson & Steiner, 2000). One criticism of these studies is that the extent of PTSD in this paediatric oncology population was low (Phipps et al., 2006).

It is worth noting that resilience or intrinsic protective factors have been further investigated. A study examining paediatric cancer survivors and their parents for 4 years found that 65% of survivors were a resilient group with good psychosocial adjustment, 23% were an at-risk group with increased internalising and attention problems, and 12% were a parent-reported at-risk group with increased parent-reported internalising, externalising, and attention problems. They also found that the resilient group differed from the other groups in child PTSD symptoms, affectivity and attachment to school, parental distress, and overprotection. In particular, positive affectivity and strong attachment to school were the resilient or protective factors for the majority of these paediatric cancer survivors (Okado et al., 2018).

Social support also appears to play a role in influencing distress outcomes in cancer survivors. PTSD has been associated with lower social support in survivors of breast cancer (Vazquez et al., 2020) and in survivors of haematological malignancies (Liu et al., 2015). Patients with various haematological malignancies who had lower levels of social support also reported higher levels of stress, anxiety, and depression than their counterparts (Santos et al., 2006). After diagnosis, social support (Andrykowski & Cordova, 1998; Mehnert & Koch, 2008; Mehnert et al., 2010) from family and friends, characterised by reassuring, comforting, and problem-solving advice, is paramount in helping cancer survivors find positive meaning in their cancer experience (Schroevers et al., 2010). In a group of long-term cancer survivors, increased emotional support 3 months after diagnosis significantly predicted a greater experience of positive consequences of the disease 8 years after diagnosis. This association remained significant even when controlling for concurrent levels of emotional support 8 years after diagnosis (Schroevers et al., 2010). On the other hand, reluctance of patients, families, partners, friends, and children to discuss concerns and emotional problems related to cancer impairs patients' adjustment to the aftermath of the diagnosis (Andrykowski et al., 2003). Reduced social support has been associated with increased PTSD symptoms (Andrykowski & Cordova, 1998; Jacobsen et al., 2002) in BMT patients (Jacobsen et al., 2002), childhood cancer survivors and their parents (Barakat et al., 1997), children of mothers with breast cancer (Brown et al., 2007), and in adults who had a parent diagnosed with cancer as a child (Wong et al., 2006).

The detrimental effect of low social support was highlighted in a study of one thousand eighty-three patients recruited through a population-based cancer registry. Forty-six per cent of women felt inadequately informed about the support offered, while 15% of all patients and 23% of patients with a possible psychiatric disorder expressed their need for psychosocial support. Lower social support predicted psychological comorbidity, along with other factors such as disease progression, lower educational level, and younger age (Mehnert & Koch, 2008). Lack of positive support also predicted psychological comorbidity and mental health in men who had undergone prostatectomy; however, the impact of social support on physical health was somewhat limited (Mehnert et al., 2010).

The buffering effect of social support appears to vary depending on the type of social support. Positive interaction as a form of social support appears to buffer the negative effects of social constraints associated with increased PTSD severity in Chinese-American breast cancer survivors. On the other hand, tangible support strengthened the association between social constraints and PTSD symptoms. Surprisingly, emotional or informational support and affectionate support played only a limited role in moderating the distress caused by social constraints (Chu et al., 2021). This surprising outcome may be related to some traditional Chinese cultural traits where showing emotion or affection is discouraged, although affectionate communication is changing among Chinese (Wu et al., 2019).

Social support appears to interact with the avoidance coping mentioned above and to influence outcomes. Among patients who had received a BMT for cancer, low levels of social support 1 month before transplant predicted an increase in PTSD symptoms at an average of 7 months after transplant, even after accounting for pre-transplant levels of psychological distress. Patients with high levels of avoidance coping and low levels of social support had the most severe symptoms (Jacobsen et al., 2002).

Other coping strategies relate to religious coping, which is particularly important for cancer patients with suicidal intent. The lack of attachment to an organised religion and spirituality has been associated with increased distress, particularly in these patients (Spencer et al., 2012). Passion also appears to be important in coping with the effects of cancer. Two types of passions have been distinguished, namely harmonious and obsessive passions. The former is a passion that results from an autonomous internalisation of an activity into one's identity. Intrinsically, people are in control, see the importance of such an activity, and are willing to engage in it. They feel that performing this activity is part of their identity. On the other hand, obsessive passion results from a controlled internalisation of an activity into one's identity. People may feel an uncontrollable urge to perform an activity because of interpersonal pressure, social acceptance, or self-esteem (Vallerand et al., 2003). Harmonious passion was associated with high levels of positive affect and lower levels of cancer worry. Obsessive passion, on the other hand, was associated with higher levels of negative affect and cancer worry (Burke et al., 2012).

Treatments for cancer-related PTSD

Despite comments from sceptics, given the previous prevalence rates, psychiatric comorbidity, and risk factors, some researchers have recognised the importance of exploring ways to treat cancer-related PTSD symptoms. This is particularly important when these symptoms can affect cancer survivors' ability to adhere to self-management behaviours and cope with comorbid illness (James et al., 2018). As mentioned in the previous chapter on PTSD in the context of cardiovascular disease, eye movement desensitisation and reprocessing (EMDR) is a widely used method that has been recommended by the National Institute for Health and Care Excellence (NICE) as an effective treatment approach for patients with PTSD, and it is not surprising that this approach has also been tested in cancer survivors. One study showed that, compared to breast cancer patients who received treatment as usual, those who received EMDR for 2–3 months no longer met criteria for PTSD after treatment. In contrast, the group treated as usual retained the diagnosis. In the EMDR patients, depressive symptoms also decreased significantly, while anxiety remained stable in all patients. This indicates that EMDR seems to cushion certain specific symptoms. The EMDR group also showed significant differences in some neurobiological features, namely delta and theta bands in the left angular and right fusiform gyrus (Carletto et al., 2019).

The EMDR Group Traumatic Episode Protocol (G-TEP), a modified form of conventional EMDR, has been used to help cancer survivors of different types. In simple terms, it is a group EMDR where all group members sit at a table with an EMDR G-TEP worksheet. The central section of the sheet represents the trauma material to be worked on and the outer sections represent past, present, and future resources (e.g. a safe place, a positive past memory, an activity, and a desirable future). During the EMD process, the desensitisation process developed by Shapiro is used. However, the processing component is considered too restrictive and focuses primarily on the content of the trauma or disturbance. During the trauma processing of the EMDR G-TEP protocol, eye movements are performed by following a hand that moves back and forth, alternately tapping certain areas on the sheet. After participating in EMDR G-TEP, PTSD, anxiety, and depression symptoms significantly decreased in these cancer patients, with medium effect sizes from pre-treatment to one-month follow-up (Roberts, 2018).

The Integrative Group Treatment Protocol adapted for ongoing traumatic stress (EMDR-IGTP-OTS) is another modified treatment protocol aimed at helping patients living with ongoing traumatic stress who do not have a post-trauma safety phase for memory consolidation. During the processing phase, patients are asked to run a mental movie of the entire event from just before it began to now and into the future, and then identify the most painful or stressful moment. One study found that this treatment protocol reduced the severity of PTSD, anxiety, and depression symptoms over time (90-day follow-up period) with large effect sizes in women with various types of cancer. The treatment group reduced the severity of PTSD, anxiety, and depression significantly more than the no-treatment group (Jarero et al., 2018).

In addition to EMDR, cognitive behavioural therapy (CBT) has also been included as a recommended treatment approach for PTSD (NICE, 2018). Not surprisingly, this intervention, which aims to alleviate distress in cancer patients, has also been explored in the literature. Internet-based cognitive behavioural therapy (iCBT) has been used to address a whole range of emotional problems associated with cancer-related distress, namely negative affect, feelings of helplessness or hopelessness, anxiety and unhelpful beliefs, i.e. fatalism in patients with early-stage cancer. A 6-week online cancer coping intervention provided patients with information, worksheets, and activities to manage physical, emotional, social, and communication difficulties following a cancer diagnosis. This intervention resulted in reductions in negative affect, helplessness/hopelessness, anxiety, and fatalism with large effect sizes (d) ranging from 0.42 to 0.64 (Beatty et al., 2011).

Internet-based interventions are increasingly used in clinical psychology or psychiatry to address the growing difficulty of meeting mental health needs through face-to-face psychological treatments. Traumatised people may not seek or use face-to-face psychological treatments due to beliefs and stigma towards psychological services or logistical difficulties (e.g. time off work) (e.g. Kulesza et al., 2015). On the other hand, telehealth services increase the likelihood that traumatised people will seek help because they feel safe accessing services in their own homes, because they are easily accessible via computer, for example, and because they are anonymous (e.g. Whealin et al.,

2015). It does not create the kind of stigma generally associated with asking a psychologist for help.

Internet-based cognitive behavioural therapy has also been combined with Internet-based stepped care (iCAN-DO) to help cancer survivors. This stepped care programme comprised two steps, namely psychoeducation and self-care strategies (step 1) and Internet-based cognitive behavioural therapy (iCBT) (step 2). It was found that iCAN-DO significantly reduced the severity of depression symptoms as well as the proportion of patients with depression symptoms after 10 months more than patients assigned to the standard care group. Patients in the standard care group received, for example, routine information about the disease and treatment, as well as basic psychosocial support from nurses, doctors, counsellors, or church groups. Interestingly, the effects on anxiety, PTSD, or health-related quality of life were limited (Hauffman et al., 2020).

Another form of cognitive behavioural therapy used with cancer survivors is telephone-administered cognitive behavioural therapy (T-CBT) for the treatment of PTSD. Forty-six patients participated in a randomised clinical trial. A higher overall therapeutic alliance score predicted a decrease in depressive symptomatology over time; a higher task score predicted a decrease in overall distress, depressive symptomatology, re-experiencing symptoms, and avoidance; and higher bond scores predicted a decrease in depressive symptomatology and re-experiencing symptoms. In other words, the therapeutic alliance should be cultivated and integrated into routine clinical care and interventions to maximise psychotherapeutic effects for cancer survivors (Applebaum et al., 2012).

In addition to Internet- or telephone-based types of CBT intervention programmes, a pilot study compared brief face-to-face cognitive behavioural stress management (CBSM) with psychoeducation in a group of patients with colorectal cancer. Overall, this study found that both CBSM and psychoeducation reduced the severity of avoidance and hyperarousal symptoms with large effect sizes (0.30 for avoidance, 0.20 for hyperarousal) (Acevedo-Ibarra et al., 2019).

The overall findings of the studies are consistent with the claims of a systematic review that EMDR and CBT are promising intervention programmes for alleviating PTSD symptoms after medical events (cardiovascular disease, cancer, HIV, multiple sclerosis, stem cell transplantation) (Haerizadeh et al., 2020). Nevertheless, the intervention approaches examined in this review differed from those mentioned above. It compared exposure-based CBT with an assessment-only control, finding that CBT reduced PTSD symptoms. It also compared imaginal exposure (another exposure-based CBT) with an attentional control, finding a trend towards reduced PTSD symptoms. The study also compared EMDR with imaginal exposure, conventional CBT and relaxation therapy, finding that EMDR was more effective in reducing distress symptoms (Haerizadeh et al., 2020).

A study that also focused on patients' cognition in relation to their own memory functions examined the effectiveness of competitive memory training (COMET) and memory specificity training (MEST) in reducing cancer-related PTSD and depressive symptoms. COMET is an intervention that aims to change dysfunctional self-representations, i.e. maladaptive cognitive–emotional networks that underlie psychological disorders, but to promote positive self-representations, partly by enabling patients to retrieve positive material from their memory, recognise faulty meanings in their thoughts, find more practical alternatives, and focus on positive traits, which in turn helps them to access positive alternative self-representations more easily. MEST the memory training method, on the other hand, is simply memory training aimed at remedying deficits in autobiographical memory. They found that the COMET group had significantly fewer PTSD and depression symptoms at post-training and follow-up assessments. However, both groups were equally effective in reducing attentional biases after training (Farahimanesh et al., 2021).

Another intervention aims to improve the ability to relax one's state of mind. An 8-week mindfulness practise helped reduce perceived stress and avoidance symptoms of PTSD and increase positive state of mind. After the mindfulness programme, cancer survivors significantly reduced more perceived stress and PTSD avoidance symptoms, but achieved more positive states of mind than a wait-list control group (Bränström et al., 2010). This mindfulness intervention programme has also been implemented for cancer patients via eHealth and mobile health. A systematic review concluded that eHealth mindfulness-based programmes (eMBPs) are a viable treatment intervention for cancer patients and are compatible with the face-to-face mindfulness programme. This eHealth tool has the potential to reduce levels of stress, anxiety, depression, fatigue, sleep disturbances, and pain, but also to promote posttraumatic growth and well-being (Matis et al., 2020).

Psychological interventions are particularly useful for highly anxious parents who are at risk for PTSS symptoms (Best et al., 2001). Based on a case study of a middle-aged man after a BMT for leukaemia, a trauma-focused intervention appears to be helpful in reducing PTSD symptoms. In addition to other strategies such as relaxation, systematic desensitisation and cognitive coping strategies, the intervention was implemented to focus on PTSD symptoms related to the transplant. Before the intervention, he had regular flashbacks related to the transplant, accompanied by physical symptoms such as sweating. The PTSD symptoms improved over time and the PTSD diagnosis was no longer maintained. This improvement continued six months later (DuHamel et al., 2000). The neuro-emotional technique, which combines conventional desensitisation principles with complementary approaches, has also been used in a small number of cases to reduce PTSD symptoms and alter physiological reactivity (heart rate and skin conductance) in cancer survivors (Monti et al., 2007).

Among breast cancer survivors in a rural community in California, a low-cost, community-based workbook journal (WBJ) was used to improve psychosocial functioning in women with primary breast cancer. Among women who received the WBJ, 74% felt emotionally supported at the 3-month follow-up, while among women who did not receive the WBJ, decreased fighting spirit but increased emotional venting and symptoms of PTSD increased. This community-based WBJ could be an effective psychosocial intervention for rural, isolated, and low-income women with breast cancer. Community involvement was critical to the success of this project (Angell et al., 2003). Another improvement to this approach is the inclusion of an additional element, namely video conferencing. This combination helped to reduce distress but increase emotional expression and self-efficacy in coping with cancer. The women felt comfortable and saw the benefit and value of forming support groups through video conferencing. They encouraged information sharing and emotional bonding with other women who shared the same illness and cancer battle. The women showed a significant decrease in symptoms of depression and PTSD (Collie et al., 2007).

Some other interventions focus on the importance of empowering cancer survivors to initiate a catharsis process through expressive writing. When breast cancer survivors wrote for 3 weeks about their deepest thoughts and feelings, their coping strategies, as well as their positive thoughts and feelings about their breast cancer experience, quality of life, fatigue, PTSD symptoms, and positive long-term effects (3 and 6 months later), improved with medium and large effect sizes (Lu et al., 2012). To further explore the effectiveness of expressive writing, another study showed how PTSD symptoms, namely re-experiencing, avoidance, and hyperarousal symptoms, interacted with each other during and after an expressive writing intervention for breast cancer survivors. Over a 6-month period, hyperarousal symptoms predicted the severity of re-experiencing and avoidance symptoms at the 1-, 3-, and 6-month assessments. In other words, hyperarousal played an important role in influencing the subsequent severity of re-experiencing and avoidance symptoms during and after the expressive writing intervention. Hyperarousal appears to be an important PTSD response that needs to be treated to improve the management of cancer-related PTSD or reduce its chronicity (Chu et al., 2020).

The Cancer Distress Coach is a mobile app designed to manage PTSD symptoms. It is designed to educate patients with lymphoma, breast, or prostate cancer about what PTSD is; to provide a self-assessment of PTSD symptoms, ways to manage their symptoms (e.g. mind-body exercises); and to provide supportive links to cancer and non-cancer professional services. One study found that 89.7% of participants were moderately satisfied with this app. The overall mean PTSD symptom score decreased significantly from baseline to weeks 4 and 8. There was also a decrease in scores on the Cancer Network Distress Thermometer from baseline to weeks 4 and 8. However, there was no significant change in self-efficacy (Smith et al., 2018).

Summary

Although much has been documented about PTSD in cancer survivors, it is controversial whether cancer should be conceptualised in terms of trauma. Some research has suggested that such conceptualisation is useful due to the sudden onset of cancer and a whole range of persistent, repetitive distressing emotional and physical symptoms from the time of diagnosis through to the aftermath of treatment, affecting daily functioning and relationships. Indeed, cancer-related PTSD has been studied using a variety of models, such as a three-symptom cluster model, a four-symptom cluster model, or a unidimensional representation of emotional distress in response to cancer risk. There are sceptics, however, who argue that PTSD is not a useful indicator for capturing the psychological changes that result from the cancer experience.

Nevertheless, studies have been conducted to examine the prevalence rates of cancer-related PTSD, which is a non-discrete clinical syndrome and is associated with other psychiatric comorbidities. Risk factors for cancer-related PTSD include demographic variables (e.g. poor financial status, unemployment, low educational attainment, and younger age), although these findings are not always consistent. Distress in both genders relates to different aspects of the cancer experience. A psychiatric history and previous traumatic life events are further risk factors. It has been suggested that a longer time since cancer diagnosis is associated with a lower number of PTSD symptoms, while a shorter waiting time for treatment is likely to increase the severity of PTSD symptoms. The pre-transplant preparation period, the duration of treatment, the intensity of treatment, and the number and type of treatments and hospitalisation experience are other factors associated with PTSD.

It is hypothesised that the subjective appraisal or perception of a life threat from cancer is associated with more severe PTSD symptoms and psychiatric comorbidity and may influence adjustment to cancer. Feeling uncertain about the impact of cancer may contribute to fear of cancer recurrence, which in turn may increase PTSD symptoms and affect quality of life. Fear of cancer progression can also affect distress and cancer-related PTSD symptoms, perceived impairment, and physical and psychological quality of life. Intrusive cancer-related rumination may carry the impact of difficulties in the emotional process on PTSD symptoms following a cancer diagnosis.

Coping strategies are also related to PTSD in cancer survivors. Avoidance coping and cognitive and behavioural avoidance coping may influence the severity of PTSD and overall distress. Peritraumatic or increased dissociative symptoms at the time of cancer diagnosis are another form of avoidance strategy associated with PTSD. Repression, on the other hand, appears to be an adaptive coping style for cancer patients. PTSD has been associated with lower levels of social support in survivors of different types of cancer. Social support from family and friends helps cancer survivors find positive meaning in their cancer experience. Other adaptive coping strategies include religious coping and passion.

Treatments for cancer-related PTSD include EMDR, the EMDR Group Traumatic Episode Protocol, the Integrative Group Treatment Protocol adapted for persistent traumatic stress, and Internet-based CBT. The Cancer Coping Online Intervention, Internet-based CBT combined with Internet-based Stepwise Care, and telephone-based CBT for PTSD have been used to support cancer survivors. Other interventions include memory training and memory specificity training, mindfulness-based programmes, neuroemotional techniques, a community-based workbook journal, expressive writing and coaching for cancer, and a mobile app developed for managing PTSD symptoms. They appear to be of benefit to people with cancer in reducing and improving various indicators of distress.

References

Aboumrad, M., Shiner, B., Mucci, L., Neupane, N., Schroeck, F. R., Klaassen, Z., Freedland, S. J., & Young-Xu, Y. (2021). Posttraumatic stress disorder and suicide among veterans with prostate cancer. *Psycho-Oncology*, *30*(4), 581–590. https://doi.org/10.1002/pon.5605

Acevedo-Ibarra, J. N., Juárez-García, D. M., Espinoza-Velazco, A., & Buenaventura-Cisneros, S. (2019). Cognitive behavioral stress management intervention in Mexican colorectal cancer patients: Pilot study. *Psycho-Oncology*, 28(7), 1445–1452. https://doi.org/10.1002/pon.5094

Allen, J., Willard, V. W., Klosky, J. L., Li, C., Srivastava, D. K., Robison, L. L., Hudson, M. M., & Phipps, S. (2018). Posttraumatic stress-related psychological functioning in adult survivors of childhood cancer. *Journal of Cancer Survivorship*, 12, 216–223. https://doi.org/10.1007/s11764-017-0660-x

Alter, C. L., Pelcovitz, D., Axelrod, A., Goldenberg, B., Harris, H., Meyers, B., Grobois, B., Mandel, F., Septimus, A., & Kaplan, S. (1996). Identification of PTSD in cancer survivors. *Psychosomatics*, 37(2), 137–143. https://doi.org/10.1016/s0033-3182(96)71580-3

American Psychiatric Association. (1994). *Diagnostic and statistical manual of mental disorders* (4th ed.).

American Psychiatric Association. (2013). *Diagnostic and statistical manual of mental disorders* (5th ed.). https://doi.org/10.1176/appi.books.9780890425596

Andrykowski, M., Carpenter, J., & Munn, R. (2003). Psychosocial sequelae of cancer diagnosis and treatment. In L. A. Schein, H. S. Bernard, H. I. Spitz, & P. R. Muskin (Eds.), *Psychosocial treatment for medical conditions: Principles and techniques* (pp. 78–130). Routledge.

Andrykowski, M. A., & Cordova, M. J. (1998). Factors associated with PTSD symptoms following treatment for breast cancer: Test of the Andersen model. *Journal of Traumatic Stress*, 11, 189–203. https://doi.org/10.1023/A:1024490718043

Andrykowski, M. A., Cordova, M. J., McGrath, P. C., Sloan, D. A., & Kenady, D. E. (2000). Stability and change in posttraumatic stress disorder symptoms following breast cancer treatment: A 1-year follow-up. *Psycho-Oncology*, 9(1), 69–78. https://doi.org/10.1002/(sici)1099-1611(200001/02)9:1<69::aid-pon439>3.0.co;2-r

Andrykowski, M. A., & Kangas, M. (2010). Posttraumatic stress disorder associated with cancer diagnosis and treatment. In *Psycho-oncology* (2nd ed., pp. 348–357). Oxford University Press. https://doi.org/10.1093/med/9780195367430.003.0047

Angell, K. L., Kreshka, M. A., McCoy, R., Donnelly, P., Turner-Cobb, J. M., Graddy, K., Kraemer, H. C., & Koopman, C. (2003). Psychosocial intervention for rural women with breast cancer. *Journal of General Internal Medicine*, 18(7), 499–507. https://doi.org/https://doi.org/10.1046/j.1525-1497.2003.20316.x

Applebaum, A. J., DuHamel, K. N., Winkel, G., Rini, C., Greene, P. B., Mosher, C. E., & Redd, W. H. (2012). Therapeutic alliance in telephone-administered cognitive–behavioral therapy for hematopoietic stem cell transplant survivors. *Journal of Consulting and Clinical Psychology*, 80, 811–816. https://doi.org/10.1037/a0027956

Baider, L., & Kaplan De-Nour, A. (1997). Psychological distress and intrusive thoughts in cancer patients. *Journal of Nervous and Mental Disease*, 185(5), 346–348. https://doi.org/10.1097/00005053-199705000-00010

Banou, E., Hobfoll, S. E., & Trochelman, R. D. (2009). Loss of resources as mediators between interpersonal trauma and traumatic and depressive symptoms among women with cancer. *Journal of Health Psychology*, 14(2), 200–214. https://doi.org/10.1177/1359105308100204

Barakat, L. P., Kazak, A. E., Meadows, A. T., Casey, R., Meeske, K., & Stuber, M. L. (1997). Families surviving childhood cancer: a comparison of posttraumatic stress symptoms with families of healthy children. *Journal of Pediatric Psychology*, 22(6), 843–859. https://doi.org/10.1093/jpepsy/22.6.843

Beatty, L., Koczwara, B., & Wade, T. (2011). 'Cancer Coping Online': A pilot trial of a self-guided CBT internet intervention for cancer-related distress. *E-Journal of Applied Psychology*, 7. https://doi.org/10.7790/ejap.v7i2.256

Best, M., Streisand, R., Catania, L., & Kazak, A. E. (2001). Parental distress during pediatric leukemia and posttraumatic stress symptoms (PTSS) after treatment ends. *Journal of Pediatric Psychology, 26*(5), 299–307. https://doi.org/10.1093/jpepsy/26.5.299

Black, E. K., & White, C. A. (2005). Fear of recurrence, sense of coherence and posttraumatic stress disorder in haematological cancer survivors. *Psycho-Oncology, 14*(6), 510–515. https://doi.org/10.1002/pon.894

Bränström, R., Kvillemo, P., Brandberg, Y., & Moskowitz, J. T. (2010). Self-report mindfulness as a mediator of psychological well-being in a stress reduction intervention for cancer patients—a randomized study. *Annals of Behavioral Medicine, 39*(2), 151–161. https://doi.org/10.1007/s12160-010-9168-6

Brown, R. T., Fuemmeler, B., Anderson, D., Jamieson, S., Simonian, S., Hall, R. K., & Brescia, F. (2007). Adjustment of children and their mothers with breast cancer. *Journal of Pediatric Psychology, 32*(3), 297–308. https://doi.org/10.1093/jpepsy/jsl015

Brown, R. T., Madan-Swain, A., & Lambert, R. (2003). Posttraumatic stress symptoms in adolescent survivors of childhood cancer and their mothers. *Journal of Trauma Stress, 16*(4), 309–318. https://doi.org/10.1023/a:1024465415620

Bruce, M. (2006). A systematic and conceptual review of posttraumatic stress in childhood cancer survivors and their parents. *Clinical Psychology Review, 26*(3), 233–256. https://doi.org/10.1016/j.cpr.2005.10.002

Brunet, A., Orr, S. P., Tremblay, J., Robertson, K., Nader, K., & Pitman, R. K. (2008). Effect of post-retrieval propranolol on psychophysiologic responding during subsequent script-driven traumatic imagery in post-traumatic stress disorder. *Journal of Psychiatric Research, 42*(6), 503–506. https://doi.org/10.1016/j.jpsychires.2007.05.006

Burke, S. M., Sabiston, C. M., & Vallerand, R. J. (2012). Passion in breast cancer survivors: examining links to emotional well-being. *Journal of Health Psychology, 17*(8), 1161–1175. https://doi.org/10.1177/1359105311429202

Bush, N. J. (2009). Post-traumatic stress disorder related to the cancer experience. *Oncology Nursing Forum, 36*(4), 395–400. https://doi.org/10.1188/09.ONF.395-400

Butler, R. W., Rizzi, L. P., & Handwerger, B. A. (1996). Brief report: the assessment of posttraumatic stress disorder in pediatric cancer patients and survivors. *Journal of Pediatric Psychology, 21*(4), 499–504. https://doi.org/10.1093/jpepsy/21.4.499

Carletto, S., Porcaro, C., Settanta, C., Vizzari, V., Stanizzo, M. R., Oliva, F., Torta, R., Fernandez, I., Moja, M. C., Pagani, M., & Ostacoli, L. (2019). Neurobiological features and response to eye movement desensitization and reprocessing treatment of posttraumatic stress disorder in patients with breast cancer. *European Journal of Psychotraumatology, 10*(1), 1600832. https://doi.org/10.1080/20008198.2019.1600832

Chu, Q., Wong, C. C. Y., & Lu, Q. (2021). Social Constraints and PTSD among Chinese American breast cancer survivors: Not all kinds of social support provide relief. *Journal of Behavioral Medicine, 44*(1), 29–37. https://doi.org/10.1007/s10865-020-00165-y

Chu, Q., Wu, I. H. C., Tang, M., Tsoh, J., & Lu, Q. (2020). Temporal relationship of posttraumatic stress disorder symptom clusters during and after an expressive writing intervention for Chinese American breast cancer survivors. *Journal of Psychosomatic Research, 135*, 110142. https://doi.org/https://doi.org/10.1016/j.jpsychores.2020.110142

Cohn, E., Lurie, I., Yang, Y. X., Bilker, W. B., Haynes, K., Mamtani, R., Shacham-Shmueli, E., Margalit, O., & Boursi, B. (2018). Posttraumatic stress disorder and cancer risk: A nested case–control study. *Journal of Trauma Stress, 31*(6), 919–926. https://doi.org/10.1002/jts.22345

Collie, K., Kreshka, M., Ferrier, S., Parsons, R., Graddy, K., Avram, S., Mannell, P., Chen, X.-H., Perkins, J., & Koopman, C. (2007). Videoconferencing for delivery of breast cancer support groups to women living in rural communities: A pilot study. *Psycho-Oncology, 16*, 778–782. https://doi.org/10.1002/pon.1145

Cordova, M. J., Andrykowski, M. A., Kenady, D. E., McGrath, P. C., Sloan, D. A., & Redd, W. H. (1995). Frequency and correlates of posttraumatic-stress-disorder-like symptoms after treatment for breast cancer. *Journal of Consulting and Clinical Psychology, 63*(6), 981–986. https://doi.org/10.1037//0022-006x.63.6.981

Cordova, M. J., Giese-Davis, J., Golant, M., Kronenwetter, C., Chang, V., & Spiegel, D. (2007). Breast cancer as trauma: Posttraumatic stress and posttraumatic growth. *Journal of Clinical Psychology in Medical Settings, 14*, 308–319. https://doi.org/10.1007/s10880-007-9083-6

Cordova, M. J., Riba, M. B., & Spiegel, D. (2017). Post-traumatic stress disorder and cancer. *Lancet Psychiatry, 4*(4), 330–338. https://doi.org/10.1016/s2215-0366(17)30014-7

Cordova, M. J., Studts, J. L., Hann, D. M., Jacobsen, P. B., & Andrykowski, M. A. (2000). Symptom structure of PTSD following breast cancer. *Journal of Traumatic Stress, 13*(2), 301–319. https://doi.org/https://doi.org/10.1023/A:1007762812848

Crochet, E., Tyc, V. L., Wang, M., Srivastava, D. K., Van Sickle, K., Nathan, P. C., Leisenring, W., Gibson, T. M., Armstrong, G. T., & Krull, K. (2019). Posttraumatic stress as a contributor to behavioral health outcomes and healthcare utilization in adult survivors of childhood cancer: A report from the Childhood Cancer Survivor Study. *Journal of Cancer Survivorship, 13*(6), 981–992. https://doi.org/10.1007/s11764-019-00822-5

Cupit-Link, M., Syrjala, K. L., & Hashmi, S. K. (2018). Damocles' syndrome revisited: Update on the fear of cancer recurrence in the complex world of today's treatments and survivorship. *Hematology/Oncology and Stem Cell Therapy, 11*(3), 129–134. https://doi.org/https://doi.org/10.1016/j.hemonc.2018.01.005

Curda, A. (2011). The Damocles Syndrome: Where we are today. *Journal of Cancer Education, 26*(2), 397–398. https://doi.org/10.1007/s13187-010-0167-x

Currier, J. M., Jobe-Shields, L. E., & Phipps, S. (2009). Stressful life events and posttraumatic stress symptoms in children with cancer. *Journal of Traumatic Stress, 22*(1), 28–35. https://doi.org/10.1002/jts.20382

Deimling, G. T., Kahana, B., Bowman, K. F., & Schaefer, M. L. (2002). Cancer survivorship and psychological distress in later life. *Psycho-Oncology, 11*(6), 479–494. https://doi.org/https://doi.org/10.1002/pon.614

DuHamel, K. N., Ostrof, J., Ashman, T., Winkel, G., Mundy, E. A., Keane, T. M., Morasco, B. J., Vickberg, S. M., Hurley, K., Burkhalter, J., Chhabra, R., Scigliano, E., Papadopoulos, E., Moskowitz, C., & Redd, W. (2004). Construct validity of the posttraumatic stress disorder checklist in cancer survivors: Analyses based on two samples. *Psychological Assessment, 16*(3), 255–266. https://doi.org/10.1037/1040-3590.16.3.255

DuHamel, K. N., Ostroff, J. S., Bovbjerg, D. H., Pfeffer, M., Morasco, B. J., Papadopoulos, E., & Redd, W. H. (2000). Trauma-focused intervention after bone marrow transplantation: A case study. *Behavior Therapy, 31*(1), 175–186. https://doi.org/https://doi.org/10.1016/S0005-7894(00)80010-6

Ehring, T., & Ehlers, A. (2014). Does rumination mediate the relationship between emotion regulation ability and posttraumatic stress disorder? *European Journal of Psychotraumatology, 5*, ArtID 23547.

Erickson, S., & Steiner, H. (1999). Somatization as an indicator of trauma adaptation in long-term pediatric cancer survivors. *Clinical Child Psychology and Psychiatry, 4*(3), 415–426. https://doi.org/10.1177/1359104599004003011

Erickson, S. J., Gerstle, M., & Montague, E. Q. (2008). Repressive adaptive style and self-reported psychological functioning in adolescent cancer survivors. *Child Psychiatry and Human Development, 39*(3), 247–260. https://doi.org/10.1007/s10578-007-0085-2

Erickson, S. J., & Steiner, H. (2000). Trauma spectrum adaptation: Somatic symptoms in long-term pediatric cancer survivors. *Psychosomatics: Journal of Consultation and Liaison Psychiatry, 41*(4), 339–346. https://doi.org/10.1176/appi.psy.41.4.339

Esser, P., Glaesmer, H., Faller, H., Koch, U., Härter, M., Schulz, H., Wegscheider, K., Weis, J., & Mehnert, A. (2019). Posttraumatic stress disorder among cancer patients—Findings from a large and representative interview-based study in Germany. *Psycho-Oncology, 28*(6), 1278–1285. https://doi.org/10.1002/pon.5079

Farahimanesh, S., Moradi, A., Sadeghi, M., & Jobson, L. (2021). Comparing the efficacy of competitive memory training (COMET) and memory specificity training (MEST) on post-traumatic stress disorder among newly diagnosed cancer patients. *Cognitive Therapy and Research, 45*(5), 918–928. https://doi.org/10.1007/s10608-020-10175-4

Fisher, P. L., McNicol, K., Cherry, M. G., Young, B., Smith, E., Abbey, G., & Salmon, P. (2018). The association of metacognitive beliefs with emotional distress and trauma symptoms in adolescent and young adult survivors of cancer. *Journal of Psychosocial Oncology, 36*(5), 545–556. https://doi.org/10.1080/07347332.2018.1440276

French-Rosas, L. N., Moye, J., & Naik, A. D. (2011). Improving the recognition and treatment of cancer-related posttraumatic stress disorder. *Journal of Psychiatric Practice, 17*(4), 270–276. https://doi.org/10.1097/01.pra.0000400264.30043.ae

Fuemmeler, B. F., Mullins, L. L., & Marx, B. P. (2001). Posttraumatic stress and general distress among parents of children surviving a brain tumor. *Children's Health Care, 30*, 169–182.

Gold, J. I., Douglas, M. M. K., Thomas, M. L., Elliott, J. E., Rao, S. M., & Miaskowski, C. (2012). The relationship between posttraumatic stress disorder, mood states, functional status, and quality of life in oncology outpatients. *Journal of Pain and Symptom Management, 44*(4), 520–531. https://doi.org/10.1016/j.jpainsymman.2011.10.014

Gonçalves, V., Jayson, G., & Tarrier, N. (2011). A longitudinal investigation of posttraumatic stress disorder in patients with ovarian cancer. *Journal of Psychosomatic Research, 70*(5), 422–431. https://doi.org/10.1016/j.jpsychores.2010.09.017

Greenberg, J., Pyszczynski, T., Solomon, S., Rosenblatt, A., Veeder, M., Kirkland, S., & Lyon, D. (1990). Evidence for terror management theory II: The effects of mortality salience on reactions to those who threaten or bolster the cultural worldview. *Journal of Personality and Social Psychology, 58*, 308–318.

Greer, J. A., Solis, J. M., Temel, J. S., Lennes, I. T., Prigerson, H. G., Maciejewski, P. K., & Pirl, W. F. (2011). Anxiety disorders in long-term survivors of adult cancers. *Psychosomatics, 52*(5), 417–423. https://doi.org/https://doi.org/10.1016/j.psym.2011.01.014

Guglietti, C. L., Rosen, B., Murphy, K. J., Laframboise, S., Dodge, J., Ferguson, S., Katz, J., & Ritvo, P. (2010). Prevalence and predictors of posttraumatic stress in women undergoing an ovarian cancer investigation. *Psychological Services, 7*, 266–274. https://doi.org/10.1037/a0020338

Haerizadeh, M., Sumner, J. A., Birk, J. L., Gonzalez, C., Heyman-Kantor, R., Falzon, L., Gershengoren, L., Shapiro, P., & Kronish, I. M. (2020). Interventions for posttraumatic stress disorder symptoms induced by medical events: A systematic review. *Journal of Psychosomatic Research, 129*, 109908. https://doi.org/10.1016/j.jpsychores.2019.109908

Hamann, H. A., Somers, T. J., Smith, A. W., Inslicht, S. S., & Baum, A. (2005). Posttraumatic stress associated with cancer history and BRCA1/2 genetic testing. *Psychosomatic Medicine, 67*(5), 766–772. https://doi.org/10.1097/01.psy.0000181273.74398.d7

Hampton, M. R., & Frombach, I. (2000). Women's experience of traumatic stress in cancer treatment. *Health Care for Women International, 21*(1), 67–76. https://doi.org/10.1080/073993300245410

Hara, E., Matsuoka, Y., Hakamata, Y., Nagamine, M., Inagaki, M., Imoto, S., Murakami, K., Kim, Y., & Uchitomi, Y. (2008). Hippocampal and amygdalar volumes in breast cancer survivors with posttraumatic stress disorder. *Journal of Neuropsychiatry and Clinical Neuroscience*, *20*(3), 302–308. https://doi.org/10.1176/jnp.2008.20.3.302

Hauffman, A., Alfonsson, S., Bill-Axelson, A., Bergkvist, L., Forslund, M., Mattsson, S., von Essen, L., Nygren, P., Igelström, H., & Johansson, B. (2020). Cocreated internet-based stepped care for individuals with cancer and concurrent symptoms of anxiety and depression: Results from the U-CARE AdultCan randomized controlled trial. *Psycho-Oncology*, *29*(12), 2012–2018. https://doi.org/https://doi.org/10.1002/pon.5489

Hobbie, W. L., Stuber, M., Meeske, K., Wissler, K., Rourke, M. T., Ruccione, K., Hinkle, A., & Kazak, A. E. (2000). Symptoms of posttraumatic stress in young adult survivors of childhood cancer. *Journal of Clinical Oncology*, *18*(24), 4060–4066. https://doi.org/10.1200/jco.2000.18.24.4060

Ingerski, L. M., Shaw, K., Gray, W. N., & Janicke, D. M. (2010). A pilot study comparing traumatic stress symptoms by child and parent report across pediatric chronic illness groups. *Journal of Developmental and Behavioral Pediatrics*, *31*(9), 713–719. https://doi.org/10.1097/DBP.0b013e3181f17c52

Jacobsen, P. B., Sadler, I. J., Booth-Jones, M., Soety, E., Weitzner, M. A., & Fields, K. K. (2002). Predictors of posttraumatic stress disorder symptomatology following bone marrow transplantation for cancer. *Journal of Consulting and Clinical Psychology*, *70*(1), 235–240. https://doi.org/10.1037//0022-006x.70.1.235

Jacobsen, P. B., Widows, M. R., Hann, D. M., Andrykowski, M. A., Kronish, L. E., & Fields, K. K. (1998). Posttraumatic stress disorder symptoms after bone marrow transplantation for breast cancer. *Psychosomatic Medicine*, *60*(3), 366–371. https://doi.org/10.1097/00006842-199805000-00026

James, J., Harris, Y. T., Kronish, I. M., Wisnivesky, J. P., & Lin, J. J. (2018). Exploratory study of impact of cancer-related posttraumatic stress symptoms on diabetes self-management among cancer survivors. *Psycho-Oncology*, *27*(2), 648–653. https://doi.org/10.1002/pon.4568

Jarero, I., Givaudan, M., & Osorio, A. (2018). Randomized controlled trial on the provision of the EMDR integrative group treatment protocol adapted for ongoing traumatic stress to female patients with cancer-related posttraumatic stress disorder symptoms. *Journal of EMDR Practice and Research*, *12*, 94–104. https://doi.org/10.1891/1933-3196.12.3.94

Kangas, M. (2013). DSM-5 trauma and stress-related disorders: Implications for screening for cancer-related stress. *Frontiers in Psychiatry*, *4*, 122. https://doi.org/10.3389/fpsyt.2013.00122

Kangas, M., Henry, J. L., & Bryant, R. A. (2002). Posttraumatic stress disorder following cancer. A conceptual and empirical review. *Clinical Psychology Review*, *22*(4), 499–524. https://doi.org/10.1016/s0272-7358(01)00118-0

Kangas, M., Henry, J. L., & Bryant, R. A. (2005a). Predictors of posttraumatic stress disorder following cancer. *Health Psychology*, *24*, 579–585. https://doi.org/10.1037/0278-6133.24.6.579

Kangas, M., Henry, J. L., & Bryant, R. A. (2005b). The relationship between acute stress disorder and posttraumatic stress disorder following cancer. *Journal of Consulting and Clinical Psychology*, *73*, 360–364. https://doi.org/10.1037/0022-006X.73.2.360

Kasparian, N. A., Sansom-Daly, U., McDonald, R. P., Meiser, B., Butow, P. N., & Mann, G. J. (2012). The nature and structure of psychological distress in people at high risk for melanoma: a factor analytic study. *Psycho-Oncology*, *21*(8), 845–856. https://doi.org/10.1002/pon.1976

Kelly, B., Raphael, B., Smithers, M., Swanson, C., Reid, C., McLeod, R., Thomson, D., & Walpole, E. (1995). Psychological responses to malignant melanoma. An investigation of traumatic stress reactions to life-threatening illness. *General Hospital Psychiatry*, *17*(2), 126–134. https://doi.org/10.1016/0163-8343(94)00098-x

Khalid, R., & Gul, A. (2000). Posttraumatic stress disorder like symptoms in breast cancer patients. *Journal of the Indian Academy of Applied Psychology, 26*, 47–55.

Kristensen, T. E., Elklit, A., & Karstoft, K.-I. (2012). Posttraumatic stress disorder after bereavement: Early psychological sequelae of losing a close relative due to terminal cancer. *Journal of Loss and Trauma, 17*(6), 508–521. https://doi.org/10.1080/15325024.2012.665304

Kulesza, M., Pedersen, E., Corrigan, P., & Marshall, G. (2015). Help-seeking stigma and mental health treatment seeking among young adult veterans. *Military Behavioral Health, 3*(4), 230–239. https://doi.org/10.1080/21635781.2015.1055866

Laubmeier, K. K., & Zakowski, S. G. (2004). The role of objective versus perceived life threat in the psychological adjustment to cancer. *Psychology and Health, 19*, 425–437. https://doi.org/10.1080/0887044042000196719

Libov, B. G., Nevid, J. S., Pelcovitz, D., & Carmony, T. M. (2002). Posttraumatic stress symptomatology in mothers of pediatric cancer survivors. *Psychology and Health, 17*, 501–511. https://doi.org/10.1080/0887044022000004975

Liu, L., Yang, Y.-L., Wang, Z.-Y., Wu, H., Wang, Y., & Wang, L. (2015). Prevalence and positive correlates of posttraumatic stress disorder symptoms among Chinese patients with hematological malignancies: A cross-sectional study. *PLoS ONE, 10*(12). https://doi.org/10.1371/journal.pone.0145103

Lu, Q., Zheng, D., Young, L., Kagawa-Singer, M., & Loh, A. (2012). A pilot study of expressive writing intervention among Chinese-speaking breast cancer survivors. *Health Psychology, 31*(5), 548–551. https://doi.org/10.1037/a0026834

Luecken, L. J., Dausch, B., Gulla, V., Hong, R., & Compas, B. E. (2004). Alterations in morning cortisol associated with PTSD in women with breast cancer. *Journal of Psychosomatic Research, 56*(1), 13–15. https://doi.org/10.1016/s0022-3999(03)00561-0

Mager, W. M., & Andrykowski, M. A. (2002). Communication in the cancer 'bad news' consultation: Patient perceptions and psychological adjustment. *Psycho-Oncology, 11*(1), 35–46. https://doi.org/10.1002/pon.563

Marusak, H. A., Elrahal, F., Peters, C. A., Kundu, P., Lombardo, M. V., Calhoun, V. D., Goldberg, E. K., Cohen, C., Taub, J. W., & Rabinak, C. A. (2018). Mindfulness and dynamic functional neural connectivity in children and adolescents. *Behavioural Brain Research, 336*, 211–218. https://doi.org/https://doi.org/10.1016/j.bbr.2017.09.010

Marusak, H. A., Martin, K. R., Etkin, A., & Thomason, M. E. (2015). Childhood trauma exposure disrupts the automatic regulation of emotional processing. *Neuropsychopharmacology, 40*(5), 1250–1258.

Matis, J., Svetlak, M., Slezackova, A., Svoboda, M., & Šumec, R. (2020). Mindfulness-based programs for patients with cancer via eHealth and mobile health: Systematic review and synthesis of quantitative research. *Journal of Medical Internet Research, 22*(11). https://doi.org/10.2196/20709

Matsuoka, Y., Yamawaki, S., Inagaki, M., Akechi, T., & Uchitomi, Y. (2003). A volumetric study of amygdala in cancer survivors with intrusive recollections. *Biological Psychiatry, 54*(7), 736–743. https://doi.org/10.1016/s0006-3223(02)01907-8

Mehnert, A., Berg, P., Henrich, G., & Herschbach, P. (2009). Fear of cancer progression and cancer-related intrusive cognitions in breast cancer survivors. *Psycho-Oncology, 18*(12), 1273–1280. https://doi.org/10.1002/pon.1481

Mehnert, A., & Koch, U. (2008). Psychological comorbidity and health-related quality of life and its association with awareness, utilization, and need for psychosocial support in a cancer register-based sample of long-term breast cancer survivors. *Journal of Psychosomatic Research, 64*(4), 383–391. https://doi.org/10.1016/j.jpsychores.2007.12.005

Mehnert, A., Lehmann, C., Graefen, M., Huland, H., & Koch, U. (2010). Depression, anxiety, post-traumatic stress disorder and health-related quality of life and its association with social support in ambulatory prostate cancer patients. *European Journal of Cancer Care (England)*, *19*(6), 736–745. https://doi.org/10.1111/j.1365-2354.2009.01117.x

Michael, T., Halligan, S. L., Clark, D. M., & Ehlers, A. (2007). *Rumination in posttraumatic stress disorder. Depression and Anxiety*, *24*(5), 307–317.

Monti, D. A., Stoner, M. E., Zivin, G., & Schlesinger, M. (2007). Short term correlates of the Neuro Emotional Technique for cancer-related traumatic stress symptoms: a pilot case series. *Journal of Cancer Survivorship*, *1*(2), 161–166. https://doi.org/10.1007/s11764-007-0018-x

Mosher, C. E., & Danoff-Burg, S. (2005). A review of age differences in psychological adjustment to breast cancer. *Journal of Psychosocial Oncology*, *23*, 101–114.

Mundy, E. A., Blanchard, E. B., Cirenza, E., Gargiulo, J., Maloy, B., & Blanchard, C. G. (2000). Posttraumatic stress disorder in breast cancer patients following autologous bone marrow transplantation or conventional cancer treatments. *Behaviour Research and Therapy*, *38*(10), 1015–1027. https://doi.org/10.1016/s0005-7967(99)00144-8

Mystakidou, K., Parpa, E., Tsilika, E., Panagiotou, I., Galanos, A., Sakkas, P., & Gouliamos, A. (2012). Posttraumatic stress disorder and preparatory grief in advanced cancer. *J BUON*, *17*(1), 155–159.

Naidich, J. B., & Motta, R. W. (2000). PTSD-related symptoms in women with breast cancer. *Journal of Psychotherapy in Independent Practice*, *1*, 35–54. https://doi.org/10.1300/J288v0 1n01_04

Nakano, T., Wenner, M., Inagaki, M., Kugaya, A., Akechi, T., Matsuoka, Y., Sugahara, Y., Imoto, S., Murakami, K., & Uchitomi, Y. (2002). Relationship between distressing cancer-related recollections and hippocampal volume in cancer survivors. *American Journal of Psychiatry*, *159*(12), 2087–2093. https://doi.org/10.1176/appi.ajp.159.12.2087

NICE. (2018). *https://www.nice.org.uk/guidance/ng116/chapter/recommendations.*

Nolen-Hoeksema, S. (1991). Responses to depression and their effects on the duration of depressive episodes. *Journal of Abnormal Psychology*, *100*(4), 569–582. https://doi.org/10.1037//0021-843x.100.4.569

Ogińska-Bulik, N., & Michalska, P. (2020). The relationship between emotional processing deficits and posttraumatic stress disorder symptoms among breast cancer patients: the mediating role of rumination. *Journal of Clinical Psychology in Medical Settings*, *27*(1), 11–21. https://doi.org/10.1007/s10880-019-09606-6

Okado, Y., Rowley, C., Schepers, S. A., Long, A. M., & Phipps, S. (2018). Profiles of adjustment in pediatric cancer survivors and their prediction by earlier psychosocial factors. *Journal of Pediatric Psychology*, *43*(9), 1047–1058. https://doi.org/10.1093/jpepsy/jsy037

Palgi, Y., Shrira, A., Haber, Y., Wolf, J. J., Goldray, O., Shacham-Shmueli, E., & Ben-Ezra, M. (2011). Comorbidity of posttraumatic stress symptoms and depressive symptoms among gastric cancer patients. *European Journal of Oncology Nursing*, *15*(5), 454–458. https://doi.org/10.1016/j.ejon.2010.11.011

Palmer, S. C., Kagee, A., Coyne, J. C., & DeMichele, A. (2004). Experience of trauma, distress, and posttraumatic stress disorder among breast cancer patients. *Psychosomatic Medicine*, *66*(2), 258–264. https://doi.org/10.1097/01.psy.0000116755.71033.10

Pelcovitz, D. (1992). Disorders of extreme stress and PTSD in cancer survivors. *Proceedings of Annual Meeting of International Society for Traumatic Stress Studies, Los Angeles, November, 1992.* https://ci.nii.ac.jp/naid/10012654932/en/

Petersen, S., Bull, C., Propst, O., Dettinger, S., & Detwiler, L. (2005). Narrative therapy to pre vent illness-related stress disorder. *Journal of Counseling and Development*, *83*(1), 41–47. https://doi.org/https://doi.org/10.1002/j.1556-6678.2005.tb00578.x

Phipps, S. (2007). Adaptive style in children with cancer: implications for a positive psychology approach. *Journal of Pediatric Psychology*, *32*(9), 1055–1066. https://doi.org/10.1093/jpepsy/jsm060

Phipps, S., Larson, S., Long, A., & Rai, S. N. (2006). Adaptive style and symptoms of post-traumatic stress in children with cancer and their parents. *Journal of Pediatric Psychology*, *31*(3), 298–309. https://doi.org/10.1093/jpepsy/jsj033

Pot-Mees, C. C., & Zeitlin, H. (1987). Psychosocial consequences of bone marrow transplantation in children. *Journal of Psychosocial Oncology*, *5*(2), 73–81. https://doi.org/10.1300/J077v05n02_07

Roberts, A. K. P. (2018). The effects of the EMDR group traumatic episode protocol with cancer survivors. *Journal of EMDR Practice and Research*, *12*(3), 105–117. https://doi.org/10.1891/1933-3196.12.3.105

Rosebrock, L. E., Arditte Hall, K. A., Rando, A., Pineles, S. L., & Liverant, G. I. (2019). Rumination and its relationship with thought suppression in unipolar depression and co-morbid PTSD. *Cognitive Therapy and Research*, *43*(1), 226–235.

Salsman, J. M., Segerstrom, S. C., Brechting, E. H., Carlson, C. R., & Andrykowski, M. A. (2009). Posttraumatic growth and PTSD symptomatology among colorectal cancer survivors: A 3-month longitudinal examination of cognitive processing. *Psycho-Oncology*, *18*(1), 30–41. https://doi.org/10.1002/pon.1367

Santos, F. R. M., Kozasa, E. H., de Lourdes L. F. Chauffaille, M., Colleoni, G. W., & Leite, J. R. (2006). Psychosocial adaptation and quality of life among Brazilian patients with different hematological malignancies. *Journal of Psychosomatic Research*, *60*(5), 505–511. https://doi.org/10.1016/j.jpsychores.2005.08.017

Schroevers, M. J., Helgeson, V. S., Sanderman, R., & Ranchor, A. V. (2010). Type of social support matters for prediction of posttraumatic growth among cancer survivors. *Psycho-Oncology*, *19*(1), 46–53. https://doi.org/10.1002/pon.1501

Schwartz, L., & Drotar, D. (2006). Posttraumatic stress and related impairment in survivors of childhood cancer in early adulthood compared to healthy peers. *Journal of Pediatric Psychology*, *31*(4), 356–366. https://doi.org/10.1093/jpepsy/jsj018

Schwartz, L. A., Kazak, A. E., Derosa, B. W., Hocking, M. C., Hobbie, W. L., & Ginsberg, J. P. (2012). The role of beliefs in the relationship between health problems and posttraumatic stress in adolescent and young adult cancer survivors. *Journal of Clinical Psychology in Medical Settings*, *19*(2), 138–146. https://doi.org/10.1007/s10880-011-9264-1

Shand, L. K., Brooker, J. E., Burney, S., Fletcher, J., & Ricciardelli, L. A. (2015). Symptoms of posttraumatic stress in Australian women with ovarian cancer. *Psycho-Oncology*, *24*(2), 190–196. https://doi.org/10.1002/pon.3627

Shelby, R. A., Golden-Kreutz, D. M., & Andersen, B. L. (2005). Mismatch of posttraumatic stress disorder (PTSD) symptoms and DSM-IV symptom clusters in a cancer sample: Exploratory factor analysis of the PTSD Checklist—Civilian Version. *Journal of Trauma Stress*, *18*(4), 347–357. https://doi.org/10.1002/jts.20033

Shelby, R. A., Golden-Kreutz, D. M., & Andersen, B. L. (2008). PTSD diagnoses, subsyndromal symptoms, and comorbidities contribute to impairments for breast cancer survivors. *Journal of Trauma Stress*, *21*(2), 165–172. https://doi.org/10.1002/jts.20316

Smith, S. K., Kuhn, E., O'Donnell, J., Koontz, B. F., Nelson, N., Molloy, K., Chang, J., & Hoffman, J. (2018). Cancer distress coach: Pilot study of a mobile app for managing posttraumatic stress. *Psycho-Oncology*, *27*(1), 350–353. https://doi.org/10.1002/pon.4363

Spencer, R. J., Ray, A., Pirl, W. F., & Prigerson, H. G. (2012). Clinical correlates of suicidal thoughts in patients with advanced cancer. *American Journal of Geriatric Psychiatry*, *20*(4), 327–336. http://easyaccess.lib.cuhk.edu.hk/login?url = http://ovidsp.ovid.com/ovidweb.cgi?T = JS&CSC = Y&NEWS = N&PAGE = fulltext&D = psyc9&AN = 2012-07694-007

Stuber, M. L., Kazak, A. E., Meeske, K., & Barakat, L. (1998). Is posttraumatic stress a viable model for understanding responses to childhood cancer? *Child and Adolescent Psychiatric Clinics of North America*, *7*(1), 169–182.

Stuber, M. L., Meeske, K. A., Leisenring, W., Stratton, K., Zeltzer, L. K., Dawson, K., Kazak, A. E., Zebrack, B., Mertens, A. C., Robison, L. L., & Krull, K. R. (2011). Defining medical posttraumatic stress among young adult survivors in the Childhood Cancer Survivor Study. *General Hospital Psychiatry*, *33*, 347–353. https://doi.org/10.1016/j.genhosppsych.2011.03.015

Stuber, M. L., Nader, K., Yasuda, P., Pynoos, R. S., & Cohen, S. (1991). Stress responses after pediatric bone marrow transplantation: Preliminary results of a prospective longitudinal study. *Journal of the American Academy of Child and Adolescent Psychiatry*, *30*(6), 952–957. https://doi.org/10.1097/00004583-199111000-00013

Swartzman, S., Booth, J. N., Munro, A., & Sani, F. (2017). Posttraumatic stress disorder after cancer diagnosis in adults: A meta-analysis. *Depression and Anxiety*, *34*(4), 327–339. https://doi.org/10.1002/da.22542

Tjemsland, L., Søreide, J. A., & Malt, U. F. (1996). Traumatic distress symptoms in early breast cancer. II: Outcome six weeks post surgery. *Psycho-Oncology*, *5*(4), 295–303. https://doi.org/https://doi.org/10.1002/(SICI)1099-1611(199612)5:4<295::AID-PON234>3.0.CO;2-9

Turner-Sack, A. M., Menna, R., Setchell, S. R., Maan, C., & Cataudella, D. (2012). Posttraumatic growth, coping strategies, and psychological distress in adolescent survivors of cancer. *Journal of Pediatric Oncology Nursing*, *29*(2), 70–79. https://doi.org/10.1177/1043454212439472

Urbaniec, O. A., Collins, K., Denson, L. A., & Whitford, H. S. (2011). Gynecological cancer survivors: Assessment of psychological distress and unmet supportive care needs. *Journal of Psychosocial Oncology*, *29*(5), 534–551. https://doi.org/10.1080/07347332.2011.599829

Vallerand, R., Blanchard, C., Mageau, G., Koestner, R., Ratelle, C., Léonard, M., Gagné, M., & Marsolais, J. (2003). Les passions de l'ame: on obsessive and harmonious passion. *Journal of Personality and Social Psychology*, *85*, 756–767. https://doi.org/10.1037/0022-3514.85.4.756

Vazquez, D., Rosenberg, S., Gelber, S., Ruddy, K. J., Morgan, E., Recklitis, C., Come, S., Schapira, L., & Partridge, A. H. (2020). Posttraumatic stress in breast cancer survivors diagnosed at a young age. *Psycho-Oncology*, *29*(8), 1312–1320. https://doi.org/https://doi.org/10.1002/pon.5438

Vuotto, S. C., Ojha, R. P., Li, C., Kimberg, C., Klosky, J. L., Krull, K. R., Srivastava, D. K., Robison, L. L., Hudson, M. M., & Brinkman, T. M. (2018). The role of body image dissatisfaction in the association between treatment-related scarring or disfigurement and psychological distress in adult survivors of childhood cancer. *Psycho-Oncology*, *27*(1), 216–222. https://doi.org/10.1002/pon.4439

Whealin, J., Seibert-Hatalsky, L., Howell, J., & Tsai, J. (2015). E-mental health preferences of Veterans with and without probable posttraumatic stress disorder. *Journal of Rehabilitation Research and Development*, *52*, 725–738. https://doi.org/10.1682/JRRD.2014.04.0113

Widows, M. R., Jacobsen, P. B., & Fields, K. K. (2000). Relation of psychological vulnerability factors to posttraumatic stress disorder symptomatology in bone marrow transplant recipients. *Psychosomatic Medicine*, *62*(6), 873–882. https://doi.org/10.1097/00006842-200011000-00018

Wiener, L., Battles, H., Bernstein, D., Long, L., Derdak, J., Mackall, C. L., & Mansky, P. J. (2006). Persistent psychological distress in long-term survivors of pediatric sarcoma: the experience at a single institution. *Psycho-Oncology*, *15*(10), 898–910. https://doi.org/10.1002/pon.1024

Wong, M., Looney, E., Michaels, J., Palesh, O., & Koopman, C. (2006). A preliminary study of peritraumatic dissociation, social support, and coping in relation to posttraumatic stress symptoms for a parent's cancer. *Psycho-Oncology*, *15*(12), 1093–1098. https://doi.org/10.1002/pon.1041

Wu, M. S., Li, B., Zhu, L., & Zhou, C. (2019). Culture change and affectionate communication in China and the United States: Evidence from Google digitized books 1960–2008. *Frontiers in Psychology, 10*(1110). https://doi.org/10.3389/fpsyg.2019.01110

Yang, X., Wu, X., Gao, M., Wang, W., Quan, L., & Zhou, X. (2020). Heterogeneous patterns of posttraumatic stress symptoms and depression in cancer patients. *Journal of Affective Disorders, 273,* 203–209.

Yu, S.-H., Chen, S.-H., & Chang, K.-J. (2008). Rumination predicting depression and PTSD symptoms in postoperative breast cancer patients. [Chinese.] *Chinese Journal of Psychology, 50*(3), 289–302.

Zhou, X., Gao, M., Wang, W., & Wu, X. (2019). Patterns of posttraumatic stress disorder symptoms among cancer patients: A latent profile analysis. *Journal of Psychosomatic Research, 125,* 109788. https://doi.org/10.1016/j.jpsychores.2019.109788

4

Posttraumatic stress disorder and cancer: Secondary victims

Cancer-related posttraumatic stress disorder (PTSD) can affect not only the patients themselves, but also their family members, each of whom has their own psychological needs (Goldwin et al., 2014). These individuals may be referred to as secondary victims, i.e. significant caregivers (e.g. parents, spouses, or children) of primary victims (i.e. individuals who have had maximum exposure to a traumatic event—in this context, the effects of cancer, whether the diagnostic or treatment aspect) (Figley & Kleber, 1995). Examining the interconnectedness or ripple effect of cancer-related PTSD is the focus of this chapter.

Why is it appropriate to examine the psychological distress of parents, children, siblings and partners of cancer survivors from a trauma perspective? According to DSM-IV (American Psychiatric Association, 1994), they have witnessed their loved ones experiencing an event (cancer) that actually threatened their physical integrity, which in turn caused their intense fear, helplessness, and horror. Such an event is not limited to cancer, but also to other frightening or potentially life-threatening diseases such as type 1 diabetes, meningococcal disease and others.

Several reviews have highlighted the relevance of a trauma framework for understanding the specific cancer experiences of secondary victims. After examining samples of children with cancer, adult cancer survivors, and parents of paediatric survivors, an earlier review concluded that cancer is a precipitating traumatic stressor (Smith et al., 1999). The diagnostic procedures and treatments can be lengthy and aversive and their traumatic impact can extend beyond the survivor to the whole family (Bruce, 2006). Another review has summarised the outcomes of cancer-related PTSD in partners (28.6%), adult children (from 13.3% to 19.4%), children siblings (22.4%), and adult siblings (2.2%) of cancer survivors (Cordova et al., 2017), despite controversial issues regarding the reliability of PTSD diagnoses in children, children's cancer

Posttraumatic Stress in Physical Illness. Man Cheung Chung, Oxford University Press. © Oxford University Press 2024.
DOI: 10.1093/oso/9780198727323.003.0004

as a distinct traumatic stressor due to its multifaceted nature, confounding factors from the direct effects of cancer, treatment, and physical late effects that influence trauma symptoms (Bruce, 2006). A recent study focusing on Turkish families facing the psychosocial impact of paediatric cancer has confirmed a whole range of psychological symptoms, namely depression, anxiety, hopelessness, posttraumatic stress, and poor quality of life among these families (Ay & Akyar, 2020). Predictors identified also include gender, previous stressful life events, perceived trauma related to the severity of the cancer and treatment, family conflict, lack of social support and emotion-focused coping, which are consistent with risk factors documented in the general trauma literature, which has strengthened the case for considering this cancer experience in the context of PTSD (Bruce, 2006).

The impact of children's cancer on parents

Children with high-risk disease tend to report the most severe symptoms (Landolt et al., 2003). Compared to physically abused adolescents, a greater proportion of adolescents with a history of cancer met criteria for lifetime PTSD (35% vs 7%). Similarly, 17% of adolescents with cancer met criteria for current PTSD compared to 11% of abused adolescents (Pelcovitz et al., 1998). PTSD is related to patients' perceived intensity of treatment, social support, and manifest anxiety (Ozawa, 2005).

At the same time, families whose loved ones have paediatric cancer also struggle with issues of acceptance and the burden of care. They rely on social support and information (Ay & Akyar, 2020). Having a child with cancer may increase the risk of parents or other family members experiencing distressing intrusive memories, hyperarousal, or avoidance symptoms (Fuemmeler et al., 2005; Kazak, Alderfer, Rourke, et al., 2004; Taïeb et al., 2003). The symptoms of re-experiencing are particularly pronounced. In 99% of cases, at least one family member suffers from this difficulty (Pelcovitz et al., 1998). Research shows that in about 20% of families where a child has survived cancer, at least one parent has current PTSD (Kazak, Alderfer, Rourke, et al., 2004). Overall, parents of children with cancer reported significantly higher levels of posttraumatic stress symptoms (PTSS) than their peers (Barakat et al., 1997). Some parents may have developed acute stress symptoms initially (e.g. one week after the child's diagnosis) that emerge over time as PTSD symptoms. This is the case for at least half of the sample in one study (Fuemmeler et al., 2005).

The traumatic effect of children with cancer is transmissible to their parents without cancer through emotional contagion (Miller et al., 1988) or the proximity effect (Verbosky & Ryan, 1988). This is possible because parents directly experience their children's suffering and are exposed to their children's PTSS. These effects would only be enhanced by the intimate, empathetic or compassionate relationship between them. Empathy would lead parents to want to understand what their children are experiencing and to identify with them and their suffering. As a result, parents might eventually experience the same traumatic reactions as their children, characterised by feelings of powerlessness, shattered assumptions of invulnerability and control, flashbacks, sleep disturbances, depression, and other symptoms. In addition, they might become exhausted (energy depletion) by the constant support of their children, i.e. parents might cope well at first but gradually develop PTSD symptoms later.

Children and their parents may experience PTSD symptoms of varying severity following a diagnosis of malignant disease, including cancer (Landolt et al., 2003). While children reported PTSD symptoms in the mild range, a proportion of parents (16% of fathers and 23.9% of mothers) met the full DSM-IV criteria for current PTSD (Landolt et al., 2003). Children and their caregivers also differ in the way they experience psychological distress symptoms over time. During the first year of treatment for paediatric cancer, children with cancer were by and large well adjusted, although they had higher levels of internalising symptoms compared to standardised samples at the time of diagnosis. On average, the children's symptoms decreased over time. Caregivers, on the other hand, were less well adjusted, with a high proportion reporting depression and anxiety symptoms over time, although the severity of their symptoms also decreased over time. This study concluded that most children adjusted well in the first year of treatment, while many caregivers continued to suffer from psychological distress symptoms (Katz et al., 2018). Indeed, it has been documented that parents of children with cancer may continue to experience PTSD symptoms for many years after their child has successfully completed treatment (Norberg, 2010; Taïeb et al., 2003).

Prevalence rates for cancer-related PTSD are estimated at 2–20% among survivors and 10–30% among parents, even many years after cancer treatment is completed (Taïeb et al., 2003). Focusing on the parents, a review study found that prevalence rates of acute stress disorder ranged from 12% to 63% and PTSD from 8% to 68% (Woolf et al., 2016). Specifically among parents of children with paediatric leukaemia (Kazak et al., 1997; Stuber et al., 1996), PTSD prevalence rates of 12.5% among survivors, between 13.7% and 39.7% among mothers and 33.3% among fathers have been found (Kazak, Alderfer, Rourke, et al., 2004; Stuber et al., 1996). Higher rates were also found among children with cancer, their mothers, and fathers, at 80%, 98%, and 93% respectively (Ozawa, 2005). This is consistent with the claim that parents are more symptomatic overall than cancer survivors, while their rates of PTSD or degree of PTSS do not necessarily differ substantially (Pelcovitz et al., 1998).

It is worth noting, however, that these prevalence rates may not tell the whole story. In one study, different groups of caregivers were found to meet different diagnostic criteria. Some (1) did not even meet the screening criteria for DSM-IV-TR (text revision, 2000) or DSM-5 (American Psychiatric Association, 2013); some (2) only met the criteria of DSM-IV-TR; and some (3) met the criteria of DSM-IV-TR and DSM-5. Group 2 had less PTSS overall than group 3, but more than group 1. In other words, there may be a 'gap group' that may have elevated PTSS but did not meet the DSM-5 screening criteria (Sharkey et al., 2018).

PTSD symptoms of parents correlate with those of their children (Barakat et al., 1997), although this association is not always consistent (Taïeb et al., 2003) and one study found no such association (Landolt et al., 2003). However, a recent study found that after controlling for covariates, depressive symptoms, perceived stress, and PTSD of Hispanic parents were positively associated with childhood cancer survivors' depression. Increased depressive symptoms and distress in parents were associated with increased depressive symptoms in childhood cancer survivors. Parental depression was associated with decreased quality of life in childhood cancer survivors. Increased perceived parental stress correlated with decreased quality of life in survivors and was associated with increased depression only in Hispanic families. It was concluded that parental mental health issues may have some negative impact on the level of depression among childhood cancer survivors or vice versa. Hispanic parents appeared to have more distress than non-Hispanic parents, suggesting that there may be ethnic differences in these psychological responses (Slaughter et al., 2020).

One might wonder whether parents' reports of their children's distress might be confounded by parents' PTSD distress. One study showed that in the cancer group, children's and parents' reports of children's PTSD symptoms were significantly correlated, with no mean differences between these two samples. By contrast, in the control group, parents reported significantly lower levels of PTSD symptoms than the children. In addition, increased parental PTSD symptomatology was associated with better concordance in the cancer group, but not in the control group. In other words, parents of children with cancer were accurate in reporting their children's distress, even with high levels of personal distress (Clawson et al., 2013).

When focusing specifically on parents of children with cancer, there appear to be differences in the way parents display PTSD symptoms. Five patterns of presenting PTSD symptoms were identified. Some parents exhibited minimal PTSD symptoms by showing below-average scores on symptoms. Some mothers, on the other hand, had higher scores than the group with minimal PTSD symptoms. Some parents had low scores on PTSD symptoms but showed high levels of cognitive and emotional disengagement. Some fathers had PTSD scores in the severe reaction range. Finally, some mothers had PTSD scores in the severe response range, while fathers had scores in the moderate response range (Alderfer et al., 2005). These patterns show that cancer-related PTSD in parents cannot be ignored and that there are individual differences in its expression. Examining these differences could provide useful information for designing family-based interventions or promoting resilience in parents of children with cancer in the future.

Viewed longitudinally, parents may maintain stable traumatic responses such as re-experiencing, avoidance, dysphoria, and hyperarousal symptoms over a 4-month period (Cernvall et al., 2011). In addition to PTSD symptoms, long-lasting (e.g. 6 months after diagnosis) symptoms such as sleep disturbances, daytime fatigue, anxiety, depression, and social isolation also occur. These long-term effects may have resulted from enduring the intense nature of PTSD symptoms (Barakat et al., 1997; Kazak, Alderfer, Rourke, et al., 2004; Ozawa, 2005), the emotional impact of the cancer diagnosis, and the intensive and prolonged treatment and aftercare (Klassen et al., 2012). Regarding the impact of the children's treatment on the parents, it is worth noting that PTSD has been associated with the timing of the children's treatment, the preparation period before bone marrow transplantation, and the failure to undergo cranial irradiation (Butler et al., 1996). Case studies of children who received a bone marrow transplant showed that parental responsiveness remained stable over time (i.e. 1 week before transplant and over 24 months after transplant). Lower parental responsiveness was associated with fewer PTSD symptoms in the children. Higher parental responsiveness was associated with more symptoms (Lee et al., 1994).

In contrast to the above studies, a longitudinal study examining family caregivers of advanced cancer patients with a follow-up period of 9 months showed that prevalence rates of PTSD and anxiety symptoms decreased over time (PTSD: 19.5% at baseline vs 12.5% at follow-up; anxiety: 32.1% at baseline vs 13% at follow-up) with varying effect sizes (small to moderate for PTSD, $d = 0.28$; moderate for anxiety, $d = 0.49$). However, depression and alcoholism remained stable over time (Rumpold et al., 2017).

The trajectory of PTSD symptoms seems to differ depending on whether the parents are bereaved parents or not. In parents of survivors of childhood cancer, a longitudinal study showed a consistent decline in PTSD symptoms in the first months after diagnosis; thereafter, the decline subsided, and from 3 months after the end of treatment, there was only a minimal decline. Five years after the end of treatment, 19% of mothers and 8% of fathers of survivors met criteria for partial PTSD. However, among bereaved parents, 20% of mothers and 35% of fathers met the same criteria 5 years after the child's death. From 3 months after the end of treatment, the level of PTSD symptoms remained stable. Bereaved parents are at particular risk for PTSD (Ljungman et al., 2015).

One study examined the association between cognitive impairment in advanced cancer patients who subsequently lost their lives and psychiatric disorders in these caregivers. It found that 12.9% of patients had mild cognitive impairment before death, which was correlated with caregiver depression. Unexpectedly, no correlation was found between patients' cognitive impairment and caregivers' generalised anxiety disorder, PTSD, panic disorder, or grief after patients' deaths. It appeared that the patients' cognitive impairment may have exacerbated the severity of the caregivers' depression during their lifetime. But this depression seemed to resolve itself after death (Meyer et al., 2013). These findings were also confirmed in a later study, which showed no significant association between patient death and caregiver psychological distress at follow-up. Rather, promoting hope and adaptive coping strategies shortly after diagnosis could help patients cushion the impact of psychiatric comorbid symptoms (Rumpold et al., 2017).

While the above has confirmed the impact of PTSD in parents of children with cancer, some studies have cast doubt on this association. One study found that rates of current (1.6%) and lifetime (7.3%) PTSD in parents of children with cancer were low and no different from those of parents of healthy children. The extent of PTSD symptoms was also not significantly different from that of the comparison parents. Parents of children diagnosed ≥5 years ago reported significantly lower PTSD symptoms than the comparison parents. One interpretation of these findings is that parents of children with cancer appeared to be resilient individuals (Phipps et al., 2015). Similarly, among parents of long-term survivors of childhood acute lymphoblastic leukaemia, only 3.9% of parents reported significant PTSD symptoms and 7.1% and 3.1% of parents reported clinically significant levels of anxiety and depression, respectively. In other words, parents of long-term survivors do not necessarily have high levels of emotional distress compared to the general population (Malpert et al., 2015).

Furthermore, parents of children with cancer did not show signs of increased PTSD symptomatology compared to parents of healthy children. Also, only parents of children who had relapsed had an increased risk of developing PTSS (Jurbergs et al., 2009). Most parents (71.5%) were indeed resilient and the remaining parents (28.5%) had increased PTSD (Sharp et al., 2021). Similarly, over a 5-year period, a large majority of children (83.5%) were resilient, with only mild PTSD symptoms initially and their symptoms decreasing significantly over 5 years, while a small group (16.5%) were classified as having increased PTSD over time. It has been argued that childhood cancer may actually strengthen the link between the parent and child in terms of their psychological functioning, although exposure to other life events for the child may weaken the bond (Okado et al., 2014). Both survivors and parents with resilience traits share some similar characteristics, namely that they tend to have higher socioeconomic status and optimism. The less resilient tend to have experienced more stressful life events and have high levels of negative affect and neuroticism. While some of these individuals are able to cope with difficult life challenges, some are likely to need intervention to recover over time (Sharp et al., 2021).

Risk factors for parents of childhood cancer survivors

Subjective appraisal or perception of the disease

Despite the resilient individuals described above, many studies have identified vulnerability and risk factors for parents at risk. While there appears to be evidence that the impact of a surviving family member is felt by other family members, such as parents, it is not always clear how this occurs (Foran-Tuller et al., 2012). Similar to research based on patients after MI-PTSD, objective medical data does not appear to contribute to PTSD symptoms in parents of childhood cancer survivors (Woolf et al., 2016). For example, time elapsed since cancer diagnosis is not predictive of persistent symptoms (Taïeb et al., 2003). More research is needed to understand the impact of objective medical factors. Regarding socioeconomic factors, primary caregivers, especially those who were not married, reported psychological maladjustment, but their financial burden did not correlate with the adjustment of their children with cancer (Galtieri et al., 2022).

On the other hand, parents' subjective perceptions of the disease appeared to play a large role in affecting their own mental health. For example, greater perceived uncertainty about the disease was associated with increased incidence of both PTSS and general psychological distress for parents (Fuemmeler et al., 2005). A path analysis also found direct and indirect effects of each subscale of illness uncertainty on the PTSS through global psychological distress among parents of children newly diagnosed with cancer. The entire model explained 47.3% of the variance in the PTSS. The ambiguity facet (e.g. the feeling of not knowing whether the child's disease will get better or worse) of illness uncertainty had a significant indirect effect on PTSS through global psychological distress. In other words, feeling unclear about their children's illness could be related to increased global psychological distress, which in turn was associated with PTSS symptoms (Tackett et al., 2016).

However, uncertainty about the illness does not influence parents' psychological distress independently of other factors. In one study, uncertainty about the illness was found to significantly mediate the impact of barriers to care on depressive symptoms in caregivers of children diagnosed with cancer. In other words, obstacles to care for their children with cancer may have increased illness uncertainty, which was then associated with parent distress. Although interventions that address illness uncertainty may help to reduce psychological distress, they also need to take account of difficulty accessing care (Perez et al., 2020).

When children received treatment, more than half of parents (55%) in one study experienced high levels of distress, in part due to the parents' perceived loss of control. This perception predicted PTSD symptoms after treatment was completed. Parents found it difficult to return to daily or pre-illness routines, financial concerns, personal emotions, and sense of identity. Although the extent of loss of control was similar for parents, it predicted more severe PTSD symptoms in mothers after their children completed treatment (Norberg & Boman, 2013). In addition, parents' subjective appraisal or perceived life threat, perceived treatment intensity and social support also played a role in predicting PTSD and other psychological distress (Kazak et al., 1998; Stuber & Shemesh, 2006; Stuber et al., 2003; Taïeb et al., 2003).

Notwithstanding, the importance of the subjective appraisal factors seems to be somewhat lower when taking into account previous life events, family functioning, post-treatment variables (time since end of treatment, child anxiety, medical sequelae) and treatment characteristics (age at diagnosis, radiotherapy, intensity of treatment) as well as trait anxiety. This anxiety emerged as the strongest predictor of PTSD symptoms in both parents (Barakat et al., 1997; Kazak et al., 1998). Similarly, a longitudinal study focusing on parents of children treated for leukaemia examined the association between parental anxiety during treatment for childhood leukaemia and PTSS after completion of treatment. The study found that anxiety during treatment was a significant predictor of later PTSS in mothers but not in fathers. Highly anxious parents are at increased risk for PTSS and may benefit from approaches that reduce anxiety during and after treatment (Best et al., 2001). In other words, personality traits may play a non-negligible role in these parents.

Looking at personality traits, one study examined subjective appraisal in relation to rumination as a trait characterised by a recurrent and repetitive way of thinking (Watkins & Nolen-Hoeksema, 2014). One study showed that parents' perceptions of the symptoms from which their children suffered can increase their distress through increased rumination. Parents' perceptions of their children's pain and nausea indirectly affected parents' PTSD symptoms through rumination. These findings persisted even after controlling for demographic variables. In other words, when parents repeatedly and passively focus on their children's suffering, they increase their own PTSD symptoms (Fisher et al., 2021).

Coping

As mentioned earlier, whereas rumination could be conceptualised as a trait, it has also been argued to be a form of cognitive avoidance strategy (Rosebrock et al., 2019) in which people avoid solving problems or changing circumstances associated with distress without taking concrete action. This preoccupation would only lead to compulsive or excessive rumination, unproductive thoughts, and negative appraisals of situations (Michael et al., 2007). Similarly, trying to avoid the disease or treatment-related distress during and immediately after a child's cancer treatment predicted PTSD symptoms in parents 1 year after their children's cancer treatment ended. For bereaved parents, avoidance during their children's treatment was a much greater risk factor than for non-bereaved parents. In other words, avoidance of reminders of distress related to their children's cancer during and immediately after their children's treatment appears to exacerbate the extent of later PTSD in both parents (Norberg et al., 2011). Confrontation and acceptance, on the other hand, should be encouraged.

Substance use is another form of avoidance coping. Although PTSD symptoms of children with cancer and parents were significantly correlated with each other, only substance misuse as a coping strategy of parents was correlated with PTSD symptoms of children. A mediation analysis showed that parental substance use mediated the impact of parental PTSD on children's PTSD symptoms. In other words, parental PTSD could trigger the increase in parental substance misuse, which then affects the child's PTSD symptoms (Stoppelbein et al., 2013).

Whereas the above research suggests that emotion-focused coping, including avoidance coping, is related to parent distress, this negative effect may not always be consistent. One study examined how parents of child cancer survivors cope with emotion-focused or problem-focused coping. The former involves efforts to reduce the discomfort associated with the stressful situation (in this case, their children's cancer) without changing the situation itself, while the latter involves planned action to change the stressful situation by acting on the environment or on oneself (Lazarus, 1993; Lazarus & Folkman, 1984). Surprisingly, reduced emotion-focused coping was associated with increased incidence of both PTSS and general psychological distress after demographic and illness variables were accounted for (Fuemmeler et al., 2005). This is unexpected, as the correlation between emotion-focused coping and psychological distress (PTSD, poor quality of life, and psychiatric comorbidity) tends to be positive (Amstadter & Vernon, 2008; Chung et al., 2005; Gross & John, 2003; Kashdan et al., 2009; Tull et al., 2007; Tull et al., 2004). In other words, lower emotion-focus should be associated with lower distress. Another reason why this finding is surprising is the assumption that lower emotion-focused coping means stronger problem-focused coping, which is not always the case. Problem-focused coping has been associated with lower caregiver distress, less depression and better adjustment (Teixeira et al., 2018).

Another surprising finding is that repression is associated with positive parent and child outcomes. Repression has been termed an adaptive style because it has been shown to benefit both parents and children with cancer. This style is defined by low levels of anxiety or repression. Children with cancer who are identified as having low levels of anxiety or repressors tend to report lower levels of PTSD than children with high levels of anxiety. Similarly, parents identified as low anxious or repressors also tend to report lower levels of PTSD than parents who are high anxious. They also tend to report lower levels of PTSD in their children (Phipps et al., 2006). The reason as to why this finding may be seem counterintuitive, as suggested at the beginning of this paragraph, is that repression is arguably another emotion-focused coping strategy, as it helps to reduce the discomfort associated with the stressful situation without changing the situation itself (Lazarus, 1993; Lazarus & Folkman, 1984).

Apart from the coping strategies described above, the regulation of anger in children is associated with increased PTSD symptoms and other psychological distress in parents in paediatric oncology. In other words, parents' psychological distress is influenced by witnessing their sick children regulate their distressing emotion of anger. Anger regulation was in turn related to children's behavioural and emotional difficulties (Davis et al., 2010). Helping children to regulate their anger could influence the severity of parental and child problems (Davis et al., 2010). Anger regulation can be an adaptive form of coping for both parents and children.

Family functioning

The implication from what has been said in relation to the impact of children's cancer on parents is that the dyadic relationship between parents and children within a family, or relational PTSD or PTSS, may be important factors in understanding cancer-related PTSD (Bruce, 2006). From the perspective of adolescents with cancer, they tend to view their parents as significantly more caring and protective than healthy adolescents or adolescents with a history of abuse (Pelcovitz et al., 1998). Increased caring by parents led to better adjustment, according to the adolescents. Overprotection, on the other hand, led to poorer adjustment outcomes (Schepers et al., 2019). Children's distress was more strongly related to their perceptions of the above factors than to their health status. These results seem to contradict previous research findings that children with cancer do not perceive parental care or overprotection differently than children without cancer. Previous research suggested that the extent of parental protection did not change whether children were seriously ill or not (Tillery et al., 2014).

Adolescent survivors of childhood cancer with PTSD are five times more likely to come from a poorly functioning family than a well-functioning family. Almost half (47%) of adolescents, a quarter (25%) of mothers, and a third (30%) of fathers were found to have poor family functioning in terms of problem-solving skills and affect. For parents, problems with affect mean that they have difficulty relating to their children at an appropriate level of affective responsiveness or engagement (Alderfer et al., 2009). Adolescents with cancer who had lifelong PTSD also rated their families as significantly more chaotic than adolescents without PTSD; 83% of these adolescents also had mothers with PTSD (Pelcovitz et al., 1998). Parental distress may lead to a relationship frustration and attachment problems and affect the relationship between them and the adolescents, which in turn may affect the adolescents' adjustment (Schepers et al., 2019). It could be suggested that the chaos in the family and the PTSD among adolescents and parents could lead to poor family functioning, which in turn would affect the adolescents' well-being.

Family functioning can also be considered in terms of perceived support and conflict within family relationships, which may influence the level of psychological distress in adolescents and young adults with cancer. Perceived family support was associated with positive affect and posttraumatic growth. On the other hand, perceived conflict within the family correlated with psychological distress and PTSD symptoms. Within other relationships (i.e. friends and medical staff), only support was associated with psychological well-being in these adolescents and young adults with cancer. Conflict did not play a role in these other relationships, but it did in family relationships (Kay et al., 2019). In other words, families where family or parent functioning is poor could benefit from improving the quality of parent–child interactions (Schepers et al., 2019). However, there is a possibility that the reason for poor family functioning is the disruption caused by childhood cancer. Psychotherapeutic treatment aimed at improving parent–child interactions must take this into account (Taïeb et al., 2003).

One study examined the interdependent, dyadic mental health of adolescent and young adult cancer patients and their caregivers. They found that the ways in which adolescent and young adult cancer patients and their caregivers experience distress and the ways in which their perceptions of illness are related to distress differ. Whereas subjective illness severity was related to objective illness severity (i.e. medical indicators) in both patients and caregivers, caregivers reported higher PTSS than patients and higher illness severity than younger patients. Caregivers' subjective illness severity was only associated with their own PTSS. Adolescent and young adult patients' subjective illness severity is the strongest predictor of their own PTSS and is significantly correlated with their caregivers' PTSS. They concluded that the illness perceptions of adolescent and young adult cancer patients and caregivers differ from each other (Juth et al., 2015).

The impact of children's cancer on mothers

To look more closely at the impact of children's cancer on parents, research has focused on the experiences of mothers. One study found that 83% of adolescents with cancer who had lifelong PTSD also had mothers who had PTSD (Pelcovitz et al., 1998); 20% and 27% of these mothers met the diagnostic criteria for current and lifelong PTSD, respectively (Libov et al., 2002), in addition to anxiety and depression (Manne et al., 1998). They showed significantly more PTSD symptoms than mothers of healthy children (Pelcovitz et al., 1996). However, mothers with a PTSD diagnosis did not necessarily fare worse than mothers without a diagnosis in terms of perceptions of the severity of the illness, family and non-family social support, and global psychological distress (Pelcovitz et al., 1996).

While mothers may exhibit severe PTSD symptoms across all symptom groups following their children's cancer diagnosis (Boman et al., 2013), they do exhibit some specific traumatic responses to childhood cancer. Similar to young adult survivors and child survivors, mothers showed PTSD symptoms, especially re-experiencing and avoidance along with intense fear, horror, and helplessness. They also tended to recall cancer-related memories and experience negative feelings when talking about their cancer experience. They were also concerned about current and potential future medical problems, difficulties, and fears associated with memories of cancer. They often talked about cancer with different people and discussed it with family members. They also experienced changes in themselves as a result of cancer, some of which were positive (Kazak et al., 2001). A qualitative study showed that protecting their children, no matter what the cost, was the most important experience that led mothers who had children with cancer to put their lives on hold and lose time with their healthy children. They felt forced to face cancer treatment, but this went against their goal of protecting their children (McEvoy & Creaner, 2021).

Mothers' distress is also reflected in some physiological data. Mothers of children who have survived cancer tend to have increased allostatic load (i.e. cumulative physiological wear and tear resulting from repeated efforts to adapt to stressors over time). Compared to mothers without PTSD symptoms, mothers with PTSD tend to have higher levels of CD4+ and lower levels of CD8+ cells, blunted natural-killer reactivity in response to acute psychological stress (Glover et al., 2005), and high levels of urinary dopamine (decreased dopamine) (Glover et al., 2003; Glover et al., 2006). High cortisol levels have been associated with higher PTSD symptoms, although post-diagnosis PTSD symptoms appeared to decrease over time in mothers who had higher cortisol levels at the time of their child's diagnosis compared to mothers who had lower cortisol levels at the time of diagnosis (Stoppelbein et al., 2010). Mothers of children diagnosed with other chronic diseases such as type I diabetes mellitus may also have higher cortisol levels than mothers of children with cancer. In other words, these mothers may be more susceptible to stress responses reflected in cortisol, a biological marker, than mothers of children with cancer. There were no racial or ethnic differences (African American vs Caucasian mothers) in the risk of PTSS among the mothers (Greening et al., 2017). However, it is difficult to determine whether this distress associated with the above physiological changes is exclusive to mothers, as caring for children with cancer has been associated with increased blood pressure, autonomic nervous system dysregulation, hypothalamic–pituitary axis, immune system changes and poor health-related behaviours (Teixeira et al., 2018).

To examine distress in children and their mothers living through a life-threatening illness (cancer) and a non-life-threatening chronic illness (juvenile rheumatoid arthritis), there are differences in psychological functioning in children in relation to age (Graziano et al., 2016). The 6–12-year-old children with cancer had more significant internalising problems and attention problems compared to healthy children, but not compared to children with juvenile rheumatoid arthritis (JRA). However, younger children with cancer aged 2–5 years showed no significant problems compared to children with JRA and healthy children. Life threat affected psychological functioning in younger children but not in older children (Graziano et al., 2016). In other words, children with cancer of different ages may manifest psychological symptoms differently. Life threat seemed to be a bigger problem for young children. Mothers of children with cancer showed higher levels of PTSD symptoms and parenting stress than mothers of children with JRA and mothers of healthy children. Similar to young children, life threat may be an important factor affecting psychological functioning and emotional adjustment in mothers of children with a chronic illness (Graziano et al., 2016; Libov et al., 2002).

Risk factors for mothers of childhood cancer survivors

The association between socio-demographic variables (single parenthood, family income, education level, race) and psychological distress in paediatric cancer survivors and their mothers is established. The ecological context of childhood cancer cannot be ignored. Some sociodemographic disadvantages affect psychological distress in these individuals (Bemis et al., 2015; Libov et al., 2002). Marital status needs to be unpacked a little. Although single mothers and married/partnered mothers did not differ significantly in terms of perceived PTSD and problem-solving skills following a child's cancer diagnosis, single mothers reported significantly more depressive symptoms. However, this difference did not become significant when maternal education was taken into account. In other words, both types of mothers did not differ too much in terms of negative affectivity and problem-solving skills after their children's cancer diagnosis (Iobst et al., 2009).

Earlier life events seem to play a role in moderating the severity of cancer-related PTSD in mothers. Mothers of children who had cancer, other debilitating illnesses (e.g. type I diabetes) or psychological disorders (e.g. depression) and had experienced stressful life events, particularly recent events or those from the past year, tended to report increased PTSD symptoms (Brown et al., 2003; Libov et al., 2002; Stoppelbein & Greening, 2007). Those meeting diagnostic criteria for PTSD tended to have experienced a greater number of high-severity events prior to diagnosis than those without a diagnosis (Pelcovitz et al., 1996). They also experienced these events significantly more often than the healthy populations (Brown et al., 2003). In particular, previous traumatic life events have been associated with increased hyper-arousal symptoms (Boman et al., 2013).

Notwithstanding, a longitudinal study has shown that stressful life events had limited impact on long-term psychological adjustment in childhood cancer survivors and their mothers. Survivors' and their mothers' appraisal of the intensity and threat of life related to cancer treatment at baseline, over and above stressful life events, predicated general adjustment approximately 18 months later. Moreover, the life events did not mediate the impact of PTSD on overall adjustment. In other words, the subjective experience of their trauma reactions to childhood cancer and its treatment, as opposed to stressful life events, affected the long-term adjustment and adaptation of survivors and mothers (Barakat et al., 2000). The concept of adjustment is complex in that parental adjustment, particularly that of the mother, may also be influenced by parental stress during treatment (Stuber, 1995) and how they perceived their children's quality of life (Kazak & Barakat, 1997).

The dyadic relationship between the mother and the adolescent with cancer is another risk factor. Adolescents' PTSD symptoms two months after cancer diagnosis were associated with their PTSD symptoms one year later. Increased maternal PTSS after their children's diagnosis predicted harsher maternal communication characterised by hostility, inconsistent discipline, and intrusiveness 3 months after diagnosis. There was an indirect effect of maternal PTSS at T1 on adolescent PTSS at T3 (1 year later) through maternal validations (the mother's validation characterised by her ability to validate, empathise, or praise the adolescent's expressions or experiences) at T2 (3 months after diagnosis). In other words, mothers' initial distress could be related to their children's lower validation 3 months after diagnosis, which was then associated with their children's increase in PTSS one year later. The study demonstrated the importance of maternal PTSS, maternal communication, and later adolescent PTSS over the course of childhood cancer treatment (Murphy et al., 2016). Similarly, maternal distress symptoms 2 months after diagnosis were associated with reductions in positive communication, characterised by warmth and positivity, and 3 months later were differentially related to negative communication, characterised by hostility or intrusiveness, withdrawal and inconsistency. Maternal posttraumatic stress and depressive symptoms each predicted the expression of negative affect (Murphy et al., 2018).

Apart from the risk factors, one must not lose sight of the fact that resilience also exists in mothers of children with cancer. They initially reported slightly elevated negative affect and PTSD symptoms, but these steadily improved over time, indicating an ability to adapt to distress (Dolgin et al., 2007). A longitudinal study over a 12-month period also showed that high levels of hardiness provided a buffer for PTSD in mothers of children with cancer, after controlling for the effect of time. These mothers also tended to experience fewer avoidance/numbing symptoms at the time of their children's cancer diagnosis and as it progressed. On the contrary, mothers with low levels of hardiness tended to report more of these symptoms (Stoppelbein et al., 2017).

A comparison between maternal and paternal experiences

The experiences of fathers who have children with cancer seem to be examined far less often than those of mothers. Research seems to suggest that fathers of children with a chronic illness may have high levels of PTSD. For example, PTSD was higher among fathers of children with a chronic illness than among fathers of children who had suffered an unintentional injury (26% at Time 1 and 21% at Time 2 for fathers of children with a chronic illness vs 12% at Time 1 and 6% at Time 2 for fathers of children with unintentional injuries). However, within six months of the child's diagnosis or accident, the severity of PTSS decreased in both groups. Follow-up reactions to PTSS were predicted by the father's initial PTSS severity, the child's medical condition and functional status, and the father's maladaptive coping strategies and neuroticism (Ribi et al., 2007).

Fathers and mothers react differently to their children's cancer (Andrykowski et al., 2003; Manne et al., 1998), with mothers being more affected than fathers. Mothers (23.9%) had higher rates of current PTSD than fathers (16%) (Landolt et al., 2003; Pöder et al., 2008), as well as higher levels of stress (Rodriguez et al., 2012). Mothers' symptoms appeared to be constant over time, while fathers' decreased (Magal-Vardi et al., 2004), although one study showed a linear, descending pattern of PTSD symptoms, with mothers reporting higher levels than fathers (Pöder et al., 2008). Mothers' elevated PTSS symptoms were related to their children's cancer diagnosis and functional status, but surprisingly not to the child with PTSS (Landolt et al., 2003). Both parents also rated the physical effects of the illness as most distressing, while the children rated role-functioning difficulties as most distressing (Rodriguez et al., 2012). The PTSS of both parents was related to each other. This might suggest that a marital relationship could exacerbate each other's distress (Landolt et al., 2003).

Similarly, one study examined distress among parents who had an infant patient or infant sibling of an older child with cancer. Mothers (47.5%) and fathers (37.5%) reported increased cancer-related PTSD symptoms, along with depression symptoms (12.2% for mothers and 12.0% for fathers) and anxiety symptoms (17.1% for mothers and 8.0% for fathers). Compared to parents of infant patients, parents of infant siblings were significantly more likely to report depressive symptoms and showed a trend towards higher rates of PTSD symptoms and anxiety symptoms (Vernon et al., 2017).

As mentioned in the section on the impact of children's cancer on parents, both parents may develop acute stress disorder (ASD) after the child's cancer diagnosis (McCarthy et al., 2012), which develops into PTSD a few months later (Fuemmeler et al., 2005; Pöder et al., 2008). Consistent with the general trend above, more mothers (63%) than fathers (60%) developed ASD, which then developed into PTSD (21% vs 16%) (McCarthy et al., 2012). Being a mother predicted ASD symptoms along with other predictors of psychosocial risk factors, trait anxiety, family functioning, and central nervous system tumour diagnoses. Younger maternal age predicted PTSD symptoms along with ASD symptom severity, trait anxiety at baseline, and child quality of life at follow-up (McCarthy et al., 2012). In other words, screening for ASD could help identify parents who are at risk for ongoing traumatic stress symptoms and who could benefit from preventive, evidence-based psychosocial interventions (McCarthy et al., 2012).

The above discussion focuses mainly on the impact of children's cancer on their parents when they are still alive. Several studies have examined how the loss of children due to cancer can have a long-term impact on the psychological well-being of parents. It was found that, 1–5 years after the loss, grieving parents experienced an increase in persistent grief, depression, PTSD symptoms, and insomnia. Mothers especially showed higher levels of prolonged grief, depression and PTSD than did fathers. Prolonged grief can be maintained by grief rumination, in which parents repeatedly think about the causes and consequences of the loss (Pohlkamp et al., 2019; Sveen et al., 2019).

The effects of a parent's cancer on family members

In addition to studies that examine the effects of a child's cancer on the parents, there are also studies that examine the effects of a parent's cancer on family members. For example, adolescents who have a parent with cancer tend to perceive their own risk of developing cancer as significantly higher than the control group (Harris & Zakowski, 2003), although the adolescents may have exacerbated this perception due to the stress of being in transition (Harris & Zakowski, 2003). There is also a tendency for children to report high levels of depression, although the level of depression appears to be mitigated by mothers' perceived social support from friends and family. That is, when children see that their parents perceive support from friends and family, they tend to show lower levels of depression. This means that the social support perceived by mothers with breast cancer could protect their children's distress (Brown et al., 2007).

As children grow older, the traumatic effects of witnessing, living with, and caring for a parent with cancer may linger. A previous review showed that adult children of cancer patients experienced PTSD, anxiety, and depression symptoms (Mosher & Danoff-Burg, 2005). Among adult children who were still caring for their parents with cancer, those who perceived greater parental dependency showed more distress, higher PTSD symptoms, greater burden of caregiving, and were less satisfied with social support. Social support partially mediated the relationship between psychological morbidity and caregiver burden (Teixeira & Pereira, 2013). Young adults whose parents had cancer in childhood (the young adults' childhood) tended to have high levels of state and trait anxiety. This increased anxiety correlated with lower current family cohesion and low satisfaction with past social support. Anxiety scores were partially moderated by the parents' cancer (Metcalf et al., 2017). These results also mirror similar findings from a previous study suggesting that family cohesion was associated with social support in terms of expressing emotions within the family, which in turn was correlated with lower anxiety (Harris & Zakowski, 2003).

In the study of adults aged 18–38 years who had a parent with cancer when they, the adults, were aged 8–17 years, 17% met diagnostic criteria for PTSD. PTSD symptoms were associated with increased peritraumatic dissociation, denial and behavioural disengagement, and lower levels of satisfied social support. Women appeared to have more severe PTSD symptoms than men. One implication from these findings is that the effects of PTSD can extend into adulthood. As children enter adulthood, they may still use a range of maladaptive avoidance strategies to cope with the effects of childhood trauma. Attention needs to be paid to this group of people whose psychological needs can be so easily neglected (Wong et al., 2006).

One might assume that children react differently to the cancer of their living parents than children who are confronted with the death of their parents. This is because children who felt content with their parents' cancer tended to show fewer PTSD symptoms than children who witnessed their parents' death. However, both groups showed similar levels of anxiety and depression. Expressive coping correlated with low levels of PTSD symptoms, anxiety, and depression in both groups. For the bereaved group, positive reinforcement and supportive communication with the surviving caregiver could be buffers against PTSD symptoms after the death of the parent (Howell et al., 2016).

When considering cancer-related PTSD from the perspective of parents, particularly mothers who have cancer, they tended to perceive more PTSD symptoms and internalised stress in their children than mothers without cancer. However, there were no significant differences in the mothers' perception of externalising symptoms in their children. In other words, maternal perceptions of children's distress varied depending on the type of symptoms in the children (Foran-Tuller et al., 2012). Research has focused specifically on female first-degree relatives of breast cancer patients, many of whom were daughters (Mosher & Danoff-Burg, 2005). Looking specifically at the relationship between daughter and mother, it appears that mothers diagnosed with cancer-related PTSD are more likely to have daughters who also suffer from PTSD symptoms (Boyer et al., 2002). In addition, mothers with high levels of cancer-related PTSD tend to have daughters who perform excessive breast self-examination, as opposed to the recommended amount. However, it may also be that daughters do not examine themselves enough. That being said, the frequency with which daughters underwent mammography was related to their own cancer-related PTSD, but not to their mothers' perceived risk of PTSD. In other words, the mother's experience may have an impact on the daughters' specific cancer-related health behaviours. Whereas the mother's cancer-related PTSD affected the daughters' propensity to self-care, i.e. to examine their own breasts, the fear of their own cancer-related PTSD motivated them to seek professional examination (Boyer & Cantor, 2005). The aforementioned health behaviour assumes that the daughter accepts and faces the likelihood of cancer. This is at odds with another study that provides some evidence of avoidance strategies. Daughters with PTSD who had a parent with cancer as a child were found to have a greater use of denial and behavioural denial (Wong et al., 2006).

The implication from the above is that knowledge of cancer in the family could have an impact on cancer-related PTSD (Cukor, 2003) and subclinical PTSD (Hamann et al., 2005; Lindberg & Wellisch, 2004) in other female family members who have not yet developed cancer. Some women who had an increased familial risk of breast cancer showed traumatic reactions similar to those of cancer patients. Four per cent reported symptoms that met criteria for a probable PTSD diagnosis, and another 7% of participants reported symptoms consistent with a potentially subclinical level of PTSD (Lindberg & Wellisch, 2004).

Some studies have examined the impact of a parent's cancer on family members in terms of family functioning. Among adult children of a parent with cancer, predictive factors for PTSD symptoms were an imbalanced family life, where family members, for example, spend too much time together or feel pressured to spend most of their free time together, and a chaotic family life, where family members, for example, never seem to be able to organise themselves in their family without knowing who is the head of the family. In addition, chaotic functioning mediated the relationship between family communication or satisfaction and PTSD symptoms. In other words, chaotic family functioning may indirectly interfere with the relationship between difficulties in positive communication within the marital or family system and feelings of being happy and fulfilled among family members and increased levels of PTSD in adult children of a parent with cancer. Adult children facing a parent's cancer with poorer family balance may need some interventions to improve family life (Teixeira & Pereira, 2016).

The above findings reflect research looking at family functioning in terms of family identification and family constraints in colorectal cancer survivors. Family identification is defined as identification with the family, focusing on a sense of belonging to the whole group and a sense of similarity with family members. Family constraints are defined as people's perception that others in the family are judgemental or avoid conversations about cancer. These two factors were stronger independent predictors of PTSD symptoms than social support. Family identification also affected PTSD symptoms through family constraints. They concluded that experiences within the family are important in predicting PTSD after cancer. In addition, a sense of belonging and similarity to the family may reduce the extent to which cancer survivors experience constraints when talking about cancer, which in turn reduces PTSD (Swartzman et al., 2017).

The effects of cancer on other family members

Patients' PTSD may also affect partners who report PTSD symptoms (Brosseau et al., 2011). The prevalence and predictors of PTSD and subclinical PTSD in people who have lost a loved one to cancer have been reported (Kristensen et al., 2012). One study showed that partners of patients with metastatic/recurrent breast cancer reported PTSD symptoms before the patients' deaths. Before the loss, partners' symptoms correlated with the level of perceived stress and expected loss. After the loss, partners' symptoms were associated with increased levels of pre-loss PTSD, previous family deaths and expected loss (Butler et al., 2005). Negative affect, social support and locus of control beliefs about the loss were associated with PTSD severity in partners (Kristensen et al., 2012). High-quality relationships between couples showed buffering effects (Brosseau et al., 2011).

Cancer may also affect siblings (Ozawa, 2005), as nearly half (49%) of adolescent siblings of adolescent cancer survivors reported mild PTSD symptoms; 32% reported moderate to severe levels. A quarter of siblings believed their sibling would die during treatment; more than half perceived the cancer experience as threatening and difficult, which correlated with PTSD symptoms. Siblings reported higher levels of PTSD symptoms than unaffected adolescents, but they all had similar levels of general anxiety (Alderfer et al., 2003). In another study, 60% of the sample (siblings of children with cancer) reported moderate-to-severe PTSD symptoms; 22% met the full diagnostic criteria for PTSD. Nearly 75% reported feeling upset when thinking about or hearing about the cancer, trying not to think about, talk about, or have feelings about the cancer. Over 60% had hyperarousal symptoms. PTSD symptoms were associated with increased difficulty in coping with everyday life in 75% of the sample and correlated with anxiety and depression (Kaplan et al., 2013).

The siblings of children with cancer had higher levels of internalising and externalising problems, as well as PTSD symptoms, than the control group who had no siblings with cancer (Hosseini et al., 2020). Both siblings and survivors of childhood cancer reported functional impairment and/or clinical distress in addition to PTSD, although survivors were more than four times more likely to have PTSD compared to siblings (Stuber et al., 2010). However, the prevalence rate of PTSD symptoms was not significantly higher in Hodgkin's lymphoma survivors (13%) compared to sibling controls (6.9%). However, 35.2% of survivors met criteria for partial PTSD compared to siblings (17.8%). In addition, 86.5% of survivors with partial PTSD had functional impairments related to PTSD symptoms (Varela et al., 2013).

However, a later study contradicted these findings and found that more than a quarter of young patients and siblings scored above the cut-off on the Impact of Event Scale—revised. There were no significant differences between patients and siblings in terms of PTSD symptom severity. Maladaptive appraisals after diagnosis and age accounted for the unique variance in PTSD scores across the sample. These appraisals reflected the idea that people's lives might change permanently and disruptively after diagnosis. For example, they felt that their lives were destroyed by cancer, that they might never have normal feelings again, and that something bad always happens (D'Urso et al., 2018).

A systematic review concluded that levels of anxiety, depression, and general adjustment were similar in siblings of children with cancer and other comparison groups, although cancer-related PTSS was common. School-age siblings were more likely to have problems with academic performance and absenteeism. Adult siblings tended to engage in risky health behaviours and had worse health outcomes than the comparison group. Low levels of social support, family functioning, and income, shorter time since diagnosis, and non-white race were some of the risk factors for poor sibling adjustment, although the results were not always consistent. It is clear that these siblings need support (Long et al., 2018).

As an aside, while most of the studies mentioned above have focused on parents and other family members such as siblings, there are also studies that include grandmothers and stepmothers, for example, although their proportion is usually much smaller. One longitudinal study looked at the stress experienced by mothers (85.4%), fathers (12.0%), grandmothers (1.7%), and stepmothers (0.9%) during the 12 months of caring for their children with cancer. Generally, the results reflected the findings presented above. Treatment-related stress, general life stress, and appraisal factors (perceived life threat and treatment intensity) were found to be associated with depression, anxiety, and PTSD symptoms and to influence caregivers' adjustment. For example, increased general life stress, treatment-related stress, perceived life threat, and treatment intensity were correlated with high levels of depression, anxiety, or PTSD symptoms over time. In addition, increased stress from general life stressors and treatment-related stressors in a given month were simultaneously associated with increased anxiety and PTSD symptoms. In other words, the psychological adjustment of these caregivers was influenced not only by the amount of stressors experienced in the first year, but also by the fluctuations in these stressors in a given month. The total frequency of general life stress and treatment-related stress most strongly predicted caregiver psychological adjustment (Gurtovenko et al., 2021).

Treatment for family members and the cancer patient

Parents of children with cancer

Since having a child with cancer is associated with an increased risk of PTSD, psychosocial interventions that specifically focus on reducing PTSD in parents of child cancer survivors are warranted (Fuemmeler et al., 2005; Pöder et al., 2008). Several studies have been conducted to examine the effectiveness of certain interventions for parents of children with cancer, including structured writing therapy. It was claimed to help parents of children with cancer cope and to improve PTSD symptoms from baseline to the end of writing therapy. However, the effects on depression were limited (Duncan et al., 2007). On the other hand, one study investigated whether structured writing about receiving a diagnosis and treatment would reduce distress in severely distressed parents of children with cancer. Using a guided disclosure protocol (GDP), parents were first asked to write chronologically about receiving the diagnosis, then explicitly state their feelings at the time of diagnosis and explain the impact of the child's illness on their lives. Finally, they were asked to reflect on their current feelings, future coping skills, and personal growth. Although distress symptoms did not change between the two baseline assessments (parents were assessed for psychological symptoms twice prior to the GDP intervention, with 1 month between each assessment), there was a significant decrease in PTSS from the first baseline to post-writing, but not in depression. This study seemed to suggest that GDP may reduce PTSS in distressed parents of children with cancer (Duncan et al., 2007).

An intervention study examined the effect of a brief problem-solving intervention for parents of children with cancer. It followed parents for 3 months after the intervention and found that there were no significant differences in improving problem-solving skills and reducing symptoms of caregiver stress and PTSD symptoms (Lamanna et al., 2018). In another study, not only was problem-solving skills training provided, but it was also combined with acceptance and commitment therapy in a programme called Take A Breath. This is a parent-focused intervention for parents of children who have received a cancer diagnosis or undergone heart surgery, in which parents were supported in adjusting to their child's diagnosis, treatment and recovery. They found that parents reported significantly fewer PTSD symptoms, less emotional distress from their children's life-threatening illness, and improved psychological flexibility and mindfulness even 6 months later (Burke et al., 2014).

The effectiveness of an Internet-based guided self-help intervention for parents of children undergoing cancer treatment was also studied. The intervention consisted of a 10-week guided self-help programme via the Internet, based on the principles of cognitive behavioural therapy. This is a psychoeducational programme that teaches strategies for coping with distress through relaxation, managing distorted thoughts and distressing feelings, behavioural experiments, problem-solving skills, structured writing therapy, values and goal setting, general self-care, and maintaining behaviour change. For those who received the treatment, PTSD symptoms, depression, and anxiety decreased over time (Cernvall et al., 2015).

Surviving Cancer Competently Intervention Programme—Newly Diagnosed is an intervention programme also based on cognitive behavioural principles combined with family therapy approaches to reduce anxiety and improve family functioning. It has been used to reduce anxiety and PTSD in caregivers of children diagnosed with cancer and to reduce intrusive thoughts in fathers and arousal among adolescent survivors (Kazak, Alderfer, Streisand, et al., 2004; Kazak et al., 2005; Kazak et al., 1999). A brief existential intervention focused on improving family functioning helps cancer patients and their families to reflect on issues of sharing personal values and philosophies, self-reflection, and growth, and to improve family cohesion and communication (Garlan et al., 2010). In addition to these interventions, providing siblings with sufficient information about the illness, treatment and the patient's condition is indeed therapeutic, reduces anxiety, and improves their ability to respond to a supportive environment (Ozawa, 2005).

Siblings of children with cancer

In supporting siblings of children with cancer, summer camps provide opportunities to address emotional issues, improve peer interaction and increase siblings' self-esteem. Camp work has also reduced PTSD symptoms and anxiety and improved the quality of life and self-esteem of cancer patients (Packman et al., 2004; Prchal & Landolt, 2009). The sibling intervention improved siblings' psychological well-being, medical knowledge, and the amount of social support they received. However, in the early phase after diagnosis, the intervention had no effect on PTSD symptoms and anxiety (Prchal et al., 2012).

A systematic review looking at the effects of psychological treatment for family members of children with cancer concluded that psychological interventions showed positive and significant differences in anxiety, problem-solving skills and, to a lesser extent, PTSS when comparing mean pre-test–post-test effects between treatment and control groups, with adjusted effect sizes (*d*) ranging from 0.22 to 0.38. However, no significant differences were found for mood, acute stress, coping skills and social support, with effect sizes ranging from –0.01 to 0.24. In other words, these treatments did not have an overall positive impact on reducing all stressors. Rather, the positive effects seemed to vary depending on the type of outcome. In addition, the study concluded that interventions with a behavioural framework appeared to be more effective. In addition, the most effective interventions appeared to be those that were of long duration, low intensity, and implemented to family members with young children who were receiving medical treatment. Overall, however, the interventions appeared to provide short-term rather than long-term benefits (Sánchez-Egea et al., 2019).

Patients and partners

A 3-month follow-up study was conducted to assess the effectiveness of mindfulness-based stress reduction plus usual care (usual care (CAU) + MBSR) for patients with lung cancer and their partners. Patients who received the CAU + MBSR reported significantly less psychological distress after the intervention and at follow-up than those who received the CAU treatment alone. Those who had more distress at baseline benefited the most from MBSR. In addition, quality of life, mindfulness skills, self-compassion, and rumination improved more after CAU + MBSR than after CAU. PTSD symptoms also improved slightly in these patients. However, no differences were found between the groups in the patients' partners. It seems that MBSR is effective in reducing psychological distress in lung cancer patients and not in their partners. This could be due to the fact that they were more concerned about their patients' well-being than their own (Schellekens et al., 2017).

A study that focused on women diagnosed with breast or gynaecological cancer and their partners examined the effectiveness of the Side by Side intervention, a cognitive behavioural approach that teaches partners individual skills and relationship skills as they grapple with issues related to the woman's breast and gynaecological cancer. In addition, this intervention was compared to the Couples Control Programme, in which couples received written educational materials about breast or gynaecological cancer. The therapists mainly listened to the women's concerns and did not teach couples dyadic skills. However, for highly distressed women or partners, the therapists were allowed to make suggestions for coping with individual distress, such as relaxation. They found that the women who participated in the Side by Side intervention showed greater reductions in fear of progression, less avoidance behaviour in dealing with the cancer, more posttraumatic growth, and better relationship skills than the Couples Control Programme. However, all the positive effects of Side by Side disappeared 16 months after diagnosis. In other words, improving couples' dyadic skills during the acute treatment phase of the disease may produce short-term rather than long-term changes in functioning (Heinrichs et al., 2012).

Summary

Cancer-related PTSD can affect both patients and their family members, the secondary victims. While some researchers rightly consider the experience of cancer as a triggering traumatic stressor, others dispute this traumatic framework. Nevertheless, there are studies showing that children's cancer can affect their parents, who show PTSD symptoms after the cancer diagnosis. Prevalence rates for PTSD are controversial. Parents' PTSD symptoms correlate with those of their children, although this relationship is not always consistent. The way parents manifest PTSD symptoms can vary, and the long-term effect is not consistent. On the contrary, some researchers have questioned the traumatic effects of PTSD in parents of children with cancer, arguing that most parents and children with cancer are in fact resilient.

Risk factors for parents of childhood cancer survivors include parents' subjective perceptions of cancer and perceived uncertainty about the disease, which may be associated with increased incidence of PTSS and general psychological distress. Parents' ambiguous feelings about their children's illness, perceived loss of control and subjective appraisal or perceived threat to life, and perceived intensity of treatment are associated with PTSD symptoms and other psychological symptoms. However, it was argued that the importance of the factors for subjective appraisal was lower when previous life events, family functioning, time since treatment ended, child anxiety, medical sequelae and treatment parameters, and trait anxiety were taken into account.

Rumination as a personality trait is another risk factor, as parents' perceptions of their children's symptoms may increase parents' distress from rumination. In terms of coping strategies, avoiding cancer or treatment-related distress during and after their children's cancer treatment may be related to PTSD symptoms in parents, even a year after treatment is completed. Surprisingly, decreasing emotion-focused coping may increase the occurrence of PTSS and general psychological distress, while increasing problem-focused coping may decrease caregiver burden, reduce depression and lead to better adjustment. Repression is considered an adaptive coping style associated with positive outcomes for parents and children. The dyadic relationship between parents and children within a family may also be a factor to consider when exploring cancer-related PTSD.

Some of the literature specifically addresses the maternal burden of childhood cancer, which is characterised by severe PTSD symptoms in addition to anxiety, depression, fear, horror, helplessness, and physiological changes. Risk factors for these mothers include sociodemographic variables, past life events, debilitating illnesses, or psychological disorders. Both fathers and mothers may react differently to their children's cancer, with mothers generally being more affected than fathers. The PTSS of both parents are interconnected.

Research has also looked at the impact of a parent's cancer on family members. The traumatic effects of witnessing, living with, and caring for a parent with cancer can be long-lasting. As children enter adulthood, they may still use maladaptive avoidance strategies to cope with the effects of childhood trauma. Regarding cancer-related PTSD from the parents' perspective, mothers who have had cancer themselves tend to perceive PTSD symptoms and internalised stress in their children and have daughters who also have PTSD symptoms. In addition to children, the literature also talks about the impact of cancer on other family members such as partners and siblings.

Interventions for parents of children with cancer have been explored. These include structured writing therapy, problem-solving training and acceptance and commitment therapy, Internet-based guided self-help for parents of children undergoing cancer treatment, the Surviving Cancer Competently Intervention Programme—Newly Diagnosed and brief existential interventions. There are other interventions aimed at siblings of children with cancer, as well as at patients and partners. These interventions showed varying effectiveness in reducing psychological distress, caregiver burden, fear of disease progression, and improving coping, problem-solving, mindfulness, and relationship skills.

References

Alderfer, M. A., Cnaan, A., Annunziato, R. A., & Kazak, A. E. (2005). Patterns of posttraumatic stress symptoms in parents of childhood cancer survivors. *Journal of Family Psychology, 19*(3), 430–440. https://doi.org/10.1037/0893-3200.19.3.430

Alderfer, M. A., Labay, L. E., & Kazak, A. E. (2003). Brief report: does posttraumatic stress apply to siblings of childhood cancer survivors? *Journal of Pediatric Psychology, 28*(4), 281–286. https://doi.org/10.1093/jpepsy/jsg016

Alderfer, M. A., Navsaria, N., & Kazak, A. E. (2009). Family functioning and posttraumatic stress disorder in adolescent survivors of childhood cancer. *Journal of Family Psychology, 23*(5), 717–725. https://doi.org/10.1037/a0015996

American Psychiatric Association. (1994). *Diagnostic and statistical manual of mental disorders* (4th ed.).

American Psychiatric Association. (2013). *Diagnostic and statistical manual of mental disorders* (5th ed.). https://doi.org/10.1176/appi.books.9780890425596

Amstadter, A. B., & Vernon, L. L. (2008). A preliminary examination of thought suppression, emotion regulation, and coping in a trauma-exposed sample. *Journal of Aggression, Maltreatment & Trauma, 17*, 279–295.

Andrykowski, M., Carpenter, J., & Munn, R. (2003). Psychosocial sequelae of cancer diagnosis and treatment. In L. A. Schein, H. S. Bernard, H. I. Spitz, & P. R. Muskin (Eds.), *Psychosocial treatment for medical conditions: Principles and techniques* (pp. 78–130). Routledge.

Ay, M. A., & Akyar, A. I. (2020). Psychosocial status of Turkish families of pediatric cancer patients. *Journal of Transcultural Nursing, 31*(3), 227–241. https://doi.org/10.1177/10436 59619849481

Barakat, L. P., Kazak, A. E., Gallagher, P. R., Meeske, K., & Stuber, M. (2000). Posttraumatic stress symptoms and stressful life events predict the long-term adjustment of survivors of childhood cancer and their mothers. *Journal of Clinical Psychology in Medical Settings, 7*(4), 189–196. https://doi.org/10.1023/A:1009516928956

Barakat, L. P., Kazak, A. E., Meadows, A. T., Casey, R., Meeske, K., & Stuber, M. L. (1997). Families surviving childhood cancer: a comparison of posttraumatic stress symptoms with families of healthy children. *Journal of Pediatric Psychology, 22*(6), 843–859. https://doi.org/ 10.1093/jpepsy/22.6.843

Bemis, H., Yarboi, J., Gerhardt, C. A., Vannatta, K., Desjardins, L., Murphy, L. K., Rodriguez, E. M., & Compas, B. E. (2015). Childhood cancer in context: Sociodemographic factors, stress, and psychological distress among mothers and children. *Journal of Pediatric Psychology, 40*(8), 733–743. https://doi.org/10.1093/jpepsy/jsv024

Best, M., Streisand, R., Catania, L., & Kazak, A. E. (2001). Parental distress during pediatric leukemia and posttraumatic stress symptoms (PTSS) after treatment ends. *Journal of Pediatric Psychology, 26*(5), 299–307. https://doi.org/10.1093/jpepsy/26.5.299

Boman, K. K., Kjällander, Y., Eksborg, S., & Becker, J. (2013). Impact of prior traumatic life events on parental early stage reactions following a child's cancer. *PLoS ONE, 8*(3). https:// doi.org/10.1371/journal.pone.0057556

Boyer, B. A., & Cantor, R. K. (2005). Posttraumatic stress among women with breast cancer and their daughters: relationship with daughters' breast cancer screening. *American Journal of Family Therapy, 33*(5), 443–460. https://doi.org/10.1080/01926180500290480

Boyer, B. A., Bubel, D., Jacobs, S. R., Knolls, M. L., Harwell, V. D., Goscicka, M., & Keegan, A. (2002). Posttraumatic stress in women with breast cancer and their daughters. *American Journal of Family Therapy, 30*(4), 323–338. https://doi.org/10.1080/01926180290033466

Brosseau, D. C., McDonald, M. J., & Stephen, J. E. (2011). The moderating effect of relationship quality on partner secondary traumatic stress among couples coping with cancer. *Families, Systems, & Health, 29*(2), 114–126. https://doi.org/10.1037/a0024155

Brown, R. T., Fuemmeler, B., Anderson, D., Jamieson, S., Simonian, S., Hall, R. K., & Brescia, F. (2007). Adjustment of children and their mothers with breast cancer. *Journal of Pediatric Psychology, 32*(3), 297–308. https://doi.org/10.1093/jpepsy/jsl015

Brown, R. T., Madan-Swain, A., & Lambert, R. (2003). Posttraumatic stress symptoms in adolescent survivors of childhood cancer and their mothers. *Journal of Traumatic Stress, 16*(4), 309–318. https://doi.org/10.1023/a:1024465415620

Bruce, M. (2006). A systematic and conceptual review of posttraumatic stress in childhood cancer survivors and their parents. *Clinical Psychology Review, 26*(3), 233–256. https://doi.org/10.1016/j.cpr.2005.10.002

Burke, K., Muscara, F., McCarthy, M., Dimovski, A., Hearps, S., Anderson, V., & Walser, R. (2014). Adapting acceptance and commitment therapy for parents of children with life-threatening illness: Pilot study. *Families, Systems, & Health, 32*(1), 122–127. https://doi.org/10.1037/fsh0000012

Butler, L. D., Field, N. P., Busch, A. L., Seplaki, J. E., Hastings, T. A., & Spiegel, D. (2005). Anticipating loss and other temporal stressors predict traumatic stress symptoms among partners of metastatic/recurrent breast cancer patients. *Psycho-Oncology, 14*(6), 492–502. https://doi.org/10.1002/pon.865

Butler, R. W., Rizzi, L. P., & Handwerger, B. A. (1996). Brief report: the assessment of posttraumatic stress disorder in pediatric cancer patients and survivors. *Journal of Pediatric Psychology, 21*(4), 499–504. https://doi.org/10.1093/jpepsy/21.4.499

Cernvall, M., Alaie, I., & von Essen, L. (2011). The factor structure of traumatic stress in parents of children with cancer: A longitudinal analysis. *Journal of Pediatric Psychology, 37*(4), 448–457. https://doi.org/10.1093/jpepsy/jsr105

Cernvall, M., Carlbring, P., Ljungman, L., Ljungman, G., & von Essen, L. (2015). Internet-based guided self-help for parents of children on cancer treatment: A randomized controlled trial. *Psycho-Oncology, 24*(9), 1152–1158. https://doi.org/10.1002/pon.3788

Chung, M. C., Dennis, I., Easthope, Y., Werrett, J., & Farmer, S. (2005). A multiple-indicator multiple-cause model for posttraumatic stress reactions: personality, coping, and maladjustment. *Psychosomatic Medicine, 67*(2), 251–259. https://doi.org/http://dx.doi.org/10.1097/01.psy.0000155675.56550.5f

Clawson, A. H., Jurbergs, N., Lindwall, J., & Phipps, S. (2013). Concordance of parent proxy report and child self-report of posttraumatic stress in children with cancer and healthy children: Influence of parental posttraumatic stress. *Psycho-Oncology, 22*(11), 2593–2600. https://doi.org/10.1002/pon.3321

Cordova, M. J., Riba, M. B., & Spiegel, D. (2017). Post-traumatic stress disorder and cancer. *Lancet Psychiatry, 4*(4), 330–338. https://doi.org/10.1016/s2215-0366(17)30014-7

Cukor, J. (2003). Posttraumatic stress in women with family histories of breast cancer (PhD thesis, Yeshiva University). ProQuest Dissertations & Theses Global (Publication Number 3376853).

D'Urso, A., Mastroyannopoulou, K., Kirby, A., & Meiser-Stedman, R. (2018). Posttraumatic stress symptoms in young people with cancer and their siblings: Results from a UK sample. *Journal of Psychosocial Oncology, 36*(6), 768–783. https://doi.org/10.1080/07347332.2018.1494664

Davis, G. L., Parra, G. R., & Phipps, S. (2010). Parental posttraumatic stress symptoms due to childhood cancer and child outcomes: Investigation of the role of child anger regulation. *Children's Health Care, 39*, 173–184. https://doi.org/10.1080/02739615.2010.493763

Dolgin, M. J., Phipps, S., Fairclough, D. L., Sahler, O. J., Askins, M., Noll, R. B., Butler, R. W., Varni, J. W., & Katz, E. R. (2007). Trajectories of adjustment in mothers of children with newly diagnosed cancer: a natural history investigation. *Journal of Pediatric Psychology, 32*(7), 771–782. https://doi.org/10.1093/jpepsy/jsm013

Duncan, E., Gidron, Y., Rabin, E., Gouchberg, L., Moser, A. M., & Kapelushnik, J. (2007). The effects of guided written disclosure on psychological symptoms among parents of children with cancer. *Journal of Family Nursing, 13*(3), 370–384. https://doi.org/10.1177/107484070 7303843

Figley, C. R., & Kleber, R. J. (1995). Beyond the "victim": Secondary traumatic stress. In R. J. Kleber, C. R. Figley, & B. P. R. Gersons (Eds.), *Beyond trauma: Cultural and societal dynamics* (pp. 75–98). Plenum Press. https://doi.org/10.1007/978-1-4757-9421-2_5

Fisher, R. S., Perez, M. N., Basile, N. L., Pepper, M., Gamwell, K. L., McNall-Knapp, R., Carter, J. C., Mayes, S., Chaney, J. M., & Mullins, L. L. (2021). Childhood cancer physical symptom burden and parent distress: The role of parent rumination. *Clinical Practice in Pediatric Psychology, 9*(3), 251–260. https://doi.org/10.1037/cpp0000403

Foran-Tuller, K., O'Hea, E. L., Moon, S., & Miller, S. J. (2012). Posttraumatic stress symptoms in children of mothers diagnosed with breast cancer. *Journal of Psychosocial Oncology, 30*(1), 41–56. https://doi.org/10.1080/07347332.2011.633979

Fuemmeler, B. F., Mullins, L. L., Van Pelt, J., Carpentier, M. Y., & Parkhurst, J. (2005). Posttraumatic stress symptoms and distress among parents of children with cancer. *Children's Health Care, 34*(4), 289–303. https://doi.org/10.1207/s15326888chc3404_4

Galtieri, L. R., Fladeboe, K. M., King, K., Friedman, D., Compas, B., Breiger, D., Lengua, L., Keim, M., Boparai, S., & Katz, L. F. (2022). Caregiver perceived financial strain during pediatric cancer treatment: Longitudinal predictors and outcomes. *Health Psychology, 41*(1), 43–52. https://doi.org/10.1037/hea0001122

Garlan, R. W., Butler, L. D., Rosenbaum, E., Siegel, A., & Spiegel, D. (2010). Perceived benefits and psychosocial outcomes of a brief existential family intervention for cancer patients/survivors. *Omega (Westport), 62*(3), 243–268. https://doi.org/10.2190/om.62.3.c

Glover, D. A., Powers, M. B., Bergman, L., Smits, J. A. J., Telch, M. J., & Stuber, M. (2003). Urinary dopamine and turn bias in traumatized women with and without PTSD symptoms. *Behavioural Brain Research, 144*(1), 137–141. https://doi.org/https://doi.org/10.1016/S0166-4328(03)00074-3

Glover, D. A., Steele, A. C., Stuber, M. L., & Fahey, J. L. (2005). Preliminary evidence for lymphocyte distribution differences at rest and after acute psychological stress in PTSD-symptomatic women. *Brain, Behavior, and Immunity, 19*(3), 243–251. https://doi.org/10.1016/j.bbi.2004.08.002

Glover, D. A., Stuber, M., & Poland, R. E. (2006). Allostatic load in women with and without PTSD symptoms. *Psychiatry, 69*(3), 191–203. https://doi.org/10.1521/psyc.2006.69.3.191

Goldwin, M., Lee, S., Afzal, K., Drossos, T., & Karnik, N. (2014). The relationship between patient and parent posttraumatic stress in pediatric oncology: A theoretical framework. *Children's Health Care, 43*(1), 1–15. https://doi.org/10.1080/02739615.2014.850855

Graziano, S., Rossi, A., Spano, B., Petrocchi, M., Biondi, G., & Ammaniti, M. (2016). Comparison of psychological functioning in children and their mothers living through a life-threatening and non life-threatening chronic disease: A pilot study. *Journal of Child Health Care, 20*(2), 174–184. https://doi.org/10.1177/1367493514563854

Greening, L., Stoppelbein, L., & Cheek, K. (2017). Racial/ethnic disparities in the risk of posttraumatic stress disorder symptoms among mothers of children diagnosed with cancer and Type-1 diabetes mellitus. *Psychological Trauma: Theory, Research, Practice, and Policy, 9*(3), 325–333. https://doi.org/10.1037/tra0000230

Gross, J. J., & John, O. P. (2003). Individual differences in two emotion regulation processes: Implications for affect, relationships, and well-being. *Journal of Personality and Social Psychology, 85*, 348–362.

Gurtovenko, K., Fladeboe, K. M., Galtieri, L. R., King, K., Friedman, D., Compas, B., Breiger, D., Lengua, L., Keim, M., Kawamura, J., & Katz, L. F. (2021). Stress and psychological adjustment in caregivers of children with cancer. *Health Psychology, 40*(5), 295–304. https://doi.org/10.1037/hea0001070

Hamann, H. A., Somers, T. J., Smith, A. W., Inslicht, S. S., & Baum, A. (2005). Posttraumatic stress associated with cancer history and BRCA1/2 genetic testing. *Psychosomatic Medicine, 67*(5), 766–772. https://doi.org/10.1097/01.psy.0000181273.74398.d7

Harris, C. A., & Zakowski, S. G. (2003). Comparisons of distress in adolescents of cancer patients and controls. *Psycho-Oncology, 12*(2), 173–182. https://doi.org/https://doi.org/10.1002/pon.631

Heinrichs, N., Zimmermann, T., Huber, B., Herschbach, P., Russell, D. W., & Baucom, D. H. (2012). Cancer distress reduction with a couple-based skills training: A randomized controlled trial. *Annals of Behavioral Medicine, 43*(2), 239–252. https://doi.org/10.1007/s12160-011-9314-9

Hosseini, F., Aghebati, A., Asgharnejad, A. A., Arjomandi Rafsanjani, K., & Ghorbani, S. (2020). Emotional behavioral problems and post traumatic stress symptoms in collaborators in children with cancer. *Iranian Journal of Psychiatry and Clinical Psychology, 26*(2), 216–227. https://doi.org/10.32598/ijpcp.26.2.2337.2

Howell, K. H., Barrett-Becker, E. P., Burnside, A. N., Wamser-Nanney, R., Layne, C. M., & Kaplow, J. B. (2016). Children facing parental cancer versus parental death: The buffering effects of positive parenting and emotional expression. *Journal of Child and Family Studies, 25*(1), 152–164. https://doi.org/10.1007/s10826-015-0198-3

Iobst, E. A., Alderfer, M. A., Sahler, O. J. Z., Askins, M. A., Fairclough, D. L., Katz, E. R., Butler, R. W., Dolgin, M. J., & Noll, R. B. (2009). Brief report: Problem solving and maternal distress at the time of a child's diagnosis of cancer in two-parent versus lone-parent households. *Journal of Pediatric Psychology, 34*, 817–821. https://doi.org/10.1093/jpepsy/jsn140

Jurbergs, N., Long, A., Ticona, L., & Phipps, S. (2009). Symptoms of posttraumatic stress in parents of children with cancer: are they elevated relative to parents of healthy children? *Journal of Pediatric Psychology, 34*(1), 4–13. https://doi.org/10.1093/jpepsy/jsm119

Juth V, Silver RC, Sender L. The shared experience of adolescent and young adult cancer patients and their caregivers. *Psychooncology.* 2015 Dec;24(12):1746–1753. doi:10.1002/pon.3785. Epub 2015 Mar 25. PMID: 25808790; PMCID: PMC4688241.

Kaplan, L. M., Kaal, K. J., Bradley, L., & Alderfer, M. A. (2013). Cancer-related traumatic stress reactions in siblings of children with cancer. *Families, Systems, & Health, 31*(2), 205–217. https://doi.org/10.1037/a0032550

Kashdan, T., Morina, N., & Priebe, S. (2009). Post-traumatic stress disorder, social anxiety disorder, and depression in survivors of the Kosovo War: experiential avoidance as a contributor to distress and quality of life. *Journal of Anxiety Disorders, 23*, 185–196.

Katz, L. F., Fladeboe, K., King, K., Gurtovenko, K., Kawamura, J., Friedman, D., Compas, B., Gruhn, M., Breiger, D., Lengua, L., Lavi, I., & Stettler, N. (2018). Trajectories of child and caregiver psychological adjustment in families of children with cancer. *Health Psychology, 37*(8), 725–735. https://doi.org/10.1037/hea0000619

Kay, J. S., Juth, V., Silver, R. C., & Sender, L. S. (2019). Support and conflict in relationships and psychological health in adolescents and young adults with cancer. *Journal of Health Psychology, 24*(4), 502–517. https://doi.org/10.1177/1359105316676629

Kazak, A. E., & Barakat, L. P. (1997). Brief report: Parenting stress and quality of life during treatment for childhood leukemia predicts child and parent adjustment after treatment ends. *Journal of Pediatric Psychology, 22*(5), 749–758. https://doi.org/10.1093/jpepsy/22.5.749

Kazak, A. E., Alderfer, M., Rourke, M. T., Simms, S., Streisand, R., & Grossman, J. R. (2004). Posttraumatic stress disorder (PTSD) and posttraumatic stress symptoms (PTSS) in families of adolescent childhood cancer survivors. *Journal of Pediatric Psychology, 29*(3), 211–219. https://doi.org/10.1093/jpepsy/jsh022

Kazak, A. E., Alderfer, M. A., Streisand, R., Simms, S., Rourke, M. T., Barakat, L. P., Gallagher, P., & Cnaan, A. (2004). Treatment of posttraumatic stress symptoms in adolescent survivors of childhood cancer and their families: A randomized clinical trial. *Journal of Family Psychology, 18*(3), 493–504. https://doi.org/10.1037/0893-3200.18.3.493

Kazak, A. E., Barakat, L. P., Alderfer, M., Rourke, M. T., Meeske, K., Gallagher, P. R., Cnaan, A., & Stuber, M. L. (2001). Posttraumatic stress in survivors of childhood cancer and mothers: development and validation of the Impact of Traumatic Stressors Interview Schedule (ITSIS). *Journal of Clinical Psychology in Medical Settings, 8*(4), 307–323. https://doi.org/10.1023/A:1011977031826

Kazak, A. E., Barakat, L. P., Meeske, K., Christakis, D., Meadows, A. T., Casey, R., Penati, B., & Stuber, M. L. (1997). Posttraumatic stress, family functioning, and social support in survivors of childhood leukemia and their mothers and fathers. *Journal of Consulting and Clinical Psychology, 65*(1), 120–129. https://doi.org/10.1037//0022–006x.65.1.120

Kazak, A. E., Simms, S., Alderfer, M. A., Rourke, M. T., Crump, T., McClure, K., Jones, P., Rodriguez, A., Boeving, A., Hwang, W. T., & Reilly, A. (2005). Feasibility and preliminary outcomes from a pilot study of a brief psychological intervention for families of children newly diagnosed with cancer. *Journal of Pediatric Psychology, 30*(8), 644–655. https://doi.org/10.1093/jpepsy/jsi051

Kazak, A. E., Simms, S., Barakat, L., Hobbie, W., Foley, B., Golomb, V., & Best, M. (1999). Surviving cancer competently intervention program (SCCIP): a cognitive-behavioral and family therapy intervention for adolescent survivors of childhood cancer and their families. *Family Process, 38*(2), 175–191. https://doi.org/10.1111/j.1545-5300.1999.00176.x

Kazak, A. E., Stuber, M. L., Barakat, L. P., Meeske, K., Guthrie, D., & Meadows, A. T. (1998). Predicting posttraumatic stress symptoms in mothers and fathers of survivors of childhood cancers. *Journal of the American Academy of Child and Adolescent Psychiatry, 37*(8), 823–831. https://doi.org/10.1097/00004583-199808000-00012

Klassen, A. F., Gulati, S., Granek, L., Rosenberg-Yunger, Z. R. S., Watt, L., Sung, L., Klaassen, R., Dix, D., & Shaw, N. T. (2012). Understanding the health impact of caregiving: A qualitative study of immigrant parents and single parents of children with cancer. *Quality of Life Research, 21*(9), 1595–1605. http://www.jstor.org/stable/41684651

Kristensen, T. E., Elklit, A., & Karstoft, K.-I. (2012). Posttraumatic stress disorder after bereavement: Early psychological sequelae of losing a close relative due to terminal cancer. *Journal of Loss and Trauma, 17*(6), 508–521. https://doi.org/10.1080/15325024.2012.665304

Lamanna, J., Bitsko, M., & Stern, M. (2018). Effects of a brief problem-solving intervention for parents of children with cancer. *Children's Health Care, 47*(1), 51–66. https://doi.org/10.1080/02739615.2016.1275638

Landolt, M. A., Vollrath, M., Ribi, K., Gnehm, H. E., & Sennhauser, F. H. (2003). Incidence and associations of parental and child posttraumatic stress symptoms in pediatric patients. *Journal of Child Psychology and Psychiatry, 44*(8), 1199–1207. https://doi.org/10.1111/1469-7610.00201

Lazarus, R. S. (1993). From psychological stress to the emotions: A history of changing outlooks. *Annual Review of Psychology, 44*, 1–21.

Lazarus, R. S., & Folkman, S. (1984). *Stress, appraisal and coping.* Springer.

Lee, M. L., Cohen, S. E., Stuber, M. L., & Nader, K. (1994). Parent–child interactions with pediatric bone marrow transplant patients. *Journal of Psychosocial Oncology, 12*, 43–60. https://doi.org/10.1300/J077V12N04_03

Libov, B. G., Nevid, J. S., Pelcovitz, D., & Carmony, T. M. (2002). Posttraumatic stress symptomatology in mothers of pediatric cancer survivors. *Psychology & Health, 17*, 501–511. https://doi.org/10.1080/0887044022000004975

Lindberg, N. M., & Wellisch, D. K. (2004). Identification of traumatic stress reactions in women at increased risk for breast cancer. *Psychosomatics, 45*(1), 7–16. https://doi.org/10.1176/appi.psy.45.1.7

Ljungman, L., Hovén, E., Ljungman, G., Cernvall, M., & Essen, L. (2015). Does time heal all wounds? A longitudinal study of the development of posttraumatic stress symptoms in parents of survivors of childhood cancer and bereaved parents. *Psycho-Oncology, 24*(12), 1792–1798. https://doi.org/10.1002/pon.3856

Long, K. A., Lehmann, V., Gerhardt, C. A., Carpenter, A. L., Marsland, A. L., & Alderfer, M. A. (2018). Psychosocial functioning and risk factors among siblings of children with cancer: An updated systematic review. *Psycho-Oncology, 27*(6), 1467–1479. https://doi.org/10.1002/pon.4669

Magal-Vardi, O., Laor, N., Toren, A., Strauss, L., Wolmer, L., Bielorai, B., Rechavi, G., & Toren, P. (2004). Psychiatric morbidity and quality of life in children with malignancies and their parents. *Journal of Nervous and Mental Disease, 192*(12), 872–875. https://doi.org/10.1097/01.nmd.0000146881.00129.ec

Malpert, A. V., Kimberg, C., Luxton, J., Mullins, L. L., Pui, C. H., Hudson, M. M., Krull, K. R., & Brinkman, T. M. (2015). Emotional distress in parents of long-term survivors of childhood acute lymphoblastic leukemia. *Psycho-Oncology, 24*(9), 1116–1123. https://doi.org/10.1002/pon.3732

Manne, S. L., Du Hamel, K., Gallelli, K., Sorgen, K., & Redd, W. H. (1998). Posttraumatic stress disorder among mothers of pediatric cancer survivors: diagnosis, comorbidity, and utility of the PTSD checklist as a screening instrument. *Journal of Pediatric Psychology, 23*(6), 357–366. https://doi.org/10.1093/jpepsy/23.6.357

McCarthy, M. C., Ashley, D. M., Lee, K. J., & Anderson, V. A. (2012). Predictors of acute and posttraumatic stress symptoms in parents following their child's cancer diagnosis. *Journal of Trauma Stress, 25*(5), 558–566. https://doi.org/10.1002/jts.21745

McEvoy, B., & Creaner, M. (2021). The experiences of mothers who have a child diagnosed with cancer. *Psychology & Health, 37*(5), 594–614. https://doi.org/10.1080/08870446.2021.1872791

Metcalf, C. A., Arch, J. J., & Greer, J. A. (2017). Anxiety and its correlates among young adults with a history of parental cancer. *Journal of Psychosocial Oncology, 35*(5), 597–613. https://doi.org/10.1080/07347332.2017.1307895

Meyer, F., Zhang, B., Gao, X., & Prigerson, H. G. (2013). Associations between cognitive impairment in advanced cancer patients and psychiatric disorders in their caregivers. *Psycho-Oncology, 22*(4), 952–955. https://doi.org/10.1002/pon.3076

Michael, T., Halligan, S. L., Clark, D. M., & Ehlers, A. (2007). Rumination in posttraumatic stress disorder. *Depression and Anxiety, 24*(5), 307–317.

Miller, K. I., Stiff, J. B., & Ellis, B. H. (1988). Communication and empathy as precursors to burnout among human service workers. *Communication Monographs, 55*, 250–265. https://doi.org/10.1080/03637758809376171

Mosher, C. E., & Danoff-Burg, S. (2005). Psychosocial impact of parental cancer in adulthood: A conceptual and empirical review. *Clinical Psychology Review, 25*(3), 365–382. https://doi.org/https://doi.org/10.1016/j.cpr.2004.12.003

Murphy, L. K., Preacher, K. J., Rights, J. D., Rodriguez, E. M., Bemis, H., Desjardins, L., Prussien, K., Winning, A. M., Gerhardt, C. A., Vannatta, K., & Compas, B. E. (2018). Maternal communication in childhood cancer: Factor analysis and relation to maternal distress. *Journal of Pediatric Psychology*, 43(10), 1114–1127. https://doi.org/10.1093/jpepsy/jsy054

Murphy, L. K., Rodriguez, E. M., Schwartz, L., Bemis, H., Desjardins, L., Gerhardt, C. A., Vannatta, K., Saylor, M., & Compas, B. E. (2016). Longitudinal associations among maternal communication and adolescent posttraumatic stress symptoms after cancer diagnosis. *Psycho-Oncology*, 25(7), 779–786. https://doi.org/10.1002/pon.3918

Norberg, A. (2010). Parents of children surviving a brain tumor: Burnout and the perceived disease-related influence on everyday life. *Journal of Pediatric Hematology/Oncology*, 32, e285–e289. https://doi.org/10.1097/MPH.0b013e3181e7dda6

Norberg, A. L., & Boman, K. K. (2013). Mothers and fathers of children with cancer: Loss of control during treatment and posttraumatic stress at later follow-up. *Psycho-Oncology*, 22(2), 324–329.

Norberg, A. L., Pöder, U., & von Essen, L. (2011). Early avoidance of disease- and treatment-related distress predicts post-traumatic stress in parents of children with cancer. *European Journal of Oncology Nursing*, 15(1), 80–84. https://doi.org/10.1016/j.ejon.2010.05.009

Okado, Y., Long, A. M., & Phipps, S. (2014). Association between parent and child distress and the moderating effects of life events in families with and without a history of pediatric cancer. *Journal of Pediatric Psychology*, 39(9), 1049–1060. https://doi.org/10.1093/jpepsy/jsu058

Ozawa, M. (2005). Psychological reaction of families with children with cancer. *Japanese Journal of Child and Adolescent Psychiatry*, 46(2), 120–127.

Packman, W., Fine, J., Chesterman, B., vanZutphen, K., Golan, R., & Amylon, M. D. (2004). Camp Okizu: Preliminary investigation of a psychological intervention for siblings of pediatric cancer patients. *Children's Health Care*, 33, 201–215. https://doi.org/10.1207/s15326888chc3303_3

Pelcovitz, D., Goldenberg, B., Kaplan, S., Weinblatt, M., Mandel, F., Meyers, B., & Vinciguerra, V. (1996). Posttraumatic stress disorder in mothers of pediatric cancer survivors. *Psychosomatics*, 37(2), 116–126. https://doi.org/10.1016/s0033-3182(96)71577-3

Pelcovitz, D., Libov, B. G., Mandel, F., Kaplan, S., Weinblatt, M., & Septimus, A. (1998). Posttraumatic stress disorder and family functioning in adolescent cancer. *Journal of Trauma Stress*, 11(2), 205–221. https://doi.org/10.1023/a:1024442802113

Perez, M. N., Traino, K. A., Bakula, D. M., Sharkey, C. M., Espeleta, H. C., Delozier, A. M., Mayes, S., McNall, R., Chaney, J. M., & Mullins, L. L. (2020). Barriers to care in pediatric cancer: The role of illness uncertainty in relation to parent psychological distress. *Psycho-Oncology*, 29(2), 304–310. https://doi.org/10.1002/pon.5248

Phipps, S., Larson, S., Long, A., & Rai, S. N. (2006). Adaptive style and symptoms of posttraumatic stress in children with cancer and their parents. *Journal of Pediatric Psychology*, 31(3), 298–309. https://doi.org/10.1093/jpepsy/jsj033

Phipps, S., Long, A., Willard, V. W., Okado, Y., Hudson, M., Huang, Q., Zhang, H., & Noll, R. (2015). Parents of children with cancer: At-risk or resilient? *Journal of Pediatric Psychology*, 40(9), 914–925. https://doi.org/10.1093/jpepsy/jsv047

Pöder, U., Ljungman, G., & von Essen, L. (2008). Posttraumatic stress disorder among parents of children on cancer treatment: a longitudinal study. *Psycho-Oncology*, 17(5), 430–437. https://doi.org/10.1002/pon.1263

Pohlkamp, L., Kreicbergs, U., & Sveen, J. (2019). Bereaved mothers' and fathers' prolonged grief and psychological health 1 to 5 years after loss—A nationwide study. *Psycho-Oncology*, 28(7), 1530–1536. https://doi.org/10.1002/pon.5112

Prchal, A., Graf, A., Bergstraesser, E., & Landolt, M. A. (2012). A two-session psychological intervention for siblings of pediatric cancer patients: A randomized controlled pilot trial. *Child Adolescent Psychiatry and Mental Health, 6*(1), 3. https://doi.org/10.1186/1753-2000-6-3

Prchal, A., & Landolt, M. A. (2009). Psychological interventions with siblings of pediatric cancer patients: A systematic review. *Psycho-Oncology, 18*(12), 1241–1251. https://doi.org/10.1002/pon.1565

Ribi, K., Vollrath, M. E., Sennhauser, F. H., Gnehm, H. E., & Landolt, M. A. (2007). Prediction of posttraumatic stress in fathers of children with chronic diseases or unintentional injuries: A six-months follow-up study. *Child and Adolescent Psychiatry and Mental Health, 1,* Art. 16. https://doi.org/10.1186/1753-2000-1-16

Rodriguez, E. M., Dunn, M. J., Zuckerman, T., Vannatta, K., Gerhardt, C. A., & Compas, B. E. (2012). Cancer-related sources of stress for children with cancer and their parents. *Journal of Pediatric Psychology, 37*(2), 185–197. https://doi.org/10.1093/jpepsy/jsr054

Rosebrock, L. E., Arditte Hall, K. A., Rando, A., Pineles, S. L., & Liverant, G. I. (2019). Rumination and its relationship with thought suppression in unipolar depression and comorbid PTSD. *Cognitive Therapy and Research, 43*(1), 226–235.

Rumpold, T., Schur, S., Amering, M., Ebert-Vogel, A., Kirchheiner, K., Masel, E., Watzke, H., & Schrank, B. (2017). Hope as determinant for psychiatric morbidity in family caregivers of advanced cancer patients. *Psycho-Oncology, 26*(5), 672–678. https://doi.org/10.1002/pon.4205

Sánchez-Egea, R., Rubio-Aparicio, M., Sánchez-Meca, J., & Rosa-Alcázar, A. I. (2019). Psychological treatment for family members of children with cancer: A systematic review and meta-analysis. *Psycho-Oncology, 28*(5), 960–969. https://doi.org/10.1002/pon.5052

Schellekens, M. P. J., van den Hurk, D. G. M., Prins, J. B., Donders, A. R. T., Molema, J., Dekhuijzen, R., van der Drift, M. A., & Speckens, A. E. M. (2017). Mindfulness-based stress reduction added to care as usual for lung cancer patients and/or their partners: A multicentre randomized controlled trial. *Psycho-Oncology, 26*(12), 2118–2126.

Schepers, S. A., Okado, Y., Russell, K., Long, A. M., & Phipps, S. (2019). Adjustment in childhood cancer survivors, healthy peers, and their parents: The mediating role of the parent–child relationship. *Journal of Pediatric Psychology, 44*(2), 186–196. https://doi.org/10.1093/jpepsy/jsy069

Sharkey, C. M., Bakula, D. M., Tackett, A. P., Mullins, A. J., Gamwell, K. L., Suorsa, K. I., Mayes, S., McNall-Knapp, R., Chaney, J. M., & Mullins, L. L. (2018). Posttraumatic stress symptomology in parents of children with cancer: Implications related to criterion changes in DSM-IV-TR to DSM-5. *Children's Health Care, 47*(4), 357–370. https://doi.org/10.1080/02739615.2017.1354295

Sharp, K., Tillery, R., Long, A., Wang, F., Pan, H., & Phipps, S. (2021). Trajectories of resilience and posttraumatic stress in childhood cancer: Consistency of child and parent outcomes. *Health Psychology* 41(4), 256–267. https://doi.org/10.1037/hea0001132

Slaughter, R. I., Hamilton, A. S., Cederbaum, J. A., Unger, J. B., Baezconde-Garbanati, L., & Milam, J. E. (2020). Relationships between parent and adolescent/young adult mental health among Hispanic and non-Hispanic childhood cancer survivors. *Journal of Psychosocial Oncology, 38*(6), 746–760. https://doi.org/10.1080/07347332.2020.1815924

Smith, M. Y., Redd, W. H., Peyser, C., & Vogl, D. (1999). Post-traumatic stress disorder in cancer: a review. *Psychooncology, 8*(6), 521–537. https://doi.org/10.1002/(sici)1099-1611(199911/12)8:6<521::aid-pon423>3.0.co;2-x

Stoppelbein, L., & Greening, L. (2007). Brief report: the risk of posttraumatic stress disorder in mothers of children diagnosed with pediatric cancer and type I diabetes. *Journal of Pediatric Psychology, 32*(2), 223–229. https://doi.org/10.1093/jpepsy/jsj120

Stoppelbein, L., Greening, L., & Fite, P. J. (2010). Brief report: Role of cortisol in posttraumatic stress symptoms among mothers of children diagnosed with cancer. *Journal of Pediatric Psychology, 35*(9), 960–965. https://doi.org/10.1093/jpepsy/jsp139

Stoppelbein, L., Greening, L., & Wells, H. (2013). Parental coping and posttraumatic stress symptoms among pediatric cancer populations: Tests of competing models. *Psycho-Oncology, 22*(12), 2815–2822. https://doi.org/10.1002/pon.3358

Stoppelbein, L., McRae, E., & Greening, L. (2017). A longitudinal study of hardiness as a buffer for posttraumatic stress symptoms in mothers of children with cancer. *Clinical Practice in Pediatric Psychology, 5*(2), 149–160. https://doi.org/10.1037/cpp0000168

Stuber, M. L. (1995). Stress responses to pediatric cancer: A family phenomenon. *Family Systems Medicine, 13*(2), 163–172. https://doi.org/10.1037/h0089256

Stuber, M. L., Christakis, D. A., Houskamp, B., & Kazak, A. E. (1996). Posttrauma symptoms in childhood leukemia survivors and their parents. *Psychosomatics, 37*(3), 254–261. https://doi.org/10.1016/s0033-3182(96)71564-5

Stuber, M. L., Meeske, K. A., Krull, K. R., Leisenring, W., Stratton, K., Kazak, A. E., Huber, M., Zebrack, B., Uijtdehaage, S. H., Mertens, A. C., Robison, L. L., & Zeltzer, L. K. (2010). Prevalence and predictors of posttraumatic stress disorder in adult survivors of childhood cancer. *Pediatrics, 125*(5), e1124–e1134. https://doi.org/10.1542/peds.2009-2308

Stuber, M. L., & Shemesh, E. (2006). Post-traumatic stress response to life-threatening illnesses in children and their parents. *Child and Adolescent Psychiatric Clinics of North America, 15*(3), 597–609. https://doi.org/10.1016/j.chc.2006.02.006

Stuber, M. L., Shemesh, E., & Saxe, G. N. (2003). Posttraumatic stress responses in children with life-threatening illnesses. *Child and Adolescent Psychiatric Clinics of North America, 12,* 195–209. https://doi.org/10.1016/S1056-4993(02)00100-1

Sveen, J., Pohlkamp, L., Kreicbergs, U., & Eisma, M. C. (2019). Rumination in bereaved parents: Psychometric evaluation of the Swedish version of the Utrecht Grief Rumination Scale (UGRS). *PLoS ONE, 14*(3), ArtID e0213152.

Swartzman, S., Sani, F., & Munro, A. J. (2017). The role of social support, family identification, and family constraints in predicting posttraumatic stress after cancer. *Psycho-Oncology, 26*(9), 1330–1335. https://doi.org/10.1002/pon.4304

Tackett, A. P., Cushing, C. C., Suorsa, K. I., Mullins, A. J., Gamwell, K. L., Mayes, S., McNall-Knapp, R., Chaney, J. M., & Mullins, L. L. (2016). Illness uncertainty, global psychological distress, and posttraumatic stress in pediatric cancer: A preliminary examination using a path analysis approach. *Journal of Pediatric Psychology, 41*(3), 309–318. https://doi.org/10.1093/jpepsy/jsv093

Taïeb, O., Moro, M. R., Baubet, T., Revah-Lévy, A., & Flament, M. F. (2003). Posttraumatic stress symptoms after childhood cancer. *European Journal of Child and Adolescent Psychiatry, 12*(6), 255–264. https://doi.org/10.1007/s00787-003-0352-0

Teixeira, R. J., & Pereira, M. G. (2013). Psychological morbidity, burden, and the mediating effect of social support in adult children caregivers of oncological patients undergoing chemotherapy. *Psycho-Oncology, 22*(7), 1587–1593. https://doi.org/10.1002/pon.3173

Teixeira, R. J., & Pereira, M. G. (2016). Posttraumatic stress disorder symptoms and family functioning in adult children facing parental cancer: A comparison study. *Research and Theory for Nursing Practice, 30*(3), 212–228. https://doi.org/10.1891/1541-6577.30.3.212

Teixeira, R. J., Applebaum, A. J., Bhatia, S., & Brandão, T. (2018). The impact of coping strategies of cancer caregivers on psychophysiological outcomes: An integrative review. *Psychology Research and Behavior Management, 11,* 207–215. https://doi.org/10.2147/PRBM.S164946

Tillery, R., Long, A., & Phipps, S. (2014). Child perceptions of parental care and overprotection in children with cancer and healthy children. *Journal of Clinical Psychology in Medical Settings, 21*(2), 165–172. https://doi.org/10.1007/s10880-014-9392-5

Tull, M. T., Gratz, K. L., Salters, K., & Roemer, L. (2004). The role of experiential avoidance in posttraumatic stress symptoms and symptoms of depression, anxiety, and somatization. *Journal of Nervous and Mental Disease, 192,* 754–761.

Tull, M. T., Jakupcak, M., Paulson, A., & Gratz, K. (2007). The role of emotional inexpressivity and experiential avoidance in the relationship between posttraumatic stress disorder symptom severity and aggressive behavior among men exposed to interpersonal violence. *Anxiety Stress & Coping, 20,* 337–351.

Varela, V. S., Ng, A., Mauch, P., & Recklitis, C. J. (2013). Posttraumatic stress disorder (PTSD) in survivors of Hodgkin's lymphoma: Prevalence of PTSD and partial PTSD compared with sibling controls. *Psycho-Oncology, 22*(2), 434–440.

Verbosky, S. J., & Ryan, D. A. (1988). Female partners of Vietnam veterans: Stress by proximity. *Issues in Mental Health Nursing, 9,* 95–104. https://doi.org/10.3109/01612848809140912

Vernon, L., Eyles, D., Hulbert, C., Bretherton, L., & McCarthy, M. C. (2017). Infancy and pediatric cancer: An exploratory study of parent psychological distress. *Psycho-Oncology, 26*(3), 361–368. https://doi.org/10.1002/pon.4141

Watkins, E. R., & Nolen-Hoeksema, S. (2014). A habit–goal framework of depressive rumination. *Journal of Abnormal Psychology, 123*(1), 24–34. https://doi.org/10.1037/a0035540

Wong, M., Looney, E., Michaels, J., Palesh, O., & Koopman, C. (2006). A preliminary study of peritraumatic dissociation, social support, and coping in relation to posttraumatic stress symptoms for a parent's cancer. *Psycho-Oncology, 15*(12), 1093–1098. https://doi.org/10.1002/pon.1041

Woolf, C., Muscara, F., Anderson, V. A., & McCarthy, M. C. (2016). Early traumatic stress responses in parents following a serious illness in their child: A systematic review. *Journal of Clinical Psychology in Medical Settings, 23*(1), 53–66. https://doi.org/10.1007/s10880-015-9430-y

5

Posttraumatic growth after cancer

The experience of cancer can be extremely stressful, but it can also be an opportunity for growth or a positive life change (e.g. Arpawong et al., 2013; Barakat et al., 2006; Cordova et al., 2007; da Silva et al., 2011; Sears et al., 2003; Stanton et al., 2006; Stuber & Kazak, 1999; Widows et al., 2005). Receiving a cancer diagnosis can be a frightening experience. However, posttraumatic growth (PTG) has been shown to have positive outcomes for cancer survivors such as adult leukaemia patients (Danhauer, Case, et al., 2013; Danhauer, Russell, et al., 2013). Sixty percent of patients in one study reported developing positive changes in themselves (Scrignaro et al., 2011), including changes in relationships with others, new possibilities, personal strength, spirituality, and appreciation of life, which are the fundamental characteristics of PTG (Tedeschi & Calhoun, 1995).

As mentioned in the chapter on cardiovascular disease, this growth phenomenon is possible because, after a trauma, people are intrinsically motivated to rebuild their assumed world in a direction guided by their innate tendency towards self-actualisation. By processing the trauma (in this case, cancer) on a cognitive–emotional level, they assimilate and accommodate (negatively or positively) the information associated with the trauma into their lives. Through positive accommodation, they actualise the positive changes in their lives, provided that the social environment can support this positive accommodative process (Joseph & Linley, 2005). This accommodative process explained a significant amount of the variance in the intrusion of the traumatic event that triggered the growth process. This process also predicted the impact of the trauma on the patient's identity, which in turn guided the rumination process towards a coping strategy (Scrignaro et al., 2011). In other words, the way people struggle with the new trauma reality can determine the extent of PTG. However, the above processes are not without controversy. While the accommodative process was correlated with increased PTG and directly predicted PTG, the assimilative process was only weakly correlated with PTG in cancer patients (Scrignaro et al., 2011).

Posttraumatic Stress in Physical Illness. Man Cheung Chung, Oxford University Press. © Oxford University Press 2024.
DOI: 10.1093/oso/9780198727323.003.0005

This coexisting double-edged phenomenon, trauma and growth, has been studied using terms such as PTG, stress-related growth, benefit finding, and adversarial growth (e.g. Antoni et al., 2001; Brunet et al., 2010; Lechner et al., 2008; Linley & Joseph, 2004; Park et al., 1996; Tedeschi & Calhoun, 1995). A clear differentiation between growth terminologies has been called for (Lechner et al., 2008) and may lead to a differentiation of growth characteristics, which in turn may be associated with specific psychological responses or processes. Even when considering growth characteristics described within the same terminology of PTG, differences may often emerge that require further refinement of the term. For example, while the experiences of women who have experienced breast cancer can be conceptualised using the terminology of PTG with the characteristics previously defined by Tedeschi and Calhoun (1995), their experience is best conceptualised as corporeal PTG for women with breast cancer experiences. It is a growth characterised by a 'reclamation' and a renewed connection to the body through an increase in appreciation of the bodily self, responsibility for one's own body and positive changes in one's health, and a new sense of positive identification with the body. The women described how they lost, regained, and relinquished control over their bodies. At the same time, they reconstructed their embodied identity and thus gained a new appreciation for their bodies. This new insight into their own bodies can play an important role in breast cancer recovery (Gorven & du Plessis, 2021). Viewing PTG from the corporeal perspective is understandable, as survivors tend to perceive the body as an integral part of their self-identity, which affects how PTG is achieved. They may be afraid of their new body and experience negative effects of chemotherapy such as fatigue and loss of desire for their body. They reconnect with their body by listening to it and perceiving their body as a barometer (Hefferon et al., 2010).

Similarly, adult survivors of childhood and adolescent cancer may also develop PTG characteristics that may be unique to their condition and similar to, but not identical to, those described in the growth model for posttraumatic stress (Tedeschi & Calhoun, 1996). Survivors developed strength characterised by psychological confidence and emotional maturity, improved intimacy with family members, and empathy for others. They developed new possibilities including a passion for working with cancer and supporting others to experience it, appreciation for life, not taking life for granted, gratitude for being alive, not forgetting, and improved spiritual development in the form of strengthened spiritual beliefs and participation in religious rituals (Zamora et al., 2017).

Some fundamental tenets of posttraumatic growth

Regardless of the various terms that can be used to describe this growth phe-nomenon, they all have some basic principles in common. First, positive life changes are paradoxical in nature. For them to occur, a stressful event, in this case cancer, must be experienced (da Silva et al., 2011). Positive life changes do not replace pain and suffering, but blend with them (Neimeyer, 2006). Cancer survivors may suffer physically and psychologically from the effects of cancer while experiencing growth (Bellizzi et al., 2010). Take an example of older adult long-term cancer survivors: when they appraised their cancer experience as stressful, distressing, and stigmatising, they also reported posttraumatic changes such as changed worldviews, a sense of vulnerability, changes in identity and decisions about what is important in life, a sense of loss, and improved maturity (Kahana et al., 2011). While most cancer patients (87%) reported at least one positive life change during their cancer treatment, half also reported negative changes in areas where growth traits tend to occur (Arpawong et al., 2013). However, it is this mixture or paradoxical situation (both positive and negative life changes) in which growth occurs that may buffer the suffering and lead people to not necessarily see their cancer as a traumatic experience (da Silva et al., 2011). This is the premise on which much of the growth research on cancer or other diseases is based.

The positive and negative changes are not necessarily linked (Schroevers et al., 2011). They are associated with specific predictors. Increased positive changes were associated with younger age at diagnosis and reduced nausea, while increased negative changes were associated with increased physical dys-function, bodily pain, and reduced psychological well-being (Arpawong et al., 2013). Increased positive change was also associated with increased positive affect, while increased negative change was associated with increased negative affect and decreased positive affect (Schroevers et al., 2011). Approach coping, characterised by positive reappraisal and renewed commitment to a goal, was associated with increased positive changes, while avoidance coping, charac-terised by self-distraction, was associated with increased negative changes. In other words, it may be important for patients to accept positive changes in their lives and approach current cancer-related situations rather than avoid them (Schroevers et al., 2011). Examining two positive and negative aspects of life changes could potentially expand our understanding of adjustment during cancer treatment (Arpawong et al., 2013).

This leads to the second principle, which is that despite differences in terminology, the stressful experience, in this case cancer, can generate resilience (Calhoun & Tedeschi, 2006; Jahn et al., 2012), which has been shown to increase life satisfaction in cancer survivors regardless of their gender, age, years since diagnosis, cancer type, and treatment (Adamkovič et al., 2022). As part of this resilience, PTG is an important component that helps patients adjust and adapt to the effects of cancer (Seiler & Jenewein, 2019). On the other hand, patients with haematopoietic cell transplantation who had low levels of resilience had higher severity of chronic graft-versus-host disease, disability, psychological distress and lower quality of life, particularly in terms of mental health (Rosenberg et al., 2015).

This notion of resilience is reflected in a 'survivor identity' that cancer survivors may develop after their stressful cancer experience (Abernathy, 2008; Sadler-Gerhardt et al., 2010). This identity is an enduring and adaptive reconstruction of the self in which cancer survivors find wisdom, change, and develop a positive sense of self (Abernathy, 2008). This identity is characterised by the ability to accept and appraise pain, suffering, and vulnerability, understand newfound strength, develop a new appreciation for life and a sense of purpose, and integrate the meaning of the stressful cancer experience into their new normal life (Abernathy, 2008; Neimeyer, 2006; Sadler-Gerhardt et al., 2010). This identity is associated with active engagement with peers and cognitive processing. Among men, adopting a survivor identity (35%) was associated with lower levels of threat appraisal, more conscious rumination, greater understanding of the cancer experience, and higher levels of PTG. Women with such survivor identity (50%) tended to post more to online support groups, perceived the group as helpful, and had fewer problems connecting with the group (Morris et al., 2014).

Notwithstanding, while we speak of PTG manifestations for people with cancer, cancer survivors are often unaware of their own unexpected personal abilities and 'life-transforming' internal resources to manage their cancer experiences, cancer-related challenges, and changes (Skeath et al., 2013). To increase the likelihood of developing PTG, cancer survivors would need to have the courage and make a conscious effort to examine and challenge their own core beliefs about personal strengths, weaknesses, human nature, relationships, the meaning of life, and religious and spiritual matters. Although this self-examination has been indirectly associated with increased PTG in people with prostate cancer (Wilson et al., 2014a), with prolongation of PTG in people with leukaemia (Danhauer, Russell, et al., 2013), and with positive and negative (e.g. PTSD) outcomes in women with breast cancer (Ramos,

Leal, et al., 2018), it may not be something that people engage with easily or naturally.

Cancer-related posttraumatic growth

In the following, the term PTG is mostly used, despite the complex issues mentioned above. This focus is an attempt to streamline and manage the considerable amount of literature in this area. It has been documented that 60–67.5% of head and neck cancer survivors (Hamdan et al., 2022; Sharp et al., 2018) have moderate to high levels of growth, although only 10% were recorded in another study (Holtmaat et al., 2017). Compared to those who had no or low levels of PTG, those with moderate to high levels reported higher health-related quality of life (Sharp et al., 2018). This positive association between PTG and health-related quality of life was confirmed in a systemic review. PTG appears to contribute to successful coping after cancer, although one needs to be cautious with this conclusion due to methodological issues or the quality of some studies. They might have influenced effect sizes and heterogeneity, which in turn affect the overall results (Z. Liu et al., 2020).

Another systematic review argues that PTG can increase hope, optimism, spirituality, and sense of purpose (Casellas-Grau et al., 2017), although in head and neck cancer survivors PTG manifested mainly in changes in relationships with others. Increased PTG was associated with lower tumour stage, fewer anxiety disorders and alcohol use, and better social functioning (Holtmaat et al., 2017). Breast cancer survivors who experienced growth tended to report positive changes in relationships with others, new possibilities, personal strength, spiritual changes, and appreciation of life (Tedeschi & Calhoun, 1995). These changes occurred regardless of age differences, type of treatment, time since diagnosis, and last treatment (Brunet et al., 2010). In addition, 83% of women who were in the early stages of their breast cancer reported at least one benefit from their illness experience (Sears et al., 2003), particularly in terms of relationships with others, appreciation of life, or spiritual changes (Cordova et al., 2001). Compared to healthy women with allostatic overload (i.e. the wear and tear on the body from repeated or chronic or cumulative effects of stressful situations in daily life that make recovery less and less complete and increasingly exhaust the body and exceed one's coping abilities), women with breast cancer had higher levels of new possibilities, personal strength, and spiritual change (Ruini et al., 2015). This supports a previous study which found that while both healthy controls and non-small-cell lung cancer survivors had PTG characteristics, the lung cancer patients reported more PTG (ES = 0.39 SD) and more PTG for three out of five subscales (relationship with others, personal strength, appreciation of life) (ES ranging from 0.34 to 0.48 SD) (Andrykowski, Steffens, et al., 2013).

Among women who had breast cancer surgery, 43% experienced high, 23% moderate, and 34% low or no PTG. Relationships with others appeared to be the most important positive change in the PTG domains (Andysz et al., 2015). This growth in social relationships may be why young adults with cancer had better social well-being after treatment than the healthy control group, despite having poorer physical and emotional well-being (Salsman et al., 2014). In addition to growth in social relationships, lung cancer survivors were also more likely to report growth in appreciation of life (Andrykowski, Steffens, et al., 2013). These two growth characteristics also occur in advanced cancer patients receiving palliative treatment, with changes in relationships with others correlated with intrusive symptoms of PTSD and appreciation of life correlated with avoidance, intrusion, and hyperarousal symptoms (Mystakidou et al., 2007).

In terms of appreciating life, this was the most prominent PTG feature in survivors of head and neck cancer (Sharp et al., 2018) and in survivors of childhood or adolescent cancer, although this finding came mainly from case studies of individuals who met criteria for partial-PTSD, as opposed to full-PTSD, where intrusive thoughts and avoidance behaviours are the predominant symptoms (Stuber & Kazak, 1999). Similarly, survivors of cancer in adolescence and young adulthood with moderate-to-high PTG reported the highest score for appreciation of life and the lowest for spiritual change (Barrett-Bernstein et al., 2020). A cross-cultural study claims that appreciation of life is particularly pronounced among Malaysian cancer patients, suggesting that it is not exclusively a Western phenomenon (Schroevers & Teo, 2008).

In terms of the course of growth change, PTG is overall a relatively stable and long-lasting phenomenon (Widows et al., 2005), with the exception of the area of relationships with others (Moore et al., 2011). Compared to healthy controls, young adults with cancer appeared to be stable in maintaining PTG after treatment (Salsman et al., 2014); young black breast cancer survivors also reported high levels of benefit-finding that persisted over time (Conley et al., 2020). One year after surgery, women who had advanced stage cancer, early stage cancer, or benign gynaecological disease reported higher levels of PTG than women who did not have cancer. Pre-surgery PTSD symptoms related to cancer and higher disease severity were associated with PTG (Posluszny et al., 2011). Similarly, adolescent cancer survivors, together with their parents, reported PTG one year after treatment. Increased perceived treatment severity and life threat were associated with PTG (Barakat et al., 2006). Even longer was a study that focused on cancer survivors nine years after haematopoietic stem cell transplantation. Despite the physical limitations of the disease, they reported high levels of physical and psychological well-being and PTG; they also reported greater personal strengths and improved interpersonal relationships. Women reported greater overall growth, while older survivors reported greater spirituality (Tallman et al., 2010). In addition, benefit finding and well-being were evident in breast cancer survivors even after they had been free of the disease for 10 years. A high percentage of them (79%) reported benefits related to relationships with others, personal strength, and appreciation of life.

It should be noted that measuring the progression of change by differences in the means of outcome variables over time risks overlooking the natural history or complexity of change on PTG. Some studies have therefore focused on 'patterns' or 'profiles' of psychological responses over time. Among women with breast cancer, longitudinal patterns of PTG were heterogeneous in nature. One study showed that three groups of women with breast cancer were stable at different levels of PTG, while two groups increased slightly over time and one group increased significantly. These groups also differed in terms of age, race, chemotherapy, disease intrusiveness, depressive symptoms, active-adaptive coping, and social support (Danhauer et al., 2015). Over the first year after breast cancer surgery, patients showed different patterns of PTG, characterised by stable high (the highest PTG and remained high over time, 27.4%), high decreasing (high at the beginning PTG but decreased somewhat over time, 39.4%), low increasing (minor increases over time, 16.9%), and low decreasing (quadratic and significant downward trend over time, 16.9%). Different patterns of PTG also brought different levels of adjustment (anxiety, depression and positive affect) over time (a 12-month period) (Wang et al., 2014). The low increasing group reported higher levels of anxiety than the other three groups; the low increasing and high decreasing groups had higher levels of depression than the stable high group. The stable high group reported higher levels of positive affect than the other three groups, while the high decreasing group reported higher levels of positive affect than the low decreasing group (Wang et al., 2014).

Also PTG was conceptualised for breast cancer patients in terms of four types of adaptation profile after cancer treatment. These were distressed (high levels of negative coping, depression, and a high likelihood of receiving a full-PTSD diagnosis), resistant (low levels of distress, growth, depression, and negative coping or positive coping), constructive growth (experiencing growth and improvements in reducing negative coping or increasing positive coping over time), and struggling growth (i.e. coexistence of high levels of distress, use of both positive and negative coping strategies and report of PTG). Most transitions between the different adaptation profiles occurred between 6 and 12 months after treatment (Pat-Horenczyk et al., 2016).

Some studies compared the course of PTG and PTSD and found that while PTG increased, psychological distress decreased 3–9 months after breast cancer diagnosis. PTG correlated with lower psychological distress. That is, 3 months after diagnosis, survivors developed PTG at a low level while receiving chemotherapy (Liu et al., 2014). However, in a later study with a shorter follow-up of 6 months, the pattern was reversed: breast cancer survivors showed an increase in their PTSS symptoms but a slight decrease in PTG (Gallagher et al., 2018). These findings mirror a previous study of adolescent and young adult cancer survivors indicating an association between increased PTSD and reduced PTG (Yi & Kim, 2014).

A recent study found further different patterns of PTSS and PTG in patients with breast cancer: resisting patients (34.6%), who reported mild levels of PTSS and PTG; growth patients (47.4%), who reported mild levels of PTSS but high PTG; and struggling patients (18.0%), who had high levels of PTSS and PTG. The growth group tended to include patients with high levels of social support, while the struggling group tended to have the highest levels of anxiety and depression. These heterogeneous posttraumatic responses may have implications for the provision of different healthcare for breast cancer patients with different patterns of response (Liu et al., 2020).

In addition to 'profiles', research has also focused on 'resources' (things that people currently own and value or plan to acquire in the future). They have been characterised in terms of hedonistic and vital resources, spiritual resources, family resources, economic and political resources, and power and prestige resources. Four latent profile classes of psoriasis patients and five classes of cancer patients were identified, all with varying levels of resources. The five classes were patients with (1) high levels of hedonic and vital resources, (2) low levels of spiritual and family resources, (3) high levels of all types of resources, (4) low levels of vital resources and power and prestige resources, and (5) low levels of all types of resources. They differed significantly in PTG, as the level of PTG was higher in the third class of cancer patients than in the fifth class of cancer patients, higher than in the third class of psoriasis patients, and higher than in the control group (no chronic diseases). The heterogeneity of this clinical sample is apparently reflected in the fact that no single pattern of PTG was found to be relevant for all individuals, even if they experienced the same type of traumatic event (Rzeszutek et al., 2020).

Some controversial issues in the relationship between PTG, PTSD and psychiatric comorbidity in cancer survivors

This double-edged sword phenomenon, where PTG and distress coexist in cancer patients, can indeed be controversial. When patients with lung cancer reported PTSD, with prevalence rates ranging from 5% to 16%, they also had PTG, which was positively correlated with PTSD (Dougall et al., 2017). Whereas increased PTSD was associated with decreased psychological well-being, increased PTG correlated with better physical health quality of life and longer survival. These associations persisted after controlling for disease variables and attrition rates due to death or illness (Dougall et al., 2017). PTG was also correlated with adjustment and positive affect in patients with cancer of the digestive system. On the other hand, PTSS correlated with reduced scores on the above outcomes but was associated with increased negative affect. Seemingly, PTG contributed to better adjustment and positive affect. It also moderated the detrimental effects of PTSS on adjustment and positive affect when patients were recovering from cancer (Ben-Zur et al., 2015). Despite the above evidence for the maladaptive and adaptive roles of PTSS and PTG respectively, the nature of these roles is not always consistent. One study showed that PTG and PTSD were associated with poorer quality of life, lack of social support, and an avoidant coping style in women with ovarian cancer, which was likely associated with distress (Shand et al., 2018).

Despite the strong association between PTSS and PTG, this relationship has not been robust in adult survivors of childhood cancer. This raises the question of whether PTSS is a prerequisite for PTG (Klosky et al., 2014). One study examined the relationship between PTSS and PTG in childhood cancer survivors and surprisingly found that the three PTSS severity groups (none, mild and moderate) did not differ significantly in PTG scores. Furthermore, no significant relationships were found between total PTSD and PTG at 12-month follow-up (Zebrack et al., 2015). Similarly, a recent study showed that there were no significant associations between PTG and the PTSS total score and the PTSS clusters (re-experiencing, avoidance, and arousal) in childhood cancer survivors. Instead, increased PTG correlated with increased fear of cancer recurrence. In other words, there was no evidence that PTG and PTSS were directly related in these survivors (Koutná et al., 2020). A systematic review also showed that among women with breast cancer, only a relatively small percentage, between 2.4% and 19%, developed PTSD, although the majority (between 83% and 98%) reported PTG. PTSD and PTG were not associated (Koutrouli et al., 2012).

Furthermore, studies demonstrating the relationship between PTSD and PTG have often suggested that this relationship is linear. This linear effect of PTSD on PTG was confirmed in a study that looked at childhood cancer survivors; a curvilinear relationship was not found (Yi & Kim, 2014). However, a later study claimed that curvilinear relationships were found between the symptom of re-experiencing and some of the domains of PTG (new possibilities, personal strengths) in young adult cancer patients (Zebrack et al., 2015). Similarly, when looking at general stress in breast cancer survivors, after controlling for confounding factors (age, education, and time since diagnosis), a curvilinear effect of general stress was found on PTG. Moderate levels of general stress were correlated with the greatest PTG (Coroiu et al., 2016).

The relationship between PTG and psychiatric comorbidity is also unclear. PTG is not necessarily related to psychological distress such as depression, general well-being (Abdullah et al., 2015; Cordova et al., 2001; Moore et al., 2011; Schroevers & Teo, 2008), anxiety, or affectivity (Abdullah et al., 2015; Koutrouli et al., 2012; Salsman et al., 2009). A meta-analysis also showed that PTG was not associated with depression when the literature as a whole was considered (Long et al., 2021). Even in those cases where PTG was associated with comorbid psychiatric symptoms, the way in which these were related was somewhat inconsistent. Among adolescent and young adult survivors of childhood cancer, those who had higher levels of PTG in young adulthood tended to have poorer health perceptions and emotional health in later adulthood. In addition, higher PTG was associated with factors such as severe chronic health conditions and cancer recurrence/relapse. Survivors with a higher PTG may experience negative effects of cancer, although the positive effects may also be felt (Weinstein et al., 2018).

Further ambiguities between PTG and psychiatric comorbidity can be found as follows. On the one hand, a systematic and critical review concluded that PTG can reduce depression and anxiety (Casellas-Grau et al., 2017). A later study confirmed this finding, showing that breast cancer survivors who recovered from depression had higher levels of PTG than those who still had depression (i.e. patients who reported depressive symptoms within 1 month of diagnosis and follow-up) and who were now depressed (patients who reported depressive symptoms only at follow-up) (Romeo et al., 2020). On the other hand, other studies showed that head and neck cancer patients had less anxiety and depression over time (6 months and 1 year), but also less PTG (Abdullah et al., 2015). In addition, young adult survivors of childhood cancer did not differ significantly from the general control group in terms of depression and anxiety, but had more PTSS and PTG than the control group (Kamibeppu et al., 2010). Although depression was more strongly associated with decreased PTG in cancer survivors than in people without cancer, certain facets of PTG were associated with increased anxiety in people without cancer, although the effect sizes for these relationships were small (Long et al., 2021).

Factors associated with posttraumatic growth in cancer

Based on the discussion in the two previous sections, it can be concluded that the relationship between PTG and psychological adjustment needs closer examination (Salsman et al., 2009). PTG is not just about reducing distress after illness; and focusing only on the relationship between PTG and psychological distress can present a rather narrow view of how growth works (Cordova et al., 2001). With this in mind, the factors that influence cancer-related PTG should be examined.

Demographic factors

Socioeconomic status (SES) may influence mental health in cancer survivors. Individuals with low SES reported poorer mental health, and the association between low SES and more positive mental health was only partially confirmed. On the other hand, high SES survivors were about 50% less likely to report anxiety and depression of clinical significance. However, when positive mental health is measured by positive self-evaluation and meaning of cancer, low SES survivors reported higher levels of these outcomes than high SES survivors. It appears that low SES cancer survivors may have both negative and positive mental health (Andrykowski, Aarts, et al., 2013).

Employment and income level are SES factors that could influence PTG in cancer survivors. Women with breast cancer who were employed or married tended to report better relationships with others, new possibility in life, and more appreciation in life. PTG was associated with life at work, with PTG being highest among survivors who were retired, PTG moderate among those who were employed, and PTG lowest among those who were on sick leave (M.-L. Wang et al., 2014). Increased growth was also associated with higher income (Cordova et al., 2001), including household income (M.-L. Wang et al., 2014). Unexpectedly, increased cancer-related financial stress correlated with increased PTG (Sharp et al., 2018). In other words, both positive and negative financial situations could play a role in stimulating growth (Bellizzi et al., 2007).

The geographic location in which cancer survivors live also plays a role in influencing PTG. Women with breast cancer who lived in rural areas differed from those who lived in non-rural areas in terms of levels of PTG. This could be due to fewer resources and available peer support groups (LeBarre & Riding-Malon, 2017). Survivors of lung cancer who lived in rural areas reported more PTG than survivors who lived in urban areas. There was a mediation effect, which was that distress (anxiety and depression) transmitted the effects of living in rural areas to PTG. Specifically, living in the countryside could have increased anxiety or depression, which in turn was associated with increased PTG. Similarly, living in the countryside might have decreased the mental health aspect of quality of life (poorer mental health), which was associated with increased PTG (Andrykowski et al., 2017).

Gender is another demographic variable that plays a role in promoting PTG. Women tend to report more overall growth than men (Sharp et al., 2018; Tallman et al., 2010; Tong et al., 2012; Yi et al., 2015). On the other hand, patients who had terminal cancer and had low-level PTG were more likely to be male (Tang et al., 2015). A more recent study confirmed the above findings and showed that men had lower levels of PTG than women (Hamdan et al., 2022). Specifically, female cancer patients reported higher levels of new possibilities, spiritual change, and appreciation of life compared to men (Bellizzi, 2004). An integrative review also argues that women with breast cancer tend to have a new perception of self, relationships with others, a new philosophy of life, and a spiritual and religious awareness of their experiences. In addition, personal characteristics (age, education, personality), disease-related factors (time since diagnosis, stage of cancer, types of treatment, perception of the disease on one's life), cognitive processing (positive attentional bias, positive cancer-related rumination, processing and seeking attribution of what happened to them), coping styles (problem-focused coping, emotion-focused coping, positive cognitive coping), social support, religious and spiritual awareness, the role of their body (how the damaged body and coping with physical suffering might affect PTG), and physical activities were all related to PTG in these women with breast cancer (Zhai et al., 2019).

Surprisingly, in mothers of breast cancer survivors, increased worry about cancer recurrence correlated with increased depression in mothers who had high levels of PTG but not in mothers with low levels of PTG. Increased cancer-related parental self-efficacy correlated with lower depression in mothers with low levels of growth. The study concluded that PTG may act as both a protective and risk factor for depression in mothers who are breast cancer survivors (Kuswanto et al., 2020).

Age also plays a role in influencing PTG. Higher PTG correlated with younger age at diagnosis and psychological distress in women with breast cancer (Koutrouli et al., 2016). Younger women with breast cancer also reported increased PTG one-and-a-half years after diagnosis (Cordova et al., 2007). A longitudinal study confirmed this finding in cancer patients who had undergone bone marrow transplantation; increased PTG in the post-transplant period was associated with younger age (Widows et al., 2005). In adult patients treated for acute leukaemia, an increase in PTG over time correlated with younger age (Danhauer, Russell, et al., 2013). In survivors of neck cancer, an increased level of PTG also correlated with younger age (Sharp et al., 2018). Notably, younger women with breast cancer (aged ≤50 years) reported higher levels of appreciation of life than older women (Andysz et al., 2015). Conversely, older patients (aged ≥55 years) reported lower levels of positive growth than younger patients (aged 26–41 and 42–54 years) (Bellizzi, 2004). Similarly, younger patients with breast cancer tended to have increased PTG (Paredes & Pereira, 2018) and approach-oriented coping; an expansive time perspective and positive mood were associated with PTG in younger women (Boyle et al., 2017). Although older women also experienced PTG, they also perceived the negative impact of the cancer experience (Boyle et al., 2017).

Furthermore, increased generativity was associated with increased PTG (Bellizzi, 2004). Generativity refers to, among other things, maintaining the well-being and welfare of the next generation and the desire to contribute to society. These are positive personality traits that are consistent with the positive orientation of growth. In this sense, it is not surprising that the two are correlated. One could even go a step further and consider the possibility of including generativity traits as part of the facets of PTG. Perhaps trauma (in this case cancer) could affect one's relationship with others (a facet of PTG) by decreasing concern for oneself but increasing concern for the continuation or improvement of the lives of others and the community as a whole. Younger cancer survivors showed more generative behaviour than older cancer survivors of different types (Bellizzi, 2004). This finding is somewhat surprising when one considers that generativity is a psychological reaction that, according to Erikson's stages of ego development, tends to occur in middle adulthood (Erikson, 1968).

However, this relationship between younger age and PTG is not always consistent. In adolescents with cancer, higher levels of PTG have been associated with older age at diagnosis (Weinstein et al., 2018). In young adult survivors of childhood cancer, older age has been associated with higher PTG (Yi & Kim, 2014; Yi et al., 2015). Similarly, older survivors after haematopoietic stem cell transplantation reported greater spirituality than younger survivors (Tallman et al., 2010). Among terminally ill cancer patients, those who had low levels PTG tended not to be middle-aged (Tang et al., 2015).

Ethnicity also plays a role in the experience of PTG, although it has been argued that help-seeking behaviour is more important for cancer survivors to cope with stress and experience of PTG than ethnicity. Such behaviour is more important than cultural background or personality. However, this claim has been contested in that cultures and ethnicity need to be taken into account as they would help us understand the psychological mechanisms of PTG and help-seeking behaviour (Matsui & Taku, 2016).

PTG was greater among non-white young adults who had survived childhood cancer (Yi et al., 2015). Hispanic women reported higher levels of new possibilities in life, personal strength, relationships with others, and spiritual change than non-Hispanic white women (Smith et al., 2008). Childhood cancer survivors who were of both Hispanic and Anglo culture were correlated with PTG, although Hispanics had the highest scores of PTG (Tobin et al., 2018). Compared to white breast cancer survivors, African American survivors reported higher scores of PTG (Bellizzi et al., 2010). Among young black cancer survivors, benefit finding correlated with greater illness intrusions, and undergoing chemotherapy (Conley et al., 2020). Patients from Taiwan had higher levels of spiritual and interpersonal PTG than people from Hong Kong, possibly due to some cultural differences and the availability of psychosocial support for cancer patients in the two countries (Ho et al., 2013).

One study examined ethnic differences in relation to acculturation discrepancy. Such a mismatch occurs when non-native parents of Hispanic children adapt to the host culture more slowly than their children. This phenomenon can also occur when children reject or have never known their parents' original home culture, while the parents maintain their culture of origin. Hispanic acculturation discrepancy was negatively correlated with psychosocial health in Hispanic survivors of childhood cancer, while Anglo-American acculturation discrepancy was positively associated with PTG and overall quality of life in Hispanic survivors of childhood cancer (Slaughter et al., 2021).

Some of the aforementioned demographic variables (ethnicity × age) interact to influence the relationship between PTG and mental and physical health. Based on patients who had cancer or HIV/AIDS, a meta-analysis shows a strong relationship between PTG and positive psychological adjustment in younger cancer survivors or mixed samples with ≥25% non-white survivors. Mixed samples with >75% white survivors or older survivors showed a stronger negative relationship between growth and psychological adjustment. Mixed samples with ≥25% non-white survivors showed a stronger relationship between PTG and physical health (Sawyer et al., 2010).

Education has also been associated with PTG (Maners & Champion, 2011) for breast cancer survivors (M.-L. Wang et al., 2014), shortly after a breast cancer diagnosis (Danhauer, Case, et al., 2013). PTG also correlated with the education of adult children of cancer patients (Teixeira & Pereira, 2013a). In particular, terminally ill cancer patients who had a low PTG tended to have low levels of education (Tang et al., 2015). On the other hand, cancer patients who underwent bone marrow transplantation and were less educated tended to have higher growth (Widows et al., 2005). Similarly, women who had breast cancer and had not attended university tended to improve their relationships with others (Bellizzi & Blank, 2006).

Past trauma

In patients with hepatobiliary carcinoma, PTG at the time of diagnosis was associated with traumatic life events in the previous 3 years. These events were related to the loss of a loved one or a serious physical injury. On the other hand, events that were not related to death or a life threat, such as divorce, separation, or sudden job change, were usually not associated with PTG (Moore et al., 2011). A relatively recent trauma related to death or life threat may have exacerbated the threat of the cancer diagnosis, which in turn triggered the experience of growth. The possibility of a cumulative or dose–trauma effect of previous trauma for PTG cannot be ruled out. Resilience could have resulted from a combination of previous stressful experiences and the effect of cancer. However, this resilience hypothesis has been challenged, as individuals with previous trauma experiences were more likely to use helpless coping strategies, while individuals without previous trauma experiences were more likely to use problem-focused coping strategies and showed greater PTG (Bellur et al., 2018).

Cancer-specific variables

While some sceptics claimed that cancer-specific stress from breast cancer, cancer site, cancer surgery, or cancer recurrence was not associated with PTG (Casellas-Grau et al., 2017; Coroiu et al., 2016), some studies have documented the opposite result, namely that PTG can be influenced by some specific cancer-related variables, but the evidence for this is mixed. The type of cancer plays a role in influencing the levels of PTG. Whereas breast cancer and prostate cancer survivors showed similar growth (Morris & Shakespeare-Finch, 2011), young adult survivors of childhood cancer who had solid or soft tissue tumours reported lower PTG (Yi et al., 2015). Women with breast cancer have been found to have higher growth than women with cervical cancer (Smith et al., 2008) and colorectal and haematological malignancies. Recurrent breast cancer has also been found to predict increased PTG (Paredes & Pereira, 2018).

Elapsed time since diagnosis and cancer stage were the other cancer-related factors that correlated with PTG (Casellas-Grau et al., 2017). On elapsed time, it was argued that disease duration could influence threat perception. Longer disease duration has been associated with increased PTG (Teixeira & Pereira, 2013a). Among breast cancer survivors, a longer time since diagnosis has been associated with greater PTG (Cordova et al., 2001; Koutrouli et al., 2016) and a stronger association between growth and positive mental health. The shorter the time since diagnosis, the stronger the association between growth and negative adjustment (Sawyer et al., 2010). Although women with breast cancer developed PTG soon after diagnosis, an increase in PTG was associated with a longer time since diagnosis (baseline assessment was conducted within 8 months of diagnosis) (Danhauer, Case, et al., 2013). In adults undergoing treatment for acute leukaemia, increases in PTG over time also correlated with a greater number of days since baseline (within 7 days of their hospital admission or diagnosis) (Danhauer, Russell, et al., 2013). It may be that the stressful effect of the cancer diagnosis needs time to subside in order for the relationship between growth and positive mental health to develop. A recent stressful diagnosis may be too overwhelming for this relationship to develop. However, these findings have been challenged in that a shorter time since cancer diagnosis has been associated with increased PTG in adult survivors of childhood cancer (Yi & Kim, 2014).

Among women with cervical cancer, advanced cancer stage was related to the totality and individual domains of PTG, that is appreciation of life, new possibilities, personal strength, relationship with others and spiritual changes

(Smith et al., 2008). This finding was also confirmed in a later study, which found that advanced cancer stage was related to overall growth in cancer patients of different types (Tong et al., 2012). However, elsewhere it was shown that women with a higher tumour stage in breast cancer had a lower benefit finding than those with a lower tumour stage at diagnosis (Mols et al., 2009). These inconsistencies may indicate that PTG can occur in cancer patients at all stages of the disease (Mols et al., 2009).

Cancer stages indicate a type of threat in cancer patients that has been associated with PTG in women with breast cancer, for example (Kolokotroni et al., 2014b). For terminally ill cancer patients, the threatening and stressful dying process might be so overwhelming that they cannot experience profound PTG (Tang et al., 2015). This could support the claim that people living with life-threatening illnesses and their family caregivers who were confronted with mortality reminders often reported lower PTG or benefit finding than the control group. In addition, a moderation effect was found, stating that mortality reminders were associated with lower PTG/benefit-finding among those who had recently received the diagnosis (Luszczynska et al., 2012). A recent diagnosis might have acted as a reminder of mortality. Apart from this, survivors' responses to PTG might depend on how patients react to the threat of death. Patients who did not let the threat of death defeat them were more likely to report PTG. On the other hand, people who were unaware of their prognosis or struggled to accept it were more likely to report little PTG (Tang et al., 2015).

The above studies mirror those examining whether PTG—particularly in the areas of relationships with others, new possibilities, and appreciation of life—is associated with patients' perceptions of the diagnosis and treatment of, for example, breast cancer as a threat to life or serious injury or a threat to physical integrity, and whether their response to the cancer experience is associated with intense fear of helplessness (i.e. the DSM-IV criteria; American Psychiatric Association, 1994). One study found that 61% of women perceived their breast cancer as a traumatic stressor, 80% viewed their cancer as a threat to life or physical integrity, and 64% responded to their cancer with fear, helplessness, or horror (Cordova et al., 2001). For breast cancer patients who did not perceive their cancer as a life-threatening traumatic experience, PTG tended to help them adjust well after their cancer diagnosis (da Silva et al., 2011), although the relationship between growth and subjective appraisal of threat from the disease is not always consistent (Thombre et al., 2010a). Notwithstanding this, it could be argued that what is ultimately at stake here is not the patient's perception of life threat. Rather, it is about the degree of intrusiveness of the disease. That is, patients' perceptions of how much their cancer diagnosis or treatment affects their work, active leisure time, relationships with loved ones and other aspects of daily life may in turn be related to PTG for cancer survivors (Danhauer, Case, et al., 2013).

Stigma can impact PTG and affect outcomes. Among lung cancer survivors who used to smoke, stigma was associated with increased psychological distress at high levels of PTG among those who stopped smoking before diagnosis. Among those who stopped smoking after diagnosis, stigma was associated with increased psychological distress among those who had low levels of PTG. Although PTG buffers the negative effects of stigma on psychological distress, this effect appears to have been found only among those who quit smoking after diagnosis (Shen et al., 2015).

Self-stigma is another form of stigma in which cancer survivors endorse negative stereotypes about people with their own stigmatised status and believe that these negative stereotypes apply to themselves. This belief may in turn affect how stigmatised survivors interact with others, for example by avoiding them or worrying about how they are perceived by others. Increased self-stigma correlated with decreased quality of life among breast cancer survivors. This relationship was influenced by intrusive thoughts and PTG. Increased intrusive thoughts and reduced PTG carried the impact of self-stigma on quality of life (Wong et al., 2019). To overcome stigma, some cancer survivors could participate in advocacy by actively demanding their rights, defending themselves, resisting, and advocating against discrimination and inappropriate treatment. This is an attempt to promote positive self-realisation through reaction rather than passively accepting the negative images of oneself. Greater participation in advocacy was associated with higher PTG (Yi & Nam, 2017).

Personality traits

Personality traits have been shown to influence PTG. A review study showed that personality traits such as openness and optimism were associated with PTG in women with breast cancer (Kolokotroni et al., 2014b). Openness to experience and feeling inward were also positively associated with growth in women with cancer. Openness refers to the ability to develop an active imagination, appreciate aesthetic beauty or experiences, accept the diversity of life, and have a sense of intellectual curiosity. The sense of innerness is an attempt to seek wholeness. People who have high levels of openness and innerness tend to increase their strength and ability to cope with adversity, to deal more calmly with difficulties or uncertainty in life, or to be at peace with themselves and the world (Jaarsma et al., 2006).

As mentioned earlier, optimism is also positively correlated with PTG (Bozo et al., 2009; Moore et al., 2011; Schwabish, 2011; Tallman et al., 2010), although this relationship is not always consistent (Smith et al., 2008). The way we cognitively process and explain why we experience good and bad events may have an impact on PTG and PTSD symptoms in cancer patients. Cultivating an optimistic explanatory style (internal, stable, and global) for good events is likely to increase self-perceived positive changes after breast cancer diagnosis and treatment. Breast cancer patients who believe that good events and positive changes can occur because of their own efforts (internal), that they can occur in many different areas of their lives (global), and that these positive changes are permanent (stable) tend to report greater growth. On the other hand, their explanation for why they experience bad events is associated with increased PTSD symptoms. Globalising the causes of good or bad events has been shown to be the most important predictor of growth or PTSD (Ho et al., 2011).

Despite the literature on the role of optimism, this personality trait does not appear to make a unique contribution to growth. It affects growth alongside other coping strategies such as social support (Tallman et al., 2010; Yi et al., 2015). Breast cancer survivors who have high levels of dispositional optimism and perceived social support are more likely to develop PTG. In particular, social support from a private individual may moderate the association between dispositional optimism and PTG (Bozo et al., 2009). In other words, optimism alone is not enough to increase growth, but feeling that you also have social support is important. Problem-focused coping also plays a role in influencing the relationship between optimism and growth in postoperative breast cancer patients. Optimistic patients are more likely to use problem-focused coping strategies, which in turn lead to the development of PTG. Emotion-focused coping, on the other hand, does not (Büyükaşik-Colak et al., 2012).

Some researchers focused on optimism as a form of positive feeling associated with PTG. However, PTG is not associated with negative feelings such as neuroticism, avoidance, anxiety, and depression. One interpretation could be that growth does not act as a buffer against negative feelings. Rather, it seems to be triggered by positive or optimistic feelings (Jaarsma et al., 2006; Maners & Champion, 2011). Although PTG may not be associated with anxiety as a negative emotion, this relationship seems to change when distinguishing between state anxiety and trait anxiety. PTG has been associated with state anxiety rather than trait anxiety (Maners & Champion, 2011). In other words, experiencing anxiety triggered by a particular situation seems to affect our sense of growth.

There have been studies looking at the link between resilience and PTG, although whether resilience should be conceptualised as a personality trait or a skill is debatable (Leys et al., 2020). Among women who had breast cancer, trait resilience was associated with high levels of perceived growth and health-related quality of life, particularly among those who used positive acceptance as a coping measure. In contrast, negative-affect coping was associated with low levels of health-related quality of life and not with perceived growth (Tu et al., 2020). It appears that resilience and positive coping interact to influence PTG and health outcomes of cancer survivors.

To examine the youth's adaptation to cancer, three profiles of resilience and growth were identified: resilient high growth (42.1%), resilient low growth (21.4%), and mild distress with growth (36.5%). The majority of these survivors were resilient, including those who experienced high levels of stress and still managed to derive some benefit from their illness. Peer relationships, demographic factors, and disease-related factors were associated with these profiles. In particular, the youth's relationships with peers played an important role in their adjustment to stressful life events (Tillery et al., 2017; Tillery et al., 2016).

A later study examined paediatric cancer survivors and identified three groups: a resilience group (65%) characterised by good psychosocial adjustment; a self-reported at-risk group (23%) characterised by subclinical elevations in self-reported internalising and attention problems; and a parent-reported at-risk group (12%) characterised by subclinical elevations in parent-reported internalising, externalising and attention problems, and self-reported attention problems. The majority of these survivors demonstrate resilience and are distinguished from the other groups by higher levels of positive affect and school connectedness and lower levels of childhood PTSD, negative affect, and parental distress and overprotection. Positive affect and strong school connectedness were among the protective factors (Okado et al., 2018). A recent study also examined PTG and emotional distress in adolescents and young adults with cancer. Four groups emerged that were resilient, resilient growth (18.8%), distressed, distressed growth (30.4%) over time. Compared to the adolescents and young adults with cancer assigned to the resilient-growth profile, the adolescents and young adults from the distressed and distressed-growth profiles reported lower levels of health-related quality of life, even after controlling for demographic, clinical and social factors (Chen et al., 2020).

Coping: rumination

It has been suggested that coping in cancer survivors such as women with breast cancer is related to PTG (Tomita et al., 2017). Rumination can be conceptualised as a type of coping in which people repeatedly and passively focus on the causes and consequences of their distress symptoms, that is do not use active coping strategies or problem-solving skills to alleviate distress symptoms (Nolen-Hoeksema, 1991). Although rumination has not been associated with PTG in women with breast cancer (Villanova Quiroga et al., 2020b), there is evidence that different types of rumination can affect PTG in different ways.

Positive cancer-related rumination mediated the relationship between dispositional hope and increased PTG for childhood cancer survivors. Negative cancer-related rumination, on the other hand, mediated the correlation between depression and anxiety (Yuen et al., 2014). However, the mediating role of rumination is not always evident. In a study focusing on women with ovarian cancer, rumination did not mediate the relationship between social support and PTG (Hill & Watkins, 2017). Despite this lack of mediation effect, a systematic review concluded that rumination and social support were related to increased PTG in women with breast cancer (Villanova Quiroga et al., 2018).

Deliberate rumination (i.e. consciously thinking about how the cancer experience affects oneself) predicted growth (Hill & Watkins, 2017; Kolokotroni et al., 2014b; Mundey et al., 2019; Ramos, Costa, et al., 2018). Deliberate rumination shortly after death in cancer patients and recent deliberate rumination mediated the impact of quality of death on PTG (Hirooka, Fukahori, Taku, et al., 2017). To help cancer survivors more effectively, it has been argued that deliberate rumination should be promoted with emotional intelligence, which was also correlated with PTG (Mundey et al., 2019). On the other hand, intrusive rumination (i.e. thoughts about the traumatic event and limited ability to stop thinking about the event) predicted increased psychological distress and decreased psychological well-being in women with ovarian cancer (Hill & Watkins, 2017) and predominantly PTSD in women with breast cancer (Ramos et al., 2018). This was at odds with a previous study suggesting that intrusive rumination was correlated with PTG in prostate cancer patients (Wilson et al., 2014b).

It has been argued that deliberate rumination and intrusive rumination are indeed linked and influence certain PTG outcomes. One study looked at people with different types of cancer and found that current deliberate ruminations mediated the effects of intrusive rumination (soon after the event) on appreciation of life and the effects of deliberate rumination (soon after the event) on changes in relationships with others (Ogińska-Bulik & Kobylarczyk, 2019). Reflective rumination about the disease (i.e. a purposeful action to turn inward to find cognitive solutions to problems) is another form of rumination that carries the impact of PTG on disease intrusion and psychological distress (Koutrouli et al., 2016). Encouraging people with cancer to ruminate can apparently facilitate growth after trauma (Ogińska-Bulik & Kobylarczyk, 2019).

Positive coping strategies

In cancer survivors, fighting spirit can be conceptualised as positive coping, which is considered the most important predictor of PTG, compared to negative coping, which is characterised by helplessness, hopelessness, anxiety and psychological distress symptoms (Ho et al., 2004). An increase in positive coping strategies over time correlated with an increase in PTG after treatment for breast cancer and after 6 months. This correlation was slightly stronger after 2 years. Five to 15 years after breast cancer diagnosis, positive coping strategies could still have a strong impact on long-term growth, which in turn was associated with psychological well-being (Lelorain et al., 2010). However, a later study contradicted this finding and claimed that the association between positive coping and PTG was no longer found 7 years after diagnosis (Hamama-Raz et al., 2019). Nevertheless, among patients with breast cancer and melanoma, PTG increased over time for both cancers. Positive coping (active coping, planning, self-distraction, positive reframing, humour, and acceptance) and emotional coping (instrumental support, use of emotional support, venting and religion) were also associated with an increase in PTG in both patient groups. Anxiety, emotional functioning as an indicator of health-related quality of life and negative coping, on the other hand, were not correlated with PTG. Substance use was associated with lower PTG 2 years after diagnosis in melanoma and breast cancer (Bourdon et al., 2019).

Positive reappraisal or reframing is also associated with PTG (Morris et al., 2007; Schroevers & Teo, 2008). In women with early breast cancer, positive reappraisal coping predicted PTG and other outcomes of positive mood and perceived health 1 year later. In other words, positive reappraisal coping has a pervasive long-term effect not only on growth but also on health (Sears et al., 2003). In cancer patients who received a bone marrow transplant, increased growth in the post-transplant period was associated with increased use of positive reappraisal of their distressing illness in the pre-transplant period (Widows et al., 2005).

Positive reappraisal or reframing is influenced by previous childhood experiences. Cancer survivors who had secure attachment tend to experience positive reframing, which in turn is related to the development of growth; insecure attachment, on the other hand, is not associated with it (Schmidt et al., 2012). It is somewhat surprising that when examining the PTG of grieving adults following the loss of a family member to cancer, grievers with high levels of attachment anxiety reported a substantial and positive relationship between grief and PTG. In contrast, those with low levels of attachment anxiety reported no such relationship. Attachment avoidance had no effect on the relationship between grief and PTG. It seems that people with high levels of attachment anxiety may benefit from the process of adjustment to loss (Xu et al., 2015).

Growth characteristics include patients' worldviews regarding social roles and relationships, religious beliefs, the meaning of life (Thombre et al., 2010b), and basic trust (i.e. the belief that the world has an unchanging order and meaning and is generally positive towards people). It is worth noting that growth can affect basic trust by positively perceiving that they trust God, live a good and valuable life and make the most of it (Trzebiński & Zięba, 2013). Basic trust was also related to an increased approach to challenges (focusing on cancer-related problems and challenges in personal, social, and professional life), positive reinterpretation of new life situations and PTG. This trust can trigger positive reinterpretation, which in turn can promote PTG after a traumatic cancer experience. Furthermore, the increase in this trust may also reduce helplessness, which in turn was associated with an increase in PTG (Trzebiński & Zięba, 2013).

Positive attentional bias (i.e. an habitual and generalised tendency to selectively focus on the positive aspects in life) and positive cancer-related rumination (i.e. actively thinking about the circumstances, understanding the cancer in different ways, and focusing on positive content of the cancer) were positively related to PTG in women with breast cancer. Neither was associated with PTSD symptoms. Cancer-related rumination partially mediated the relationship between attentional bias and growth. This means that after cancer diagnosis and treatment, survivors' habitual bias towards the positive aspect of life may have led them to think more about, make sense of, and focus on the positive aspect of cancer. This in turn led to more growth. On the other hand, negative attentional biases and negative cancer-related rumination were associated with an increase in PTSD symptoms after cancer diagnosis and treatment, but not with growth (Chan et al., 2011). Positive cognitive processing also appeared to be important in the emergence of PTG after cancer. Positive cognitive processes, together with depression, anxiety, and perceived threat, explained 42.7% of the variance of PTG (Caspari et al., 2017).

Problem-solving is another positive coping. Following bone marrow transplantation, patients who increased their growth in the post-transplant period tended to use many problem-solving skills and seek alternative rewards in the pre-transplant period. Paradoxically, increased growth in the post-transplant period was also associated with increased stressful appraisals of aspects of the transplant experience and increased negatively biased memories of pre-transplant psychological distress (Widows et al., 2005). In other words, although cancer patients perceived their transplant as stressful, they were still able to experience positive changes in their lives provided they acquired problem-solving skills prior to transplantation. Furthermore, there is evidence that problem-solving coping interacts with secure attachment and influences growth. In contrast, there was no association with PTG in individuals with insecure attachment (Schmidt et al., 2012).

Problem-focused coping, which includes problem-solving skills, plays an important role in the development of PTG, for example in postoperative breast cancer patients. Emotion-focused coping, on the other hand, does not (Büyükaşik-Colak et al., 2012). In breast cancer survivors, focusing on improving their situation (problem-focused coping) has been associated with growth (Bellizzi & Blank, 2006; Kolokotroni et al., 2014a; Maners & Champion, 2011), particularly in terms of relationships with others, new possibilities, and appreciation of life (Bellizzi & Blank, 2006; Maners & Champion, 2011). This type of coping may also moderate the links between dyadic adjustment (the quality of marriage) and PTG, social support from family and PTG, and self-efficacy and PTG (Bellur et al., 2018).

Adopting a positive problem orientation (i.e. perceiving problems as challenges, optimistically believing that these problems are solvable, and believing that one has the ability to solve problems) and minimising impulsive or careless problem-solving styles may have an impact on PTG (Markman et al., 2020). This has provided further evidence to support the claim that challenge appraisal (i.e. appraising cancer as a challenge) directly correlates with PTG in people with prostate cancer (Wilson et al., 2014a). Patients recovering from haematopoietic cell transplantation who used this positive-problem oriented coping to face their difficulties—which presumably included distressing emotions related to their disease—reported higher levels of PTG at follow-up (6 and 12 months) than pre-transplant levels. The use of emotional engagement was also associated with the post-transplant period PTG. In contrast, the use of emotional avoidance was not correlated with PTG. Treatment-related factors or post-transplant complications were also not related to PTG. In other words, confronting and dealing with difficult emotions may facilitate PTG in people who have received haematopoietic cell transplantation (Schwartz et al., 2022).

The above findings on the relationship between problem-solving skills, problem-focused coping and PTG are not surprising when one considers that, as mentioned earlier, resilience, strength, the acceptance of pain and suffering, the construction of new meanings, the transformation of oneself, and the development of a positive sense of self form the basis for growth. All this requires the ability to use positive, active, and purposeful problem-focused coping strategies. What follows is a sense of mastery which is also linked to PTG (Schwabish, 2011).

It has been suggested that the positive approaches described above can also be extended to patients' perceptions of whether they are living satisfying lives with positive affect. Women with cancer who perceived or appraised themselves as living satisfying lives tended to report higher levels of PTG than women who did not (Mols et al., 2009). Positive affect was associated with growth, which in turn was associated with the psychological aspect of quality of life and happiness in breast cancer patients (Lelorain et al., 2010).

Coping: Social support

It has been postulated that the incidence of positive change resulting from the cancer experience can range from 30% to 90%, with social support playing an important role (Ogińska-Bulik, 2013). Social support is associated with increased PTG (Bozo et al., 2009; Kolokotroni et al., 2014b; Love & Sabiston, 2011; Morris et al., 2007; Sharp et al., 2018; Tallman et al., 2010; Tomita et al., 2017; Tong et al., 2012). In cancer patients recovering from haematopoietic cell transplantation, increased social support prior to transplantation was found to be associated with increased PTG over time (Schwartz et al., 2022). Even in a study showing that social support was not correlated with overall PTG in women with ovarian cancer, social support was nevertheless associated with increased relationships with others (a PTG domain), lower psychological distress and higher psychological well-being (Hill & Watkins, 2017).

PTG developed soon after diagnosis and increased PTG have been associated with increased social support in women with breast cancer (Danhauer, Case, et al., 2013). Talking to someone about breast cancer before diagnosis is also likely to increase growth (Cordova et al., 2001). In addition, breast cancer-specific social support and cancer worry were associated with increased PTG, while increased general social support and reduced general stress were associated with improved subjective well-being. It appears that two different types of social support influence different psychological outcomes (McDonough et al., 2014).

Benefit finding over time was associated with increased social support in young black breast cancer survivors. A one-point increase in social support correlated with a 0.05 per year increase in benefit finding (Conley et al., 2020). Another study examined PTG in people after prostate cancer and found that factors of peer support correlated directly with PTG. Connecting with peers and gaining an understanding of the cancer experience through peers was important in facilitating PTG (Wilson et al., 2014a).

In young adult cancer survivors, social support predicted psychological growth and stress, with the first prediction stronger than the second. Moreover, social support interacted with physical activity to additionally explain about 13% of the variance in growth. It follows that young adult cancer survivors should seek social support and engage in regular physical activity after their diagnosis and treatment to promote psychological growth (Love & Sabiston, 2011). On the other hand, patients who had low levels PTG tended to have severe distress and receive inadequate social support, be functionally dependent, and be unaware of or have difficulty accepting their prognosis (Tang et al., 2015).

Relational coping is associated with growth (Lelorain et al., 2010), which was more pronounced in patients with a spouse than those without (Leong Abdullah et al., 2019; Tong et al., 2012). Among women who had breast cancer, the presence of a husband/partner correlated with PTG (Villanova Quiroga et al., 2020a). The relationship quality between couples and the spouse's self-esteem and subjective distress could influence PTG in breast cancer survivors. In other words, it is important for breast cancer survivors and their spouses to maintain solidarity in their relationship, which thereby provides healthy relationship support and promotes PTG (Lee et al., 2017). Similarly, breast cancer patients who recently completed treatment tended to report higher levels of marital intimacy than survivors. A higher appreciation of life as a PTG domain was associated with lower anxiety through higher levels of marital intimacy. In other words, greater marital intimacy carried the impact of valuing life on reducing anxiety. Regardless of disease stage, positive changes after breast cancer, particularly in terms of greater appreciation of life, appeared to be associated with greater intimacy, which in turn was associated with lower anxiety (Canavarro et al., 2015).

Emotional and instrumental social support (tangible help with housework, transport or financial matters) and venting are among the characteristics of relational coping (Lelorain et al., 2010). PTG has been shown to be associated with emotional and instrumental social support in survivors of haematopoietic stem cell transplantation (Nenova et al., 2013). While instrumental support was a unique social context predictor of increased growth in survivors of haematopoietic stem cell transplantation, surprisingly, emotional support was found to be unrelated to growth in some studies (Schroevers & Teo, 2008). Notwithstanding this finding, one study found that receiving emotional support 3 months after diagnosis was related to increased PTG 8 years after diagnosis. The effect of receiving actual social support was stronger than the effect of perceived availability of, or dissatisfaction with, social support (Schroevers et al., 2010). In other words, growth was closely related to patients' actual experience of receiving reassuring, comforting, and problem-solving types of emotional support from family or friends, rather than to subjective perceptions of support, that is whether it would be available or how good it would be (Schroevers et al., 2010).

The venting of emotions is associated with the growth dimensions of new possibilities and relationships with others (Schroevers & Teo, 2008). This result is somewhat surprising, as emotion venting is not problem-focused but emotion-focused. It aims to avoid dealing with the problem (Morris et al., 2007) but to offload distressing emotions. In this way, negative or distressing emotions are indeed maintained. But seemingly there is also growth when one avoids active or problem-focused coping strategies and instead uses passive coping strategies by allowing such distressing emotions to linger. This could be why the use of humour is also associated with increased PTG (Schroevers & Teo, 2008). It aims to deflect or mitigate the confrontation with the stress associated with cancer, which also means that the stress is not resolved but is maintained. The same argument can apply to cognitive avoidance, which is also associated with growth (Carboon et al., 2005).

It is possible that these somewhat surprising findings simply reflect the paradoxical nature of PTG, i.e. the coexistence of distress and growth. Even when distress is maintained or left unresolved, it is still the foundation from which growth is sought. Alternatively, some survivors have learned to accept the cancer rather than actively change it. The coping strategies of acceptance predict high levels of PTG. Among adolescents who had completed cancer treatment 2–10 years prior to the study, those who accepted and came to terms with the current situation and expected the worst, that is the possibility of relapse, reported increased growth (Turner-Sack et al., 2012). Similarly, among adolescents with cancer, higher levels of PTG were associated with cancer recurrence (Weinstein et al., 2018). The belief that they might relapse and the use of acceptance coping strategies were also associated with increased PTG (Turner-Sack et al., 2013).

Overall, while the above findings have conveyed the message that social support and PTG are interrelated, social support does not appear to contribute alone but interacts with other factors to influence PTG. In women with breast cancer, PTG along with perceived social support and positive coping reduced depressive symptoms. On the other hand, the use of self-restraining coping increased depressive symptoms (Tomita et al., 2017). Similarly, perceived social support and resilience correlated with increased PTG in colorectal cancer survivors with permanent intestinal ostomies. Resilience carried the impact of perceived social support at PTG. These survivors experienced moderate-to-high PTG, and improving social support and resilience appeared to be important in facilitating PTG (Dong et al., 2017). It was also claimed that adaptive coping carried the influence of social support on growth and the influence of uncontrollability (patients' perception of the degree of uncontrollability of the disease after diagnosis) on growth. It appears that both internal factors such as cognitive appraisal and coping and external factors such as social support are required for growth to occur (Cao et al., 2018).

Participation in a support programme and confiding in health care providers have also been associated with higher PTG for breast cancer survivors. There appear to be ethnic differences, as PTG was higher among non-Hispanic whites and African Americans who participated in the programme, but not among Hispanics/Latinas. Confiding in a health care provider was associated with PTG only among non-Hispanic whites (Kent et al., 2013). Similarly, breast cancer survivors were found to have psychological and social wellbeing related to their subjective experience of social relationships and support, help and mutual support developed through a dragon boat programme (McDonough et al., 2011). PTG was also associated with the amount of help cancer patients gave to other cancer patients and healthy people. There were different motivations for giving help: they helped because they were empathetic and compassionate or because they intended to strengthen their self by helping others or identifying with others; they helped because they had previously been helped by others and now wanted to give back to others. They also helped others to find meaning in life (Trzmielewska et al., 2019).

Though the above studies argue for a link between social support and increased PTG, this relationship is not always consistent (Schmidt et al., 2012). Somewhat surprisingly, there is evidence that how patients perceive the willingness of others (e.g. friends and family members) to express or discuss cancer-related thoughts and feelings is more likely to be related to PTSD symptoms than to growth. Similarly, social inhibition to disclose one's cancer experience has not been found to be related to growth (Nenova et al., 2013). On the other hand, inhibition is related to an increase in PTSD symptoms (Cordova et al., 2007). These studies seem to suggest that survivors' perceptions of others' externally observable attitudes towards their disease or perceptions of their loved ones' degree of willingness to talk about their cancer may influence distress symptoms more than PTG.

Religious coping or spirituality

Higher levels of religious coping or spirituality are associated with increased growth (Conley et al., 2020; Lelorain et al., 2010; Leong Abdullah et al., 2019; Sherman & Simonton, 2007; Smith et al., 2008). Among women with breast cancer (Tomita et al., 2017; Villanova Quiroga et al., 2020a) and bereaved family members of cancer patients (Hirooka et al., 2018), religious belief was associated with PTG; moderate attendance at religious services correlated with high PTG scores (Tobin et al., 2018). Muslims and Buddhists have been shown to have higher levels of PTG than people of other religious beliefs (Hamdan et al., 2022). Religious coping and growth have been associated with psychological well-being and happiness in women who were free of breast cancer 5–15 years after diagnosis (Lelorain et al., 2010). As noted earlier, African American breast cancer survivors reported higher levels of growth than white survivors. The former also used religious coping more than the latter. Religious coping mediated the relationship between racial differences and growth. In other words, survivors from different racial backgrounds may use different levels of religious coping to facilitate different levels of growth (Bellizzi et al., 2010).

However, the types of religious coping may relate differently to PTG. While negative religious coping, characterised by strain and an ominous worldview, was associated with greater distress and lower PTG, positive religious coping, characterised by a sense of love, compassion, and partnership with God, was associated with greater growth (Trevino et al., 2012). It follows that growth may need to be fostered in an environment of safety, security, connectedness, tranquillity, and hope. This could explain why religion influences growth especially in survivors who have a secure attachment experience (Schmidt et al., 2012). The experience of security in childhood may have increased their propensity to experience this sense of safety, connectedness, hope, or even faith in God, which in turn promotes growth. It is perhaps worth noting that hope is the most important predictor of PTG in cancer patients (Leong Abdullah et al., 2019). Depositional hope is a protective factor for childhood cancer survivors and has been associated with PTG, increased positive cancer-related thoughts, and better psychological adjustment (less depression and anxiety) (Yuen et al., 2014). In fact, increased hope was also associated with increased PTG in parents who cared for their children with cancer. Specifically, hope was associated with increases in developing relationships with others, new possibilities, personal strength, and appreciation of life. It appears that hope during a child's cancer may promote PTG in parents (Hullmann et al., 2014).

As mentioned earlier, cancer survivors can promote their growth by accepting their cancer situation and anticipating the worse outcome that will follow. In this way, cancer survivors can accept control over their lives and surrender it to God. As a result, their trust in and dependence on God grows—a sense of divine peace and connection with this higher being during cancer—which subsequently helps them overcome the fear of death. Their spiritual strengthening may be accompanied by increased spiritual support from family, friends, and people from their faith community. As a result, they feel they have the courage to share their spirituality with others, which in turn has a positive impact on the spirituality of their family and friends (Denney et al., 2011).

It has been argued that the important role of peace should not be underestimated. One study examined changes in spiritual well-being, characterised by faith, meaning and peace, and psychological well-being in ovarian cancer survivors. It found that greater peace was associated with lower levels of depression, anxiety, and mood disturbance at 1 year, although meaning and faith were unexpectedly not associated with these outcomes. On the other hand, changes in peace moderated the impact of stressful life events on depression, anxiety and mood disturbance. Specifically, those who had a higher number of life events and lower levels of peace reported the worst psychological outcomes after 1 year. The sense of peace appears to be the most adaptive aspect of spiritual growth in cancer patients (Davis et al., 2018).

As for spirituality, this predicted increased PTG in breast cancer patients. It seems that spirituality should be part of the intervention for women with breast cancer (Paredes & Pereira, 2018). On the other hand, in patients undergoing treatment for acute leukaemia, increased distress was associated with lower spiritual well-being (Danhauer, Russell, et al., 2013). In adult cancer survivors, spiritual well-being at baseline was positively correlated with some aspects of psychological adjustment 1 year later. Spiritual struggle at baseline, on the other hand, correlated with lower psychological adjustment 1 year later. Spiritual well-being and struggle played an important role in psychological adjustment one year later, even when demographic and cancer-related variables were controlled. Spiritual well-being at baseline, but not spiritual struggle, was also associated with increased perceived PTG 1 year later (Park & Cho, 2017).

The link between growth and spirituality has been shown to increase quality of life, psychological adjustment, and positive affect, and to reduce physical discomfort and dysfunction following a cancer diagnosis (Carver & Antoni, 2004; Cotton et al., 1999; Krupski et al., 2006). Furthermore, PTG has been linked not only to spirituality, but also to the use of active–adaptive coping strategies and mental health (Danhauer, Case, et al., 2013). This may be consistent with the claim that having a faith (although being spiritual does not necessarily mean having a religious faith) and using adaptive coping strategies were correlated with PTG in women with breast cancer (Villanova Quiroga et al., 2020a).

It is not surprising that spirituality plays a role in influencing PTG and psychological distress. Spirituality is a general life orientation system that aims to order one's experiences and give direction to life. It offers a way of coping for people who turn inward and focus on faith to respond to a medical crisis such as cancer by praying for strength, seeking support from the church community, and understanding the meaning behind suffering. This affects the quality of one's spiritual life or spiritual well-being, which is characterised by a sense of harmony or purpose after cancer (Sherman & Simonton, 2007).

Meaning-making

It has been postulated that the religious dimension of PTG is related to the process of meaning-making, more specifically the process of integrating the meaning of the traumatic event into one's life. This relationship is stronger than the association between meaning-making and relationship with others as another dimension of growth (Eva, 2006). Meaning-making could motivate women with breast cancer to understand and explore the possible reasons or causes for their breast cancer, which in turn increases growth over time (Cohen & Numa, 2011). One study showed that cancer survivors who put effort into finding meaning behind their cancer experience found their lives meaningful, restored beliefs in a just world, and experienced PTG, which in turn influenced psychological adjustment. It is worth noting that these were young and middle-aged adult cancer survivors (Park et al., 2008) who began the process of meaning-making before later adulthood (Erikson, 1963). However, the tendency to make meaning is not limited to old age, rather to an increased sense of one's own mortality. For Erikson, engaging in the process of meaning-making implies coming to terms with one's own death. In this sense, it is not surprising that adult cancer survivors in young and middle age also engage with this process.

Notwithstanding, emotional processing, which involved exploring the meaning behind their feelings, did not predict PTG, whereas emotional expression (e.g. expressing inner feelings) did. For growth, the expression of emotions over time seems to be more important than a good understanding of the meaning behind those emotions (Cohen & Numa, 2011; Manne et al., 2004). This was also confirmed by another study which showed that PTG was positively related to the expression of emotions about the illness (Jaarsma et al., 2006). However, one study showed that emotion expression was associated with lower resilience, while emotion processing was associated with higher levels of PTG and resilience in young adults with cancer. An interaction effect was also found, which was that low levels of emotional expression were associated with low levels of fear of cancer recurrence, particularly among those who had high levels of emotion processing. It appears that interventions aimed at promoting emotion-regulating coping strategies may be useful in helping young adults adapt and grow in coping with their illness (Darabos et al., 2021).

In examining the relationship between meaning-making and PTG, research has explored this relationship in relation to other variables. For example, some researchers are looking at meaning and purpose and how these might relate to PTG. Meaning, characterised by a sense of understanding and significance in life, and purpose, characterised by defined goals and direction in life, were strongly correlated in cancer patients. During follow-up, meaning correlated with increased PTG and decreased posttraumatic depreciation, while purpose correlated with decreased intrusive thoughts related to cancer. Meaning at follow-up (1 year) correlated with spirituality at baseline, while purpose at follow-up correlated with social support at baseline in cancer patients (George & Park, 2013).

In addition to purpose, research also examined meaning and social support and found that PTG was associated with women with ovarian cancer using meaning and social support to cope with their experiences (Shand et al., 2018). Other studies have examined all of the above constructs together by examining the concept of eudaimonic well-being, which encompasses meaning and purpose in life. They found that it was associated with higher PTG, greater social support, and lower fear of cancer recurrence. Hedonic well-being (e.g. happiness, life satisfaction) was associated with lower levels of sleep disturbance, fatigue, and depressive symptoms (Moreno et al., 2018).

The link between PTG and the sense of coherence, characterised by an integration of meaningfulness, comprehensibility, and manageability of an illness (in this case cancer), was also investigated. High levels of PTG and sense of coherence, as well as the absence of cancer metastases, were associated with less depression in adult cancer patients. Specifically, an increased sense of coherence was associated with lower depression <1 year and >1 year after diagnosis for different types of cancer. That is, being able to understand, integrate, cope with, and make sense of one's cancer can prevent depression in the short and long term (Aderhold et al., 2019).

Other coping strategies

Other forms of coping strategies include information seeking. Whereas PTSD was correlated with increased time spent searching for cancer-related online information (both medical and psychosocial) in breast cancer survivors, PTG was not related to time spent but to searching for information mainly about the psychosocial aspect of cancer. The psychological impact of online information was associated with increased levels of PTG and/or PTSS. PTG was related to lower hope among women. PTSS was associated with lower awareness or insufficient information about the disease, which in turn exacerbated feelings of distress (Casellas-Grau et al., 2018).

An attitude of gratitude can impact PTG and psychological distress. Gratitude correlated with all domains of PTG, psychological well-being, symptom relief, and contentment, and was associated with reduced anxiety, depression, and hostility–irritability. Breast cancer survivors with high and low gratitude differed in PTG and symptoms, but surprisingly not in psychological well-being, with women with high gratitude having higher levels of PTG, positive affect and lower symptomatology (Ruini & Vescovelli, 2013).

Some studies examined emotion regulation (expressive revealing vs expressive suppression) and found that positive affect partially mediated the effects of expressive revealing and general self-efficacy on PTG, and fully mediated the effects of expressive suppression on PTG. Cancer survivors benefited more from expressive revealing than from expressive suppression, as the former was positively correlated with PTG, while the latter was not correlated with PTG in the mediation analysis. In other words, cancer survivors who have high self-efficacy and use effective emotion regulation strategies (expressive revealing) would report more positive affect, which in turn would promote PTG (Yu et al., 2014).

Some other studies focused on PTG and beliefs about oneself. Cancer survivors' sense of meaningfulness or predictability of events in terms of justice and personal luck predicted increased PTG. Belief in a predictable, just world (i.e. people get what they deserve and they deserve what they get; e.g. cancer had happened to them because of some terrible things they had done) was associated with stronger growth. Therapeutically, it would be beneficial for survivors to believe that things would usually turn out well despite different situations or circumstances. This would provide a sense of predictability in uncontrollable circumstances such as cancer. A link was also found between PTG and self-worth. Higher self-worth predicted an increase in the PTG domain of new possibilities. Lower self-worth, as well as completion of treatment, affected the PTG domain of relationships with others. It is somewhat surprising that in patients with haematological cancer, cognitive avoidance and low self-worth and self-control facilitated PTG in the early stages of cancer (Carboon et al., 2005). In addition to looking at self-worth from a cognitive perspective, one study also examined physical self-worth. It showed that physical self-worth predicted persistent stressors. The combination of physical self-worth and persistent stressors explained all dimensions of PTG for breast cancer survivors (Castonguay et al., 2015).

Posttraumatic growth in family caregivers of cancer survivors

The experience of cancer can be extremely stressful not only for the survivors themselves, but also for the family members who care for them. Cancer can affect the entire family, including children or spouses, with each member having their own psychological needs (Levesque & Maybery, 2012). Caring for cancer survivors can impact on psychophysiological outcomes, including increased blood pressure, dysregulation of the autonomic nervous system and hypothalamic–pituitary axis, altered immune function, and poor health-related behaviours (Teixeira et al., 2018).

Notwithstanding this, parents of children with cancer reported positive changes in care at least 6 months after diagnosis, as they appreciated their children and family much more. They also showed more compassion, empathy, patience, inner strength, and perspective on life. However, they also reported some health problems, including sleep disturbances, fatigue, anxiety, depression, social isolation, and changes in social roles. These problems were thought to be due to the distress associated with the cancer diagnosis, the intensive and lengthy treatment, and aftercare (Klassen et al., 2012).

Family caregivers of patients with chronic illnesses, including cancer, may increase positive affect, which correlates with PTG (Hamama & Sharon, 2013). Among parents of children with cancer or type 1 diabetes, 62.7% reported moderate levels of PTG three years after diagnosis (Hungerbuehler et al., 2011). Although carers of cancer survivors with head and neck cancer may experience significant psychological distress in the post-treatment phase of the disease (e.g. worries about the cancer and increased financial burden of caring for their cancer survivor), these carers could also experience PTG and change their self-concept and social world (Balfe et al., 2016). Similarly, carers who cared for their loved ones following haematopoietic stem cell transplantation were able to experience more PTG, which was associated with increased resilience, social support and a positive coping style. Resilience mediated the effects of positive coping style on PTG. On the other hand, lower PTG was related to a passive coping style (Luo et al., 2020).

This mirrors previous research that focused on coping styles: problem-focused coping was adaptive, or positive coping that was associated with lower caregiver burden, lower depression, and better adjustment (Teixeira et al., 2018). Specifically, following a diagnosis of advanced cancer (e.g. hepatobiliary carcinoma) in a loved one (Moore et al., 2011), family caregivers have shown that PTG is associated with increased use of positive religious coping and decreased use of negative coping (Thombre et al., 2010b), with increased benevolent religious reappraisal (positive religious reappraisal) and decreased punishing God reappraisal (negative religious coping) being the strongest predictors. Other predictors were stronger spiritual connection and lower spiritual discontent. One conclusion is that constructing meaning from one's relationship with God is important to foster growth in family caregivers (Thombre et al., 2010b).

Posttraumatic growth also occurred in parents of adolescent survivors 1 year after treatment. PTG was found to be associated with a decrease in anxiety among mothers within 12 months of the end of treatment (Nakayama et al., 2017). For mothers, 58% reported a positive impact on the way they related to others and 50% on how cautious they had become. For fathers, 62% reported changes in their outlook on life. Almost half also reported positive changes in their relationships with others. While factors associated with mothers' growth were limited, time since treatment ended and perceived treatment intensity correlated with fathers' PTG (Barakat et al., 2006). A later study shed further light on the PTG responses of mothers of children with cancer, finding that optimism, disrupted core beliefs, social support, and deliberate rumination explained 41.4% of the variance in mothers' PTG. Social support and deliberate rumination directly influenced PTG in mothers of children with cancer (Kim, 2017).

The study of PTG among family caregivers of cancer survivors should not be conducted independently of the survivors themselves. In one study, about half of the samples—patients with advanced colorectal cancer and family caregivers—reported at least one identical positive change. Patients and caregivers experienced positive changes in the form of closer relationships with others, a greater appreciation of life and faith, a clarification of life priorities, and more empathy for others. Carers also improved their health habits after a cancer diagnosis (Mosher et al., 2017). Another study found differences in PTG between patients and their caregivers. Compared to patients, caregivers reported higher levels of 'personal strength', alongside an association between caregiver anxiety and depression with the same distress outcomes as patients. Younger caregivers were better than older ones in terms of physical activity, vitality, mental health, and social activities (Cormio et al., 2014).

At the time of diagnosis, based on the interclass correlation, there was high agreement (between 0.34 and 0.74) in the level of PTG, particularly in the areas of relationship with others, spiritual change and personal strength, between the rating from patients with hepatobiliary carcinoma and the rating from their family caregivers. Based on patients' and carers' own assessment of growth, significant correlations were also found in relation to spirituality and personal strength (Moore et al., 2011).

For the young childhood cancer survivors, the parent–child relationship played an important role in mediating the impact of parental distress on the adjustment of these young survivors. Increased caregiving was associated with better adolescent adjustment, whereas increased overprotection was associated with poorer adjustment outcomes. For parents, increased relational frustration and reduced attachment mediated the impact of parental distress/ growth on adolescent adjustment. It appears that parental distress and the parent–child relationship played a role in adolescents' adjustment (Schepers et al., 2019).

Caring for cancer survivors could also lead to growth in patients with a serious illness (Loiselle et al., 2011) and their family members without a chronic illness (Hamama & Sharon, 2013), although there could be differences in how both groups of individuals anticipate growth. For survivors, anticipation of growth as a coping process is an important precursor to later development of PTG (Tallman, 2013). They tended to anticipate growth more than collaterals (e.g. spouses, family members, close friends). Family members, however, tended to under-anticipated it (Tallman et al., 2014).

Increased growth in parents and children was related to the level of psychological distress in the parents, the medical characteristics of the children 1 month after diagnosis, and the female gender of the parents (Hungerbuehler et al., 2011). Increased depressive symptoms and stress in parents were also related to increased depressive symptoms in their cancer-surviving children. Parental depression correlated with reduced quality of life in survivors; their perceived stress was also related to reduced quality of life in survivors' PTG. Greater parental psychological distress could have a negative impact on the level of depression in childhood cancer survivors, while lower poor parental health was associated with positive outcomes for childhood cancer survivors' mental health (Slaughter et al., 2020).

When examining caregivers' resilience in caring for their children who received childhood cancer treatment, caregivers had moderate levels of PTG, but high levels of distress and low PTSS compared to norms. Somewhat surprisingly, PTG was not related to PTSS or distress, while PTSS and distress were related (Barakat et al., 2021). These results may have been influenced by family psychosocial risk (in terms of resource needs, social support, problems with the child, family problems and acute stress), which was associated with resilience at the end of treatment. Perceived social support, healthcare self-efficacy, and psychosocial services provided were associated with resilience. In other words, resilience and psychosocial risk at diagnosis most strongly predicted caregiver resilience outcomes at the end of childhood cancer treatment (Barakat et al., 2021).

Children's perceptions of their parents' PTG could also influence the parent–child relationship at PTG (Koutná & Blatný, 2020). Compared to young people who had reported a non-cancer event, young people who had experienced a cancer-related event tended to perceive their parents as responding to the cancer burden with more support, reassurance or distraction. Increased PTG was associated with perceived parental support, reassurance/distraction and increases in adolescent distress. Young people perceived that their parents responded differently to cancer or non-cancer distress, which in turn was associated with their perceptions of growth. In addition, parental support and reassurance or distraction appeared to play a role in promoting resilience and growth in these young people (Howard Sharp et al., 2017).

This could be the reason why conflicts within family relationships as well as perceived support with psychological health and interactions between family members were strongly correlated with psychological distress in young adults with cancer (Kay et al., 2019). This is also why family resilience is so important. As families had increased their family resilience since diagnosis, breast cancer survivors also exhibited moderate levels of PTG, while caregivers reported moderate levels of distress. Family resilience was associated with increased PTG and decreased distress. In other words, family resilience may influence breast cancer survivors' PTG and caregiver burden. To help these survivors, it is important to promote family resilience PTG in these survivors and reduce caregiver burden (Liu et al., 2018).

As cancer survivors and their families live through and process the illness, they tend to come to know themselves and the world more deeply and with new meaning (Duran, 2013). By processing the illness, they see and understand their situation differently, gain some understanding and meaning of the event, reformulate their beliefs and life goals, and integrate this understanding into their global meaning system. They realised that life is fragile and precious and changed their attitude towards life. They also overcame their weaknesses and developed their self-improvement. They improved their self-esteem and felt that they had become better people. Families came together, became more cohesive and integrated, and felt more able to share their feelings with each other. They felt they had something to give back to society because they received help and support from others in coping with their cancer (Duran, 2013).

It is worth noting that although much research has been conducted on the role of the parent–child relationship, other individuals are also involved in the experience of PTG in cancer survivors. For example, one study examined siblings of children with cancer and found that siblings experienced difficult emotions and experienced changes in their lives during cancer, including increased empathy and resilience, improved family relationships, disrupted routines, increased responsibility, and perceived changes in the child with cancer (D'Urso et al., 2017). Female siblings of cancer survivors in particular have been shown to have greater PTG than the control group (Kamibeppu et al., 2010).

Non-family members, such as close friends or medical staff, may also play a role in cancer survivors' experience of PTG. Research showed that interaction with friends was correlated with PTG as well as with PTSD and positive affect. Support from close friends and medical staff appeared to be an important factor associated with psychological health in young adults with cancer (Kay et al., 2019). Similarly, PTG was positively correlated in paediatric cancer survivors not only with their PTSS symptoms, religious coping by parents, strong family relationships, but also with their relationship with their oncologists. Disease-related distress was also associated with increased patient PTSS, increased parent psychological distress, and decreased nurse trust in the family. In other words, both family members and professionals can influence the experience of PTG (Wilson et al., 2016).

Most of the above studies focused on family caregivers of patients who are still alive, whereas some studies looked at bereaved family members. One study found that 47% and 15% of family carers of cancer patients in the palliative care unit were prone to major depressive disorder (MDD) before and after the loss, respectively; about 90% of family carers prone to MDD after the loss were also affected by MDD before the loss. After controlling for background variables, family caregivers' pre-loss depression interacted with resilience to predict post-loss depression. Pre-loss resilience moderated post-loss depressive symptoms, especially among family caregivers who were at high risk of developing depression prior to loss (Shimizu et al., 2021). PTG among family caregivers appeared to be related to quality of life at the end of life in cancer patients. PTG correlated with a good death (i.e. end-of-life care from the family caregiver's perspective), which was correlated with satisfaction with overall care. On the other hand, a good death and PTG were not associated with any health outcomes in bereaved caregivers (Hatano et al., 2015).

Posttraumatic growth in children of parents with cancer

It has been documented that adult children of parents with cancer can show symptoms of distress as well as PTG. Adult children whose parents had cancer and had probable PTSD showed increased PTG. PTSD symptoms were correlated with increased PTG after controlling for demographic and clinical variables (Teixeira & Pereira, 2013b). Elevated PTG for these adult children, with females having higher PTG, correlated with elevated PTSD, parental dependence, and family functioning (Teixeira & Pereira, 2013a).

Among adult children whose parents had terminal cancer or no cancer in childhood, 44% reported different levels of PTG (Wong et al., 2009). Positive changes included improved relationships with their parents, increased emphasis on family, changed life priorities, and personal development (Levesque & Maybery, 2012). Growth was also seen in adolescents coping with their parents' breast cancer. Positive growth responses included a greater appreciation of life, improved interpersonal relationships, a stronger sense of personal strengths, and changed life priorities (Kissil et al., 2010). In addition, these young people noted that their health behaviours and attitudes had changed

(Kissil et al., 2010). This is interesting in that growth is not only associated with changes in the classic PTG areas (e.g. personal relationships, strength, etc.), but also with improved health care for oneself (Tallman et al., 2010). This information may be useful for some adult children (60%) who coped with their parents' cancer in childhood and reported negative consequences, one of which is worry about their own health. Other negative consequences include feelings of loss and emptiness, negative changes in outlook on life, and negative effects on personal relationships (Wong et al., 2009). Other studies also show that both PTG and negative affects often exist in parallel for cancer survivors. Young adults whose parents had cancer in childhood reported more state and trait anxiety than others. Parental cancer outcome or survivorship status predicted the number of cancer-related life changes and moderated the relationship between anxiety and PTG (Metcalf et al., 2017). One study specifically looked at the factors associated with PTG in adolescents who have lost their parents to cancer. Engaging in some ritualistic behaviours helps them cope with the loss. Joining palms in front of their parents' picture or an altar, visiting their parents' graves, and spending time with friends have been associated with increased PTG (Hirooka, Fukahori, Akita, et al., 2017).

Posttraumatic growth in partners or spouses

A cancer such as breast cancer can also be stressful for the partner/husband and may have an impact on the development of PTG (Weiss, 2002; Zwahlen et al., 2010). In breast cancer patients, the patient's PTG was associated with the significant other's cognitive and emotional processing of the breast cancer. The partner's PTG was predicted by more intrusive thoughts and greater use of positive reappraisal and emotional processing (Manne et al., 2004).

The more women with breast cancer perceived their husbands as supportive, the more they reported PTG, which in turn influenced their husband's growth (Weiss, 2004). Husbands' growth was influenced by the increased depth of marital commitment, the increased amount of growth their wives experienced, and whether the severity of the breast cancer met criteria for posttraumatic stress DSM-IV (Weiss, 2004). Although breast cancer patients reported more PTG than their husbands, the patients' marital adjustment was positively associated with their own PTG and their husbands' PTG. In other words, promoting marital adjustment is important in facilitating PTG for cancer patients and their husbands (Suo et al., 2022). Among women with breast cancer, the partner's attachment security was correlated with PTG in both couples, while their own attachment security was not associated with their own PTG in either couple. In other words, couple attachment is an inter-dependent phenomenon (Ávila et al., 2017).

Among caring husbands of breast cancer survivors, after controlling for covariates, it was found that higher levels of PTG were associated with higher caregiving burden, higher marital satisfaction, higher challenge appraisal towards the impact of breast cancer, and seeking social support. There was an interaction effect in that positive reframing was associated with higher levels of PTG among those with higher caregiving burdens. In other words, accounting for caregiving husbands' marital satisfaction, challenge appraisal toward the impact of breast cancer and need to seek social support is important in facilitating their PTG. For husbands who had a higher caregiving burden, positive reframing is one way that could help them facilitate their PTG (Yeung et al., 2020).

Following treatment for prostate cancer 1 year after surgery, high levels of negative affect before surgery, the use of positive reframing, and emotional support were associated with high levels of growth after surgery. Partner growth was predicted by younger age, increased intrusive thoughts, and greater use of positive reappraisal and emotional processing. Among partners, PTG after patient surgery was also higher only among those who were employed, had lower levels of education, and had higher cancer-specific avoidance symptoms of stress before surgery, and among those who used positive reappraisal. Interestingly, quality of life was not associated with PTG among patients and partners (Thornton & Perez, 2006).

Based on the above studies, it is not surprising that in patients with different types of cancer, gender, role (patient vs partner), and dyadic relationship were associated with PTG, with dyadic relationship being the strongest factor. Patients reported higher levels of PTG than partners; female participants reported higher growth than males. The type of couple also appeared to have an impact on the results, with male patients and female partner couples reporting a greater association in PTG than female patients and male partner couples (Zwahlen et al., 2010). Regarding the dyadic relationship between couples which may have an important function in the experience of PTG (Zwahlen et al., 2010), the importance of couples facing cancer together and sharing not only the pain but also the potential for gain from trauma cannot be underestimated (Weiss, 2004). The importance of the quality of family relationships (Hungerbuehler et al., 2011), marital satisfaction (Kausar & Saghir, 2010), or a family approach to understanding the positive psychological impact of cancer cannot be overemphasised (Zwahlen et al., 2010).

The facilitation of posttraumatic growth

As adverse consequences and growth characteristics coexist in cancer patients and their loved ones, it is important to minimise these consequences while facilitating PTG (Wong et al., 2009). This is consistent with a post-diagnosis care model for cancer patients with different types which aims to facilitate adaptation during this cancer period (Morris & Shakespeare-Finch, 2011). In addition to the timely identification and management of psychological distress, improving PTG is also important in influencing the long-term quality of life of cancer patients (Wittmann et al., 2017). In other words, PTG is not only a concept of positive psychology that can expand our understanding of human functioning beyond negative, pathological states; it also has important implications for rehabilitation psychology (Ehde, 2010).

Despite claims that evidence for the effectiveness of specific interventions to facilitate growth in cancer patients is limited (Calhoun & Tedeschi, 2000), evidence for the effectiveness of specific interventions for cancer survivors is emerging. Posttraumatic growth along with distress or dysfunction has been found in women who have received chemotherapy or radiotherapy for breast cancer. Increased negative perceptions of the impact of breast cancer have been associated with increased emotional distress and impaired physical and psychological quality of life. However, this depended on the extent of PTG that individuals had experienced due to their cancer. The growth thus acted as a stress buffer, particularly against the stress that affected psychological and social quality of life and depression. It follows that psychosocial intervention programmes should be implemented to facilitate PTG, which in turn should promote better adjustment (Silva et al., 2012). The lack of PTG, on the other hand, has been advocated as having a negative impact on life satisfaction in long-term survivors of adolescent cancer. It has also been associated with impaired overall and health-related life satisfaction (Seitz et al., 2011).

One study examined breast cancer survivors who participated in a resilience-building intervention related to coping and PTG. More than half of the participants improved PTG after 6 months. Compared to the control group (no intervention), those who participated in the intervention reported greater increases in PTG and positive coping. In addition, the proportion of constructive PTG, as opposed to illusory PTG, was higher in the intervention group (89.3%) than in the control group (56.3%) (Pat-Horenczyk et al., 2015).

It was suggested that parents of children with leukaemia who had high levels of anxiety and were at risk of PTSD benefited from interventions aimed at reducing anxiety during and after treatment. At the same time, the aim was to increase self-efficacy in caring for their children after treatment and to focus on the positive changes resulting from the traumatic experiences. This should be the treatment regime for family members of children with cancer (Best et al., 2001).

Although the transition of the cancer experience can be stressful, it is an opportunity to promote personal growth through psychosocial interventions. While dispositional mindfulness in cancer patients predicted psychological distress and PTG and was associated with distress outcomes and adjustment in cancer patients (Omid et al., 2017), an intervention such as a mindfulness-based stress reduction (MBSR) programme has been advocated to potentially alleviate the distressing symptoms associated with cancer diagnosis and treatment. In this way, patients and their family members can improve their ability to adapt and adjust to the disease and its consequences (Carlson et al., 2009). One study found that cancer patients who participated in MBSR improved their spirituality, PTG, and mindfulness. The change in all facets of mindfulness mediated the effect of MBSR on spirituality and PTG. The mindfulness skills that emerged from MBSR may promote a sense of purpose, peace, connectedness, and personal growth in cancer patients (Labelle et al., 2015). In particular, it has been suggested that spirituality and PTG can be promoted (Lechner & Antoni, 2004; Linley & Joseph, 2004) as they have been shown to improve quality of life, positive affect, psychological adjustment, and physical well-being in cancer patients (Carver & Antoni, 2004; Cotton et al., 1999; Krupski et al., 2006).

The effectiveness of mindfulness meditation training in men with prostate cancer was studied. They were randomly assigned to either a mindfulness or an attention control group. In the mindfulness group, prostate cancer anxiety and uncertainty intolerance decreased. On the other hand, scores for mindfulness, global mental health, and PTG increased. Interestingly, mindfulness also increased over time for participants in the control group. But the increase in PTG was greater in the mindfulness group over time than in the control group (Victorson et al., 2017).

This study looked at breast cancer survivors and found that there were no differences between two groups (the MBSR group and the usual care group) before the intervention. Compared to the usual care group, the MBSR group had a higher PTG level after the 8-week intervention and follow-up (3 months later). At the same time, feelings of stress and anxiety decreased after the intervention and 3 months later. Seemingly, MBSR could enhance PTG and reduce perceived stress and anxiety, and the effects lasted for 3 months after the intervention (Zhang et al., 2017).

A randomised controlled trial demonstrated the effectiveness of a mindfulness-based Tai Chi Chuan (MTCC) programme on PTG and psychological distress (perceived stress and anxiety) in breast cancer patients. After the intervention and follow-up, the MTCC group reported higher levels of PTG than the wait-list control group. The intervention group increased the level of PTG, which persisted for 1 year after the intervention. After the intervention, perceived stress and anxiety decreased over time (Zhang et al., 2022).

A meta-analysis also concluded that in terms of the effectiveness of psychosocial interventions for PTG in cancer patients, the intervention groups had higher overall scores compared to the control group PTG. Mindfulness-based interventions were the most effective and were used most frequently. In particular, psychosocial interventions had a greater effect on breast cancer patients than on patients with other types of cancer. In other words, psychosocial interventions for cancer patients were effective in facilitating PTG (Li et al., 2020). A systematic review also examined the literature on mindfulness-based programmes for cancer patients. It showed that eHealth mindfulness-based programmes (eMBPs) can improve not only PTG, but also mental health (stress, anxiety, depression), fatigue, sleep problems and pain, as well as general health. The effectiveness of eMBP is comparable to that of face-to-face MBPs. It seems that eMBP is a viable method to help cancer patients (Matis et al., 2020).

Studies have been conducted to examine the effectiveness of meaning-centred group psychotherapy for cancer survivors (MCGP-CS). They found that, compared to a usual care group, this intervention showed stronger treatment effects on personal meaning, goal orientation, positive relationships, life purpose and fighting spirit (post-intervention), helplessness/hopelessness at 3-month follow-up, and distress and depression at 6-month follow-up. Compared to supportive group psychotherapy, results showed a stronger effect of MCGP-CS on personal growth at 3-month follow-up and environmental mastery at 6-month follow-up. It appears that MCGP-CS was effective for cancer survivors in improving personal meaning, psychological well-being and psychological adjustment to cancer in the short term and in reducing psychological distress in the long term (van der Spek et al., 2017). Another randomised controlled trial with a 2-year follow-up also showed that survivors who received this intervention improved more in positive relationships over time as an indicator of psychological well-being than survivors who received care as a usual intervention; they also reported more personal growth as another indicator of psychological well-being than those who completed supportive group psychotherapy over time (Holtmaat et al., 2020).

This meaning-centred approach is also reflected in a recent finding indicating a positive relationship between PTG, the presence of and search for meaning in life, and life satisfaction. There was a mediation effect in that the presence of meaning in life carried the impact of PTG on life satisfaction. Seemingly, it is essential to promote PTG, meaning in life and life satisfaction, which will ultimately protect survivors' daily functioning (Mostarac & Brajković, 2021). However, a network analysis showed that among cancer survivors, life satisfaction was only marginally associated with PTG (Adamkovič et al., 2022).

Other studies also examined other forms of intervention aimed at facilitating PTG. For example, one study examined a psychosocial intervention at PTG for Chinese American breast cancer survivors. Those who received the group support intervention (Joy Luck Academy (JLA)) were compared with Chinese American breast cancer survivors who received routine care. Those who participated in the JLA intervention improved their PTG, particularly in terms of meaningful interpersonal relationships, appreciation of life, finding new possibilities in life and personal strength over time. On the other hand, routine care participants reported no significant change in any of these outcome variables. It appears that such psychosocial intervention may promote PTG in cancer survivors (Chu et al., 2022).

However, a systematic review showed that both exercise and psychosocial interventions have limited effects on patients with bladder cancer. One to three studies found positive effects of exercise on physical fitness, health-related quality of life (HRQoL), personal activities of daily living, and muscle strength. Psychosocial interventions showed positive effects on anxiety, fatigue, depression, HRQoL and PTG, especially in one study. The conclusion from this review is that the evidence for the effects of exercise on patients with bladder cancer is limited, and is even less for psychosocial interventions (Rammant et al., 2018).

The above findings were somewhat surprising given that exercise most strongly predicted the positive association with PTG in breast cancer survivors (M.-L. Wang et al., 2014). It has also been shown that for lung cancer survivors, due to their older age, poor functional status, and reduced lung capacity, it may be beneficial to reduce sedentary time but to increase physical activity at a low intensity (Vallance et al., 2018). Among gynaecological cancer survivors, increases in physical activity (i.e. the extent to which the cancer diagnosis itself led to changes in the amount, type, or nature of exercise activities) were significantly associated with PTG. The physical activity increase items explained 37.2% of the variance in PTG, 19.9% of the variance in the positive impact of cancer, and 23% of the variance in benefit finding. Apparently, for these survivors who want to increase PTG, it may be important to change the amount, type, and/or nature of their physical activity after diagnosis (Crawford et al., 2015). Another study also showed that wall climbing can facilitate some aspects of PTG, particularly in terms of discovering new possibilities, personal strength, and psychological well-being for gynaecological cancer survivors (Crawford et al., 2016).

Furthermore, women with primary breast cancer who received psycho-spiritual integrative therapy reported short-term improvements (1 month after treatment) in, for example, physical, emotional, and functional well-being, as well as mood, depression, anger, and fatigue. They also became more spiritually aware, and more aware of new possibilities in life and personal strength (Garlick et al., 2011). Women with breast cancer who participated in dragon boat programmes reported benefits in terms of social support, shared challenges and understanding of survivorship, a sense of personal control, the development of a new identity as an athlete, and the ability to overcome physical challenges, all of which contributed to an increase in psychological growth (Sabiston et al., 2007).

Other interventions have also been documented. People with advanced cancer and nurses who delivered the intervention appeared to be satisfied with the life review intervention (Revie ⊕ intervention), which focused on developing strength and resources for patients (da Rocha Rodrigues et al., 2019). After the motivational interviewing-based self-efficacy intervention, lung cancer patients did not differ in terms of PTG from the group receiving usual care. However, they reduced anxiety and depression, improved self-efficacy, quality of life, confrontational coping, social support, and functional capacity more than the group receiving usual care (Huang et al., 2018).

Similarly, a multiple health behaviour change intervention (CanChange) for colorectal cancer survivors showed significant intervention effects for PTG at 6 and 12 months, for spirituality and acceptance at 6 months, and for quality of life at both 6 and 12 months (Hawkes et al., 2014). After positive psychotherapy for cancer, cancer survivors reported greater reductions in distress and PTSD symptoms compared to the control group, but an increase in PTG over time (3 and 12 month periods) (Ochoa et al., 2017). Parents of children with cancer also appeared to benefit from the Thank You–Sorry–Love (TSL˚) programme at PTG and cortisol levels. Cortisol levels were found to differ at post-test between mothers of children with cancer who had received the programme and those who had not (Choi & Kim, 2018). This is consistent with previous research showing an association between PTG and diurnal cortisol slope (i.e. a relationship between positive psychological changes and healthier endocrine function) in women with metastatic breast cancer. It appears that people with PTG have more normal (i.e. steeper) diurnal cortisol patterns in response to cancer-related stress (Diaz et al., 2014).

Though facilitating PTG is highly advocated in the literature, there is a warning that the relationship between growth and adjustment may be much more complex than previously thought. Individuals with high or low growth at baseline had fewer depressive symptoms than those with moderate growth. People with high or low growth had better physical health 3 months later than people with moderate levels of growth. The high-growth group did find the cancer distressing and reported intrusive thoughts about their diagnosis, but interpreted it more positively than the other groups. The low-growth group found the cancer less stressful and had less intrusive thoughts than the other groups. The moderate-growth group, however, perceived the cancer as more stressful and had more intrusive thoughts, especially compared to the low-growth group. Increased growth may not always have better therapeutic effects on patients (Tomich & Helgeson, 2012).

Similarly, breast cancer survivors who volunteered to work with newly diagnosed breast cancer patients were compared to non-volunteers. Although both groups reported significant levels of PTG, there were no significant differences in growth between them. The volunteers reported a higher level of health outcomes, which surprisingly was not related to growth. On the other hand, better health was associated with higher growth among the non-volunteers (Cohen & Numa, 2011). The relationship between growth and adjustment is complex (Tomich & Helgeson, 2012) and requires further clarification.

Some researchers have even questioned the real or illusory nature of growth and its adaptive value (Sumalla et al., 2009). The motivation behind the study of PTG in cancer patients is partly influenced by the attempt to include severe illness as events that might trigger PTSD symptoms, to view cancer experiences from a positive psychological perspective, and to encourage patients to engage in a fighting spirit. However, it is quite difficult to clearly define the processes involved in this subjective sense of growth after a serious illness such as cancer. Consequently, the illusory nature of growth is a possibility that cannot be denied (Sumalla et al., 2009). A longitudinal study (7 years) shows that women with breast cancer who used helplessness–hopelessness coping strategies and had low levels of depression at baseline were more likely to report illusory growth than constructive growth over time. In other words, illusory growth may be a type of coping rather than positive change (Cheng et al., 2020).

Summary

Although cancer is an extremely stressful experience, it can also be an opportunity for growth. After a cancer diagnosis, people can experience both positive and negative changes in themselves. The positive changes are sometimes referred to as PTG, stress-related growth, benefit finding, or adversarial growth. Regardless, they have some basic principles in common: paradoxically, a stressful event such as cancer must be experienced for positive life changes to emerge from adversity. Resilience can emerge from stressful experiences as part of a survival identity or an adaptive reconstruction of the self.

The link between PTG and cancer experiences of various kinds has been demonstrated in the literature. By and large, PTG is a relatively stable and long-lasting phenomenon. Growth has been examined in terms of patterns or profiles of growth related to different levels of distress, adjustment, adaptation, and negative or positive coping strategies used over time. While there is a wealth of evidence linking cancer and PTG, how PTG, PTSD/PTSS and psychiatric comorbidity interact to affect cancer survivors is somewhat controversial. Despite this controversy, factors have been documented to be associated with cancer-related PTG. These factors include demographic variables such as socioeconomic status, employment, income level, place of residence, age, ethnicity, education and gender differences, with men showing lower growth.

Previous trauma is another risk factor; the type of trauma or how long ago the trauma occurred appears to have an impact on cancer PTG. Cancer survivors may become resilient because of their past stressful experiences combined with their cancer experiences. Cancer-specific variables are not always consistent as risk factors influencing PTG after diagnosis. Nevertheless, cancer types appear to play a role in influencing PTG. Longer disease duration also tends to be associated with increased PTG. Whether cancer stage increases PTG is somewhat controversial and may depend on survivors' perception of life threat. Stigma was also found to be related to different levels of psychological distress and PTG.

In terms of personality: openness, optimism, and resilience are overall related to increased PTG. Different types of rumination can have different effects on PTG. Positive cancer-related rumination is associated with increased PTG, whereas negative cancer-related rumination is not. Deliberate rumination is also thought to be useful in promoting PTG. Intrusive rumination, on the other hand, is associated with distress. PTG may influence cancer intrusion and distress through reflective rumination. Positive coping, positive reappraisal or reframing strategies and positive attentional biases are associated with increased PTG overtime. Overall, social support is associated with increased PTG. The quality of the relationship or intimacy between spouses or partners can also provide healthy relational support and promote PTG. Emotional and instrumental social support, as well as venting emotions, are also associated with increased PTG, although the effect of emotional support on PTG is not always consistent. Religious coping (positive religious coping), spirituality, and meaning making have also been found to be useful in improving PTG. Other coping strategies associated with PTG include information seeking, gratitude, emotion regulation, and self-worth.

In addition to cancer survivors, PTG is also important for family caregivers of cancer survivors. Parents of children with cancer may report positive changes or PTG as a result of caring for their loved ones with cancer, although they also report some health difficulties and psychological distress. PTG appears to manifest differently in mothers and fathers. The parent–child relationship may influence the adjustment of childhood cancer survivors. Parents' level of psychological distress is often related to that of their child cancer survivors. The way the two groups influence each other may be the reason for the emphasis on family resilience. In addition to parents, other family members can be affected by PTG, including siblings of children with cancer.

Research has also focused on PTG in children of parents with cancer. They too may report PTG as well as changes in health behaviours and attitudes. Similarly, PTG may also manifest in the partners or spouses of loved ones with cancer. Survivors' perceptions of support from their spouses and survivors' reported growth may be related to their spouses' growth. Promoting marital adjustment is important to facilitate PTG for cancer survivors and their spouses. Several factors are involved in predicting partner growth, with the dyadic relationship being the strongest factor.

The studies reviewed above suggest that promoting PTG can benefit both cancer survivors and their family members, as PTG can act as a stress buffer. Intervention programmes include a resilience-building programme for coping and PTG, a mindfulness-based programme, a meaning-centred intervention, and psycho-spiritual integrative therapy, which have been shown to have varying degrees of effectiveness. Other programmes include a dragon boat programme, a life review intervention, a motivational interviewing-based self-efficacy enhancing intervention, a multiple health behaviour change intervention, a positive psychotherapy for cancer, and a programme targeting PTG and cortisol levels. They all showed varying levels of improvement in psychological distress, quality of life, PTG, and self-efficacy.

References

Abdullah, M. F. I. L., Jaafar, N. R. N., Zakaria, H., Rajandram, R. K., Mahadevan, R., Yunus, M. R. M., & Shah, S. A. (2015). Posttraumatic growth, depression and anxiety in head and neck cancer patients: Examining their patterns and correlations in a prospective study. *Psycho-Oncology*, *24*(8), 894–900. https://doi.org/10.1002/pon.3740

Abernathy, B. (2008). Who am I now? Helping trauma clients find meaning, wisdom, and a renewed sense of self. In G. Walz, J. Bleuer, & R. Yep (Eds.), *Compelling counseling interventions: Celebrating VISTAS' fifth anniversary* (pp. 199–208). American Counseling Association.

Adamkovič, M., Fedáková, D., Kentoš, M., Bozogáňová, M., Havrillová, D., Baník, G., Dědová, M., & Piterová, I. (2022). Relationships between satisfaction with life, posttraumatic growth, coping strategies, and resilience in cancer survivors: A network analysis approach. *Psycho-Oncology*, *31*(11), 1913–1921. https://doi.org/10.1002/pon.5948

Aderhold, C., Morawa, E., Paslakis, G., & Erim, Y. (2019). Protective factors of depressive symptoms in adult cancer patients: The role of sense of coherence and posttraumatic growth in different time spans since diagnosis. *Journal of Psychosocial Oncology*, *37*(5), 616–635. https://doi.org/10.1080/07347332.2019.1631931

American Psychiatric Association. (1994). *Diagnostic and statistical manual of mental disorders* (4th ed.).

Andrykowski, M. A., Aarts, M. J., van de Poll-Franse, L. V., Mols, F., Slooter, G. D., & Thong, M. S. Y. (2013). Low socioeconomic status and mental health outcomes in colorectal cancer survivors: Disadvantage? Advantage? ... Or both? *Psycho-Oncology*, *22*(11), 2462–2469. https://doi.org/10.1002/pon.3309

Andrykowski, M. A., Steffens, R. F., Bush, H. M., & Tucker, T. C. (2013). Reports of 'growth' in survivors of non-small cell lung cancer and healthy controls: What is the value-added by the cancer experience? *Psycho-Oncology*, *22*(10), 2214–2219.

Andrykowski, M. A., Steffens, R. F., Bush, H. M., & Tucker, T. C. (2017). Posttraumatic growth and benefit-finding in lung cancer survivors: The benefit of rural residence? *Journal of Health Psychology*, *22*(7), 896–905. https://doi.org/10.1177/1359105315617820

Andysz, A., Najder, A., Merecz-Kot, D., & Wójcik, A. (2015). Posttraumatic growth in women after breast cancer surgery—Preliminary results from a study of Polish patients. *Health Psychology Report*, *3*(4), 336–344. https://doi.org/10.5114/hpr.2015.52383

Antoni, M. H., Lehman, J. M., Kilbourn, K. M., Boyers, A. E., Culver, J. L., Alferi, S. M., Yount, S. E., McGregor, B. A., Arena, P. L., Harris, S. D., Price, A. A., & Carver, C. S. (2001). Cognitive-behavioral stress management intervention decreases the prevalence of depression and enhances benefit finding among women under treatment for early-stage breast cancer. *Health Psychology*, *20*(1), 20–32. https://doi.org/10.1037//0278-6133.20.1.20

Arpawong, T. E., Richeimer, S. H., Weinstein, F., Elghamrawy, A., & Milam, J. E. (2013). Posttraumatic growth, quality of life, and treatment symptoms among cancer chemotherapy outpatients. *Health Psychology*, *32*(4), 397–408. https://doi.org/10.1037/a0028223

Ávila, M., Coimbra, J. L., Park, C. L., & Matos, P. M. (2017). Attachment and posttraumatic growth after breast cancer: A dyadic approach. *Psycho-Oncology*, *26*(11), 1929–1935. https://doi.org/10.1002/pon.4409

Balfe, M., O'Brien, K., Timmons, A., Butow, P., O'Sullivan, E., Gooberman-Hill, R., & Sharp, L. (2016). What factors are associated with posttraumatic growth in head and neck cancer carers? *European Journal of Oncology Nursing*, *21*, 31–37. https://doi.org/10.1016/j.ejon.2015.11.005

Barakat, L., Alderfer, M., & Kazak, A. (2006). Posttraumatic growth in adolescent survivors of cancer and their mothers and fathers. *Journal of Pediatric Psychology, 31*, 413–419. https://doi.org/10.1093/jpepsy/jsj058

Barakat, L. P., Madden, R. E., Vega, G., Askins, M., & Kazak, A. E. (2021). Longitudinal predictors of caregiver resilience outcomes at the end of childhood cancer treatment. *Psycho-Oncology, 30*(5), 474–755. https://doi.org/10.1002/pon.5625

Barrett-Bernstein, M., Wurz, A., & Brunet, J. (2020). Posttraumatic growth and its correlates among survivors of adolescent and young adult cancer: A brief report. *Journal of Psychosocial Oncology, 38*(2), 228–234. https://doi.org/10.1080/07347332.2019.1664702

Bellizzi, K. M. (2004). Expressions of generativity and posttraumatic growth in adult cancer survivors. *International Journal of Aging and Human Development, 58*(4), 267–287. https://doi.org/10.2190/dc07-cpvw-4uve-5gk0

Bellizzi, K. M., & Blank, T. O. (2006). Predicting posttraumatic growth in breast cancer survivors. *Health Psychology, 25*(1), 47–56. https://doi.org/10.1037/0278-6133.25.1.47

Bellizzi, K. M., Miller, M. F., Arora, N. K., & Rowland, J. H. (2007). Positive and negative life changes experienced by survivors of non-Hodgkin's lymphoma. *Annals of Behavioral Medicine, 34*(2), 188–199. https://doi.org/10.1007/BF02872673

Bellizzi, K. M., Smith, A. W., Reeve, B. B., Alfano, C. M., Bernstein, L., Meeske, K., Baumgartner, K. B., & Ballard-Barbash, R. R. (2010). Posttraumatic growth and health-related quality of life in a racially diverse cohort of breast cancer survivors. *Journal of Health Psychology, 15*(4), 615–626. https://doi.org/10.1177/1359105309356364

Bellur, Z., Aydın, A., & Alpay, E. H. (2018). Mediating role of coping styles in personal, environmental and event related factors and posttraumatic growth relationships in women with breast cancer. *Klinik Psikiyatri Dergisi: The Journal of Clinical Psychiatry, 21*(1), 38–51. https://doi.org/10.5505/kpd.2018.65365

Ben-Zur, H., Cohen, M., & Gouzman, J. (2015). Posttraumatic growth moderates the effects of posttraumatic stress symptoms on adjustment and positive affective reactions in digestive system cancer patients. *Psychology, Health & Medicine, 20*(6), 685–696. https://doi.org/10.1080/13548506.2014.969747

Best, M., Streisand, R., Catania, L., & Kazak, A. E. (2001). Parental distress during pediatric leukemia and posttraumatic stress symptoms (PTSS) after treatment ends. *Journal of Pediatric Psychology, 26*(5), 299–307. https://doi.org/10.1093/jpepsy/26.5.299

Bourdon, M., Blanchin, M., Campone, M., Quéreux, G., Dravet, F., Sébille, V., & Bonnaud Antignac, A. (2019). A comparison of posttraumatic growth changes in breast cancer and melanoma. *Health Psychology, 38*(10), 878–887. https://doi.org/10.1037/hea0000766

Boyle, C. C., Stanton, A. L., Ganz, P. A., & Bower, J. E. (2017). Posttraumatic growth in breast cancer survivors: Does age matter? *Psycho-Oncology, 26*(6), 800–807. https://doi.org/10.1002/pon.4091

Bozo, O., Gündogdu, E., & Büyükasik-Colak, C. (2009). The moderating role of different sources of perceived social support on the dispositional optimism—Posttraumatic growth relationship in postoperative breast cancer patients. *Journal of Health Psychology, 14*(7), 1009–1020. https://doi.org/10.1177/1359105309342295

Brunet, J., McDonough, M. H., Hadd, V., Crocker, P. R., & Sabiston, C. M. (2010). The Posttraumatic Growth Inventory: An examination of the factor structure and invariance among breast cancer survivors. *Psycho-Oncology, 19*(8), 830–838. https://doi.org/10.1002/pon.1640

Büyükaşik-Colak, C., Gündoğdu-Aktürk, E., & Bozo, O. (2012). Mediating role of coping in the dispositional optimism–posttraumatic growth relation in breast cancer patients. *Journal of Psychology, 146*(5), 471–483. https://doi.org/10.1080/00223980.2012.654520

Calhoun, L. G., & Tedeschi, R. G. (2000). Early posttraumatic interventions: Facilitating possibilities for growth. In J. M. Violanti, D. Paton, & C. Dunning (Eds.), *Posttraumatic stress intervention: Challenges, issues, and perspectives* (pp. 135–152). Charles C. Thomas.

Calhoun, L. G., & Tedeschi, R. G. (2006). *The handbook of posttraumatic growth: Research and practice*. Lawrence Erlbaum Associates.

Canavarro, M. C., Silva, S., & Moreira, H. (2015). Is the link between posttraumatic growth and anxious symptoms mediated by marital intimacy in breast cancer patients? *European Journal of Oncology Nursing, 19*(6), 673–679. https://doi.org/10.1016/j.ejon.2015.04.007

Cao, W., Qi, X., Cai, D. A., & Han, X. (2018). Modeling posttraumatic growth among cancer patients: The roles of social support, appraisals, and adaptive coping. *Psycho-Oncology, 27*(1), 208–215. https://doi.org/10.1002/pon.4395

Carboon, I., Anderson, V. A., Pollard, A., Szer, J., & Seymour, J. F. (2005). Posttraumatic growth following a cancer diagnosis: Do world assumptions contribute? *Traumatology, 11*, 269–283. https://doi.org/10.1177/153476560501100406

Carlson, L. E., Labelle, L. E., Garland, S. N., Hutchins, M. L., & Birnie, K. (2009). Mindfulness-based interventions in oncology. In F. Didonna (Ed.), *Clinical handbook of mindfulness* (pp. 383–404). Springer. https://doi.org/10.1007/978-0-387-09593-6_21

Carver, C. S., & Antoni, M. H. (2004). Finding benefit in breast cancer during the year after diagnosis predicts better adjustment 5 to 8 years after diagnosis. *Health Psychology, 23*(6), 595–598. https://doi.org/10.1037/0278-6133.23.6.595

Casellas-Grau, A., Ochoa, C., & Ruini, C. (2017). Psychological and clinical correlates of posttraumatic growth in cancer: A systematic and critical review. *Psycho-Oncology, 26*(12), 2007–2018. https://doi.org/10.1002/pon.4426

Casellas-Grau, A., Sumalla, E. C., Lleras, M., Vives, J., Sirgo, A., León, C., Rodríguez, A., Campos, G., Valverde, Y., Borràs, J. M., & Ochoa, C. (2018). The role of posttraumatic stress and posttraumatic growth on online information use in breast cancer survivors. *Psycho-Oncology, 27*(8), 1971–1978. https://doi.org/10.1002/pon.4753

Caspari, J. M., Raque-Bogdan, T. L., McRae, C., Simoneau, T. L., Ash-Lee, S., & Hultgren, K. (2017). Posttraumatic growth after cancer: The role of perceived threat and cognitive processing. *Journal of Psychosocial Oncology, 35*(5), 561–577. https://doi.org/10.1080/07347 332.2017.1320347

Castonguay, A. L., Crocker, P. R. E., Hadd, V., McDonough, M. H., & Sabiston, C. M. (2015). Linking physical self-worth to posttraumatic growth in a sample of physically active breast cancer survivors. *Journal of Applied Biobehavioral Research, 20*(2), 53–70. https://doi.org/10.1111/jabr.12042

Chan, M. W. C., Ho, S. M. Y., Tedeschi, R. G., & Leung, C. W. L. (2011). The valence of attentional bias and cancer-related rumination in posttraumatic stress and posttraumatic growth among women with breast cancer. *Psycho-Oncology, 20*(5), 544–552.

Chen, J., Zebrack, B., Embry, L., Freyer, D. R., Aguilar, C., & Cole, S. (2020). Profiles of emotional distress and growth among adolescents and young adults with cancer: A longitudinal study. *Health Psychology, 39*(5), 370–380. https://doi.org/10.1037/hea0000843.

Cheng, C.-T., Ho, S. M. Y., Hou, Y.-C., Lai, Y., & Wang, G.-L. (2020). Constructive, illusory, and distressed posttraumatic growth among survivors of breast cancer: A 7-year growth trajectory study. *Journal of Health Psychology, 25*(13–14), 2233–2243. https://doi.org/10.1177/1359105318793199

Choi, K., & Kim, J. Y. (2018). Evaluation of the TSL® program for parents of children with cancer. *Research on Social Work Practice, 28*(2), 146–153. https://doi.org/10.1177/104973151 6637121

Chu, Q., Tang, M., Chen, L., Young, L., Loh, A., Wang, C., & Lu, Q. (2022). Evaluating a pilot culturally sensitive psychosocial intervention on posttraumatic growth for Chinese American breast cancer survivors. *Behavioral Medicine*, 48(4), 251–260. https://doi.org/10.1080/08964 289.2020.1845600

Cohen, M., & Numa, M. (2011). Posttraumatic growth in breast cancer survivors: A comparison of volunteers and non-volunteers. *Psycho-Oncology*, 20(1), 69–76. https://doi.org/ 10.1002/pon.1709

Conley, C. C., Small, B. J., Christie, J., Hoogland, A. I., Augusto, B. M., Garcia, J. D., Pal, T., & Vadaparampil, S. T. (2020). Patterns and covariates of benefit finding in young Black breast cancer survivors: A longitudinal, observational study. *Psycho-Oncology*, 29(7), 1115–1122. https://doi.org/10.1002/pon.5398

Cordova, M. J., Cunningham, L. L., Carlson, C. R., & Andrykowski, M. A. (2001). Posttraumatic growth following breast cancer: A controlled comparison study. *Health Psychol*, 20(3), 176–185.

Cordova, M. J., Giese-Davis, J., Golant, M., Kronenwetter, C., Chang, V., & Spiegel, D. (2007). Breast cancer as trauma: Posttraumatic stress and posttraumatic growth. *Journal of Clinical Psychology in Medical Settings*, 14, 308–319. https://doi.org/10.1007/s10880-007-9083-6

Cormio, C., Romito, F., Viscanti, G., Turaccio, M., Lorusso, V., & Mattioli, V. (2014). Psychological well-being and posttraumatic growth in caregivers of cancer patients. *Frontiers in Psychology*, 5. https://doi.org/10.3389/fpsyg.2014.01342

Coroiu, A., Körner, A., Burke, S., Meterissian, S., & Sabiston, C. M. (2016). Stress and posttraumatic growth among survivors of breast cancer: A test of curvilinear effects. *International Journal of Stress Management*, 23(1), 84–97. https://doi.org/10.1037/a0039247

Cotton, S. P., Levine, E. G., Fitzpatrick, C. M., Dold, K. H., & Targ, E. (1999). Exploring the relationships among spiritual well-being, quality of life, and psychological adjustment in women with breast cancer. *Psycho-Oncology*, 8(5), 429–438. https://doi.org/10.1002/(sici)1099-1611(199909/10)8:5<429::aid-pon420>3.0.co;2-p

Crawford, J. J., Holt, N. L., Vallance, J. K., & Courneya, K. S. (2015). Prevalence and interest in extreme/adventure activities among gynecologic cancer survivors: Associations with posttraumatic growth. *Mental Health and Physical Activity*, 9, 35–40. https://doi.org/10.1016/j.mhpa.2015.09.001

Crawford, J. J., Vallance, J. K., Holt, N. L., Steed, H., & Courneya, K. S. (2016). A phase I/II pilot study assessing the preliminary efficacy of wall climbing for improving posttraumatic growth and quality of life in gynecologic cancer survivors. *Mental Health and Physical Activity*, 11, 60–66. https://doi.org/10.1016/j.mhpa.2016.10.002

D'Urso, A., Mastroyannopoulou, K., & Kirby, A. (2017). Experiences of posttraumatic growth in siblings of children with cancer. *Clinical Child Psychology and Psychiatry*, 22(2), 301–317. https://doi.org/10.1177/1359104516660749

da Rocha Rodrigues, M. G., Pautex, S., & Zumstein-Shaha, M. (2019). Revie ⊕: An intervention promoting the dignity of individuals with advanced cancer: A feasibility study. *European Journal of Oncology Nursing*, 39, 81–89. https://doi.org/10.1016/j.ejon.2019.01.006

da Silva, S. I. M., Moreira, H., & Canavarro, M. C. (2011). Growing after breast cancer: A controlled comparison study with healthy women. *Journal of Loss and Trauma*, 16, 323–340. https://doi.org/10.1080/15325024.2011.572039

Danhauer, S. C., Case, L. D., Tedeschi, R., Russell, G., Vishnevsky, T., Triplett, K., Ip, E. H., & Avis, N. E. (2013). Predictors of posttraumatic growth in women with breast cancer. *Psycho-Oncology*, 22(12), 2676–2683. https://doi.org/10.1002/pon.3298

Danhauer, S. C., Russell, G., Case, L. D., Sohl, S. J., Tedeschi, R. G., Addington, E. L., Triplett, K., Van Zee, K. J., Naftalis, E. Z., Levine, B., & Avis, N. E. (2015). Trajectories of posttraumatic growth and associated characteristics in women with breast cancer. *Annals of Behavioral Medicine*, 49(5), 650–659. https://doi.org/10.1007/s12160-015-9696-1

Danhauer, S. C., Russell, G. B., Tedeschi, R. G., Jesse, M. T., Vishnevsky, T., Daley, K., Carroll, S., Triplett, K. N., Calhoun, L. G., Cann, A., & Powell, B. L. (2013). A longitudinal investigation of posttraumatic growth in adult patients undergoing treatment for acute leukemia. *Journal of Clinical Psychology in Medical Settings, 20*(1), 13–24. https://doi.org/10.1007/s10 880-012-9304-5

Darabos, K., Renna, M. E., Wang, A. W., Zimmermann, C. F., & Hoyt, M. A. (2021). Emotional approach coping among young adults with cancer: Relationships with psychological distress, posttraumatic growth, and resilience. *Psycho-Oncology, 30*(5), 728–735. https://doi.org/10.1002/pon.5621

Davis, L. Z., Cuneo, M., Thaker, P. H., Goodheart, M. J., Bender, D., & Lutgendorf, S. K. (2018). Changes in spiritual well-being and psychological outcomes in ovarian cancer survivors. *Psycho-Oncology, 27*(2), 477–483. https://doi.org/10.1002/pon.4485

Denney, R. M., Aten, J. D., & Leavell, K. (2011). Posttraumatic spiritual growth: A phenomenological study of cancer survivors. *Mental Health, Religion & Culture, 14*(4), 371–391. https://doi.org/10.1080/13674671003758667

Diaz, M., Aldridge-Gerry, A., & Spiegel, D. (2014). Posttraumatic growth and diurnal cortisol slope among women with metastatic breast cancer. *Psychoneuroendocrinology, 44*, 83–87. https://doi.org/10.1016/j.psyneuen.2014.03.001

Dong, X., Li, G., Liu, C., Kong, L., Fang, Y., Kang, X., & Li, P. (2017). The mediating role of resilience in the relationship between social support and posttraumatic growth among colorectal cancer survivors with permanent intestinal ostomies: A structural equation model analysis. *European Journal of Oncology Nursing, 29*, 47–52. https://doi.org/10.1016/j.ejon.2017.04.007

Dougall, A. L., Swanson, J., Kyutoku, Y., Belani, C. P., & Baum, A. (2017). Posttraumatic symptoms, quality of life, and survival among lung cancer patients. *Journal of Applied Biobehavioral Research, 22*(3), 1–23. https://doi.org/10.1111/jabr.12065

Duran, B. (2013). Posttraumatic growth as experienced by childhood cancer survivors and their families: A narrative synthesis of qualitative and quantitative research. *Journal of Pediatric Oncology Nursing, 30*(4), 179–197. https://doi.org/10.1177/1043454213487433

Ehde, D. M. (2010). Application of positive psychology to rehabilitation psychology. In R. G. Frank, M. Rosenthal, & B. Caplan (Eds.), *Handbook of rehabilitation psychology* (2nd ed., pp. 417–424). American Psychological Association. https://doi.org/10.1037/15972-029

Erikson, E. H. (1963). *Childhood and society*. Norton.

Erikson, E. H. (1968). *Identity: Youth and crisis*. Norton.

Eva, K. (2006). Possible positive posttraumatic reactions in cancer patients. *Cogniție Creier Comportament, 10*(1), 133–150.

Gallagher, M. W., Long, L. J., Tsai, W., Stanton, A. L., & Lu, Q. (2018). The unexpected impact of expressive writing on posttraumatic stress and growth in Chinese American breast cancer survivors. *Journal of Clinical Psychology, 74*(10), 1673–1686. https://doi.org/10.1002/jclp.22636

Garlick, M., Wall, K., Corwin, D., & Koopman, C. (2011). Psycho-spiritual integrative therapy for women with primary breast cancer. *Journal of Clinical Psychology in Medical Settings, 18*(1), 78–90. https://doi.org/10.1007/s10880-011-9224-9

George, L. S., & Park, C. L. (2013). Are meaning and purpose distinct? An examination of correlates and predictors. *Journal of Positive Psychology, 8*(5), 365–375. https://doi.org/10.1080/17439760.2013.805801

Gorven, A., & du Plessis, L. (2021). Corporeal posttraumatic growth as a result of breast cancer: An interpretative phenomenological analysis. *Journal of Humanistic Psychology, 61*(4), 561–590. https://doi.org/10.1177/0022167818761997

Hamama-Raz, Y., Pat-Horenczyk, R., Roziner, I., Perry, S., & Stemmer, S. M. (2019). Can posttraumatic growth after breast cancer promote positive coping?—A cross-lagged study. *Psycho-Oncology, 28*(4), 767–774. https://doi.org/10.1002/pon.5017

Hamama, L., & Sharon, M. (2013). Posttraumatic growth and subjective well-being among caregivers of chronic patients: A preliminary study. *Journal of Happiness Studies, 14*, 1717–1737. https://doi.org/10.1007/s10902-012-9405-8

Hamdan, N. A., Abd Hamid, N., & Leong Bin Abdullah, M. F. I. (2022). A longitudinal investigation of posttraumatic growth and its associated factors among head and neck cancer survivors. *Psycho-Oncology, 31*(3), 504–511. https://doi.org/10.1002/pon.5835

Hatano, Y., Fujimoto, S., Hosokawa, T., & Fukui, K. (2015). Association between 'Good Death' of cancer patients and post-traumatic growth in bereaved caregivers. *Journal of Pain and Symptom Management, 50*(2), e4–e6. https://doi.org/10.1016/j.jpainsymman.2015.05.002

Hawkes, A. L., Pakenham, K. I., Chambers, S. K., Patrao, T. A., & Courneya, K. S. (2014). Effects of a multiple health behavior change intervention for colorectal cancer survivors on psychosocial outcomes and quality of life: A randomized controlled trial. *Annals of Behavioral Medicine, 48*(3), 359–370. https://doi.org/10.1007/s12160-014-9610-2

Hefferon, K., Grealy, M., & Mutrie, N. (2010). Transforming from cocoon to butterfly: The potential role of the body in the process of posttraumatic growth. *Journal of Humanistic Psychology, 50*, 224–247. https://doi.org/10.1177/0022167809341996

Hill, E. M., & Watkins, K. (2017). Women with ovarian cancer: Examining the role of social support and rumination in posttraumatic growth, psychological distress, and psychological well-being. *Journal of Clinical Psychology in Medical Settings, 24*(1), 47–58.

Hirooka, K., Fukahori, H., Akita, Y., & Ozawa, M. (2017). Posttraumatic growth among Japanese parentally bereaved adolescents: A Web-based survey. *American Journal of Hospice & Palliative Medicine, 34*(5), 442–448.

Hirooka, K., Fukahori, H., Taku, K., Togari, T., & Ogawa, A. (2017). Quality of death, rumination, and posttraumatic growth among bereaved family members of cancer patients in home palliative care. *Psycho-Oncology, 26*(12), 2168–2174. https://doi.org/10.1002/pon.4446

Hirooka, K., Fukahori, H., Taku, K., Togari, T., & Ogawa, A. (2018). Examining posttraumatic growth among bereaved family members of patients with cancer who received palliative care at home. *American Journal of Hospice & Palliative Medicine, 35*(2), 211–217.

Ho, R. T. H., Chan, C. L. W., & Ho, S. M. Y. (2004). Emotional control in Chinese female cancer survivors. *Psycho-Oncology, 13*, 808–817.

Ho, S. M., Chan, M. W., Yau, T. K., & Yeung, R. M. (2011). Relationships between explanatory style, posttraumatic growth and posttraumatic stress disorder symptoms among Chinese breast cancer patients. *Psychology & Health, 26*(3), 269–285. https://doi.org/10.1080/08870440903287926

Ho, S. M. Y., Law, L. S. C., Wang, G. L., Shih, S. M., Hsu, S. H., & Hou, Y. C. (2013). Psychometric analysis of the Chinese version of the Posttraumatic Growth Inventory with cancer patients in Hong Kong and Taiwan. *Psycho-Oncology, 22*(3), 715–719. https://doi.org/10.1002/pon.3024

Holtmaat, K., Spek, N., Cuijpers, P., Leemans, C. R., & Verdonck-de Leeuw, I. M. (2017). Posttraumatic growth among head and neck cancer survivors with psychological distress. *Psycho-Oncology, 26*(1), 96–101. https://doi.org/10.1002/pon.4106

Holtmaat, K., van der Spek, N., Lissenberg-Witte, B., Breitbart, W., Cuijpers, P., & Verdonck-de Leeuw, I. (2020). Long-term efficacy of meaning-centered group psychotherapy for cancer survivors: 2-year follow-up results of a randomized controlled trial. *Psycho-Oncology, 29*(4), 711–718. https://doi.org/10.1002/pon.5323

Howard Sharp, K. M., Willard, V. W., Barnes, S., Tillery, R., Long, A., & Phipps, S. (2017). Emotion socialization in the context of childhood cancer: Perceptions of parental support promotes posttraumatic growth. *Journal of Pediatric Psychology, 42*(1), 95–103.

Huang, F.-F., Yang, Q., Zhang, J., Han, X. Y., Zhang, J.-P., & Ye, M. (2018). A self-efficacy enhancing intervention for pulmonary rehabilitation based on motivational interviewing for postoperative lung cancers patients: Modeling and randomized exploratory trial. *Psychology, Health & Medicine, 23*(7), 804–822. https://doi.org/10.1080/13548506.2018.1434216

Hullmann, S. E., Fedele, D. A., Molzon, E. S., Mayes, S., & Mullins, L. L. (2014). Posttraumatic growth and hope in parents of children with cancer. *Journal of Psychosocial Oncology, 32*(6), 696–707. https://doi.org/10.1080/07347332.2014.955241

Hungerbuehler, I., Vollrath, M. E., & Landolt, M. A. (2011). Posttraumatic growth in mothers and fathers of children with severe illnesses. *Journal of Health Psychology, 16*(8), 1259–1267. https://doi.org/10.1177/1359105311405872

Jaarsma, T. A., Pool, G., Sanderman, R., & Ranchor, A. V. (2006). Psychometric properties of the Dutch version of the posttraumatic growth inventory among cancer patients. *Psycho-Oncology, 15*(10), 911–920. https://doi.org/10.1002/pon.1026

Jahn, A. L., Herman, L., Schuster, J., Naik, A., & Moye, J. (2012). Distress and resilience after cancer in veterans. *Research in Human Development, 9*(3), 229–247. https://doi.org/10.1080/15427609.2012.705555

Joseph, S., & Linley, P. A. (2005). Positive adjustment to threatening events: An organismic valuing theory of growth through adversity. *Review of General Psychology, 9*(3), 262–280. https://doi.org/10.1037/1089-2680.9.3.262

Kahana, B., Kahana, E., Deimling, G., Sterns, S., & VanGunten, M. (2011). Determinants of altered life perspectives among older-adult long-term cancer survivors. *Cancer Nursing, 34*(3), 209–218. https://doi.org/10.1097/NCC.0b013e3181fa56b0

Kamibeppu, K., Sato, I., Honda, M., Ozono, S., Sakamoto, N., Iwai, T., Okamura, J., Asami, K., Maeda, N., Inada, H., Kakee, N., Horibe, K., & Ishida, Y. (2010). Mental health among young adult survivors of childhood cancer and their siblings including posttraumatic growth. *Journal of Cancer Survivorship, 4*(4), 303–312. https://doi.org/10.1007/s11764-010-0124-z

Kausar, R., & Saghir, S. (2010). Posttraumatic growth and marital satisfaction after breast cancer: Patient and spouse perspective. *Pakistan Journal of Social and Clinical Psychology, 8*, 3–17.

Kay, J. S., Juth, V., Silver, R. C., & Sender, L. S. (2019). Support and conflict in relationships and psychological health in adolescents and young adults with cancer. *Journal of Health Psychology, 24*(4), 502–517. https://doi.org/10.1177/1359105316676629

Kent, E. E., Alfano, C. M., Smith, A. W., Bernstein, L., McTiernan, A., Baumgartner, K. B., & Ballard-Barbash, R. (2013). The roles of support seeking and race/ethnicity in posttraumatic growth among breast cancer survivors. *Journal of Psychosocial Oncology, 31*(4), 393–412. https://doi.org/10.1080/07347332.2013.798759

Kim, M. Y. (2017). Factors influencing posttraumatic growth in mothers of children with cancer. *Journal of Pediatric Oncology Nursing, 34*(4), 250–260. https://doi.org/10.1177/1043454217697021

Kissil, K., Niño, A., Jacobs, S., Davey, M., & Tubbs, C. Y. (2010). 'It has been a good growing experience for me': Growth experiences among African American youth coping with parental cancer. *Families, Systems, & Health, 28*(3), 274–289. https://doi.org/10.1037/a0020001

Klassen, A. F., Gulati, S., Granek, L., Rosenberg-Yunger, Z. R. S., Watt, L., Sung, L., Klaassen, R., Dix, D., & Shaw, N. T. (2012). Understanding the health impact of caregiving: A qualitative study of immigrant parents and single parents of children with cancer. *Quality of Life Research, 21*(9), 1595–1605. http://www.jstor.org/stable/41684651

Klosky, J. L., Krull, K. R., Kawashima, T., Leisenring, W., Randolph, M. E., Zebrack, B., Stuber, M. L., Robison, L. L., & Phipps, S. (2014). Relations between posttraumatic stress and post-traumatic growth in long-term survivors of childhood cancer: A report from the Childhood Cancer Survivor Study. *Health Psychology*, *33*(8), 878–882. https://doi.org/10.1037/hea 0000076

Kolokotroni, P., Anagnostopoulos, F., & Tsikkinis, A. (2014a). Psychosocial factors related to posttraumatic growth in breast cancer survivors: A review. *Women & Health*, *54*(6), 569–592. https://doi.org/10.1080/03630242.2014.899543

Kolokotroni, P., Anagnostopoulos, F., & Tsikkinis, A. (2014b). Psychosocial factors related to posttraumatic growth in breast cancer survivors: A review. *Women & Health*, *54*(6), 569–592.

Koutná, V., & Blatný, M. (2020). Socialization of coping in pediatric oncology settings: Theoretical consideration on parent–child connections in posttraumatic growth. *Frontiers in Psychology*, *11*, 554325. https://doi.org/10.3389/fpsyg.2020.554325

Koutná, V., Blatný, M., & Jelínek, M. (2020). Posttraumatic stress and growth in childhood cancer survivors: Considering the pathways for relationship. *Journal of Psychosocial Oncology*, *39*(1), 105–117. https://doi.org/10.1080/07347332.2020.1789907

Koutrouli, N., Anagnostopoulos, F., Griva, F., Gourounti, K., Kolokotroni, F., Efstathiou, V., Mellon, R., Papastylianou, D., Niakas, D., & Potamianos, G. (2016). Exploring the relationship between posttraumatic growth, cognitive processing, psychological distress, and social constraints in a sample of breast cancer patients. *Women & Health*, *56*(6), 650–667.

Koutrouli, N., Anagnostopoulos, F., & Potamianos, G. (2012). Posttraumatic stress disorder and posttraumatic growth in breast cancer patients: A systematic review. *Women & Health*, *52*(5), 503–516. https://doi.org/10.1080/03630242.2012.679337

Krupski, T. L., Kwan, L., Fink, A., Sonn, G. A., Maliski, S., & Litwin, M. S. (2006). Spirituality influences health related quality of life in men with prostate cancer. *Psycho-Oncology*, *15*, 121–131. https://doi.org/10.1002/pon.929

Kuswanto, C. N., Sharp, J., Stafford, L., & Schofield, P. (2020). Posttraumatic growth as a buffer and a vulnerability for psychological distress in mothers who are breast cancer survivors. *Journal of Affective Disorders*, *275*, 31–37. https://doi.org/10.1016/j.jad.2020.06.013

Labelle, L. E., Lawlor-Savage, L., Campbell, T. S., Faris, P., & Carlson, L. E. (2015). Does self-report Mindfulness-Based Stress Reduction (MBSR) on spirituality and posttraumatic growth in cancer patients? *Journal of Positive Psychology*, *10*(2), 153–166. https://doi.org/ 10.1080/17439760.2014.927902

LeBarre, S., & Riding-Malon, R. (2017). Posttraumatic growth in breast cancer survivors: Sources of support in rural and non-rural areas. *Journal of Rural Mental Health*, *41*(1), 54–65. https://doi.org/10.1037/rmh0000069

Lechner, S. C., & Antoni, M. H. (2004). Posttraumatic growth and group-based interventions for persons dealing with cancer: What have we learned so far? *Psychological Inquiry*, *15*, 35–41.

Lechner, S. C., Stoelb, B. L., & Antoni, M. H. (2008). Group-based therapies for benefit finding in cancer. In S. Joseph & P. A. Linley (Eds.), *Trauma, recovery, and growth* (pp. 207–231). Wiley. https://doi.org/https://doi.org/10.1002/9781118269718.ch11

Lee, M., Kim, K., Lim, C., & Kim, J. S. (2017). Posttraumatic growth in breast cancer survivors and their husbands based on the actor–partner interdependence model. *Psycho-Oncology*, *26*(10), 1586–1592. https://doi.org/10.1002/pon.4343

Lelorain, S., Bonnaud-Antignac, A., & Florin, A. (2010). Long term posttraumatic growth after breast cancer: Prevalence, predictors and relationships with psychological health. *Journal of Clinical Psychology in Medical Settings*, *17*(1), 14–22. https://doi.org/10.1007/s10 880-009-9183-6

Leong Abdullah, M. F. I., Hami, R., Appalanaido, G. K., Azman, N., Mohd Shariff, N., & Md Sharif, S. S. (2019). Diagnosis of cancer is not a death sentence: Examining posttraumatic growth and its associated factors in cancer patients. *Journal of Psychosocial Oncology, 37*(5), 636–651. https://doi.org/10.1080/07347332.2019.1574946

Levesque, J. V., & Maybery, D. (2012). Parental cancer: Catalyst for positive growth and change. *Qualitative Health Research, 22*(3), 397–408. https://doi.org/10.1177/1049732311421617

Leys, C., Arnal, C., Wollast, R., Rolin, H., Kotsou, I., & Fossion, P. (2020). Perspectives on resilience: Personality trait or skill? *European Journal of Trauma & Dissociation, 4*(2), 100074. https://doi.org/https://doi.org/10.1016/j.ejtd.2018.07.002

Li, J., Peng, X., Su, Y., He, Y., Zhang, S., & Hu, X. (2020). Effectiveness of psychosocial interventions for posttraumatic growth in patients with cancer: A meta-analysis of randomized controlled trials. *European Journal of Oncology Nursing, 48*, 101798. https://doi.org/10.1016/j.ejon.2020.101798

Linley, P. A., & Joseph, S. (2004). Positive change following trauma and adversity: A review. *Journal of Trauma Stress, 17*(1), 11–21. https://doi.org/10.1023/B:JOTS.0000014671.27856.7e

Liu, J. E., Wang, H. Y., Wang, M. L., Su, Y. L., & Wang, P. L. (2014). Posttraumatic growth and psychological distress in Chinese early-stage breast cancer survivors: A longitudinal study. *Psycho-Oncology, 23*(4), 437–443. https://doi.org/10.1002/pon.3436

Liu, X., Zhang, Q., Yu, M., & Xu, W. (2020). Patterns of posttraumatic stress disorder and posttraumatic growth among breast cancer patients in China: A latent profile analysis. *Psycho-Oncology, 29*(4), 743–750. https://doi.org/10.1002/pon.5332

Liu, Y., Li, Y., Chen, L., Li, Y., Qi, W., & Yu, L. (2018). Relationships between family resilience and posttraumatic growth in breast cancer survivors and caregiver burden. *Psycho-Oncology, 27*(4), 1284–1290. https://doi.org/10.1002/pon.4668

Liu, Z., Doege, D., Thong, M. S. Y., & Arndt, V. (2020). The relationship between posttraumatic growth and health-related quality of life in adult cancer survivors: A systematic review. *Journal of Affective Disorders, 276*, 159–168. https://doi.org/10.1016/j.jad.2020.07.044

Loiselle, K. A., Devine, K. A., Reed-Knight, B., & Blount, R. L. (2011). Posttraumatic growth associated with a relative's serious illness. *Families, Systems, & Health, 29*, 64–72. https://doi.org/10.1037/a0023043

Long, L. J., Phillips, C. A., Glover, N., Richardson, A. L., D'Souza, J. M., Cunningham-Erdogdu, P., & Gallagher, M. W. (2021). A meta-analytic review of the relationship between posttraumatic growth, anxiety, and depression. *Journal of Happiness Studies, 22*, 3703–3728. https://doi.org/10.1007/s10902-021-00370-9

Love, C., & Sabiston, C. M. (2011). Exploring the links between physical activity and posttraumatic growth in young adult cancer survivors. *Psycho-Oncology, 20*(3), 278–286. https://doi.org/10.1002/pon.1733

Luo, R.-Z., Zhang, S., & Liu, Y.-H. (2020). Short report: Relationships among resilience, social support, coping style and posttraumatic growth in hematopoietic stem cell transplantation caregivers. *Psychology, Health & Medicine, 25*(4), 389–395. https://doi.org/10.1080/13548506.2019.1659985

Luszczynska, A., Durawa, A. B., Dudzinska, M., Kwiatkowska, M., Knysz, B., & Knoll, N. (2012). The effects of mortality reminders on posttraumatic growth and finding benefits among patients with life-threatening illness and their caregivers. *Psychology & Health, 27*(10), 1227–1243. https://doi.org/10.1080/08870446.2012.665055

Maners, A., & Champion, V. L. (2011). Coping and quality of life outcomes in younger breast cancer survivors. *Western Journal of Nursing Research, 33*(8), 1106–1107. https://doi.org/10.1177/0193945911413673

Manne, S., Ostroff, J., Winkel, G., Goldstein, L., Fox, K., & Grana, G. (2004). Posttraumatic growth after breast cancer: Patient, partner, and couple perspectives. *Psychosomatic Medicine*, *66*(3), 442–454. https://doi.org/10.1097/01.psy.0000127689.38525.7d

Markman, E. S., McClure, K. S., McMahon, C. E., Zelikovsky, N., Macone, B. W., & Bullock, A. J. (2020). Social problem solving and posttraumatic growth new possibilities in postoperative breast cancer survivors. *Journal of Clinical Psychology in Medical Settings*, *27*(3), 518–526. https://doi.org/10.1007/s10880-019-09641-3

Matis, J., Svetlak, M., Slezackova, A., Svoboda, M., & Šumec, R. (2020). Mindfulness-based programs for patients with cancer via eHealth and mobile health: Systematic review and synthesis of quantitative research. *Journal of Medical Internet Research*, *22*(11). https://doi.org/10.2196/20709

Matsui, T., & Taku, K. (2016). A review of posttraumatic growth and help-seeking behavior in cancer survivors: Effects of distal and proximate culture. *Japanese Psychological Research*, *58*(1), 142–162. https://doi.org/10.1111/jpr.12105

McDonough, M. H., Sabiston, C. M., & Ullrich-French, S. (2011). The development of social relationships, social support, and posttraumatic growth in a dragon boating team for breast cancer survivors. *Journal of Sport and Exercise Psychology*, *33*(5), 627–648. https://doi.org/10.1123/jsep.33.5.627

McDonough, M. H., Sabiston, C. M., & Wrosch, C. (2014). Predicting changes in posttraumatic growth and subjective well-being among breast cancer survivors: The role of social support and stress. *Psycho-Oncology*, *23*(1), 114–120. https://doi.org/10.1002/pon.3380

Metcalf, C. A., Arch, J. J., & Greer, J. A. (2017). Anxiety and its correlates among young adults with a history of parental cancer. *Journal of Psychosocial Oncology*, *35*(5), 597–613. https://doi.org/10.1080/07347332.2017.1307895

Mols, F., Vingerhoets, A. J., Coebergh, J. W., & van de Poll-Franse, L. V. (2009). Well-being, posttraumatic growth and benefit finding in long-term breast cancer survivors. *Psychology & Health*, *24*(5), 583–595. https://doi.org/10.1080/08870440701671362

Moore, A. M., Gamblin, T. C., Geller, D. A., Youssef, M. N., Hoffman, K. E., Gemmell, L., Likumahuwa, S. M., Bovbjerg, D. H., Marsland, A., & Steel, J. L. (2011). A prospective study of posttraumatic growth as assessed by self-report and family caregiver in the context of advanced cancer. *Psycho-Oncology*, *20*(5), 479–487. https://doi.org/10.1002/pon.1746

Moreno, P. I., Dooley, L. N., & Bower, J. E. (2018). Unique associations of eudaimonic and hedonic wellbeing with psychosocial adjustment in breast cancer survivors. *Journal of Psychosocial Oncology*, *36*(5), 649–657. https://doi.org/10.1080/07347332.2018.1471564

Morris, B. A., & Shakespeare-Finch, J. (2011). Cancer diagnostic group differences in posttraumatic growth: Accounting for age, gender, trauma severity, and distress. *Journal of Loss and Trauma*, *16*(3), 229–242. https://doi.org/10.1080/15325024.2010.519292

Morris, B. A., Lepore, S. J., Wilson, B., Lieberman, M. A., Dunn, J., & Chambers, S. K. (2014). Adopting a survivor identity after cancer in a peer support context. *Journal of Cancer Survivorship*, *8*(3), 427–436. https://doi.org/10.1007/s11764-014-0355-5

Morris, B. A., Shakespeare-Finch, J., & Scott, J. L. (2007). Coping processes and dimensions of posttraumatic growth. *Australasian Journal of Disaster and Trauma Studies*, *(1)*.

Mosher, C. E., Adams, R. N., Helft, P. R., O'Neil, B. H., Shahda, S., Rattray, N. A., & Champion, V. L. (2017). Positive changes among patients with advanced colorectal cancer and their family caregivers: A qualitative analysis. *Psychology & Health*, *32*(1), 94–109. https://doi.org/10.1080/08870446.2016.1247839

Mostarac, I., & Brajković, L. (2021). Life after facing cancer: Posttraumatic growth, meaning in life and life satisfaction. *Journal of Clinical Psychology in Medical Settings*, *29*, 92–102. https://doi.org/10.1007/s10880-021-09786-0

Mundey, K. R., Nicholas, D., Kruczek, T., Tschopp, M., & Bolin, J. (2019). Posttraumatic growth following cancer: The influence of emotional intelligence, management of intrusive rumination, and goal disengagement as mediated by deliberate rumination. *Journal of Psychosocial Oncology*, *37*(4), 456–477.

Mystakidou, K., Parpa, E., Tsilika, E., Pathiaki, M., Galanos, A., & Vlahos, L. (2007). Traumatic distress and positive changes in advanced cancer patients. *American Journal of Hospice and Palliative Medicine*, *24*(4), 270–276. https://doi.org/10.1177/1049909107299917

Nakayama, N., Mori, N., Ishimaru, S., Ohyama, W., Yuza, Y., Kaneko, T., Kanda, E., & Matsushima, E. (2017). Factors associated with posttraumatic growth among parents of children with cancer. *Psycho-Oncology*, *26*(9), 1369–1375. https://doi.org/10.1002/pon.4307

Neimeyer, R. A. (2006). Re-storying loss: Fostering growth in the posttraumatic narrative. In L. G. Calhoun & R. G. Tedeschi (Eds.), *Handbook of posttraumatic growth: Research & practice* (pp. 68–80). Lawrence Erlbaum Associates.

Nenova, M., DuHamel, K., Zemon, V., Rini, C., & Redd, W. H. (2013). Posttraumatic growth, social support, and social constraint in hematopoietic stem cell transplant survivors. *Psycho-Oncology*, *22*(1), 195–202. https://doi.org/10.1002/pon.2073

Nolen-Hoeksema, S. (1991). Responses to depression and their effects on the duration of depressive episodes. *Journal of Abnormal Psychology*, *100*(4), 569–582. https://doi.org/10.1037//0021-843x.100.4.569

Ochoa, C., Casellas-Grau, A., Vives, J., Font, A., & Borràs, J.-M. (2017). Positive psychotherapy for distressed cancer survivors: Posttraumatic growth facilitation reduces posttraumatic stress. *International Journal of Clinical and Health Psychology*, *17*(1), 28–37. https://doi.org/10.1016/j.ijchp.2016.09.002

Ogińska-Bulik, N. (2013). The role of social support in posttraumatic growth in people struggling with cancer. *Health Psychology Report*, *1*, 1–8. https://doi.org/10.5114/hpr.2013.40464

Ogińska-Bulik, N., & Kobylarczyk, M. (2019). The role of rumination in posttraumatic growth in people struggling with cancer. *Journal of Psychosocial Oncology*, *37*(5), 652–664. https://doi.org/10.1080/07347332.2019.1600628

Okado, Y., Rowley, C., Schepers, S. A., Long, A. M., & Phipps, S. (2018). Profiles of adjustment in pediatric cancer survivors and their prediction by earlier psychosocial factors. *Journal of Pediatric Psychology*, *43*(9), 1047–1058. https://doi.org/10.1093/jpepsy/jsy037

Omid, A., Mohammadi, A. S., Jalaeikhoo, H., & Taghva, A. (2017). Dispositional mindfulness, psychological distress, and posttraumatic growth in cancer patients. *Journal of Loss and Trauma*, *22*(8), 681–688. https://doi.org/10.1080/15325024.2017.1384783

Paredes, A. C., & Pereira, M. G. (2018). Spirituality, distress and posttraumatic growth in breast cancer patients. *Journal of Religion and Health*, *57*(5), 1606–1617. https://doi.org/10.1007/s10943-017-0452-7

Park, C. L., & Cho, D. (2017). Spiritual well-being and spiritual distress predict adjustment in adolescent and young adult cancer survivors. *Psycho-Oncology*, *26*(9), 1293–1300. https://doi.org/10.1002/pon.4145

Park, C. L., Cohen, L. H., & Murch, R. L. (1996). Assessment and prediction of stress-related growth. *Journal of Personality*, *64*, 71–105. https://doi.org/10.1111/j.1467-6494.1996.tb00815.x

Park, C. L., Edmondson, D., Fenster, J. R., & Blank, T. O. (2008). Meaning making and psychological adjustment following cancer: The mediating roles of growth, life meaning, and restored just-world beliefs. *Journal of Consulting and Clinical Psychology*, *76*(5), 863–875. https://doi.org/10.1037/a0013348

Pat-Horenczyk, R., Perry, S., Hamama-Raz, Y., Ziv, Y., Schramm-Yavin, S., & Stemmer, S. M. (2015). Posttraumatic growth in breast cancer survivors: Constructive and illusory aspects. *Journal of Traumatic Stress*, *28*(3), 214–222. https://doi.org/10.1002/jts.22014

Pat-Horenczyk, R., Saltzman, L. Y., Hamama-Raz, Y., Perry, S., Ziv, Y., Ginat-Frolich, R., & Stemmer, S. M. (2016). Stability and transitions in posttraumatic growth trajectories among cancer patients: LCA and LTA analyses. *Psychological Trauma: Theory, Research, Practice, and Policy, 8*(5), 541–549. https://doi.org/10.1037/tra0000094

Posluszny, D. M., Baum, A., Edwards, R. P., & Dew, M. A. (2011). Posttraumatic growth in women one year after diagnosis for gynecologic cancer or benign conditions. *Journal of Psychosocial Oncology, 29*(5), 561–572. https://doi.org/10.1080/07347332.2011.599360

Rammant, E., Decaestecker, K., Bultijnck, R., Sundahl, N., Ost, P., Pauwels, N. S., Deforche, B., Pieters, R., & Fonteyne, V. (2018). A systematic review of exercise and psychosocial rehabilitation interventions to improve health-related outcomes in patients with bladder cancer undergoing radical cystectomy. *Clinical Rehabilitation, 32*(5), 594–606. https://doi.org/10.1177/0269215517746472

Ramos, C., Costa, P. A., Rudnicki, T., Maroco, A. L., Leal, I., Guimaraes, R., Fougo, J. L., & Tedeschi, R. G. (2018). The effectiveness of a group intervention to facilitate posttraumatic growth among women with breast cancer. *Psycho-Oncology, 27*(1), 258–264.

Ramos, C., Leal, I., Costa, P. A., Tapadinhas, A. R., & Tedeschi, R. G. (2018). An item-level analysis of the Posttraumatic Stress Disorder Checklist and the Posttraumatic Growth Inventory and its associations with challenge to core beliefs and rumination. *Frontiers in Psychology, 9*, ArtID 2346.

Romeo, A., Di Tella, M., Ghiggia, A., Tesio, V., Torta, R., & Castelli, L. (2020). Posttraumatic growth in breast cancer survivors: Are depressive symptoms really negative predictors? *Psychological Trauma: Theory, Research, Practice, and Policy, 12*(3), 244–250. https://doi.org/10.1037/tra0000508

Rosenberg, A. R., Syrjala, K. L., Martin, P. J., Flowers, M. E., Carpenter, P. A., Salit, R. B., Baker, K. S., & Lee, S. J. (2015). Resilience, health, and quality of life among long-term survivors of hematopoietic cell transplantation. *Cancer, 121*(23), 4250–4257. https://doi.org/10.1002/cncr.29651

Ruini, C., & Vescovelli, F. (2013). The role of gratitude in breast cancer: Its relationships with post-traumatic growth, psychological well-being and distress. *Journal of Happiness Studies, 14*(1), 263–274. https://doi.org/10.1007/s10902-012-9330-x

Ruini, C., Offidani, E., & Vescovelli, F. (2015). Life stressors, allostatic overload, and their impact on posttraumatic growth. *Journal of Loss and Trauma, 20*(2), 109–122. https://doi.org/10.1080/15325024.2013.830530

Rzeszutek, M., Zawadzka, A., Pięta, M., Houn, A., Pankowski, D., & Kręcisz, B. (2020). Profiles of resources and posttraumatic growth among cancer and psoriatic patients compared to non-clinical sample. *International Journal of Clinical and Health Psychology, 20*(3), 222–231. https://doi.org/10.1016/j.ijchp.2020.07.004

Sabiston, C. M., McDonough, M. H., & Crocker, P. R. (2007). Psychosocial experiences of breast cancer survivors involved in a dragon boat program: Exploring links to positive psychological growth. *Journal of Sport and Exercise Psychology, 29*(4), 419–438. https://doi.org/10.1123/jsep.29.4.419

Sadler-Gerhardt, C. J., Reynolds, C. A., Britton, P. J., & Kruse, S. D. (2010). Women breast cancer survivors: Stories of change and meaning. *Journal of Mental Health Counseling, 32*, 265–282. https://doi.org/10.17744/mehc.32.3.q14777j84kx3285x

Salsman, J. M., Garcia, S. F., Yanez, B., Sanford, S. D., Snyder, M. A., & Victorson, D. (2014). Physical, emotional, and social health differences between posttreatment young adults with cancer and matched healthy controls. *Cancer, 120*(15), 2247–2254. https://doi.org/10.1002/cncr.28739

Salsman, J. M., Segerstrom, S. C., Brechting, E. H., Carlson, C. R., & Andrykowski, M. A. (2009). Posttraumatic growth and PTSD symptomatology among colorectal cancer survivors: A

3-month longitudinal examination of cognitive processing. *Psycho-Oncology*, *18*(1), 30–41. https://doi.org/10.1002/pon.1367

Sawyer, A., Ayers, S., & Field, A. (2010). Posttraumatic growth and adjustment among individuals with cancer or HIV/AIDS: A meta-analysis. *Clinical Psychology Review*, *30*, 436–447. https://doi.org/10.1016/j.cpr.2010.02.004

Schepers, S. A., Okado, Y., Russell, K., Long, A. M., & Phipps, S. (2019). Adjustment in childhood cancer survivors, healthy peers, and their parents: The mediating role of the parent–child relationship. *Journal of Pediatric Psychology*, *44*(2), 186–196. https://doi.org/10.1093/jpepsy/jsy069

Schmidt, S. D., Blank, T. O., Bellizzi, K. M., & Park, C. L. (2012). The relationship of coping strategies, social support, and attachment style with posttraumatic growth in cancer survivors. *Journal of Health Psychology*, *17*(7), 1033–1040. https://doi.org/10.1177/1359105311429203

Schroevers, M. J., & Teo, I. (2008). The report of posttraumatic growth in Malaysian cancer patients: Relationships with psychological distress and coping strategies. *Psycho-Oncology*, *17*(12), 1239–1246. https://doi.org/10.1002/pon.1366

Schroevers, M. J., Helgeson, V. S., Sanderman, R., & Ranchor, A. V. (2010). Type of social support matters for prediction of posttraumatic growth among cancer survivors. *Psycho-Oncology*, *19*(1), 46–53. https://doi.org/10.1002/pon.1501

Schroevers, M. J., Kraaij, V., & Garnefski, N. (2011). Cancer patients' experience of positive and negative changes due to the illness: Relationships with psychological well-being, coping, and goal reengagement. *Psycho-Oncology*, *20*, 165–172. https://doi.org/10.1002/pon.1718

Schwabish, S. D. (2011). Cognitive adaptation theory as a means to PTSD reduction among cancer pain patients. *Journal of Psychosocial Oncology*, *29*(2), 141–156. https://doi.org/10.1080/07347332.2010.548440

Schwartz, J. R., Thomas, E. B. K., Juckett, M. B., & Costanzo, E. S. (2022). Predictors of posttraumatic growth among hematopoietic cell transplant recipients. *Psycho-Oncology*, *31*(6), 1013–1021. https://doi.org/10.1002/pon.5892

Scrignaro, M., Barni, S., Bonetti, M. L., & Magrin, M. E. (2011). Studying predictors of posttraumatic growth in cancer patients. In I. Brdar (Ed.), *The human pursuit of well-being: A cultural approach* (pp. 83–91). Springer. https://doi.org/10.1007/978-94-007-1375-8_8

Sears, S. R., Stanton, A. L., & Danoff-Burg, S. (2003). The yellow brick road and the emerald city: Benefit finding, positive reappraisal coping and posttraumatic growth in women with early-stage breast cancer. *Health Psychology*, *22*(5), 487–497. https://doi.org/10.1037/0278-6133.22.5.487

Seiler, A., & Jenewein, J. (2019). Resilience in cancer patients. *Frontiers in Psychiatry*, *10*, 208. https://doi.org/10.3389/fpsyt.2019.00208

Seitz, D. C., Hagmann, D., Besier, T., Dieluweit, U., Debatin, K. M., Grabow, D., Kaatsch, P., Henrich, G., & Goldbeck, L. (2011). Life satisfaction in adult survivors of cancer during adolescence: What contributes to the latter satisfaction with life? *Quality of Life Research*, *20*(2), 225–236. https://doi.org/10.1007/s11136-010-9739-9

Shand, L. K., Brooker, J. E., Burney, S., Fletcher, J., & Ricciardelli, L. A. (2018). Psychosocial factors associated with posttraumatic stress and growth in Australian women with ovarian cancer. *Journal of Psychosocial Oncology*, *36*(4), 470–483. https://doi.org/10.1080/07347332.2018.1461728

Sharp, L., Redfearn, D., Timmons, A., Balfe, M., & Patterson, J. (2018). Posttraumatic growth in head and neck cancer survivors: Is it possible and what are the correlates? *Psycho-Oncology*, *27*(6), 1517–1523. https://doi.org/10.1002/pon.4682

Shen, M. J., Coups, E. J., Li, Y., Holland, J. C., Hamann, H. A., & Ostroff, J. S. (2015). The role of posttraumatic growth and timing of quitting smoking as moderators of the relationship between stigma and psychological distress among lung cancer survivors who are former smokers. *Psycho-Oncology*, *24*(6), 683–690. https://doi.org/10.1002/pon.3711

Sherman, A., & Simonton, S. (2007). Spirituality and cancer. In T. Plante & C. Thoresen (Eds.), *Spirit, science, and health: How the spiritual mind fuels physical wellness* (pp. 157–175). Praeger Publishers/Greenwood Publishing Group.

Shimizu, Y., Hayashi, A., Maeda, I., Miura, T., Inoue, A., Takano, M., Aoyama, M., Matsuoka, Y. J., Morita, T., Kizawa, Y., Tsuneto, S., Shima, Y., Masukawa, K., & Miyashita, M. (2021). Changes in depressive symptoms among family caregivers of patients with cancer after bereavement and their association with resilience: A prospective cohort study. *Psycho-Oncology*, *31*(1), 86–97. https://doi.org/10.1002/pon.5783

Silva, S. M., Moreira, H. C., & Canavarro, M. C. (2012). Examining the links between perceived impact of breast cancer and psychosocial adjustment: The buffering role of posttraumatic growth. *Psycho-Oncology*, *21*(4), 409–418. https://doi.org/10.1002/pon.1913

Skeath, P., Norris, S., Katheria, V., White, J., Baker, K., Handel, D., Sternberg, E., Pollack, J., Groninger, H., Phillips, J., & Berger, A. (2013). The nature of life-transforming changes among cancer survivors. *Qualitative Health Research*, *23*(9), 1155–1167. https://doi.org/ 10.1177/1049732313499074

Slaughter, R. I., Hamilton, A. S., Cederbaum, J. A., Unger, J. B., Baezconde-Garbanati, L., & Milam, J. E. (2020). Relationships between parent and adolescent/young adult mental health among Hispanic and non-Hispanic childhood cancer survivors. *Journal of Psychosocial Oncology*, *38*(6), 746–760. https://doi.org/10.1080/07347332.2020.1815924

Slaughter, R. I., Hamilton, A. S., Cederbaum, J. A., Unger, J. B., Baezconde-Garbanati, L., & Milam, J. E. (2021). Acculturation discrepancy and mental health associations among Hispanic childhood cancer survivors and their parents. *Psycho-Oncology*, *31*(5), 761–769. https://doi.org/10.1002/pon.5860

Smith, B. W., Dalen, J., Bernard, J. F., & Baumgartner, K. B. (2008). Posttraumatic growth in non-Hispanic White and Hispanic women with cervical cancer. *Journal of Psychosocial Oncology*, *26*(4), 91–109. https://doi.org/10.1080/07347330802359768

Stanton, A., Bower, J., & Low, C. (2006). Posttraumatic growth after cancer. In L. Calhoun, & R. Tedeschi (Eds.), *Handbook of posttraumatic growth: Research and practice* (pp. 138–175). Routledge.

Stuber, M., & Kazak, A. (1999). The developmental impact of cancer diagnosis and treatment for adolescents. In M. Sugar (Ed.), *Trauma and adolescence* (pp. 143–162). International Universities Press, Inc.

Sumalla, E. C., Ochoa, C., & Blanco, I. (2009). Posttraumatic growth in cancer: Reality or illusion? *Clinical Psychology Review*, *29*(1), 24–33. https://doi.org/10.1016/j.cpr.2008.09.006

Suo, R., Ye, F., Xie, M., Zhang, X., Li, M., Zhang, Y., Xiong, C., & Yan, J. (2022). The relationship of marital adjustment and posttraumatic growth in female breast cancer patients and their husbands. *Psychology, Health & Medicine*, *28*(2), 401–407. https://doi.org/10.1080/13548 506.2022.2067339

Tallman, B., Shaw, K., Schultz, J., & Altmaier, E. (2010). Well-being and posttraumatic growth in unrelated donor marrow transplant survivors: A nine-year longitudinal study. *Rehabilitation Psychology*, *55*(2), 204–210. https://doi.org/10.1037/a0019541

Tallman, B. A. (2013). Anticipated posttraumatic growth from cancer: The roles of adaptive and maladaptive coping strategies. *Counselling Psychology Quarterly*, *26*(1), 72–88. https://doi. org/10.1080/09515070.2012.728762

Tallman, B. A., Lohnberg, J., Yamada, T. H., Halfdanarson, T. R., & Altmaier, E. M. (2014). Anticipating posttraumatic growth from cancer: Patients' and collaterals' experiences. *Journal of Psychosocial Oncology*, *32*(3), 342–358. https://doi.org/10.1080/07347 332.2014.897291

Tang, S. T., Lin, K. C., Chen, J. S., Chang, W. C., Hsieh, C. H., & Chou, W. C. (2015). Threatened with death but growing: Changes in and determinants of posttraumatic growth over the dying process for Taiwanese terminally ill cancer patients. *Psycho-Oncology*, 24(2), 147–154. https://doi.org/10.1002/pon.3616

Tedeschi, R. G., & Calhoun, L. G. (1995). *Trauma & transformation: Growing in the aftermath of suffering*. Sage Publications. https://doi.org/10.4135/9781483326931

Tedeschi, R. G., & Calhoun, L. G. (1996). The Posttraumatic Growth Inventory: Measuring the positive legacy of trauma. *Journal of Traumatic Stress*, 9, 455–472. https://doi.org/10.1002/jts.2490090305

Teixeira, R. J., & Pereira, M. G. (2013a). Factors contributing to posttraumatic growth and its buffering effect in adult children of cancer patients undergoing treatment. *Journal of Psychosocial Oncology*, 31(3), 235–265. https://doi.org/10.1080/07347332.2013.778932

Teixeira, R. J., & Pereira, M. G. (2013b). Growth and the cancer caregiving experience: Psychometric properties of the Portuguese Posttraumatic Growth Inventory. *Families, Systems, & Health*, 31(4), 382–395. https://doi.org/10.1037/a0032004

Teixeira, R. J., Applebaum, A. J., Bhatia, S., & Brandão, T. (2018). The impact of coping strategies of cancer caregivers on psychophysiological outcomes: An integrative review. *Psychology Research and Behavior Management*, 11, 207–215. https://doi.org/10.2147/PRBM.S164946

Thombre, A., Sherman, A. C., & Simonton, S. (2010a). Posttraumatic growth among cancer patients in India. *Journal of Behavioral Medicine*, 33(1), 15–23. https://doi.org/10.1007/s10865-009-9229-0

Thombre, A., Sherman, A. C., & Simonton, S. (2010b). Religious coping and posttraumatic growth among family caregivers of cancer patients in India. *Journal of Psychosocial Oncology*, 28(2), 173–188.

Thornton, A. A., & Perez, M. A. (2006). Posttraumatic growth in prostate cancer survivors and their partners. *Psycho-Oncology*, 15(4), 285–296. https://doi.org/10.1002/pon.953

Tillery, R., Cohen, R., Berlin, K. S., Long, A., & Phipps, S. (2017). Youth's adjustment to cancer: Examination of patterns of adjustment and the role of peer relations. *Journal of Pediatric Psychology*, 42(10), 1123–1132. https://doi.org/10.1093/jpepsy/jsx067

Tillery, R., Sharp, K. M. H., Okado, Y., Long, A., & Phipps, S. (2016). Profiles of resilience and growth in youth with cancer and healthy comparisons. *Journal of Pediatric Psychology*, 41(3), 290–297. https://doi.org/10.1093/jpepsy/jsv091

Tobin, J. L., Allem, J.-P., Slaughter, R., Unger, J. B., Hamilton, A. S., & Milam, J. E. (2018). Posttraumatic growth among childhood cancer survivors: Associations with ethnicity, acculturation, and religious service attendance. *Journal of Psychosocial Oncology*, 36(2), 175–188. https://doi.org/10.1080/07347332.2017.1365799

Tomich, P. L., & Helgeson, V. S. (2012). Posttraumatic growth following cancer: Links to quality of life. *Journal of Trauma Stress*, 25(5), 567–573. https://doi.org/10.1002/jts.21738

Tomita, M., Takahashi, M., Tagaya, N., Kakuta, M., Kai, I., & Muto, T. (2017). Structural equation modeling of the relationship between posttraumatic growth and psychosocial factors in women with breast cancer. *Psycho-Oncology*, 26(8), 1198–1204. https://doi.org/10.1002/pon.4298

Tong, Y., Zhou, Y., Yang, Y., Qian, M., Zhang, J., & Gao, J. (2012). A prevalence survey on posttraumatic growth and influencing factors of cancer patients. *Chinese Journal of Clinical Psychology*, 20(1), 76–79.

Trevino, K. M., Archambault, E., Schuster, J., Richardson, P., & Moye, J. (2012). Religious coping and psychological distress in military veteran cancer survivors. *Journal of Religion and Health*, 51(1), 87–98. https://doi.org/10.1007/s10943-011-9526-0

Trzebiński, J., & Zięba, M. (2013). Basic trust and posttraumatic growth in oncology patients. *Journal of Loss and Trauma*, 18(3), 195–209. https://doi.org/10.1080/15325024.2012.687289

Trzmielewska, W., Zięba, M., Boczkowska, M., Rak, T., & Wrześniowski, S. (2019). Motivation of cancer patients to help others and the relation between posttraumatic growth and helping. *Current Issues in Personality Psychology*, 7(3), 232–241. https://doi.org/10.5114/cipp.2019.86231

Tu, P.-C., Yeh, D.-C., & Hsieh, H.-C. (2020). Positive psychological changes after breast cancer diagnosis and treatment: The role of trait resilience and coping styles. *Journal of Psychosocial Oncology*, 38(2), 156–170. https://doi.org/10.1080/07347332.2019.1649337

Turner-Sack, A. M., Menna, R., Setchell, S. R., Maan, C., & Cataudella, D. (2012). Posttraumatic growth, coping strategies, and psychological distress in adolescent survivors of cancer. *Journal of Pediatric Oncology Nursing*, 29(2), 70–79. https://doi.org/10.1177/1043454212439472

Turner-Sack, A. M., Menna, R., Setchell, S. R., Maan, C., & Cataudella, D. (2013). 'Posttraumatic growth, coping strategies, and psychological distress in adolescent survivors of cancer': Corrigendum. *Journal of Pediatric Oncology Nursing*, 30(4), 70–79. https://doi.org/10.1177/1043454213494352

Vallance, J. K., Bebb, G. D., Boyle, T., Johnson, S. T., Gardiner, P. A., & D'Silva, A. (2018). Psychosocial health is associated with objectively assessed sedentary time and light intensity physical activity among lung cancer survivors. *Mental Health and Physical Activity*, 14, 61–65. https://doi.org/10.1016/j.mhpa.2018.02.002

van der Spek, N., Vos, J., van Uden-Kraan, C. F., Breitbart, W., Cuijpers, P., Holtmaat, K., Witte, B. I., Tollenaar, R. A. E. M., & Verdonck-de Leeuw, I. M. (2017). Efficacy of meaning-centered group psychotherapy for cancer survivors: A randomized controlled trial. *Psychological Medicine*, 47(11), 1990–2001. https://doi.org/10.1017/S0033291717000447

Victorson, D., Hankin, V., Burns, J., Weiland, R., Maletich, C., Sufrin, N., Schuette, S., Gutierrez, B., & Brendler, C. (2017). Feasibility, acceptability and preliminary psychological benefits of mindfulness meditation training in a sample of men diagnosed with prostate cancer on active surveillance: Results from a randomized controlled pilot trial. *Psycho-Oncology*, 26(8), 1155–1163. https://doi.org/10.1002/pon.4135

Villanova Quiroga, C., Fritzen Binfare, L., Rudnicki, T., & Iracema de Lima Argimon, I. (2018). Rumination and social support as predictors of posttraumatic growth in women with breast cancer: A systematic review. *Psicooncologia*, 15(2), 301–314.

Villanova Quiroga, C., Raquel Bridi Dacroce, L., Rudnicki, T., & Iracema de Lima Argimon, I. (2020a). Posttraumatic growth and predictor variables in Brazilian women with breast cancer. *Psicooncología*, 17(1), 91–103. https://doi.org/10.5209/psic.68243

Villanova Quiroga, C., Raquel Bridi Dacroce, L., Rudnicki, T., & Iracema de Lima Argimon, I. (2020b). Posttraumatic growth and predictor variables in Brazilian women with breast cancer. *Psicooncologia*, 17(1), 91–103.

Wang, A. W. T., Chang, C. S., Chen, S. T., Chen, D. R., & Hsu, W. Y. (2014). Identification of posttraumatic growth trajectories in the first year after breast cancer surgery. *Psycho-Oncology*, 23(12), 1399–1405. https://doi.org/10.1002/pon.3577

Wang, M.-L., Liu, J.-E., Wang, H.-Y., Chen, J., & Li, Y.-Y. (2014). Posttraumatic growth and associated socio-demographic and clinical factors in Chinese breast cancer survivors. *European Journal of Oncology Nursing*, 18(5), 478–483. https://doi.org/10.1016/j.ejon.2014.04.012

Weinstein, A. G., Henrich, C. C., Armstrong, G. T., Stratton, K. L., King, T. Z., Leisenring, W. M., & Krull, K. R. (2018). Roles of positive psychological outcomes in future health perception and mental health problems: A report from the Childhood Cancer Survivor Study. *Psycho-Oncology*, 27(12), 2754–2760. https://doi.org/10.1002/pon.4881

Weiss, T. (2002). Posttraumatic growth in women with breast cancer and their husbands. *Journal of Psychosocial Oncology*, 20(2), 65–80. https://doi.org/10.1300/J077v20n02_04

Weiss, T. (2004). Correlates of posttraumatic growth in husbands of breast cancer survivors. *Psycho-Oncology, 13*(4), 260–268. https://doi.org/10.1002/pon.735

Widows, M. R., Jacobsen, P. B., Booth-Jones, M., & Fields, K. K. (2005). Predictors of posttraumatic growth following bone marrow transplantation for cancer. *Health Psychology, 24*(3), 266–273. https://doi.org/10.1037/0278-6133.24.3.266

Wilson, B., Morris, B. A., & Chambers, S. (2014a). A structural equation model of posttraumatic growth after prostate cancer. *Psycho-Oncology, 23*(11), 1212–1219. https://doi.org/10.1002/pon.3546

Wilson, B., Morris, B. A., & Chambers, S. (2014b). A structural equation model of posttraumatic growth after prostate cancer. *Psycho-Oncology, 23*(11), 1212–1219.

Wilson, J. Z., Marin, D., Maxwell, K., Cumming, J., Berger, R., Saini, S., Ferguson, W., & Chibnall, J. T. (2016). Association of posttraumatic growth and illness-related burden with psychosocial factors of patient, family, and provider in pediatric cancer survivors. *Journal of Traumatic Stress, 29*(5), 448–456. https://doi.org/10.1002/jts.22123

Wittmann, V., Látos, M., Horváth, Z., Simonka, Z., Paszt, A., Lázár, G., & Csabai, M. (2017). What contributes to long-term quality of life in breast cancer patients who are undergoing surgery? Results of a multidimensional study. *Quality of Life Research, 26*(8), 2189–2199. https://doi.org/10.1007/s11136-017-1563-z

Wong, C. C. Y., Pan-Weisz, B. M., Pan-Weisz, T. M., Yeung, N. C. Y., Mak, W. W. S., & Lu, Q. (2019). Self-stigma predicts lower quality of life in Chinese American breast cancer survivors: Exploring the mediating role of intrusive thoughts and posttraumatic growth. *Quality of Life Research, 28*(10), 2753–2760. https://doi.org/10.1007/s11136-019-02213-w

Wong, M. L., Cavanaugh, C. E., Macleamy, J. B., Sojourner-Nelson, A., & Koopman, C. (2009). Posttraumatic growth and adverse long-term effects of parental cancer in children. *Families, Systems, & Health, 27*(1), 53–63. https://doi.org/10.1037/a0014771

Xu, W., Fu, Z., He, L., Schoebi, D., & Wang, J. (2015). Growing in times of grief: Attachment modulates bereaved adults' posttraumatic growth after losing a family member to cancer. *Psychiatry Research, 230*(1), 108–115. https://doi.org/10.1016/j.psychres.2015.08.035

Yeung, N. C. Y., Zhang, Y., Ji, L., Lu, G., & Lu, Q. (2020). Finding the silver linings: Psychosocial correlates of posttraumatic growth among husbands of Chinese breast cancer survivors. *Psycho-Oncology, 29*(10), 1646–1654. https://doi.org/10.1002/pon.5484

Yi, H. J., & Nam, S. I. (2017). The effect of advocacy for overcoming stigma on posttraumatic growth: Focusing on childhood cancer survivors. *Social Work in Health Care, 56*(9), 840–854. https://doi.org/10.1080/00981389.2017.1353569

Yi, J., & Kim, M. A. (2014). Postcancer experiences of childhood cancer survivors: How is posttraumatic stress related to posttraumatic growth? *Journal of Traumatic Stress, 27*(4), 461–467.

Yi, J., Zebrack, B., Kim, M. A., & Cousino, M. (2015). Posttraumatic growth outcomes and their correlates among young adult survivors of childhood cancer. *Journal of Pediatric Psychology, 40*(9), 981–991. https://doi.org/10.1093/jpepsy/jsv075

Yu, Y., Peng, L., Tang, T., Chen, L., Li, M., & Wang, T. (2014). Effects of emotion regulation and general self-efficacy on posttraumatic growth in Chinese cancer survivors: Assessing the mediating effect of positive affect. *Psycho-Oncology, 23*(4), 473–478.

Yuen, A. N. Y., Ho, S. M. Y., & Chan, C. K. Y. (2014). The mediating roles of cancer-related rumination in the relationship between dispositional hope and psychological outcomes among childhood cancer survivors. *Psycho-Oncology, 23*(4), 412–419.

Zamora, E. R., Yi, J., Akter, J., Kim, J., Warner, E. L., & Kirchhoff, A. C. (2017). 'Having cancer was awful but also something good came out': Post-traumatic growth among adult survivors of pediatric and adolescent cancer. *European Journal of Oncology Nursing, 28*, 21–27. https://doi.org/10.1016/j.ejon.2017.02.001

Zebrack, B., Kwak, M., Salsman, J., Cousino, M., Meeske, K., Aguilar, C., Embry, L., Block, R., Hayes-Lattin, B., & Cole, S. (2015). The relationship between posttraumatic stress and posttraumatic growth among adolescent and young adult (AYA) cancer patients. *Psycho-Oncology, 24*(2), 162–168. https://doi.org/10.1002/pon.3585

Zhai, J., Newton, J., & Copnell, B. (2019). Posttraumatic growth experiences and its contextual factors in women with breast cancer: An integrative review. *Health Care for Women International, 40*(5), 554–580. https://doi.org/10.1080/07399332.2019.1578360

Zhang, J.-Y., Li, S.-S., Meng, L.-N., & Zhou, Y.-Q. (2022). Effectiveness of a nurse-led mindfulness-based Tai Chi Chuan (MTCC) program on posttraumatic growth and perceived stress and anxiety of breast cancer survivors. *European Journal of Psychotraumatology, 13*(1). https://doi.org/10.1080/20008198.2021.2023314

Zhang, J.-Y., Zhou, Y.-Q., Feng, Z.-W., Fan, Y.-N., Zeng, G.-C., & Wei, L. (2017). Randomized controlled trial of mindfulness-based stress reduction (MBSR) on posttraumatic growth of Chinese breast cancer survivors. *Psychology, Health & Medicine, 22*(1), 94–109. https://doi.org/10.1080/13548506.2016.1146405

Zwahlen, D., Hagenbuch, N., Carley, M. I., Jenewein, J., & Buchi, S. (2010). Posttraumatic growth in cancer patients and partners—Effects of role, gender and the dyad on couples' posttraumatic growth experience. *Psycho-Oncology, 19*(1), 12–20. https://doi.org/10.1002/pon.1486

6

Posttraumatic stress disorder associated with human immunodeficiency virus/acquired immunodeficiency syndrome

People infected with HIV/AIDS are significantly more distressed and have more psychiatric disorders than the general population (Beyer et al., 2007). Some of the psychiatric disorders first appeared after HIV diagnosis or during the course of the disease. The severity seems to be consistent: in one study, 56% of patients initially met the diagnostic criteria for a psychiatric disorder. Six months later, 48% still had at least one psychiatric disorder (Olley et al., 2006). People with HIV alone or with another illness would express their psychiatric symptoms differently. One study looked at adult patients with HIV, tuberculosis, or both. Rates of suicidality (34.8%) and panic disorder (4.1%) were highest in the tuberculosis–HIV group, whereas rates of anxiety disorder (37.8%), generalised anxiety disorder (13.3%), obsessive–compulsive disorder (7.6%), and PTSD (7.4%) were highest in the HIV group (van den Heuvel et al., 2013).

Among psychiatric outpatients, 1.2% had HIV infection, which is about four times the frequency of HIV infection in the general population (Beyer et al., 2007). More than one-third of these patients had two or more co-occurring psychological disorders (Israelski et al., 2007), including mood disorders, personality disorders, bipolar disorder, acute stress disorder, and suicidality (Beyer et al., 2007; Haller & Miles, 2003; Israelski et al., 2007; Myer et al., 2008; Pence et al., 2006). Among psychiatric patients with HIV who had suicidal ideation, more than half reported comorbid psychiatric symptoms such as depression, substance abuse, and depressive personality disorder (Haller & Miles, 2003). Men with generalised anxiety disorder were ten times more likely to be diagnosed with HIV (adjusted odds ratio (aOR): 10.3) than

Posttraumatic Stress in Physical Illness. Man Cheung Chung, Oxford University Press. © Oxford University Press 2024.
DOI: 10.1093/oso/9780198727323.003.0006

men without generalised anxiety disorder. Women with generalised anxiety disorder were five times more likely to be diagnosed with HIV (aOR: 5.01) than women without such an anxiety diagnosis (Brown et al., 2020).

PTSD, psychiatric comorbidity in people with HIV/ AIDS

Posttraumatic stress disorder is another condition that has been identified in people with HIV/AIDS. For example, among people with HIV/AIDS who were exposed to trauma, 34% met diagnostic criteria for PTSD (Gonzalez et al., 2016). The potential impact of past trauma on disease progression cannot be underestimated (Kimerling et al., 1999). A trauma model has been postulated as a way to care for and treat people with HIV/AIDS. The reason for this assertion is that trauma rates are high and variable among people with HIV infection. Many people living with HIV are also trauma victims who endure negative health consequences. Such trauma can also increase HIV risk behaviours and thus transmission and acquisition of the virus, and is associated with negative factors mediating the impact of poor health status on risky HIV behaviours, poor treatment adherence, poor HIV-related health, and other health outcomes, and is particularly evident among some vulnerable groups of people such as sex workers and victims of abuse (Brezing et al., 2015).

When addressing PTSD in this HIV/AIDS population, one cannot focus only on PTSD. Syndemic conditions (i.e. coexisting, interrelated biological, or psychological epidemics that impact the health of a population or community) are common in this population. This is consistent with the argument made in the previous chapter that PTSD is not a clinical syndrome in its own right, but that it often manifests itself through other clinical problems. In the context of HIV/AIDS, different combinations of medical conditions and psychiatric symptoms can impact HIV-related psychiatric outcomes and increase HIV risk behaviours (e.g. condom negotiation and sex without condoms) and HIV/AIDS severity (Singer, 1996; Singer & Clair, 2003).

PTSD and depression are common among HIV/AIDS patients, ranging from 2% to 34% among the former and from 14% to 76% among the latter (Cohen et al., 2009). Among people living with HIV in the Gambia, prevalence rates for PTSD and depressive symptoms were 43.2% and 40.9%, respectively (Klis et al., 2011). In South Africa, PTSD and depression were most prevalent among HIV-positive patients over time (baseline: approximately 15% and 35%; 6-month follow-up: 20% and 26%). Although there was evidence of symptom reduction in half of the patients, new cases of depression (8%) and PTSD (71%) also occurred at follow-up (Olley et al., 2006). Another study found that 34% had PTSD, 38% had depression and 43% had acute stress disorder. In addition, they found that 38% met the diagnostic criteria for two or more disorders (Israelski et al., 2007). Among people seeking HIV testing in South Africa, prevalence rates appeared to be lower: 8.04% met diagnostic criteria for PTSD (Kagee, Bantjes, et al., 2017).

PTSD and depression symptoms can affect general psychological well-being, social functioning (e.g. work performance), and pain tolerance, and may increase pain levels in HIV patients (Leserman et al., 2005; O'Cleirigh et al., 2009; Tsao et al., 2004). It has been shown that patients with HIV/AIDS and high rates of PTSD, depression, and acute stress disorder tend to use public health services (Israelski et al., 2007). The severity of these symptoms may have been responsible for health care utilisation over and above the severity of HIV symptoms or other HIV-related indicators (Leserman et al., 2005; O'Cleirigh et al., 2009). PTSD has been specifically associated with an increased risk of bed confinement, hospitalisation, emergency room visits, and outpatient visits, especially among those who had experienced trauma such as sexual or physical abuse in the past (Leserman et al., 2005).

In addition to depression (14.2%), PTSD (4.9%) was also reported alongside generalised anxiety disorder (5.0%) (Kagee, Saal, et al., 2017), death anxiety (Safren et al., 2003), decreased life satisfaction (Oniszczenko et al., 2019), and alcohol use disorder (19.8%) (Kagee, Saal, et al., 2017). Specifically, PTSD, depression, insomnia, alcohol and substance use disorders (i.e. cocaine abuse and dependence, opioid abuse and dependence, cannabis abuse, other psychoactive substance abuse and dependence, and polysubstance use disorders) were each positively associated with suicidal ideation/behaviour in people living with HIV. Alcohol and cocaine dependence, depression, and PTSD were the most significant predictors (Brown et al., 2021). A large cohort study examined just over 139,000 veterans with dually diagnosed PTSD and co-morbid substance use disorders, finding that HIV was one of the medical diagnoses strongly associated with this dual diagnosis (Bowe & Rosenheck, 2015).

The above findings on substance use are perhaps not too surprising, as it has been shown to be a common form of avoidance coping among trauma victims. For example, about half (50.5%) of HIV-positive adults exposed to the Haiti earthquake met criteria for PTSD. Individuals with greater alcohol problems, women, younger participants, and those who had lost all belongings during the earthquake were more likely to report PTSD symptoms. Individuals who felt the need to reduce their alcohol consumption and who sought distraction through behavioural disengagement were more likely to meet criteria for PTSD (Dévieux et al., 2013).

HIV patients with a lifetime of trauma and PTSD symptoms also tend to have neurocognitive impairment (OR: 6.12) (Deiss et al., 2019) and poorer cognitive functioning, in addition to physical and social functioning, than their comparison group (Leserman et al., 2005). Compared to healthy controls, people with HIV had lower scores on executive function and autobiographical recall (semantic and episodic), along with higher scores on PTSD and depressive symptoms. They were less able to recall specific autobiographical memories than the control group. Caregivers of people living with HIV also had lower scores on episodic recall, fewer specific memories, and higher levels of depression than the healthy control group (Moradi et al., 2013).

Neurocognitive impairment especially is a problem among older people with HIV. One study showed that 40% suffered from mild cognitive impairment and 12% from PTSD, along with lack of social support (60%), loneliness (58%), depression (55%), falls (40%), and poor or mediocre quality of life (30%) (John et al., 2016). People who develop neurological and cognitive changes, which can result from deficits in executive function, initiation, and perseveration difficulties, are more prone to rumination, which can lead to impaired ability to cope with the stresses associated with HIV. In addition, pre-existing conditions such as PTSD can lead these older adults to exacerbate neurological and cognitive problems, which in turn can trigger further rumination and increase the severity of depression and suicidal ideation (Vance et al., 2008). Not only do adults living with HIV exhibit coexisting psychiatric problems, but so do adolescents living with HIV. Violence leading to PTSD, depression, and anxiety has been found among inner-city HIV-positive adolescents (Martinez et al., 2009), with these prevalence rates identified: PTSD, 20.6%; depression, 35%; anxiety, 25.7% (Lynn et al., 2018).

It is worth pointing out that most, if not all, of these prevalence rates may have been the by-product of different types of screening instruments. For example, among adults in Africa with varying HIV status (44.6% positive, 49% negative, and HIV status for the rest unknown), the Posttraumatic Stress Disorder Checklist—5 validated 74.5% as a sensitivity score, 70.6% as a specificity score, and 0.92 as a Cronbach's alpha; 0.78 was the value for the area under the receiver operating characteristic curve (Verhey et al., 2018). Similarly, among HIV test seekers in South Africa, the Posttraumatic Stress Scale—Self-Report version has been shown to be effective in screening for PTSD, distinguishing those who meet the diagnostic criteria for PTSD from those who do not. This scale had a sensitivity, specificity, and internal consistency of 0.76, 0.78, and 0.95, respectively, and was compared to the Structured

Clinical Interview for the *Diagnostic and statistical manual of mental disorders* as the gold standard measure (Kagee et al., 2019).

The short version of the Hopkins Symptom Checklist (HSCL-25) was found to be moderately accurate in identifying common psychological disorders in these individuals, with a sensitivity of 69% and a specificity of 71%. It also performed better than the Beck Depression Inventory in identifying depressive disorders and was equally as good as the Beck Anxiety Inventory and the Posttraumatic Stress Scale—Self-Report in identifying generalised anxiety disorders and PTSD cases. However, as a transdiagnostic screening measure in the HIV setting, the HSCL-25 did not perform well, especially in identifying alcohol use disorders (Bantjes et al., 2020). While these prevalence rates might identify some individual psychological disorders associated with HIV, they do not provide a clear picture of the underlying vulnerabilities they all share.

It is noteworthy that PTSD and comorbid psychological disorders are also associated with biological markers. For example, significant associations have been found between depression, anxiety, and CD4 count (T-cells or T-helper cells that prevent infection by activating our immune system when viruses or bacteria are detected) and anxiety and viral load (VL) (Lynn et al., 2019). Traumatic stressors were also associated with lower ratios of CD4 to CD8 T-cells (a marker of disease progression) over time, while a PTSD diagnosis was specifically related to lower ratios of CD4 to CD8 t-cells over time (Kimerling et al., 1999). In addition, depression and PTSD predicted other biological markers, with the former predicting detectable viral load (Boarts et al., 2006), while the latter predicted lower morning salivary cortisol levels (Delahanty et al., 2004). Depression has also been associated with low CD4 cell count (Boarts et al., 2006; Cohen et al., 2009; Klis et al., 2011; Olley et al., 2006; Sledjeski et al., 2005), although this association is not always consistent (Fincham et al., 2008).

PTSD due to HIV-related events

It is worth noting that, in most of the studies mentioned above, PTSD symptoms were due to previous trauma unrelated to the HIV event. However, a case study was presented on the development of PTSD in a male institutional worker who was bitten by an HIV-positive inmate. Interestingly, the PTSD reactions did not result from the bite, but from the threat of being infected by AIDS (Geller, 1989). Subsequently, several case studies emerged examining PTSD symptoms associated with HIV disease progression (Kimerling et al., 1999) and contact with persons believed to have HIV-positive blood (Howsepian, 1998).

The impact of HIV diagnosis can also be psychologically distressing, leading some people (30%) to meet diagnostic criteria for PTSD (PTSD–HIV). More than one-third of patients with PTSD show a delayed-onset PTSD response, i.e. ≥6 months after the initial HIV diagnosis. PTSD-HIV has been associated with depression occurring after HIV diagnosis, with a diagnosis prior to PTSD–HIV resulting from previous trauma, with psychiatric disorders prior to HIV diagnosis and with neuroticism (Kelly et al., 1998). Similarly, another study showed that adolescents and young adults reported an average of six traumatic events in their lives. Most of them (93%) found the diagnosis of having HIV traumatic. Of these patients, 13% met criteria for PTSD, while 20% met criteria for partial PTSD (Radcliffe et al., 2007). Another study also showed that patients experienced an average of six different types of trauma in their lives. Receiving an HIV diagnosis was also considered one of the most distressing experiences, with almost 54% meeting the criteria for PTSD. These individuals also tended to report greater pain intensity and pain-related impairment in daily functioning (e.g. working and sleeping) than those who did not meet the PTSD diagnosis (Smith et al., 2002). PTSD–HIV Severity may have been exacerbated by feelings of guilt, shame or regret about taking sexual risks, although this finding is not always consistent (Theuninck et al., 2010).

However, without repeating the arguments discussed in Chapter 1, the question arises whether the diagnosis of HIV can be treated as a traumatic event. That being said, it is not unreasonable to assume a certain level of 'trauma' when one learns that one has HIV, even though this may not fit the official diagnostic definition. It could therefore be argued that understanding traumatic responses needs to take into account the impact of such a diagnosis, while recognising that using HIV diagnosis as the official trauma index or focusing solely on the psychological impact may not be sufficient. A broader approach is needed. For example, one study examined the impact of diagnosis, treatment, physical symptoms, disclosure of HIV-positive status, and the experience of HIV-related death on the development of PTSD. Patients' experiences of medical treatment, experiencing physical symptoms and witnessing HIV-related death were strongly related to HIV-PTSD symptoms. In other words, several potentially traumatic factors may play a role in the different stages of HIV screening, assessment, and treatment (Theuninck et al., 2010).

Risk factors

Among the risk factors influencing the relationships between PTSD and psychiatric comorbidity in people living with HIV/AIDS, gender differences, stigma, and coping strategies appear to play a role.

Women's responses

It has been suggested that trauma and PTSD disproportionately affect HIV-positive women. A meta-analysis showed that the prevalence of PTSD among these women was 30%, more than five times higher than among women without HIV (Machtinger, Wilson, et al., 2012). Their psychological distress was related to multiple traumas (Delany-Brumsey et al., 2013). Among African American women living with HIV, 67% reported clinically significant PTSD symptoms (Andu et al., 2018), while in another study 36% met screening criteria for PTSD and 37% had depression (Battaglia et al., 2015). This rate of depression was compatible (36%) with HIV-positive women in South Africa, 70% of whom met screening criteria for PTSD due to past trauma (Yemeke et al., 2020).

Compared to uninfected women, HIV-positive women in South Africa were significantly more likely to report depressive symptoms and PTSD in addition to alcohol abuse (Hansrod et al., 2015). They also tended to report more PTSD, depression and anxiety symptoms than non-abused women (Axelrod et al., 1999). Another study focused on HIV-infected mothers with young children, most of whom were African American and Latina. It found that the prevalence rates of major depression and PTSD were 58% and 38%, respectively. PTSD correlated with prior substance use and the number of traumas experienced correlated with psychiatric and psychological functioning (Mellins et al., 1997).

In terms of the nature of trauma, intimate partner violence (IPV) appears to be particularly common among HIV-positive women, with an estimated prevalence rate of 55%—more than double that of women without HIV (Machtinger, Wilson, et al., 2012). Women exposed to IPV and living with HIV had more severe mental health symptoms than those who did not suffer from either problem (Kaufman et al., 2020). Some of these women may also be involved with illicit substances. Women with experiences of HIV, IPV, and substance abuse tended to have more severe posttraumatic stress symptoms

(PTSS), especially among those who had experienced more than one of the above events. However, the impact of these trauma reactions can be mitigated by social support. For women who had higher levels of support, experiencing any of the above adversities was associated with lower PTSS. Conversely, for women with lower levels of support, experiencing more than one of these adversities was associated with higher PTSS. In other words, social support may apparently be a protective factor for these women (Howell et al., 2020).

One study also showed that in addition to IPV (75%), 51% of respondents also reported a history of sexual abuse (Yemeke et al., 2020). Sexual trauma appeared to be more prevalent among European American and African American women than among Latina women (Paxton et al., 2004). HIV-infected women also had higher rates of childhood trauma, which mediated the impact of intimate partner violence on PTSD. In other words, these HIV-positive women's experiences of IPV may have triggered their childhood trauma experiences, which in turn increased the severity of their PTSD (Hansrod et al., 2015).

PTSD has also been found in Rwandan women exposed to the 1994 genocide. Fifty-eight per cent of HIV-positive and 66% of HIV-negative women met diagnostic criteria for PTSD resulting from the genocide. HIV-positive women (81%) showed more depressive symptoms than HIV-negative women (65%). Increased depression was associated with increased PTSD symptoms (Cohen et al., 2009). Although trauma symptoms decreased over time (18 months) and prevalence rates for PTSD decreased significantly from 61% at baseline to 24%, there were individual differences in improvement of PTSD symptoms. Those who had initially suffered high levels of trauma related to the genocide appeared to have improved the most in PTSD symptoms. In contrast, those who initially had high levels of depression tended to have less improvement in PTSD symptoms, suggesting that initial depression levels may have acted as a barrier to improvement in PTSD symptoms. Severity of HIV infection and antiretroviral treatment were not consistently associated with improvement in PTSD symptoms (Cohen et al., 2011).

Among these Rwandan genocide survivors, women with more severe PTSD reported poorer health-related quality of life and overall quality of life than women with fewer PTSD symptoms, even after controlling for depression and HIV disease progression (Gard et al., 2013). In addition, women with HIV, notably those with the lowest CD4 levels, reported poorer health-related quality of life and overall quality of life than women without HIV (Gard et al., 2013). This finding is consistent with research suggesting that HIV-positive women tend to have a low quality of life and low CD4 count but a high HIV viral load (Rose et al., 2010).

While the above studies focused on women with positive or negative HIV infection or on specific trauma types, it has been argued that, regardless of HIV status or trauma types, the impact of cumulative trauma and the extent of victimisation or aggression are the important factors to focus on. Cumulative trauma exposure is positively associated with increased psychological distress. However, this association is partly mediated by various factors, e.g. impaired psychosocial resources (Delany-Brumsey et al., 2013). Women who experienced more victimisation and aggression were more likely to report PTSD and depressive symptoms, regardless of the type of trauma (Weiss et al., 2017).

Men's responses

A large epidemiological study has shown that experiencing family violence in childhood was related to HIV infection in men. This life event can lead to the development of PTSD, which in turn affects HIV infection (Reisner et al., 2011). Similar to women, childhood trauma also appears to be prevalent, as in one study more than one-third and one-half of the sample, respectively, reported childhood sexual abuse and met diagnostic criteria for PTSD. The severity of dissociation was associated with the experience of abuse and the severity of PTSD symptoms, suggesting that these HIV-positive men may be dissociative PTSD subtypes (Kamen et al., 2012). These findings were confirmed in a later study, which showed that sexual revictimisation was correlated with the severity of current PTSD symptoms in a group of HIV-positive men. They were also prone to peritraumatic dissociation, which increases the risk of PTSD and worsening HIV-related health (Yiaslas et al., 2014).

Studies have been conducted specifically looking at men who have sex with men (MSM). One study found that PTSD and major depressive disorder, as well as substance use disorders and major depressive disorder, can co-occur and synergistically increase HIV risk. Surprisingly, however, substance use and PTSD did not appear to have a significant association (Batchelder et al., 2019). This finding was surprising as the relationship between these two constructs has been demonstrated in the trauma literature (Vujanovic et al., 2018), suggesting that the relationship between PTSD and substance use may vary by trauma type. Other studies also examined associations between PTSD symptoms, posttraumatic cognitions, and alcohol intoxication among sexually risky HIV-uninfected MSM who reported a history of childhood sexual abuse. They found that higher levels of PTSD symptoms and posttraumatic cognitions were associated with increased intoxication, accounting for 2.6%

and 5.2% of the variance above demographics, respectively. Higher PTSD symptom severity was indirectly associated with more frequent alcohol intoxication through cognitions about the self and the world. PTSD due to past trauma was associated with distorted perceptions and appraisals of the world as dangerous, which may have exacerbated the desire to use alcohol as a form of self-medication among MSM with a history of childhood sexual abuse (Banerjee et al., 2018).

Another study examined PTSD in sexual minority adult men. It compared emerging adult sexual minority men (aged 18–29 years) with sexual minority men of older age on PTSD and other mental health and substance use. There was a higher likelihood of PTSD (OR: 0.57), panic disorder (OR: 0.36), and cocaine use (OR: 0.50) among older sexual minority men. At the same time, they found a higher likelihood of alcohol intoxication (OR: 5.60), cannabis use (OR: 3.09), and non-HIV-related sexually transmitted infections (OR: 3.03) among emerging adult men. These findings revealed some complex associations of health risks among sexual minority men in general and emerging adult sexual minority men in particular (Boroughs et al., 2018).

Gender comparison

It has been postulated that, by and large, HIV-infected women have worse health or psychological outcomes than men (Rose et al., 2010). For example, women with HIV reported higher scores on all PTSS dimensions than men with HIV (Rzeszutek et al., 2017a). Women also need more social support than men and had actually received more support than men. Furthermore, a positive relationship between support received and global trauma score was only found in women (Rzeszutek et al., 2017a). Regardless, one could argue that the focus should not be on which gender is a risky one. Rather, the focus should be on how they differ in the manifestation of psychological symptoms. For example, anxiety and mood disorders were highly likely in men infected with HIV/AIDS, while depression and PTSD were prevalent in women (Myers & Durvasula, 1999). In men, major depression was fully associated with physical/psychological abuse and sexual abuse, as well as HIV/STI (sexually transmitted infection). For women, major depression fully mediated physical/psychological abuse and parental violence. For men, IPV fully mediated sexual abuse and HIV/STI. For women, IPV perpetration was not a mediator (Brown et al., 2017).

Among people who were willing to undergo HIV testing, men were 1.64 and 4.88 times more likely than women to have an alcohol problem and substance abuse, respectively. PTSD and anxiety and depression were associated with alcohol abuse, while PTSD accounted for 23.5% of the variance in substance use (Kagee et al., 2018). Among female homeless youth, experiencing PTSD due to sexual victimisation was associated with HIV risk behaviours, whereas male youth were more likely to use drugs (Harris et al., 2017).

Stigmatisation

Stigma can arise from HIV/AIDS diagnoses, mental health diagnoses, or misconceptions about one's behaviour (Schneider et al., 2018). It is a factor that can exacerbate trauma-related psychopathology and hinder symptom improvement. Stigma was strongly associated with increased rates of lifetime and current PTSD and decreased likelihood of spontaneous remission, and this effect was stronger than the effect of trauma exposure (Katz & Nevid, 2005; Schneider et al., 2018). After controlling for gender, age, education and number of traumatic events, internalised HIV stigma remained positively associated with overall PTSD symptom severity and severity of re-experiencing and hyperarousal, but not with trauma avoidance in people living with HIV/AIDS (Gonzalez et al., 2016).

One study showed that more than a quarter of the sample met criteria for HIV stigma-related PTSD after at least one intense HIV-related stigmatising event or situation. Risk factors included low levels of social support, psychological disorders, as well as low self-esteem. The presence of these risk factors could increase the likelihood of HIV stigma-related PTSD by two to nine times. It has been suggested that stigma should be considered when designing a rehabilitation strategy for HIV patients (Adewuya et al., 2009). When considering rehabilitation for these patients, it is important not to overlook the protective or resilience factors that may also be present in some of these individuals. For example, while internalised HIV stigma may be a vulnerability factor for PTSD symptom severity, older age and higher education have been shown to be protective (Andu et al., 2018).

Adolescents-may also experience the effects of stigma on their mental health. Among HIV-affected adolescents in South Africa, after adjusting for mental health symptoms and demographic characteristics at baseline, internalised stigma at baseline was associated with worse outcomes on all psychological measures (depression, anxiety, posttraumatic stress, bullying victimisation) in the long term (18 months later). Bullying victimisation was indirectly associated with all psychological measures through internalised stigma. In other words, bullying may have triggered internalised stigma, which in turn was associated with psychological symptoms over time (Boyes et al., 2020).

Similarly, AIDS orphaned youth may experience higher levels of stigma in the community than non-orphaned youth or youth orphaned by causes other than AIDS (Cluver et al., 2008). Stigma has been found to mediate the relationship between AIDS orphanhood and psychological distress. While this could mean that AIDS orphanhood results in high levels of stigma, which in turn increases psychological distress, it could also be argued that improving stigma might in turn reduce psychological distress for these young people (Cluver et al., 2008). It is understandable that these young people needed support. One study showed that those with high levels of perceived social support tended to have lower PTSD symptoms, which were due to varying levels of trauma exposure. Such support could be provided by caregivers, school staff, and friends (Cluver et al., 2009).

A problem closely related to stigma is that of discrimination. Among black women living with HIV, after controlling for age, education, and income, higher gender-based racial microaggression (i.e. daily insults experienced by black women based on skin colour and gender) and HIV-related discrimination were associated with increased PTSD symptoms, although only gender-based racial microaggression uniquely contributed to both total PTSD symptoms and total posttraumatic cognitions (Dale & Safren, 2019).

Coping

In examining the coping strategies of HIV/AIDS patients, the literature seems to indicate that one should not focus only on the individual strategies. Instead, consideration should be given to how these strategies may interact with each other and influence the outcome of distress. For example, in HIV/AIDS patients, attachment may be particularly effective in reducing trauma-related symptoms in adults living with HIV/AIDS (Gore-Felton et al., 2013). However, attachment should not be considered alone. Avoidant attachment and emotion-focused coping (e.g. venting emotions or avoidance coping) have been associated with increased PTSD symptoms. Those who exhibited a strong avoidant attachment style tended to have more PTSD symptoms. However, those who practised a great deal of emotion-focused coping and who had low levels of avoidant attachment or secure attachment (i.e. insecure attachment) tended to have higher levels of PTSD (Gore-Felton et al., 2013).

The interrelationship between attachment, coping, and distress can also be influenced by social support. Patients with avoidant and insecure attachment styles who receive varying levels of social support may influence the impact of emotion-focused coping on increased PTSD symptoms. For example, research shows that people who are highly avoidant are less likely to seek social support to cope with distress and therefore the extent of their emotion-focused coping may not affect distress. On the other hand, people who are not of the avoidant type are more likely to seek social support and rely on this relational support to cope with stress, which is likely to be influenced by their level of emotion-focused coping (Gore-Felton et al., 2013). Similarly, a study found that attachment anxiety, rather than insecure attachment, was associated with PTSD symptoms in people with HIV/AIDS through levels of social support and resilience (Wang et al., 2018).

In terms of social support, although HIV–PTSD has been associated with lower perceived social support (Katz & Nevid, 2005), personality traits must also be considered. One study focused on these patients, as well as on patients with chronic pain, finding that temperament traits (emotional reactivity, perseveration, and sensory sensitivity) and dimensions of social support (perceived support, need for support, seeking support, and actual support received) predicted trauma symptoms in participants. These traits and social support did not appear to interact to influence outcomes. There were significant differences between trauma symptom severity, temperament, and social support between HIV/AIDS and chronic pain patients (Rzeszutek et al., 2016).

Patients' coping styles may change from maladaptive to adaptive coping behaviours over a 6-month period, with the use of denial and ventilation decreasing over time. Meanwhile, the use of instrumental and emotional support, positive reframing, planning, and acceptance increased (Olley et al., 2006). Some researchers took a positive psychology approach and focused on 'adaptive' coping strategies. For example, mindfulness has been shown to buffer the severity of PTSD symptoms. Acting with awareness can protect oneself and act as a resilient factor (Gonzalez et al., 2016). It has been suggested that coping self-efficacy appraisals in HIV-seropositive patients influence psychological and physiological functioning. Greater endorsement of this self-efficacy contributed to reductions in emotional distress, PTSD symptoms, and to norepinephrine:cortisol ratios in HIV patients (Benight et al., 1997). However, for many patients, this positive approach may be hindered by their distorted view of their own health, as they become preoccupied with various illnesses and symptoms of illness (Botha, 1996), while they may have difficulty expressing their associated emotions. This in turn contributed to their low quality of life, i.e. reduced physical and psychological well-being, as well as lower overall social functioning (Olley & Bolajoko, 2008).

Other risk factors

Among women living with HIV, high spirituality was associated with increased mental health symptoms. However, among those not living with HIV, high spirituality was associated with lower levels of mental health symptoms (Kaufman et al., 2020). Similarly, religious fundamentalism was positively correlated with PTSD intensity (Oniszczenko et al., 2019). These findings seemed to have supported the claim that spirituality is associated with mental health problems to varying degrees especially among women facing adversity. It could be that these women have heightened their awareness of spiritual or religious matters when faced with a life-threatening illness and the associated psychological problems (Kaufman et al., 2020).

PTSD, psychiatric comorbidity and the risk behaviour for HIV/AIDS

Whereas the foregoing literature focuses on the relationship between PTSD and psychiatric comorbidity in people with HIV/AIDS, other literature specifically addresses risk factors for increased risk behaviours for HIV/AIDS. Past trauma or negative life events and psychiatric disorders have been shown to be risk factors (Katz & Nevid, 2005; Kelly et al., 1998). Past trauma prior to HIV infection may have influenced HIV risk behaviour or transmission risk (Machtinger, Haberer, et al., 2012) before a diagnosis of HIV was made. PTSD has been associated with decreased sexual control, which in turn led to an increase in unprotected sex (Munroe et al., 2010).

One study examined young gay and bisexual men and found that PTSD from past trauma was associated with a higher risk of sexual transmission behaviours in younger but not older men, regardless of stage of HIV disease or treatment status (O'Cleirigh et al., 2013). PTSD increased the likelihood of engaging in risky sexual behaviour by 5.1% (Paxton et al., 2004).

Hyperarousal symptom severity predicted risky sexual behaviour above and beyond age and all other PTSD symptom clusters. In other words, PTSD, especially hyperarousal symptoms, may heighten certain HIV risk behaviours (Weiss et al., 2013). An alternative explanation is that engaging in these behaviours would likely lead to increased feelings of anxiety or hyperarousal.

Hyperarousal is a symptom that overlaps with anxiety disorder symptoms (Zoellner et al., 2011).

Among young people who inject drugs, although PTSD did not appear to be related to syringe sharing, which is known to increase the likelihood of risky injecting behaviour (i.e. syringe sharing) and thus HIV risk, substance-induced depression across the life course and in the past year and borderline personality disorder were significantly associated with a higher likelihood of such risky behaviour (Mackesy-Amiti et al., 2014). The lack of an association between PTSD and injecting drug use was also found in a previous study that focused on adults (Weiss et al., 2013).

Soldiers who had both PTSD and depressive disorders were very likely to report increased HIV risk behaviours (adjusted odds ratio: 2.75) and a greater risk of HIV infection (Marshall et al., 2013). A history of PTSD along with other psychological problems (e.g. substance abuse) could increase the risk of HIV infection by almost 12-fold compared to individuals without any of these problems (Hoff et al., 1997). In addition to the psychiatric disorders mentioned above, experiences of child abuse also appear to play a role. MSM with a history of childhood sexual abuse has been found to dissociate, carrying the severity of lifelong PTSD symptoms to condomless sex episodes. It appears that dissociation in traumatised MSM with a history of childhood sexual abuse distorted their perception of sexual risk and safety and increased vulnerability to HIV infection (Coleman et al., 2022). This echoes a previous study that a cycle of unprocessed early trauma may contribute to early and sexual risk behaviours and thus HIV risk among club drug users (Narvaez et al., 2019). Traumatic stress due to racial discrimination is another factor influencing sexual risk behaviour. Among urban black heterosexually identified men, PTSS was found to mediate the relationship between everyday racial discrimination and sexual risk behaviour. In other words, traumatic stress due to racial discrimination could lead to an increase in sexual risk behaviour among black heterosexual men (Bowleg et al., 2014).

Focusing on women's experiences, women who exhibited PTSD symptoms due to previous trauma tended to engage in HIV risk behaviours, including sexual relationships with multiple people or high-risk partners, violent experiences related to condom use, injection drug use, prostitution, needle sharing, and anal intercourse (El-Bassel et al., 2011; Hutton et al., 2001). Compared to women without recent trauma, women with trauma were more than four times as likely to report antiretroviral failure (aOR: 4.3), more than three times as likely to report having sex with a partner with HIV-negative or unknown serostatus (aOR: 3.9) and more than four times as likely to report not always using condoms with these partners (aOR: 4.5) (Machtinger, Haberer, et al., 2012).

It has been postulated that risk behaviours, including HIV risk behaviours, are more common among women who have experienced sexual victimisation, particularly aggression (Weiss et al., 2017). One study examined women with protection orders against violent partners in South Africa and found that a high proportion (51.9%) suffered from PTSD and depression (66.4%). Severe physical and sexual intimate partner violence and PTSD increased HIV risk, e.g. never having used a condom in the last 3 months (Pengpid & Peltzer, 2013). Similarly, almost 75% of women with partner violence, substance abuse, risky alcohol use, depression, and PTSD also showed fear of negotiating and using condoms, which would increase the likelihood of sexual risk. These psychiatric conditions were mostly correlated with each other and the severity of the symptoms correlated with the aforementioned fear (Peasant et al., 2017). Another study has shown that single homeless women with childhood abuse experiences may increase the risk of HIV/sexually transmitted infections through a combination of PTSD and borderline personality disorder (Houston et al., 2013).

Several studies have been conducted to examine women in forensic settings. Among African American female juvenile offenders, trauma in the community was found to be associated with PTSD over time and HIV/STI-associated sexual risk factors and behaviours such as unprotected sex and having a sexual partner with a correctional/juvenile justice history. In addition, trauma in the community was also associated with sexual sensation seeking, marijuana use, and affiliation with deviant peers. The findings highlight the influence of community-level factors and co-occurring health problems, particularly among vulnerable populations (Seth et al., 2017). When examining HIV risk behaviours among rural women drug users in prison, almost 80% of women reported symptoms of depression, and more than 60% reported anxiety and PTSD symptoms. Mental health problems correlated significantly with the severity of certain types of drug use, as well as with risky sexual activity. Among women who suffered from anxiety and PTSD, injecting drug use moderated the association between mental health and risky sexual activity. In other words, the impact of mental health on risky sexual activity varies by type of injecting drug use (Staton-Tindall et al., 2015).

Women prison inmates and adolescents who have PTSD due to childhood abuse may engage in high-risk behaviours and are at higher risk of acquiring HIV (Cotter et al., 2006). Among women on probation with a lifetime history of victimisation, substance use also correlated with most of their HIV risks, including lifetime sexual partners and sexual partners in the past 12 months.

Lifetime traumatic experiences were associated with specific HIV risks along with age, race/ethnicity, homelessness, regular use of alcohol leading to intoxication and other drugs, functional social support, and substance use in the past 12 months (Engstrom et al., 2017).

PTSD, psychiatric comorbidity and medication adherence

PTSD and depression can also affect adherence to medication among HIV-infected individuals, which in turn has implications for the management of the disease. People with PTSD and depression are less likely to adhere to their medications and to highly active antiretroviral therapy (HAART) (Boarts et al., 2006; Chernoff, 2007; Delahanty et al., 2004; Sledjeski et al., 2005; Wagner et al., 2012). Thus, they could become resistant to the drugs and tend to have deteriorating immune systems, which in turn would increase the chances of infection (Delahanty et al., 2004). This problem of non-adherence could be due to the 'spectrum of posttraumatic disturbance' that we discussed in Chapter 2. As part of their PTSD symptoms, patients wanted to avoid being reminded of HIV/AIDS and could therefore avoid adherence to medication. However, this theoretical postulate is challenged when high levels of perceived vulnerability to HIV and PTSD symptoms have been shown to increase the likelihood of HIV test acceptance (Ratcliff et al., 2012). That is, if HIV patients avoid being reminded of their HIV disease by not adhering to medication as part of their PTSD reactions, they should also avoid being tested for a possible case of HIV/AIDS. However, the above study suggests otherwise.

There is evidence that discrimination plays an important role in medication non-adherence. People living with HIV are often discriminated against (e.g. because of their HIV status and sexual orientation), which can be traumatic and is seen as a kind of hate crime. Different types of discrimination have been associated with increased PTSD symptoms and decreased adherence (Wagner et al., 2012). In other words, to pick up on the spectrum of posttraumatic disturbance hypothesis, PTSD affects non-adherence, but indirectly through the type of discrimination. From the perspective of disease progression, this is a serious problem. Allowing this non-adherence behaviour to be perpetuated by unaddressed PTSD or discrimination is ultimately destructive to the patient. It is a form of 'self-defeating and self-destructive behavioural manifestations of PTSD' (Cohen et al., 2001). Discrimination can also reduce perceived general health and satisfaction with health care (Bird et al., 2004), but exacerbate symptoms of PTSD and depression (Bogart et al., 2011).

Secondary victims of HIV/AIDS

HIV/AIDS affects not only patients themselves, but also those who are closely associated with them in one way or another (i.e. secondary victims). These may be formal or informal caregivers. Formal carers include AIDS or frontline staff who are often distressed by caring for patients with AIDS. These staff may exhibit thoughts and feelings associated with PTSD. Measures need to be taken to identify those who may be at risk, to prevent them from falling into this distress and to support those who need it (Wade et al., 1996).

There are also informal caregivers who spend a lot of time caring for their loved ones with AIDS. As a result, they too may exhibit PTSD symptoms. After the death of their sons due to AIDS, mothers who had spent a lot of time caring were more likely to show PTSD symptoms than those who had not taken on the role of a caregiver. These symptoms occurred alongside other problems such as divorce/separation, job loss, nightmares, violence, psychosomatic illness and panic attacks (Trice, 1988). One study examined the psychosocial difficulties facrfed by Japanese bereaved families of HIV-infected haemophiliacs. The survivors continued to express feelings of grief, sadness, resentment, anger, guilt, regret, fear of discrimination, and loneliness. A large majority (95%) of mothers regretted 'having given birth to a haemophilic child'. About 70% of the respondents continued to restrict their daily activities due to the stigma or fear of discrimination; 59% showed PTSD-like symptoms (Mizota et al., 2006).

Similarly, 19% of adults caring for AIDS-orphaned children reported clinically significant PTSS in an HIV-endemic South African community; caregivers of AIDS orphans and other orphaned children were significantly more likely to meet threshold criteria for PTSD (28%) than caregivers of non-orphaned children (10%) (Kuo et al., 2013). Conversely, secondary victims could include the children of caregivers (e.g. parents) who have HIV/AIDS. It was estimated that 18.4 million children in sub-Saharan Africa had been orphaned by AIDS in 2010 (Cluver et al., 2008). One study showed that they live with and are traumatised by AIDS caregiver illness or orphanhood through AIDS. AIDS illness and AIDS orphanhood have been associated with increased depression, anxiety, and PTSD in the long term. Both could have a cumulative psychological effect on these young people. However, their psychological distress was not related to caregiver illness or death from causes other than AIDS (Cluver et al., 2012). Orphans from Tanzania were significantly more likely to report neglect, depressive symptoms, PTSD symptoms, and aggression than non-orphans. Perceived stigma was also associated with mental health problems (Hermenau et al., 2015).

A study looking at children affected by HIV in China examined paternal (children who lost their fathers) and maternal (children who lost their mothers) orphans who had lost a parent to HIV. There were no significant differences between maternal and paternal orphans, except that paternal orphans reported better trusting relationships with caregivers than maternal orphans. Children with an ill parent had worse scores for depression, loneliness, post-traumatic stress, and social support than children with a healthy surviving parent (Zhao et al., 2010).

Interventions for PTSD, psychiatric comorbidity in people with HIV/AIDS

The foregoing suggests that HIV-infected patients have complex psychological issues related to past trauma, psychological disorders, discrimination, lack of medication adherence, and other factors (Whetten et al., 2008). Medical professionals should therefore not only focus on the physical treatment of HIV/AIDS. Rather, psychological treatments should also be considered to address the impact of PTSD symptoms or other psychological disorders on the course of the disease (Kimerling et al., 1999; Ricart et al., 2002; Samuels et al., 2011). However, among HIV/AIDS patients with at least one psychological disorder, almost half (43%) reported that they had not received psychological treatment (Israelski et al., 2007). This is particularly worrying as the evidence above suggests that it is important to provide psychological treatment alongside physical treatment (Olley et al., 2006; Pence et al., 2006).

Exposure therapy and cognitive behavioural therapy

Nevertheless, a number of studies have been published examining the effectiveness of a range of interventions for people living with HIV/AIDS. These studies relied on prescriptive forms of therapy, i.e. prescribing tasks for patients to perform as part of their treatment (Barkham et al., 1996; Stiles et al., 1988). For example, one study examined the effectiveness of prolonged exposure in reducing PTSD symptoms and comorbidities (depression, negative posttraumatic cognitions, and substance abuse) in HIV-infected individuals. Those who received prolonged exposure tended to report fewer PTSD symptoms and negative posttraumatic cognitions, and achieved better functioning over time than those who did not receive treatment. However, the effects of prolonged exposure on substance abuse were limited (Pacella et al., 2012).

Further supporting these findings, another study found that PTSD symptoms in people living with HIV decreased throughout the prolonged exposure. Experiencing several previous types of traumatic events was associated with slower change in PTSD symptoms. Also, people with a non-HIV-related, as opposed to an HIV-related, index trauma had a slower rate of change in PTSD symptoms over the course of prolonged exposure. The years since HIV diagnosis did not affect the change in PTSD symptoms (Junglen et al., 2017).

Another study examined the effectiveness of cognitive behavioural therapy for trauma and self-care (CBT–TSC) in men who have sex with men and who have a history of child sexual abuse (CAS). This study focused on the effect of this intervention not only on PTSD but also on child abuse symptoms. It was found that CBT–TSC reduced the likelihood (approximately 60%) of sero-discordant condomless anal/vaginal sex and reduced child abuse symptoms more than HIV voluntary counselling and testing (VCT only) after treatment. The CBT–TSC group also reported greater reductions in overall PTSD and avoidance symptoms. At follow-up (6 and 9 months after randomisation), the CBT–TSC group showed a significant reduction in CAS symptoms. However, for PTSD symptoms, only avoidance behaviour remained significantly different from VCT only. CBT–TSC is a potentially effective approach to address HIV risk among MSM with a history of childhood sexual abuse (O'Cleirigh et al., 2019).

A qualitative study suggests that sexual minority men appear to positively benefit from the cognitive behavioural therapy for trauma and sexual health intervention (CBT-TSH), which aims to reduce PTSD associated with child sexual abuse. They felt motivated to participate in the intervention, to process their abuse experiences, and to address the trauma symptoms associated with these experiences, although they still had many issues with their anger and perceived changes in themselves or their own behaviour (Taylor et al., 2018).

The above studies seem to reflect the observations noted in a systematic review that, in addition to eye movement desensitisation and reprocessing (EMDR), approaches based on the principles of CBT appear to show promise in reducing PTSD symptoms resulting from illnesses such as HIV, cancer, cardiovascular disease and multiple sclerosis (Haerizadeh et al., 2020). While the above prescriptive therapies should reduce the severity of psychological symptoms, some researchers have focused on the previously discussed problems associated with treatment non-adherence. A psychodynamic approach has been advocated. The therapeutic orientation of this approach contrasts with behavioural therapy programmes, which focus mainly on improving patients' behaviour or their ability to care for themselves. A psychodynamic approach allows patients to confront their past struggles and in this way gain a better understanding of the underlying unconscious issues related to the lack of treatment adherence. This unconscious past could relate to early or late childhood trauma (emotional, physical and sexual), early abandonment or trauma in adulthood leading to PTSD and non-compliance with risk reduction and HIV treatment (Ricart et al., 2002).

Group therapy

One study examined the effectiveness of group psychotherapy in reducing feelings of shame and guilt in women who had been sexually abused in childhood and who were at risk of HIV, and whether such a reduction in feelings of shame and guilt affected the impact of treatment on symptoms of PTSD. The women were randomly assigned to a trauma-focused group, a present-focused group, or a waiting group. This was a 6-month follow-up study. Both treatment groups reported a reduction in shame and guilt. The treatment effect on PTSD symptoms was mediated by changes in shame, but was not related to changes in guilt. In other words, when treating the PTSD symptoms of victims of childhood sexual abuse who were at risk of HIV, feelings of shame should not be ignored as they are often associated with these symptoms (Ginzburg et al., 2009).

Expressive writing

Based on the emotional disclosure hypothesis (Pennebaker, 1995, 1997), the researchers found that expressive writing (four 30-minute expressive writing sessions) was useful as a form of intervention for HIV-infected men and women. Through writing, patients processed issues related to past trauma, self-worth, and problem solving. Although expressive writing as a group did not show significant treatment effects, there appeared to be gender-specific effects, with women experiencing significant reductions in PTSD symptoms, depression, and HIV-related physical symptoms. Notably, the benefits of writing seemed to be much greater in women who had elevated PTSD symptoms at the beginning of the study, whereas men did not benefit from writing about the trauma—in fact, they did not improve on any of the outcome variables compared to the control group (Ironson et al., 2013).

The collaborative care model

Instead of implementing individualised or group therapy programmes for HIV patients, some studies have developed community-based intervention programmes. The collaborative care model (CCM), for example, is an HIV primary care clinic and evidence-based integrated care model that aims to improve the identification and treatment of patients (in this case HIV patients) with depressive symptoms. It includes routine screening for depression, measurement-based care, proactive disease management, behavioural health coordination, and case consultation by the behavioural health care manager with a psychiatrist. In one study, patients presenting for HIV care were screened for depression. Four latent profiles of people with HIV were identified, namely those with improving (58.4%), worsening (9.4%), highly responsive (19.5%), and persistently severe (12.7%) depressive symptoms. The group that responded very well to treatment had an average decrease in depressive symptoms of >50%. Trauma, PTSD, lower educational attainment and fewer HIV and psychiatry clinic visits were associated with worsening or persistently severe depressive symptoms (Gunzler et al., 2020).

Supervised injection facility

There are other community-based intervention programmes that target HIV risk behaviours. For example, some researchers have studied the effectiveness of supervised injection facilities. One study looked at people who injected drugs and had a range of chronic conditions, including HIV, finding that willingness to use such a facility correlated with PTSD diagnosis (OR: 3.27) (León et al., 2018).

SAFE-IPV and AWARE

A number of programmes targeting women have been documented. One of them is the safe alternatives for empowered sex for intimate partner violence (SAFE-IPV) intervention. One study showed that women who participated in this programme reported significantly fewer unprotected vaginal and anal sexual contacts 3 months after leaving the shelter and higher motivation to engage in risk-preventive behaviour than in the 3 months before the shelter. Other HIV risk factors also improved at the 3-month follow-up, i.e. emotional, physical, and sexual harm from the perpetrator, PTSS, and risky alcohol and drug use (Johnson et al., 2017).

Another programme, Asian women's action for resilience and empowerment (AWARE), aims to reduce depressive symptoms, suicidality, substance use, and HIV, and sexual risk behaviours among Asian American women. This programme targets women who meet the criteria for PTSD or who have been exposed to interpersonal violence. It is based on theoretical models such as fractured identity theory, empowerment theory, CBT, mindfulness-based techniques and the AIDS risk reduction model (ARRM). A qualitative study suggested further exploration of feelings, improving the provision of technology, focusing on learning and practising coping skills, developing more cultural sensitivity to sexual health, reducing the number of sessions but increasing the time per session (Hahm et al., 2017).

Patient navigation

Another study looked at HIV patients' experiences of patient navigation. This is a patient-centred model of care in which health workers (patient navigators) support patients to overcome barriers and access disconnected health systems. They engage in advocacy, health education, case management and social work, peer support, and community-based programmes. In other words, patient navigation aims to connect and re-engage people living with HIV to health care. Patients who participated in navigation reported, among other things, that they recognised the importance of this client–navigator relationship, that they were reluctant to discontinue the navigation programme, and that they felt self-efficacy, hope, and psychological change as a result of their navigation experience. Further research is needed to examine how participation in this navigation affects patients' self-efficacy and resilience, and improves posttraumatic growth, which in turn could influence HIV outcomes (Roland et al., 2020).

Posttraumatic growth after HIV/AIDS

When patients are confronted with a life-threatening disease like HIV/AIDS, they do not always lose their courage to live and their ability to enjoy life. For some scientists, looking at patients' experiences from a pathological perspective is not the way to go. Instead, they argue for a rehabilitation psychology based on positive psychological principles (Ehde, 2010). Posttraumatic growth (PTG) can develop in patients and their caregivers after a diagnosis of HIV/AIDS. More than half of the patients in one study experienced PTG (Milam, 2004), although the emergence of PTG does not mean the end of pain and suffering due to HIV. Whereas PTG can influence the way people adapt to their illness—from infection to disease progression/stability and the idea of death—it can also serve as a form of defence, i.e. a way to protect oneself through perceived increases in personal strength, improvement in personal relationships, and discovery of new possibilities (Luszczynska et al., 2012; Milam, 2006a), even though people may also report depression, anxiety, fear, helplessness and guilt (Milam, 2006a). Although PTG gives HIV patients hope and reassurance, it does not replace grief (Gorman, 2010).

Nonetheless, the evidence that PTG has positive effects on distress cannot be overlooked. Women living with HIV have claimed that their lives have been transformed into what has been described as a 'gift' (Lennon-Dearing, 2022) or a kind of positive change consistent with the concept of PTG described by Tedeschi and Calhoun (1995). Younger individuals tended to experience higher growth associated with less alcohol abuse, depression, or pessimism (Milam, 2004). PTG was mostly not associated with disease status over time, but correlated positively with CD4 count in Hispanic participants (compared to non-Hispanic participants) among those with low (compared to high) levels of optimism. On the other hand, PTG correlated negatively with CD4 count among those with high levels of optimism. PTG correlated negatively with viral load among those with low (vs high) levels of pessimism (Milam, 2006b). A meta-analysis concluded that, following an HIV/AIDS or cancer diagnosis, growth was associated with more positive and less negative mental health and better subjective physical health (Sawyer et al., 2010). The associations found in that meta-analysis may be influenced by patient demographic information (age, ethnicity), time since the event, and by the nature of the negative mental health outcomes (Sawyer et al., 2010). When studying HIV/AIDS patients over a period of more than 1.6 years, PTG was prevalent in 59% of participants who reported moderate positive changes since diagnosis. At baseline, PTG was negatively correlated with age, alcohol use, depression, and pessimism, and positively associated with African American ethnicity (compared to white), female gender, healthy eating, and optimism. At follow-up, religiosity was positively correlated with PTG. The experience of PTG was associated with lower depression over time (Milam, 2004).

However, the association between PTG and positive health outcomes described above is not always consistent. When examining the impact of mortality reminders on PTG in patients with HIV or other life-threatening illnesses such as cancer, those exposed to mortality reminders reported lower PTG or benefit finding compared to controls, especially among those who had recently received the diagnosis (Luszczynska et al., 2012).

Another study examined the course of PTG and posttraumatic depreciation (PTD) (i.e. negative cognitive changes in the domains of self, relationship with others, and philosophy of life) in people with HIV every 6 months in three consecutive assessments. Surprisingly, a positive relationship was found between PTG and PTD. Following the person-centred approach, specific PTG/PTD clusters were also found among people with different levels of resilience and HIV/AIDS stigma. The first cluster consisted of people with average levels of PTG and PTD, the second cluster of high levels of PTG and PTD, the third cluster of average levels of PTG and high levels of PTD, and the final cluster of high levels of PTG and average levels of PTD (Pięta & Rzeszutek, 2023). Gaining resources (i.e. psychosocial resources due to living with HIV) was associated with a PTG trajectory, whereas losing resources was associated with PTD. This study concluded that PTG and PTD could influence the growth processes in people living with HIV (Pięta & Rzeszutek, 2022).

Personal variables

Posttraumatic growth is related to some personal factors of people living with HIV/AIDS. Regarding personality, as mentioned earlier, growth was negatively associated with viral load in those with low levels of pessimism (Milam, 2006b). On the contrary, optimism was associated with psychological and immunological status in HIV-infected men, as high levels of optimism were associated with lower levels of depression, global distress, PTSD related to a recent traumatic life event (e.g. a natural disaster), and lower antibody levels to Epstein-Barr Virus and Human Herpes Virus-6, suggesting more effective cellular immunological control over these viruses. Optimism led to less depression, which in turn led to lower Epstein-Barr Virus status (Cruess et al., 2000). It has also been claimed that extraversion and life satisfaction are the most important factors associated with PTG in people living with HIV (Rzeszutek et al., 2019). A previous study found an association between PTG and life satisfaction after controlling for stigma and regret about disclosure (i.e. disclosure of HIV status) (Dibb, 2018). The relationship between life satisfaction and PTG was influenced by neuroticism and socio-medical variables (antiretroviral treatment, education, relationship status) (Rzeszutek et al., 2019).

On a cognitive level, the way people living with HIV/AIDS centralise the traumatic event may influence PTG. Those who positively centralise their traumatic experiences tend to experience PTG, while those who negatively centralise their traumatic experiences are more likely to experience PTSD symptoms (Ugwu et al., 2021). There could be common and separate pathways from the traumatic stressor (HIV) to psychological distress and PTG, with the pathways mediated by cognitive processing. HIV as a traumatic stressor was associated with intrusive cognitive processing in the past (e.g. shortly after learning of their HIV diagnosis, they thought about it even though they did not want to), which affected psychological distress via current intrusive cognitive processing. In contrast, HIV as a traumatic stressor was negatively associated with past deliberate cognitive processing (e.g. shortly after learning of their HIV diagnosis, they recalled some benefits of adjusting to the diagnosis), which impacted on PTG through current deliberate cognitive processing (Nightingale et al., 2010). Similarly, when people perceive themselves as stigmatised, this can affect PTG. One study examined the interrelationship between stigma, social support, and PTG. Both stigma and social support were associated with PTG following an HIV diagnosis, with no interaction between them (Zeligman et al., 2016). Internalised HIV-related stigma was associated with poorer outcomes in the PTG domains of veridical growth (i.e. personal strength, relating to others, and new possibilities). Mode of HIV transmission was associated with outcomes in all PTG domains, with the least stigmatised mode of transmission being associated with the greatest growth. Thus, stigma is a relevant concept for clinicians seeking to promote the growth of people living with HIV (Murphy & Hevey, 2013).

PTG and social support

Several studies have highlighted the link between posttraumatic growth (PTG) and social support. In one study, half of HIV-positive individuals reported high levels of PTSD symptoms, while the majority also reported medium- or high-level PTG. Seeking emotional support was positively correlated with PTG and was considered the leading predictor of PTG (Ogińska-Bulik & Kraska, 2017). Disclosure to sexual partners and emotional support were also associated with higher levels of PTG, although HIV-related stigma was associated with lower levels of PTG. In other words, interventions should empower people living with HIV to disclose their HIV status to sexual partners and increase social support for them (Kamen et al., 2016). A longitudinal study showed that after controlling for socio-medical variables (gender, employment, higher education, committed relationship, and HIV/AIDS status) for people living with HIV, social support was positively correlated with PTG. Positive affect also carried the effects of social support on PTG. In other words, promoting positive affect should be part of the intervention strategy for people living with HIV (Rzeszutek, 2017). However, it was argued that social support had a limited impact on PTG as it only related to the area of relationships with other HIV patients who had experienced a natural disaster (Cieslak et al., 2009).

The role of social support on PTG was also studied in relation to resilience. Social support and resilience were positively correlated with PTG in HIV-infected individuals (Rzeszutek et al., 2017b). In particular, a positive correlation was found between resilience and the two domains (personal strength and appreciation of life) of PTG (Murphy & Hevey, 2013). Among children of HIV-infected parents, social support was also positively correlated with resilience and PTG. Increased resilience and PTG were associated with lower hopelessness, which in turn was associated with less depression. Improving social support for children affected by HIV is therefore important for improving their mental health (Mo et al., 2014). For women living with HIV, PTG correlated positively not only with resilience, but also with social support from family, intimacy from partner, and empathy from doctors. However, there was a negative correlation with support from friends. Seemingly, the types of support play a role in influencing PTG. Resilience partially mediated the effects of family support or partner intimacy on PTG, explaining 13.6–14.2% of the variance (Yang et al., 2020).

PTG and coping strategies

When looking at HIV-infected men who have sex with men (MSM), a negative association was found between PTSD and PTG after controlling for sociodemographic and HIV-related variables. A randomised controlled trial examined the effectiveness of a group intervention programme aimed at improving psychological well-being and adaptive coping strategies in HIV-infected MSM. Compared to the control group, the number of problem-focused coping strategies and PTG significantly increased in the intervention group and PTSD symptoms decreased after the completion of the intervention.

Changes in problem-focused coping strategies play a role in influencing the intervention effect on increased PTG. Problem solving and self-blame also mediated the impact of PTSD on PTG. It seems important that to promote growth, one should enhance problem-solving skills while minimising self-blame (Ye et al., 2018). Similarly, among HIV patients who had experienced a natural disaster, higher levels of coping self-efficacy were associated with higher growth, particularly among those who suffered from more intense PTSD symptoms as a result of the disaster (Cieslak et al., 2009). This sense of self-efficacy was reflected in a case study of a patient who, through metacognitive interpersonal therapy, overcame her PTSD symptoms, developed a more benevolent self-image, regained her sense of being a person and her ability to plan for the future with strength and dignity, participated in social activities after years of avoidance and isolation, and felt accepted by society, thereby developing PTG (Dimaggio et al., 2017).

Among newly diagnosed HIV-positive young homosexual men, focusing on the negative aspect of adversity was associated with depression and PTSD, with low levels of resilience serving as a mediator. On the other hand, focusing on the positive aspect of adversity was associated with PTG, with resilience serving as a mediator. In other words, resilience plays a role in influencing the relationship between positive or negative perceptions of adversity and positive growth or distress outcomes (Yu et al., 2017). HIV-related resilience was associated with rumination, emotional expression, positive thinking, internalised stigma, and perceived prior resilience 8 months after diagnosis. At the same time, positive thinking, internalised stigma, perceived prior resilience along with isolation, self-blame, thought avoidance, and help-seeking predicted PTG (changes in life philosophy, perceptions of personal strength, interpersonal relationships) 8 months after diagnosis. These findings suggest that it is important for people living with HIV-positive people to reduce stigma and promote adaptive coping strategies (Garrido-Hernansaiz et al., 2017).

Religiosity appeared to be associated with increased growth (Milam, 2004). Turning to religion and acceptance were also positively correlated with PTG among HIV-positive people (Ogińska-Bulik & Kraska, 2017), which contradicts existing literature suggesting that returning to religion as a coping strategy was negatively correlated with PTG among people with HIV (Rzeszutek et al., 2017b). This finding is somewhat surprising given that changes in faith are a component of growth.

Posttraumatic growth may also develop in patients' caregivers (Cadell, 2007; Cadell & Sullivan, 2006). Caregivers of patients who had died from complications related to HIV/AIDS also reported PTG as well as coping strategies such as humour, social support, and spirituality, although distress and fear of death were also part of their psychological state (Cadell, 2007; Cadell et al., 2003). Even those who had low scores on PTG could still report positive outcomes (Cadell & Sullivan, 2006).

The results of the above studies were included in a systematic review, which showed that PTG was positively correlated with optimism, resilience, positive reappraisal coping, positive affect, self-efficacy, and social support in people living with HIV. On the other hand, PTG correlated negatively with HIV-related stress, which was characterised by depression, substance use, PTSD, and HIV stigma. Sociodemographic and HIV-related clinical variables, on the other hand, were not related to PTG (Rzeszutek & Gruszczyńska, 2018).

Summary

People with HIV/AIDS may suffer from PTSD, which is often associated with other psychiatric disorders. HIV patients with a lifetime of trauma and PTSD symptoms also tend to have neurocognitive impairment, poor cognitive function, and poor physical and social functioning. These PTSD and comorbid psychological disorders are related to biological markers. It is controversial whether receiving an HIV diagnosis can be considered a traumatic event. It has been argued that the treatment regime, distressing physical symptoms, and witnessing HIV-related death may be other traumatic stressors that can be considered.

According to the literature, risk factors for the association between PTSD and psychiatric comorbidity in people living with HIV/AIDS include gender differences, stigma, and coping strategies. Trauma or PTSD can disproportionately affect HIV-positive women. In men, family violence in childhood can trigger PTSD, which in turn can influence HIV infection. Similar to women, they have also experienced trauma in childhood and show dissociation. Comparing women and men infected with HIV, the former generally face worse health or mental health problems than the latter. Women also need more social support than men. There appear to be gender differences in the types of psychiatric symptoms experienced by men and women.

Stigma associated with HIV/AIDS can exacerbate trauma-related psychiatric symptoms, bullying and discrimination, and reduce the likelihood of remission. In terms of coping strategies, avoidant attachment may interact with emotion-focused coping to influence PTSD. Social support may also influence the impact of avoidant and insecure attachment styles on PTSD. In addition to social support, personality traits (temperament traits) may also influence trauma symptoms in patients with HIV-PTSD and patients with chronic pain. Instead of focusing on maladaptive coping strategies, some researchers emphasise the importance of adaptive coping strategies such as mindfulness or self-efficacy in coping.

The risk factors for increased risk behaviours for HIV/AIDS have been identified. Previous trauma prior to HIV infection may influence HIV risk behaviour or transmission risk, high-risk sexual behaviour and ultimately HIV risk behaviour in patients. PTSD, substance abuse, major depression, borderline personality disorder, child abuse and racial discrimination-based traumatic stress may also be related to increases in HIV risk behaviour or risk of HIV infection. Women who have experienced sexual victimisation, aggression, and psychiatric disorders are more prone to HIV risk behaviours.

Research has also covered interventions for PTSD and psychiatric co-morbidity in people with HIV/AIDS. Generally, people with HIV/AIDS can benefit from exposure therapy, although its effectiveness may be affected by cumulative trauma. CBT for trauma and self-care also appears to be effective in reducing symptoms of PTSD, HIV risk behaviours, and child abuse. Psychodynamic therapy may be helpful for patients to examine their past struggles and explore underlying unconscious issues from the past related to medication non-adherence. Women may benefit from a trauma-informed group and a present-focused group, which are associated with a reduction in shame and guilt. Women may also benefit from expressive writing. Through the collaborative care model, HIV patients who responded well to the group also reduced their depressive symptoms. Other interventions include supervised injection facilities; the SAFE-IPV and AWARE interventions also aim to help women reduce their HIV risk behaviours as well as abuse symptoms, PTSS, substance use, depression, and suicidality. Patient navigation aims to reconnect people living with HIV to care by helping them overcome barriers and gain access to disconnected health systems.

After HIV/AIDS diagnosis, patients and caregivers may develop PTG and other psychological distress symptoms. PTG is associated with viral load in people with low levels of pessimism. Extraversion and life satisfaction are associated with PTG in people living with HIV. Cognitive processing may affect how HIV as a traumatic stressor affects psychological distress and PTG. Internalised HIV-related stigma and social support may also be related to PTG following an HIV diagnosis. Seeking social support and resilience are correlated with PTG. Other factors associated with PTG in people living with HIV/AIDS include problem-focused coping and coping self-efficacy. Focusing on the positive aspect of adversity is associated with PTG in HIV-positive men with different levels of resilience. Religiosity is also associated with increased growth.

References

Adewuya, A. O., Afolabi, M. O., Ola, B. A., Ogundele, O. A., Ajibare, A. O., Oladipo, B. F., & Fakande, I. (2009). Post-traumatic stress disorder (PTSD) after stigma related events in HIV infected individuals in Nigeria. *Social Psychiatry and Psychiatric Epidemiology*, 44(9), 761–766. https://doi.org/10.1007/s00127-009-0493-7

Andu, E., Wagenaar, B. H., Kemp, C. G., Nevin, P. E., Simoni, J. M., Andrasik, M., Cohn, S. E., French, A. L., & Rao, D. (2018). Risk and protective factors of posttraumatic stress disorder among African American women living with HIV. *AIDS Care*, 30(11), 1393–1399. https://doi.org/10.1080/09540121.2018.1466981

Axelrod, J., Myers, H. F., Durvasula, R. S., Wyatt, G. E., & Cheng, M. (1999). The impact of relationship violence, HIV, and ethnicity on adjustment in women. *Cultural Diversity and Ethnic Minority Psychology*, 5(3), 263–275. https://doi.org/10.1037/1099-9809.5.3.263

Banerjee, N., Ironson, G., Fitch, C., Boroughs, M. S., Safren, S. A., Powell, A., & O'Cleirigh, C. (2018). The indirect effect of posttraumatic stress disorder symptoms on current alcohol use through negative cognitions in sexual minority men. *Journal of Traumatic Stress*, 31(4), 602–612. https://doi.org/10.1002/jts.22304

Bantjes, J., Kagee, A., & Saal, W. (2020). The utility of the Hopkins Symptom Checklist as a trans-diagnostic screening instrument for common mental disorders among persons seeking HIV testing. *AIDS and Behavior*, 24(2), 629–636. https://doi.org/10.1007/s10461-019-02524-6

Barkham, M., Rees, A., Shapiro, D. A., Stiles, W. B., Agnew, R. M., Halstead, J., Culverwell, A., & Harrington, V. M. G. (1996). Outcomes of time-limited psychotherapy in applied settings: Replicating the Second Sheffield Psychotherapy Project. *Journal of Consulting and Clinical Psychology*, 64, 1079–1085. https://doi.org/10.1037/0022-006X.64.5.1079

Batchelder, A. W., Choi, K., Dale, S. K., Pierre-Louis, C., Sweek, E. W., Ironson, G., Safren, S. A., & O'Cleirigh, C. (2019). Effects of syndemic psychiatric diagnoses on health indicators in men who have sex with men. *Health Psychology*, 38(6), 509–517. https://doi.org/10.1037/hea0000724

Battaglia, T. A., Gunn, C. M., McCoy, M. E., Mu, H. H., Baranoski, A. S., Chiao, E. Y., Kachnic, L. A., & Stier, E. A. (2015). Beliefs about anal cancer among HIV-infected women: Barriers and motivators to participation in research. *Women's Health Issues*, 25(6), 720–726.

Benight, C. C., Antoni, M. H., Kilbourn, K., Ironson, G., Kumar, M. A., Fletcher, M. A., Redwine, L., Baum, A., & Schneiderman, N. (1997). Coping self-efficacy buffers psychological and physiological disturbances in HIV-infected men following a natural disaster. *Health Psychology*, 16(3), 248–255.

Beyer, J. L., Taylor, L., Gersing, K. R., & Krishnan, K. R. (2007). Prevalence of HIV infection in a general psychiatric outpatient population. *Psychosomatics*, 48(1), 31–37. https://doi.org/10.1176/appi.psy.48.1.31

Bird, S. T., Bogart, L. M., & Delahanty, D. L. (2004). Health-related correlates of perceived discrimination in HIV care. *AIDS Patient Care and STDS*, 18(1), 19–26. https://doi.org/10.1089/108729104322740884

Boarts, J. M., Sledjeski, E. M., Bogart, L. M., & Delahanty, D. L. (2006). The differential impact of PTSD and depression on HIV disease markers and adherence to HAART in people living with HIV. *AIDS and Behavior*, 10(3), 253–261. https://doi.org/10.1007/s10461-006-9069-7

Bogart, L. M., Wagner, G. J., Galvan, F. H., Landrine, H., Klein, D. J., & Sticklor, L. A. (2011). Perceived discrimination and mental health symptoms among Black men with HIV. *Cultural Diversity & Ethnic Minority Psychology, 17*(3), 295–302. https://doi.org/10.1037/a0024056

Boroughs, M. S., Ehlinger, P. P., Batchelder, A. W., Safren, S. A., & O'Cleirigh, C. (2018). Posttraumatic stress symptoms and emerging adult sexual minority men: Implications for assessment and treatment of childhood sexual abuse. *Journal of Traumatic Stress, 31*(5), 665–675. https://doi.org/10.1002/jts.22335

Botha, K. F. (1996). Posttraumatic stress disorder and illness behaviour in HIV+ patients. *Psychological Reports, 79*(3 Pt 1), 843–845. https://doi.org/10.2466/pr0.1996.79.3.843

Bowe, A., & Rosenheck, R. (2015). PTSD and substance use disorder among veterans: Characteristics, service utilization and pharmacotherapy. *Journal of Dual Diagnosis, 11*(1), 22–32. https://doi.org/10.1080/15504263.2014.989653

Bowleg, L., Fitz, C. C., Burkholder, G. J., Massie, J. S., Wahome, R., Teti, M., Malebranche, D. J., & Tschann, J. M. (2014). Racial discrimination and posttraumatic stress symptoms as pathways to sexual HIV risk behaviors among urban Black heterosexual men. *AIDS Care, 26*(8), 1050–1057. https://doi.org/10.1080/09540121.2014.906548

Boyes, M. E., Pantelic, M., Casale, M., Toska, E., Newnham, E., & Cluver, L. D. (2020). Prospective associations between bullying victimisation, internalised stigma, and mental health in South African adolescents living with HIV. *Journal of Affective Disorders, 276*, 418–423. https://doi.org/10.1016/j.jad.2020.07.101

Brezing, C., Ferrara, M., & Freudenreich, O. (2015). The syndemic Illness of HIV and trauma: Implications for a trauma-informed model of care. *Psychosomatics: Journal of Consultation and Liaison Psychiatry, 56*(2), 107–118. https://doi.org/10.1016/j.psym.2014.10.006

Brown, L. A., Majeed, I., Mu, W., McCann, J., Durborow, S., Chen, S., & Blank, M. B. (2021). Suicide risk among persons living with HIV. *AIDS Care, 33*, 616–622. https://doi.org/10.1080/09540121.2020.1801982

Brown, M. J., Cohen, S. A., & DeShazo, J. P. (2020). Psychopathology and HIV diagnosis among older adults in the United States: Disparities by age, sex, and race/ethnicity. *Aging & Mental Health, 24*(10), 1746–1753. https://doi.org/10.1080/13607863.2019.1636201

Brown, M. J., Masho, S. W., Perera, R. A., Mezuk, B., Pugsley, R. A., & Cohen, S. A. (2017). Sex disparities in adverse childhood experiences and HIV/STIs: Mediation of psychopathology and sexual behaviors. *AIDS and Behavior, 21*(6), 1550–1566. https://doi.org/10.1007/s10461-016-1553-0

Cadell, S. (2007). The sun always comes out after it rains: Understanding posttraumatic growth in HIV caregivers. *Health & Social Work, 32*(3), 169–176. https://doi.org/10.1093/hsw/32.3.169

Cadell, S., & Sullivan, R. (2006). Posttraumatic growth and HIV bereavement: Where does it start and when does it end? *Traumatology, 12*(1), 45–59. https://doi.org/10.1177/153476560601200104

Cadell, S., Regehr, C., & Hemsworth, D. (2003). Factors contributing to posttraumatic growth: a proposed structural equation model. *American Journal of Orthopsychiatry, 73*(3), 279–287. https://doi.org/10.1037/0002-9432.73.3.279

Chernoff, R. A. (2007). Treating an HIV/AIDS patient's PTSD and medication nonadherence with cognitive-behavioral therapy: a principle based approach. *Cognitive and Behavioral Practice, 14*(1), 107–117. https://doi.org/https://doi.org/10.1016/j.cbpra.2006.09.001

Cieslak, R., Benight, C., Schmidt, N., Luszczynska, A., Curtin, E., Clark, R. A., & Kissinger, P. (2009). Predicting posttraumatic growth among Hurricane Katrina survivors living with HIV: The role of self-efficacy, social support, and PTSD symptoms. *Anxiety, Stress & Coping, 22*(4), 449–463.

Cluver, L., Fincham, D. S., & Seedat, S. (2009). Posttraumatic stress in AIDS-orphaned children exposed to high levels of trauma: the protective role of perceived social support. *Journal of Traumatic Stress, 22*(2), 106–112. https://doi.org/10.1002/jts.20396

Cluver, L. D., Gardner, F., & Operario, D. (2008). Effects of stigma on the mental health of adolescents orphaned by AIDS. *Journal of Adolescent Health, 42*(4), 410–417. https://doi.org/https://doi.org/10.1016/j.jadohealth.2007.09.022

Cluver, L. D., Orkin, M., Boyes, M. E., Gardner, F., & Nikelo, J. (2012). AIDS-orphanhood and caregiver HIV/AIDS sickness status: effects on psychological symptoms in South African youth. *Journal of Pediatric Psychology, 37*(8), 857–867. https://doi.org/10.1093/jpepsy/jss004

Cohen, M. A., Alfonso, C. A., Hoffman, R. G., Milau, V., & Carrera, G. (2001). The impact of PTSD on treatment adherence in persons with HIV infection. *General Hospital Psychiatry, 23*(5), 294–296. https://doi.org/10.1016/s0163-8343(01)00152-9

Cohen, M. H., Fabri, M., Cai, X., Shi, Q., Hoover, D. R., Binagwaho, A., Culhane, M. A., Mukanyonga, H., Karegeya, D. K., & Anastos, K. (2009). Prevalence and predictors of posttraumatic stress disorder and depression in HIV-infected and at-risk Rwandan women. *Journal of Women's Health (Larchmt), 18*(11), 1783–1791. https://doi.org/10.1089/jwh.2009.1367

Cohen, M. H., Shi, Q., Fabri, M., Mukanyonga, H., Cai, X., Hoover, D. R., Binagwaho, A., & Anastos, K. (2011). Improvement in posttraumatic stress disorder in postconflict Rwandan women. *Journal of Women's Health (Larchmt), 20*(9), 1325–1332. https://doi.org/10.1089/jwh.2010.2404

Coleman, J. N., Batchelder, A. W., Kirakosian, N., Choi, K. W., Shipherd, J. C., Bedoya, C. A., Safren, S. A., Ironson, G., & O'Cleirigh, C. (2022). Indirect effects of dissociation on the relationship between lifetime PTSD symptoms and condomless sex among men who have sex with men with a history of childhood sexual abuse. *Journal of Trauma & Dissociation, 23*, 279–295. https://doi.org/10.1080/15299732.2021.1989118

Cotter, A., Potter, J. E., & Tessler, N. (2006). Management of HIV/AIDS in women. In J. Beal, J. J. Orrick, & K. Alfonso, *HIV/AIDS: Primary care guide* (pp. 533–546). Crown House Publishing.

Cruess, S., Antoni, M., Kilbourn, K., Ironson, G., Klimas, N., Fletcher, M. A., Baum, A., & Schneiderman, N. (2000). Optimism, distress, and immunologic status in HIV-infected gay men following hurricane Andrew. *International Journal of Behavioral Medicine, 7*(2), 160–182. https://doi.org/10.1207/S15327558IJBM0702_5

Dale, S. K., & Safren, S. A. (2019). Gendered racial microaggressions predict posttraumatic stress disorder symptoms and cognitions among Black women living with HIV. *Psychological Trauma: Theory, Research, Practice, and Policy, 11*(7), 685–694. https://doi.org/10.1037/tra0000467

Deiss, R., Campbell, C. J., Watson, C. W.-M., Moore, R. C., Crum-Cianflone, N. F., Wang, X., Ganesan, A., Okulicz, L. C. J., Letendre, S., Maves, R. C., Moore, D. J., & Agan, B. K. (2019). Posttraumatic stress disorder and neurocognitive impairment in a US military cohort of persons living with HIV. *Psychiatry: Interpersonal and Biological Processes, 82*(3), 228–239. https://doi.org/10.1080/00332747.2019.1586503

Delahanty, D. L., Bogart, L. M., & Figler, J. L. (2004). Posttraumatic stress disorder symptoms, salivary cortisol, medication adherence, and CD4 levels in HIV-positive individuals. *AIDS Care, 16*(2), 247–260. https://doi.org/10.1080/09540120410001641084

Delany-Brumsey, A., Joseph, N. T., Myers, H. F., Ullman, J. B., & Wyatt, G. E. (2013). Modeling the relationship between trauma and psychological distress among HIV-positive and HIV-negative women. *Psychological Trauma: Theory, Research, Practice, and Policy, 5*(1), 69–76. https://doi.org/10.1037/a0022381

Dévieux, J. G., Malow, R. M., Attonito, J. M., Jean-Gilles, M., Rosenberg, R., Gaston, S., Saint-Jean, G., & Deschamps, M.-M. (2013). Post-traumatic stress disorder symptomatology and alcohol use among HIV-seropositive adults in Haiti. *AIDS Care, 25*(10), 1210–1218. https://doi.org/10.1080/09540121.2013.763894

Dibb, B. (2018). Assessing stigma, disclosure regret and posttraumatic growth in people living with HIV. *AIDS and Behavior, 22*(12), 3916–3923. https://doi.org/10.1007/s10461-018-2230-2

Dimaggio, G., Conti, C., Lysaker, P. H., Popolo, R., Salvatore, G., & Sofia, S. A. (2017). Reauthoring one's own life in the face of being HIV+: Promoting healthier narratives with metacognitive interpersonal therapy. *Journal of Constructivist Psychology, 30*(4), 388–403. https://doi.org/10.1080/10720537.2016.1238788

Ehde, D. M. (2010). Application of positive psychology to rehabilitation psychology. In R. G. Frank, M. Rosenthal, & B. Caplan (Eds.), *Handbook of rehabilitation psychology*, 2nd ed. (pp. 417–424). American Psychological Association. https://doi.org/10.1037/15972-029

El-Bassel, N., Gilbert, L., Vinocur, D., Chang, M., & Wu, E. (2011). Posttraumatic stress disorder and HIV risk among poor, inner-city women receiving care in an emergency department. *American Journal of Public Health, 101*(1), 120–127. https://doi.org/10.2105/ajph.2009.181842

Engstrom, M., Winham, K. M., Golder, S., Higgins, G., Renn, T., & Logan, T. K. (2017). Correlates of HIV risks among women on probation and parole. *AIDS Education and Prevention, 29*(3), 256–273. https://doi.org/10.1521/aeap.2017.29.3.256

Fincham, D., Smit, J., Carey, P., Stein, D. J., & Seedat, S. (2008). The relationship between behavioural inhibition, anxiety disorders, depression and CD4 counts in HIV-positive adults: a cross-sectional controlled study. *AIDS Care, 20*(10), 1279–1283. https://doi.org/10.1080/09540120801927025

Gard, T. L., Hoover, D. R., Shi, Q., Cohen, M. H., Mutimura, E., Adedimeji, A. A., & Anastos, K. (2013). The impact of HIV status, HIV disease progression, and post-traumatic stress symptoms on the health-related quality of life of Rwandan women genocide survivors. *Quality of Life Research, 22*(8), 2073–2084. https://doi.org/10.1007/s11136-012-0328-y

Garrido-Hernansaiz, H., Murphy, P. J., & Alonso-Tapia, J. (2017). Predictors of resilience and posttraumatic growth among people living with HIV: A longitudinal study. *AIDS and Behavior, 21*(11), 3260–3270. https://doi.org/10.1007/s10461-017-1870-y

Geller, J. L. (1989). A bite of AIDS? Institutional line staff and the fear of HIV contagion. *Psychiatric Quarterly, 60*(3), 243–251. https://doi.org/10.1007/bf01064800

Ginzburg, K., Butler, L. D., Giese-Davis, J., Cavanaugh, C. E., Neri, E., Koopman, C., Classen, C. C., & Spiegel, D. (2009). Shame, guilt, and posttraumatic stress disorder in adult survivors of childhood sexual abuse at risk for human immunodeficiency virus: outcomes of a randomized clinical trial of group psychotherapy treatment. *Journal of Nervous and Mental Disease, 197*(7), 536–542. https://doi.org/10.1097/NMD.0b013e3181ab2ebd

Gonzalez, A., Locicero, B., Mahaffey, B., Fleming, C., Harris, J., & Vujanovic, A. A. (2016). Internalized HIV stigma and mindfulness: Associations with PTSD symptom severity in trauma-exposed adults with HIV/AIDS. *Behavior Modification, 40*(1–2), 144–163. https://doi.org/10.1177/0145445515615354

Gore-Felton, C., Ginzburg, K., Chartier, M., Gardner, W., Agnew-Blais, J., McGarvey, E., Weiss, E., & Koopman, C. (2013). Attachment style and coping in relation to posttraumatic stress disorder symptoms among adults living with HIV/AIDS. *Journal of Behavioral Medicine, 36*(1), 51–60. https://doi.org/10.1007/s10865-012-9400-x

Gorman, E. (2010). Adaptation, resilience, and growth after loss. In D. L. Harris (Ed.), *Counting our losses: Reflecting on change, loss, and transition in everyday life* (pp. 225–237). Routledge. https://doi.org/10.4324/9780203860731

Gunzler, D., Lewis, S., Webel, A., Lavakumar, M., Gurley, D., Kulp, K., Pile, M., El-Hayek, V., & Avery, A. (2020). Depressive symptom trajectories among people living with HIV in a collaborative care program. *AIDS and Behavior*, 24(6), 1765–1775. https://doi.org/10.1007/s10 461-019-02727-x

Haerizadeh, M., Sumner, J. A., Birk, J. L., Gonzalez, C., Heyman-Kantor, R., Falzon, L., Gershengoren, L., Shapiro, P., & Kronish, I. M. (2020). Interventions for posttraumatic stress disorder symptoms induced by medical events: A systematic review. *Journal of Psychosomatic Research*, 129, 109908. https://doi.org/10.1016/j.jpsychores.2019.109908

Hahm, H. C., Chang, S. T.-H., Lee, G. Y., Tagerman, M. D., Lee, C. S., Trentadue, M. P., & Hien, D. A. (2017). Asian women's action for resilience and empowerment intervention: Stage I pilot study. *Journal of Cross-Cultural Psychology*, 48(10), 1537–1553. https://doi.org/ 10.1177/0022022117730815

Haller, D. L., & Miles, D. R. (2003). Suicidal ideation among psychiatric patients with HIV: psychiatric morbidity and quality of life. *AIDS and Behavior*, 7(2), 101–108. https://doi.org/ 10.1023/a:1023985906166

Hansrod, F., Spies, G., & Seedat, S. (2015). Type and severity of intimate partner violence and its relationship with PTSD in HIV-infected women. *Psychology, Health & Medicine*, 20(6), 697–709. https://doi.org/10.1080/13548506.2014.967702

Harris, T., Rice, E., Rhoades, H., Winetrobe, H., & Wenzel, S. (2017). Gender differences in the path from sexual victimization to HIV risk behavior among homeless youth. *Journal of Child Sexual Abuse*, 26(3), 334–351. https://doi.org/10.1080/10538712.2017.1287146

Hermenau, K., Eggert, I., Landolt, M. A., & Hecker, T. (2015). Neglect and perceived stigmatization impact psychological distress of orphans in Tanzania. *European Journal of Psychotraumatology*, 6. https://doi.org/10.3402/ejpt.v6.28617

Hoff, R. A., Beam-Goulet, J., & Rosenheck, R. A. (1997). Mental disorder as a risk factor for human immunodeficiency virus infection in a sample of veterans. *Journal of Nervous and Mental Disease*, 185(9), 556–560. https://doi.org/10.1097/00005053-199709000-00004

Houston, E., Sandfort, T. G. M., Watson, K. T., & Caton, C. L. M. (2013). Psychological pathways from childhood sexual and physical abuse to HIV/sexually transmitted infection outcomes among homeless women: The role of posttraumatic stress disorder and borderline personality disorder symptoms. *Journal of Health Psychology*, 18(10), 1330–1340. https:// doi.org/10.1177/1359105312464674

Howell, K. H., Schaefer, L. M., Hasselle, A. J., & Thurston, I. B. (2020). Social support as a moderator between syndemics and posttraumatic stress among women experiencing adversity. *Journal of Aggression, Maltreatment & Trauma*, 30(6), 828–843. https://doi.org/10.1080/ 10926771.2020.1783732

Howsepian, A. A. (1998). Post-traumatic stress disorder following needle-stick contaminated with suspected HIV-positive blood. *General and Hospital Psychiatry*, 20(2), 123–124. https:// doi.org/10.1016/s0163-8343(97)00118-7

Hutton, H. E., Treisman, G. J., Hunt, W. R., Fishman, M., Kendig, N., Swetz, A., & Lyketsos, C. G. (2001). HIV risk behaviors and their relationship to posttraumatic stress disorder among women prisoners. *Psychiatric Services*, 52(4), 508–513. https://doi.org/10.1176/appi. ps.52.4.508

Ironson, G., O'Cleirigh, C., Leserman, J., Stuetzle, R., Fordiani, J., Fletcher, M., & Schneiderman, N. (2013). Gender-specific effects of an augmented written emotional disclosure intervention on posttraumatic, depressive, and HIV-disease-related outcomes: A randomized, controlled trial. *Journal of Consulting and Clinical Psychology*, 81(2), 284–298. https://doi.org/ 10.1037/a0030814

Israelski, D. M., Prentiss, D. E., Lubega, S., Balmas, G., Garcia, P., Muhammad, M., Cummings, S., & Koopman, C. (2007). Psychiatric co-morbidity in vulnerable populations receiving primary care for HIV/AIDS. *AIDS Care*, 19(2), 220–225. https://doi.org/10.1080/095401 20600774230

John, M. D., Greene, M., Hessol, N. A., Zepf, R., Parrott, A. H., Foreman, C., Bourgeois, J., Gandhi, M., & Hare, C. B. (2016). Geriatric assessments and association with VACS index among HIV-infected older adults in San Francisco. *Journal of Acquired Immune Deficiency Syndromes*, 72(5), 534–541.

Johnson, D. M., Johnson, N. L., Beckwith, C. G., Palmieri, P. A., & Zlotnick, C. (2017). Rapid human immunodeficiency virus testing and risk prevention in residents of battered women's shelters. *Women's Health Issues*, 27(1), 36–42. https://doi.org/10.1016/j.whi.2016.10.007

Junglen, A. G., Smith, B. C., Coleman, J. A., Pacella, M. L., Boarts, J. M., Jones, T., Feeny, N. C., Ciesla, J. A., & Delahanty, D. L. (2017). A multi-level modeling approach examining PTSD symptom reduction during prolonged exposure therapy: Moderating effects of number of trauma types experienced, having an HIV-related index trauma, and years since HIV diagnosis among HIV-positive adults. *AIDS Care*, 29(11), 1391–1398. https://doi.org/10.1080/ 09540121.2017.1300625

Kagee, A., Bantjes, J., & Saal, W. (2017). Prevalence of traumatic events and symptoms of PTSD among South Africans receiving an HIV test. *AIDS and Behavior*, 21(11), 3219–3227. https:// doi.org/10.1007/s10461-017-1730-9

Kagee, A., Bantjes, J., Saal, W., & Sefatsa, M. (2019). Utility of the Posttraumatic Stress Scale–Self-report version in screening for posttraumatic stress disorder among persons seeking HIV testing. *South African Journal of Psychology*, 49(1), 136–147. https://doi.org/ 10.1177/0081246318779191

Kagee, A., Saal, W., & Bantjes, J. (2018). The relationship between symptoms of common mental disorders and drug and alcohol misuse among persons seeking an HIV test. *AIDS Care*, 30(2), 219–223. https://doi.org/10.1080/09540121.2017.1361510

Kagee, A., Saal, W., De Villiers, L., Sefatsa, M., & Bantjes, J. (2017). The prevalence of common mental disorders among South Africans seeking HIV testing. *AIDS and Behavior*, 21(6), 1511–1517. https://doi.org/10.1007/s10461-016-1428-4

Kamen, C., Bergstrom, J., Koopman, C., Lee, S., & Gore-Felton, C. (2012). Relationships among childhood trauma, posttraumatic stress disorder, and dissociation in men living with HIV/ AIDS. *Journal of Trauma Dissociation*, 13(1), 102–114. https://doi.org/10.1080/15299 732.2011.608629

Kamen, C., Vorasarun, C., Canning, T., Kienitz, E., Weiss, C., Flores, S., Etter, D., Lee, S., & Gore-Felton, C. (2016). The impact of stigma and social support on development of post-traumatic growth among persons living with HIV. *Journal of Clinical Psychology in Medical Settings*, 23(2), 126–134. https://doi.org/10.1007/s10880-015-9447-2

Katz, S., & Nevid, J. S. (2005). Risk factors associated with posttraumatic stress disorder symp-tomatology in HIV-infected women. *AIDS Patient Care and STDS*, 19(2), 110–120. https:// doi.org/10.1089/apc.2005.19.110

Kaufman, C. C., Thurston, I. B., Howell, K. H., & Crossnine, C. B. (2020). Associations between spirituality and mental health in women exposed to adversity. *Psychology of Religion and Spirituality*, 12(4), 400–408. https://doi.org/10.1037/rel0000254

Kelly, B., Raphael, B., Judd, F., Perdices, M., Kernutt, G., Burnett, P., Dunne, M., & Burrows, G. (1998). Posttraumatic stress disorder in response to HIV infection. *General Hospital Psychiatry*, 20(6), 345–352. https://doi.org/10.1016/s0163-8343(98)00042-5

Kimerling, R., Calhoun, K. S., Forehand, R., Armistead, L., Morse, E., Morse, P., Clark, R., & Clark, L. (1999). Traumatic stress in HIV-infected women. *AIDS Education and Prevention*, 11(4), 321–330.

Klis, S., Velding, K., Gidron, Y., & Peterson, K. (2011). Posttraumatic stress and depressive symptoms among people living with HIV in the Gambia. *AIDS Care*, *23*(4), 426–434. https://doi.org/10.1080/09540121.2010.507756

Kuo, C., Reddy, M. K., Operario, D., Cluver, L., & Stein, D. J. (2013). Posttraumatic stress symptoms among adults caring for orphaned children in HIV-endemic South Africa. *AIDS and Behavior*, *17*(5), 1755–1763. https://doi.org/10.1007/s10461-013-0461-9

Lennon-Dearing, R. (2022). "HIV is a gift": Posttraumatic growth in women with HIV. *Illness, Crisis & Loss*, *30*(2), 224–239. https://doi.org/10.1177/1054137320906559

León, C., Cardoso, L., Mackin, S., Bock, B., & Gaeta, J. M. (2018). The willingness of people who inject drugs in Boston to use a supervised injection facility. *Substance Abuse*, *39*(1), 95–101. https://doi.org/10.1080/08897077.2017.1365804

Leserman, J., Whetten, K., Lowe, K., Stangl, D., Swartz, M. S., & Thielman, N. M. (2005). How trauma, recent stressful events, and PTSD affect functional health status and health utilization in HIV-infected patients in the South. *Psychosomatic Medicine*, *67*(3), 500–507. https://doi.org/10.1097/01.psy.0000160459.78182.d9

Luszczynska, A., Durawa, A. B., Dudzinska, M., Kwiatkowska, M., Knysz, B., & Knoll, N. (2012). The effects of mortality reminders on posttraumatic growth and finding benefits among patients with life-threatening illness and their caregivers. *Psychology & Health*, *27*(10), 1227–1243. https://doi.org/10.1080/08870446.2012.665055

Lynn, C., Bradley-Klug, K., Chenneville, T. A., Walsh, A. S. J., Dedrick, R., & Rodriguez, C. (2018). Mental health screening in integrated care settings: Identifying rates of depression, anxiety, and posttraumatic stress among youth with HIV. *Journal of HIV/AIDS & Social Services*, *17*(3), 239–245. https://doi.org/10.1080/15381501.2018.1437585

Lynn, C., Chenneville, T., Bradley-Klug, K., Walsh, A. S. J., Dedrick, R. F., & Rodriguez, C. A. (2019). Depression, anxiety, and posttraumatic stress as predictors of immune functioning: Differences between youth with behaviorally and perinatally acquired HIV. *AIDS Care*, *31*(10), 1261–1270. https://doi.org/10.1080/09540121.2019.1587354

Machtinger, E. L., Haberer, J. E., Wilson, T. C., & Weiss, D. S. (2012). Recent trauma is associated with antiretroviral failure and HIV transmission risk behavior among HIV-positive women and female-identified transgenders. *AIDS and Behavior*, *16*(8), 2160–2170. https://doi.org/10.1007/s10461-012-0158-5

Machtinger, E. L., Wilson, T. C., Haberer, J. E., & Weiss, D. S. (2012). Psychological trauma and PTSD in HIV-positive women: a meta-analysis. *AIDS and Behavior*, *16*(8), 2091–2100. https://doi.org/10.1007/s10461-011-0127-4

Mackesy-Amiti, M. E., Donenberg, G. R., & Ouellet, L. J. (2014). Psychiatric correlates of injection risk behavior among young people who inject drugs. *Psychology of Addictive Behaviors*, *28*(4), 1089–1095. https://doi.org/10.1037/a0036390

Marshall, B. D. L., Prescott, M. R., Liberzon, I., Tamburrino, M. B., Calabrese, J. R., & Galea, S. (2013). Posttraumatic stress disorder, depression, and HIV risk behavior among Ohio Army Rational Guard Soldiers. *Journal of Traumatic Stress*, *26*(1), 64–70. https://doi.org/10.1002/jts.21777

Martinez, J., Hosek, S. G., & Carleton, R. A. (2009). Screening and assessing violence and mental health disorders in a cohort of inner city HIV-positive youth between 1998–2006. *AIDS Patient Care and STDS*, *23*(6), 469–475. https://doi.org/10.1089/apc.2008.0178

Mellins, C. A., Ehrhardt, A. A., & Grant, W. F. (1997). Psychiatric symptomatology and psychological functioning in HIV-infected mothers. *AIDS and Behavior*, *1*(4), 233–245. https://doi.org/10.1023/A:1026227418721

Milam, J. (2006a). Positive changes attributed to the challenge of HIV/AIDS. In L. G. Calhoun, & R. G. Tedeschi (Eds.), *Handbook of posttraumatic growth: Research & practice* (pp. 214–224). Lawrence Erlbaum Associates.

Milam, J. (2006b). Posttraumatic growth and HIV disease progression. *Journal of Consulting and Clinical Psychology*, *74*(5), 817–827. https://doi.org/10.1037/0022-006x.74.5.817

Milam, J. E. (2004). Posttraumatic growth among HIV/AIDS patients. *Journal of Applied Social Psychology*, *34*, 2353–2376. https://doi.org/10.1111/j.1559-1816.2004.tb01981.x

Mizota, Y., Ozawa, M., Yamazaki, Y., & Inoue, Y. (2006). Psychosocial problems of bereaved families of HIV-infected hemophiliacs in Japan. *Social Science & Medicine*, *62*(10), 2397–2410. https://doi.org/10.1016/j.socscimed.2005.10.032

Moradi, A. R., Miraghaei, M. A., Parhon, H., Jabbari, H., & Jobson, L. (2013). Posttraumatic stress disorder, depression, executive functioning, and autobiographical remembering in individuals with HIV and in carers of those with HIV in Iran. *AIDS Care*, *25*(3), 281–288.

Munroe, C. D., Kibler, J. L., Ma, M., Dollar, K. M., & Coleman, M. (2010). The relationship between posttraumatic stress symptoms and sexual risk: Examining potential mechanisms. *Psychological Trauma: Theory, Research, Practice, and Policy*, *2*, 49–53. https://doi.org/10.1037/a0018960

Murphy, P. J., & Hevey, D. (2013). The relationship between internalised HIV-related stigma and posttraumatic growth. *AIDS and Behavior*, *17*(5), 1809–1818. https://doi.org/10.1007/s10461-013-0482-4

Myer, L., Smit, J., Roux, L. L., Parker, S., Stein, D. J., & Seedat, S. (2008). Common mental disorders among HIV-infected individuals in South Africa: prevalence, predictors, and validation of brief psychiatric rating scales. *AIDS Patient Care and STDS*, *22*(2), 147–158. https://doi.org/10.1089/apc.2007.0102

Myers, H. F., & Durvasula, R. S. (1999). Psychiatric disorders in African American men and women living with HIV/AIDS. *Cultural Diversity and Ethnic Minority Psychology*, *5*, 249–262. https://doi.org/10.1037/1099-9809.5.3.249

Narvaez, J. C. d. M., Remy, L., Bermudez, M. B., Scherer, J. N., Ornell, F., Surratt, H., Kurtz, S. P., & Pechansky, F. (2019). Re-traumatization cycle: Sexual abuse, post-traumatic stress disorder and sexual risk behaviors among club drug users. *Substance Use & Misuse*, *54*(9), 1499–1508. https://doi.org/10.1080/10826084.2019.1589521

Nightingale, V. R., Sher, T. G., & Hansen, N. B. (2010). The impact of receiving an HIV diagnosis and cognitive processing on psychological distress and posttraumatic growth. *Journal of Traumatic Stress*, *23*(4), 452–460.

O'Cleirigh, C., Safren, S. A., Taylor, S. W., Goshe, B. M., Bedoya, C. A., Marquez, S. M., Boroughs, M. S., & Shipherd, J. C. (2019). Cognitive behavioral therapy for trauma and self-care (CBT-TSC) in men who have sex with men with a history of childhood sexual abuse: A randomized controlled trial. *AIDS and Behavior*, *23*(9), 2421–2431. https://doi.org/10.1007/s10461-019-02482-z

O'Cleirigh, C., Skeer, M., Mayer, K. H., & Safren, S. A. (2009). Functional impairment and health care utilization among HIV-infected men who have sex with men: the relationship with depression and post-traumatic stress. *Journal of Behavioral Medicine*, *32*(5), 466–477. https://doi.org/10.1007/s10865-009-9217-4

O'Cleirigh, C., Traeger, L., Mayer, K. H., Magidson, J. F., & Safren, S. A. (2013). Anxiety specific pathways to HIV sexual transmission risk behavior among young gay and bisexual men. *Journal of Gay & Lesbian Mental Health*, *17*(3), 314–326. https://doi.org/10.1080/19359705.2012.755142

Ogińska-Bulik, N., & Kraska, K. (2017). Posttraumatic stress disorder and posttraumatic growth in HIV-infected patients—The role of coping strategies. *Health Psychology Report*, *5*(4), 323–332. https://doi.org/10.5114/hpr.2017.68017

Olley, B. O., & Bolajoko, A. J. (2008). Psychosocial determinants of HIV-related quality of life among HIV-positive military in Nigeria. *Int J STD AIDS*, *19*(2), 94–98. https://doi.org/10.1258/ijsa.2007.007134

Olley, B. O., Seedat, S., & Stein, D. J. (2006). Persistence of psychiatric disorders in a cohort of HIV/AIDS patients in South Africa: a 6-month follow-up study. *Journal of Psychosomatic Research*, 61(4), 479–484. https://doi.org/10.1016/j.jpsychores.2006.03.010

Oniszczenko, W., Rzeszutek, M., & Firląg-Burkacka, E. (2019). Religious fundamentalism, satisfaction with life and posttraumatic stress symptoms intensity in a Polish sample of people living with HIV/AIDS. *Journal of Religion and Health*, 58(1), 168–179. https://doi.org/10.1007/s10943-018-0615-1

Pacella, M. L., Armelie, A., Boarts, J., Wagner, G., Jones, T., Feeny, N., & Delahanty, D. L. (2012). The impact of prolonged exposure on PTSD symptoms and associated psychopathology in people living with HIV: a randomized test of concept. *AIDS and Behavior*, 16(5), 1327–1340. https://doi.org/10.1007/s10461-011-0076-y

Paxton, K. C., Myers, H. F., Hall, N. M., & Javanbakht, M. (2004). Ethnicity, serostatus, and psychosocial differences in sexual risk behavior among HIV-seropositive and HIV-seronegative women. *AIDS and Behaviour*, 8(4), 405–415. https://doi.org/10.1007/s10461-004-7325-2

Peasant, C., Sullivan, T. P., Weiss, N. H., Martinez, I., & Meyer, J. P. (2017). Beyond the syndemic: Condom negotiation and use among women experiencing partner violence. *AIDS Care*, 29(4), 516–523. https://doi.org/10.1080/09540121.2016.1224296

Pence, B. W., Miller, W. C., Whetten, K., Eron, J. J., & Gaynes, B. N. (2006). Prevalence of DSM-IV-defined mood, anxiety, and substance use disorders in an HIV clinic in the Southeastern United States. *Journal of Acquired Immune Deficiency Syndromes*, 42(3), 298–306. https://doi.org/10.1097/01.qai.0000219773.82055.aa

Pengpid, S., & Peltzer, K. (2013). Mental health, partner violence and HIV risk among women with protective orders against violent partners in Vhembe district, South Africa. *Asian Journal of Psychiatry*, 6(6), 494–499. https://doi.org/10.1016/j.ajp.2013.06.005

Pennebaker, J. W. (1995). *Emotion, disclosure & health*. American Psychological Association.

Pennebaker, J. W. (1997). Writing about emotional experiences as a therapeutic process. *Psychological Science*, 8, 162–166.

Pięta, M., & Rzeszutek, M. (2022). Trajectories of posttraumatic growth and posttraumatic depreciation: A one-year prospective study among people living with HIV. *PLoS ONE*, 17(9), e0275000. https://doi.org/10.1371/journal.pone.0275000

Pięta, M., & Rzeszutek, M. (2023). Posttraumatic growth and posttraumatic depreciation among people living with HIV: the role of resilience and HIV/AIDS stigma in the person-centered approach. *AIDS Care*, 35(2), 230–237. https://doi.org/10.1080/09540121.2022.2141184

Radcliffe, J., Fleisher, C. L., Hawkins, L. A., Tanney, M., Kassam-Adams, N., Ambrose, C., & Rudy, B. J. (2007). Posttraumatic stress and trauma history in adolescents and young adults with HIV. *AIDS Patient Care and STDS*, 21(7), 501–508. https://doi.org/10.1089/apc.2006.0144

Ratcliff, T. M., Zlotnick, C., Cu-Uvin, S., Payne, N., Sly, K., & Flanigan, T. (2012). Acceptance of HIV antibody testing among women in domestic violence shelters. *Journal of HIV AIDS & Social Services*, 11(3), 291–304. https://doi.org/10.1080/15381501.2012.703555

Reisner, S. L., Falb, K. L., & Mimiaga, M. J. (2011). Early life traumatic stressors and the mediating role of PTSD in incident HIV infection among US men, comparisons by sexual orientation and race/ethnicity: results from the NESARC, 2004–2005. *Journal of Acquired Immune Deficiency Syndromes*, 57(4), 340–350. https://doi.org/10.1097/QAI.0b013e31821d36b4

Ricart, F., Cohen, M. A., Alfonso, C. A., Hoffman, R. G., Quiñones, N., Cohen, A., & Indyk, D. (2002). Understanding the psychodynamics of non-adherence to medical treatment in persons with HIV infection. *General Hospital Psychiatry*, 24(3), 176–180. https://doi.org/10.1016/s0163-8343(02)00172-x

Roland, K. B., Higa, D. H., Leighton, C. A., Mizuno, Y., DeLuca, J. B., & Koenig, L. J. (2020). Client perspectives and experiences with HIV patient navigation in the United States: A qualitative meta-synthesis. *Health Promotion Practice, 21*(1), 25–36. https://doi.org/10.1177/1524839919875727

Rose, R. C., House, A. S., & Stepleman, L. M. (2010). Intimate partner violence and its effects on the health of African American HIV-positive women. *Psychological Trauma: Theory, Research, Practice, and Policy, 2,* 311–317. https://doi.org/10.1037/a0018977

Rzeszutek, M. (2017). Social support and posttraumatic growth in a longitudinal study of people living with HIV: The mediating role of positive affect. *European Journal of Psychotraumatology, 8*(1). https://doi.org/10.1080/20008198.2017.1412225

Rzeszutek, M., & Gruszczyńska, E. (2018). Posttraumatic growth among people living with HIV: A systematic review. *Journal of Psychosomatic Research, 114,* 81–91. https://doi.org/10.1016/j.jpsychores.2018.09.006

Rzeszutek, M., Oniszczenko, W., & Firląg-Burkacka, E. (2017a). Gender differences in posttraumatic stress symptoms and social support in a sample of HIV-positive individuals. *Women & Health, 57*(7), 792–803. https://doi.org/10.1080/03630242.2016.1206057

Rzeszutek, M., Oniszczenko, W., & Firląg-Burkacka, E. (2017b). Social support, stress coping strategies, resilience and posttraumatic growth in a Polish sample of HIV-infected individuals: Results of a 1 year longitudinal study. *Journal of Behavioral Medicine, 40*(6), 942–954. https://doi.org/10.1007/s10865-017-9861-z

Rzeszutek, M., Oniszczenko, W., & Gruszczyńska, E. (2019). Satisfaction with life, big-five personality traits and posttraumatic growth among people living with HIV. *Journal of Happiness Studies, 20*(1), 35–50. https://doi.org/10.1007/s10902-017-9925-3

Rzeszutek, M., Oniszczenko, W., Schier, K., Biernat-Kałuża, E., & Gasik, R. (2016). Temperament traits, social support, and trauma symptoms among HIV/AIDS and chronic pain patients. *International Journal of Clinical and Health Psychology, 16*(2), 137–146. https://doi.org/10.1016/j.ijchp.2015.10.001

Safren, S. A., Gershuny, B. S., & Hendriksen, E. (2003). Symptoms of posttraumatic stress and death anxiety in persons with HIV and medication adherence difficulties. *AIDS Patient Care and STDS, 17*(12), 657–664. https://doi.org/10.1089/108729103771928717

Samuels, E., Khalife, S., Alfonso, C. A., Alvarez, R., & Cohen, M. A. (2011). Early childhood trauma, posttraumatic stress disorder, and non-adherence in persons with AIDS: a psychodynamic perspective. *Journal of the American Academy of Psychoanalysis and Dynamic Psychiatry, 39*(4), 633–650. https://doi.org/10.1521/jaap.2011.39.4.633

Sawyer, A., Ayers, S., & Field, A. (2010). Posttraumatic growth and adjustment among individuals with cancer or HIV/AIDS: A meta-analysis. *Clinical Psychology Review, 30,* 436–447. https://doi.org/10.1016/j.cpr.2010.02.004

Schneider, A., Conrad, D., Pfeiffer, A., Elbert, T., Kolassa, I.-T., & Wilker, S. (2018). Stigmatization is associated with increased PTSD risk after traumatic stress and diminished likelihood of spontaneous remission—A study with East-African conflict survivors. *Frontiers in Psychiatry, 9.* https://doi.org/10.3389/fpsyt.2018.00423

Seth, P., Jackson, J. M., DiClemente, R. J., & Fasula, A. M. (2017). Community trauma as a predictor of sexual risk, marijuana use, and psychosocial outcomes among detained African-American female adolescents. *Vulnerable Children and Youth Studies, 12*(4), 353–359. https://doi.org/10.1080/17450128.2017.1325547

Singer, M. (1996). A dose of drugs, a touch of violence, a case of AIDS: Conceptualizing the SAVA syndemic. *Free Inquiry in Creative Sociology, 24,* 99 110.

Singer, M., & Clair, S. (2003). Syndemics and public health: reconceptualizing disease in biosocial context. *Medical Anthropology Quarterly, 17*(4), 423–441. http://www.jstor.org/stable/3655345

Sledjeski, E. M., Delahanty, D. L., & Bogart, L. M. (2005). Incidence and impact of posttraumatic stress disorder and comorbid depression on adherence to HAART and CD4+

counts in people living with HIV. *AIDS Patient Care and STDS, 19*(11), 728–736. https://doi. org/10.1089/apc.2005.19.728

Smith, M. Y., Egert, J., Winkel, G., & Jacobson, J. (2002). The impact of PTSD on pain experience in persons with HIV/AIDS. *Pain, 98*(1–2), 9–17. https://doi.org/10.1016/ s0304-3959(01)00431-6

Staton-Tindall, M., Harp, K. L. H., Minieri, A., Oser, C., Webster, J. M., Havens, J., & Leukefeld, C. (2015). An exploratory study of mental health and HIV risk behavior among drug-using rural women in jail. *Psychiatric Rehabilitation Journal, 38*(1), 45–54. https://doi.org/10.1037/ prj0000107

Stiles, W. B., Shapiro, D. A., & Firth-Cozens, J. A. (1988). Do sessions of different treatments have different impacts? *Journal of Counseling Psychology, 35*(4), 391–396. https://doi.org/ 10.1037/0022-0167.35.4.391

Taylor, S. W., Goshe, B. M., Marquez, S. M., Safren, S. A., & O'Cleirigh, C. (2018). Evaluating a novel intervention to reduce trauma symptoms and sexual risk taking: Qualitative exit interviews with sexual minority men with childhood sexual abuse. *Psychology, Health & Medicine, 23*(4), 454–464. https://doi.org/10.1080/13548506.2017.1348609

Tedeschi, R. G., & Calhoun, L. G. (1995). *Trauma & transformation: Growing in the aftermath of suffering.* Sage Publications. https://doi.org/10.4135/9781483326931

Theuninck, A. C., Lake, N., & Gibson, S. (2010). HIV-related posttraumatic stress disorder: investigating the traumatic events. *AIDS Patient Care and STDS, 24*(8), 485–491. https://doi.org/10.1089/apc.2009.0231

Trice, A. D. (1988). Posttraumatic stress syndrome-like symptoms among AIDS caregivers. *Psychological Reports, 63*(2), 656-658.

Tsao, J. C., Dobalian, A., & Naliboff, B. D. (2004). Panic disorder and pain in a national sample of persons living with HIV. *Pain, 109*(1–2), 172–180. https://doi.org/10.1016/ j.pain.2004.02.001

Ugwu, L. I., Onu, D. U., Nnadozie, E. E., & Iorfa, S. K. (2021). Psychometric validation of the Centrality of Events Scale in a Nigerian clinical sample. *Journal of Psychology in Africa, 31*(2), 167–176. https://doi.org/10.1080/14330237.2021.1910410

van den Heuvel, L., Chishinga, N., Kinyanda, E., Weiss, H., Patel, V., Ayles, H., Harvey, J., Cloete, K. J., & Seedat, S. (2013). Frequency and correlates of anxiety and mood disorders among TB- and HIV-infected Zambians. *AIDS Care, 25*(12), 1527–1535. https://doi.org/ 10.1080/09540121.2013.793263

Vance, D. E., Moneyham, L., & Farr, K. F. (2008). Suicidal ideation in adults aging with HIV. *Journal of Psychosocial Nursing and Mental Health Services, 46*(11), 33–38.

Verhey, R., Chibanda, D., Gibson, L., Brakarsh, J., & Seedat, S. (2018). Validation of the Posttraumatic Stress Disorder Checklist—5 (PCL-5) in a primary care population with high HIV prevalence in Zimbabwe. *BMC Psychiatry, 18*(1), 109. https://doi.org/10.1186/s12 888-018-1688-9

Vujanovic, A. A., Farris, S. G., Bartlett, B. A., Lyons, R. C., Haller, M., Colvonen, P. J., & Norman, S. B. (2018). Anxiety sensitivity in the association between posttraumatic stress and substance use disorders: A systematic review. *Clinical Psychology Review, 62*, 37–55. https://doi. org/10.1016/j.cpr.2018.05.003

Wade, K., Beckerman, N., & Stein, E. J. (1996). Risk of posttraumatic stress disorder among AIDS social workers: Implications for organizational response. *The Clinical Supervisor, 14*(2), 85–97. https://doi.org/10.1300/J001v14n02_07

Wagner, G. J., Bogart, L. M., Galvan, F. H., Banks, D., & Klein, D. J. (2012). Discrimination as a key mediator of the relationship between posttraumatic stress and HIV treatment adherence among African American men. *Journal of Behavioral Medicine, 35*(1), 8–18. https://doi.org/ 10.1007/s10865-011-9320-1

Wang, Q., Zhou, T., Gao, J., Xu, K., Qu, W., & Yang, Y. (2018). Attachment, social support, resilience and posttraumatic stress disorder symptoms in Chinese adults living with HIV/AIDS. *Journal of Loss and Trauma, 23*(2), 113–127. https://doi.org/10.1080/15325 024.2017.1419803

Weiss, N. H., Dixon-Gordon, K. L., Peasant, C., Jaquier, V., Johnson, C., & Sullivan, T. P. (2017). A latent profile analysis of intimate partner victimization and aggression and examination of between-class differences in psychopathology symptoms and risky behaviors. *Psychological Trauma: Theory, Research, Practice, and Policy, 9*(3), 370–378. https://doi.org/10.1037/tra 0000202

Weiss, N. H., Tull, M. T., Borne, M. E. R., & Gratz, K. L. (2013). Posttraumatic stress disorder symptom severity and HIV-risk behaviors among substance-dependent inpatients. *AIDS Care, 25*(10), 1219–1226. https://doi.org/10.1080/09540121.2013.764381

Whetten, K., Reif, S., Whetten, R., & Murphy-McMillan, L. K. (2008). Trauma, mental health, distrust, and stigma among HIV-positive persons: implications for effective care. *Psychosomatic Medicine, 70*(5), 531–538. https://doi.org/10.1097/PSY.0b013e31817749dc

Yang, X., Wang, Q., Wang, X., Mo, P. K. H., Wang, Z., Lau, J. T. F., & Wang, L. (2020). Direct and indirect associations between interpersonal resources and posttraumatic growth through resilience among women living with HIV in China. *AIDS and Behavior, 24*(6), 1687–1700. https://doi.org/10.1007/s10461-019-02694-3

Ye, Z., Chen, L., & Lin, D. (2018). The relationship between posttraumatic stress disorder symptoms and posttraumatic growth among HIV-infected men who have sex with men in Beijing, China: The mediating roles of coping strategies. *Frontiers in Psychology, 9*. https://doi.org/ 10.3389/fpsyg.2018.01787

Yemeke, T. T., Sikkema, K. J., Watt, M. H., Ciya, N., Robertson, C., & Joska, J. A. (2020). Screening for traumatic experiences and mental health distress among women in HIV care in Cape Town, South Africa. *Journal of Interpersonal Violence, 35*(21–22), 4842–4862. https://doi.org/10.1177/0886260517718186

Yiaslas, T. A., Kamen, C., Arteaga, A., Lee, S., Briscoe-Smith, A., Koopman, C., & Gore-Felton, C. (2014). The relationship between sexual trauma, peritraumatic dissociation, posttraumatic stress disorder, and HIV-related health in HIV-positive men. *Journal of Trauma & Dissociation, 15*(4), 420–435. https://doi.org/10.1080/15299732.2013.873376

Yu, N. X., Chen, L., Ye, Z., Li, X., & Lin, D. (2017). Impacts of making sense of adversity on depression, posttraumatic stress disorder, and posttraumatic growth among a sample of mainly newly diagnosed HIV-positive Chinese young homosexual men: The mediating role of resilience. *AIDS Care, 29*(1), 79–85. https://doi.org/10.1080/09540121.2016.1210073

Zeligman, M., Barden, S. M., & Hagedorn, W. B. (2016). Posttraumatic growth and HIV: A study on associations of stigma and social support. *Journal of Counseling & Development, 94*(2), 141–149. https://doi.org/10.1002/jcad.12071

Zhao, Q., Li, X., Fang, X., Zhao, G., Zhao, J., Lin, X., & Stanton, B. (2010). Difference in psychosocial well-being between paternal and maternal AIDS orphans in rural China. *Journal of the Association of Nurses in AIDS Care, 21*(4), 335–344. https://doi.org/10.1016/ j.jana.2009.12.001

Zoellner, L. A., Rothbaum, B. O., & Feeny, N. C. (2011). PTSD not an anxiety disorder? DSM committee proposal turns back the hands of time. *Depression and Anxiety, 28*(10), 853–856. https://doi.org/10.1002/da.20899

7

Posttraumatic stress disorder in vascular and neurological diseases

Haemorrhage is the loss of blood from a damaged blood vessel inside or outside the body (internal or external bleeding). It can occur suddenly and unexpectedly in any part of the body and can be life-threatening and traumatic. Nevertheless, a study looking at patients who suffered from variceal haemorrhage found that only one of the thirty patients studied met the diagnostic criteria for posttraumatic stress disorder (PTSD), even though most of them found the experience distressing. It was concluded that PTSD is indeed quite rare in patients who have survived a life-threatening variceal haemorrhage (O'Carrol et al., 1999).

PTSD and haemorrhage

However, the above claim is not without controversy. In one study, 32% of patients with a subarachnoid haemorrhage (SAH) met the diagnostic criteria for PTSD (post-SAH PTSD), and 50% suffered from anxiety (Berry, 1998). While recovering from SAH, patients often live with PTSD symptoms alongside prolonged fatigue, anxiety about their condition, fear of recurrent SAH, depression, sleep disturbance, cognitive and physical impairment, headaches, and inadequate information about their illness (Kutlubaev et al., 2012; McKenna & Neil-Dwyer, 1993). As a result, their quality of life and life satisfaction have also decreased (Kutlubaev et al., 2012). To alleviate their great anxiety, appropriate and informed counselling is of utmost importance (McKenna & Neil-Dwyer, 1993).

In another study, patients with subarachnoid haemorrhage were examined. Of these, 68.4% reported a cerebral aneurysm as the cause of their SAH. The prevalence of PTSD was even higher, as 44.4% met the diagnostic criteria. Similar to the above studies, anxiety was of clinical significance in 68.8% and depression was of clinical significance in 45.2%. Despite these psychological

Posttraumatic Stress in Physical Illness. Man Cheung Chung, Oxford University Press. © Oxford University Press 2024.
DOI: 10.1093/oso/9780198727323.003.0007

needs, 47% of distressed patients had not been examined for post-SAH distress and 55% had not been treated (Noble & Schenk, 2014).

Regarding the progression of PTSD symptoms, a longitudinal study examined patients suffering from aneurysmal subarachnoid haemorrhage and assessed patients over a one-year period (3, 6, and 12 months). There were no differences in the level of PTSD related to the haemorrhage over time in the group, although significant changes in PTSD over time were observed at the individual level. The study found that 8.5% met the cut-off for PTSD at all three assessments; 14.9% at 3 months, then recovered later. However, 12.8% showed delayed PTSD (Huenges Wajer et al., 2018). In another longitudinal study that focused on a different type of haemorrhage, intracerebral haemorrhage (ICH), patients were assessed at 3 and 12 months after the onset of ICH. When assessed at 3 months, 23.4% of patients met the diagnostic criteria for post-ICH PTSD of whom 43% had recovered one year later (Jiang, 2020). Compared to patients without PTSD, patients with PTSD were more likely to be female, to have received minimally invasive surgery, to have poorer quality of life, higher levels of anxiety and depression, and to have stroke-related disability and greater endorsement of maladaptive coping strategies (Jiang, 2020). An important observation from these findings is that examining changes in PTSD symptoms over time by looking only at group differences over time would overlook some important individual differences in response to the traumatic effects of haemorrhage. These differences would raise the question of what explains patients with chronic symptoms or delayed symptoms and explain the resilience of some patients who did not develop or recover from PTSD.

PTSD and stroke

A stroke is a life-threatening condition that occurs when the blood supply to part of the brain is restricted or cut off. As a result, brain cells begin to die, which can lead to disability and possibly death. The two main causes of stroke are ischaemic, when the blood supply is cut off, for example, by a blood clot, and haemorrhagic, when a blood vessel supplying the brain bursts.

The posttraumatic effects of stroke have been studied in the literature. A longitudinal study showed that 30% of stroke patients met diagnostic criteria for full PTSD at baseline (post-stroke PTSD), and 23.1% three months after. Although post-stroke PTSD did not change significantly within 3 months, psychiatric comorbid symptoms decreased significantly (Wang et al., 2011). As the follow-up period for this study was relatively short, it focused only on the short-term trajectory of post-stroke PTSD. In terms of long-term changes, a meta-analytic review suggests that one in four patients with stroke or transient ischaemic attack (TIA) (the blood supply to the brain is temporarily interrupted) develop post-stroke or post-TIA PTSD. The prevalence of PTSD depends on length of time after the stroke/TIA, and the rate is estimated to be 23% within one year of the event but 11% one year after (Edmondson et al., 2013). Similar to PTSD associated with other health conditions, PTSD associated with stroke is not a stand-alone clinical condition but a comorbidity with other disorders such as post-stroke depression, all of which can affect recovery, medical outcomes, quality of life, recurrence of ischaemic events, treatment adherence, and ultimately the likelihood of mortality (Kronenberg et al., 2017). Attention has also been drawn to the fact that depression may be associated with panic attacks and PTSD in patients with TIA (Chardavoyne & Frechette, 2006).

In terms of risk factors, alexithymia, particularly difficulty in identifying feelings, correlated with post-stroke PTSD and psychiatric comorbidity at baseline. However, there was no correlation with distress scores at follow-up. In other words, patients' difficulty in identifying feelings might influence short-term rather than long-term PTSD and comorbid psychiatric symptoms (Wang et al., 2011). In addition, cognitive appraisals or a certain way of thinking about oneself also seemed to play a role in influencing post-stroke PTSD. In one study, stroke patients were examined during hospitalisation and 3 months after discharge. Significant correlations were found between negative cognitions about the self and the world and severity of PTSD symptoms during hospitalisation and after discharge. However, considering prediction, cognitive appraisal—especially negative cognitions about the self—explained a significant proportion of the variance in PTSD symptom severity during hospitalisation, but not the additional variance in PTSD severity after discharge (Field et al., 2008). This study mirrors the findings of the previous study: stroke patients appear to respond differently to short- or long-term PTSD. Similarly, for caregivers (i.e. family members or close associates) of stroke patients, negative cognitions about themselves and the world and self-blame correlated with PTSD in relation to their experiences with stroke survivors (Carek et al., 2010).

This may explain why intervention programmes such as 'recovering together', in which stroke patients and their family caregivers work together to prevent chronic psychological distress for both parties and to support patients' recovery, have been proposed. This programme is based on the assumption that patients can experience suffering in dependence on family members in the dyad, but can adapt to adversity or illness, develop coping skills through the dyad's relationship systems within the family, and develop resilience. Cognitive–behavioural principles, dialectical–behavioural therapy principles, and mind–body approaches are embedded in the programme to help patients develop resilience and improve interpersonal communication skills in the acute phase of their illness during hospitalisation and after discharge at home or in rehabilitation centres (Meyers et al., 2020).

To shed light on the impact of the dyad relationship on recovery, one study examined the impact of cohabiting partners in patients who came to the emergency department for a stroke or TIA. It found that having a cohabiting partner only cushioned distress in patients who experienced a low level of threat during their visit to the emergency department. When the threat level was high, a partner was not a protective factor (Cornelius et al., 2021).

To conclude this section on PTSD and stroke, Moyamoya disease has also been suggested as a condition associated with PTSD. This is a rare blood vascular disorder in which the carotid artery in the skull becomes blocked or narrowed, leading to a reduction in blood flow to the brain. As a result, small blood vessels form at the base of the brain to supply blood to the brain. This disease can lead to TIA, stroke, cognitive, and developmental disabilities or delays. Research found that 47.5% of these patients reported PTSD, 46.7% reported depression, and 50% reported anxiety. PTSD and anxiety correlated with increased neurological disability, while depression and anxiety correlated with increased cognitive deficits. PTSD was the only risk factor for neurological disability, while depression and anxiety were risk factors for cognitive impairment (Liu et al., 2019).

PTSD and neurological diseases

It has been widely documented that trauma can alter brain structure in traumatised people with PTSD. Abnormalities in the hippocampus or hippocampal atrophy, for example, may be the result of stressors associated with PTSD, depression and borderline personality disorder (Sala et al., 2004). A meta-analysis shows that patients with PTSD have more consistent reductions in grey matter in the anterior cingulate cortex, ventromedial prefrontal cortex, left temporal pole/middle temporal gyrus, and left hippocampus than patients without PTSD. The grey matter deficit overlaps with the brain networks of emotion processing, fear extinction, and emotion regulation, which are problematic for people with PTSD (Kühn & Gallinat, 2013).

In this sense, neuropsychiatric disorders have been described as those related to stress, including PTSD. Constant distress can influence the development of some neurological diseases. In these diseases, inflammatory responses can exacerbate cell damage. While physical and psychological stressors such as PTSD, depression, and sleep deprivation can trigger an inflammatory response that increases disease risk (Kendall-Tackett, 2010), the response to stress can also activate anti-inflammatory pathways in our brain. This creates a kind of defence against excessive inflammation. In other words, stress can cause a dual response in our brain, both pro-inflammatory and anti-inflammatory, or both damaging and protective (García-Bueno et al., 2008). However, this dual response is much less well known than the link between distress and neurological functions.

PTSD and epilepsy

As mentioned earlier, trauma can affect neurological function. Some researchers have studied the link between PTSD and epilepsy. Since this book is about PTSD in physical illness, this section of the chapter will only address epilepsy, which is characterised by a predisposition to recurrent unprovoked epileptic seizures ≥24 h apart, and not post-traumatic seizures and post-traumatic epilepsy, which are lifelong complications of traumatic brain injury such as car accidents, falls, sports injuries and assaults. The seizures that occur in these conditions are thought to be caused by the trauma itself or non-degenerative damage to the brain from external mechanical forces.

A PTSD diagnosis as a psychiatric comorbidity with epilepsy consistently corresponded with low levels of quality of life, followed by depression (Zeber et al., 2007). Based on a case study, posttraumatic stress-sensitive epilepsy was introduced with the intention of emphasising the association between stress-induced epilepsy or seizures. However, this proposed clinical syndrome was based on only one case study and requires further systematic investigation (Zijlmans et al., 2017).

Although an association between PTSD and epilepsy has been suggested, when considering the studies comparing patients with epilepsy to those with non-epileptic seizures or psychogenic non-epileptic seizures (PNES) this association is indeed somewhat tenuous. It remains to be seen whether there is a unique contribution of PTSD to epilepsy. For example, one study compared patients with epileptic seizures (ES) with those with non-epileptic seizures (NES). It turned out that all patients with NES had experienced trauma before the onset of the seizures and had suffered physical or sexual assaults in the past. In contrast, for patients with ES, 55.2% reported pre-seizure trauma and 67.6% reported assaultive trauma (Dikel et al., 2003). Compared to patients with ES, patients with NES had higher rates of PTSD (70.6% vs 32.4%) and child sexual abuse (70.6% vs 32.4%) and higher levels of dissociation. PTSD, dissociation, and child sexual abuse were prevalent among women in both ES and NES (Dikel et al., 2003). To shed further light on the patients with NES, 56.5% had motor manifestations and 10% were flaccid and unresponsive. Only patients with motor manifestations had a history of sexual and physical abuse (Abubakr et al., 2003).

Other studies compared patients who had ES with patients who had psychogenic non-epileptic seizures (PNES). Before reporting the findings, it is noteworthy that despite the variation in the expression of PNES across cultural groups (Ho et al., 2019), people with PNES had a history of trauma (69%) and sexual trauma (29%), with generalised anxiety disorder (76%), major depressive disorder (64%), and PTSD (22%) being the most common psychiatric diagnoses. They also reported comorbid symptoms such as anxiety (90%), dissociative symptoms (51%), headaches (76%), and gastrointestinal problems (36%) (Taylor et al., 2020).

Returning to the comparison between ES and PNES individuals, the literature has broadly shown that PNES patients experienced more traumatic events in the past and had higher levels of PTSD symptoms than the ES group, although both groups had equal severity of suicidal ideation (Guillen et al., 2019). One study found that 58% of PNES and 13.5% of ES among veterans met diagnostic criteria for PTSD. PTSD was the only significant psychiatric diagnosis (odds ratio: 9.2) that contributed significantly to the classification of seizure types. Although depression and alcohol abuse were common, they did not differ between the two groups (Salinsky et al., 2012). A follow-up study examined veterans' health-related quality of life and found that the PNES group was also significantly more likely to report PTSD than the ES group. Veterans with PNES reported lower levels of quality of life than the sample of ES. Regardless of seizure type, psychological factors such as PTSD and depression explained most of the variance in quality of life and also explained the difference between the two groups (Salinsky et al., 2019). A later study showed that in people with PNES, PTSD, depression, anxiety, alexithymia, and dissociation were associated with poor quality of life at the time of diagnosis, while the number of seizures and co-occurrence of epilepsy were not related to quality of life (Gagny et al., 2021).

Another study showed that patients with behavioural spells (synonymous with PNES) and those with ES did not differ in the extent of past sexual trauma, with 38% as an approximate estimate for each group. Of those with behavioural spells, 27.8% reported three or more PTSD symptoms than 13% of those with ES. Past physical abuse, as opposed to sexual abuse, was more likely to predict a diagnosis of spells rather than epilepsy (Koby et al., 2010).

To expand the control groups, adolescents with PNES were compared with adolescents with ES and healthy controls. Those with PNES were more likely to report traumatic past events, including abuse, as well as parental conflict, interpersonal relationship problems with siblings/peers, and school difficulties. Those with PNES were significantly more likely to report comorbid psychiatric disorders (64.7%) than the ES group (47.8%). PNES also had higher levels of PTSD than the healthy group, although attention deficit/hyperactivity disorder and depressive disorders were common in both the PNES and ES groups. In addition, adolescents with PNES reported significantly lower self-esteem than the other groups (Say et al., 2014).

People with ES were also compared with people with PNES and others with non-epileptic seizures (oNES). While all reported PTSD, depression, and anxiety symptoms, people with PNES reported higher levels of these symptoms, with the exception of anxiety, than people with ES and the ES and oNES groups combined. No significant differences were found between the PNES and ES groups, or between the PNES and combined groups, on any of the Big Five personality subscales (Vilyte & Pretorius, 2019).

Another study compared patients with PNES only and patients with PNES and coexisting epilepsy. They found that the PNES-only group reported significantly more PTSD and dissociative disorders than the other group, while both groups were similar in terms of frequency of suicide attempts, antiepileptic therapy, and conversive, affective, and personality disorders (D'Alessio et al., 2006). Another study compared the two groups, finding high and similar rates of psychiatric disorders: 79.1% of patients with PNES only and 76.2% of patients with PNES + epilepsy had at least one psychiatric disorder. However, compared to patients with PNES + epilepsy (16.7%), patients with PNES-only had higher rates of PTSD (32.9%). They did not differ in terms of age of first trauma, types of trauma, number of patients with single traumas and patients with repeated traumatic experiences. The level of experience of child abuse was high in both groups and did not differ between the groups. In other words, both types of patients seemed to be similar in terms of psychopathological characteristics and negative life experiences (Labudda, Frauenheim, et al., 2018).

Similarly, patients with PNES and patients with drug-resistant epilepsy (DRE) were compared: the PNES group reported significantly more history of trauma (24.5% vs 48.57%), PTSD (4.08% vs 22.85%), anxiety disorders (16.32% vs 40%), and personality disorders (18.37% vs 42.86%) than the DRE group. However, patients with DRE reported more psychotic disorders (20.4% vs 2.85%) than the PNES group. The groups did not differ in terms of depression (Scévola et al., 2013).

Given the above studies pointing to the psychological problems of patients with PNES and their poor quality of life, psychological interventions including cognitive processing therapy are of paramount importance for these people (Gagny et al., 2021). A case study has shown that a patient with PNES who had experienced repeated domestic sexual assault as an adult had significantly less PTSD and depressive symptoms and reduced the number of psychogenic non-epileptic seizures after treatment with this therapy (Partlow & Birkley, 2022). Similarly, in a patient with PNES and PTSD, seizure frequency, quality of life, PTSD symptoms, suicidal ideation, and anxiety improved after prolonged exposure therapy, although there were no changes in alexithymia, anger, depression, and trait anxiety (Myers et al., 2021). While these treatment approaches seem to reflect some promising approaches for patients with PNES and PTSD, they only reflect treatment effects from case studies. It is clear that more research with large samples is needed before a conclusion can be reached about the effectiveness of these interventions.

Given the comparative studies between people with ES and PNES, and given the evidence about the generally poor health of people with PNES, it was concluded that PTSD was not among the most prominent pre-existing predictors in older adults with new-onset epilepsy, whereas substance abuse/dependence and psychosis were (Martin et al., 2014).

PTSD, epilepsy, and psychiatric comorbidity

Patients with epilepsy often have psychiatric comorbidity and report an average of 21% lower quality of life or poorer health than epilepsy patients without psychiatric comorbidity (Zeber et al., 2007). Notwithstanding this, a national survey also estimated that lifetime epilepsy with psychiatric comorbid symptoms such as PTSD, panic attacks, conduct disorder, and substance abuse was only 1.8%. Although these comorbid disorders could explain the association between epilepsy and impairment, epilepsy was the most important factor for work disability, cognitive impairment, and days of role impairment (Kessler et al., 2012). A systematic review and meta-analysis compared the prevalence rates of PTSD in different medical populations. It concluded that epilepsy has the lowest rate of 4.5%. The highest prevalence of PTSD over a period of 24 months or longer was found in people with intraoperative awareness (18.5%). This is a condition in which patients who have been under general anaesthesia can remember their surroundings or an event during surgery, or even pain related to their surgery (Cyr et al., 2021). The type of epilepsy could also have an impact on the incidence of PTSD. In patients with refractory focal epilepsy, one study found that only 1% suffered from PTSD, while less than 10% of them also suffered from other psychiatric comorbidities: social phobia (7.2%), specific phobia (6.2%), panic disorder (5.1%) and generalised anxiety disorder (3.1%), unspecified anxiety disorder (2.1%), and obsessive–compulsive disorder (1.0%) (Brandt et al., 2010).

On the contrary, case studies have shown that children with epilepsy may have comorbid psychiatric disorders including PTSD in addition to depression, anxiety, and obsessive–compulsive disorders (Papavasiliou et al., 2004). In particular, children aged 13 and 14 years who had both generalised and partial epilepsy were at high risk for PTSD (44.6%) and other psychiatric disorders. This percentage was the highest among all other disorders, followed by 32.4% for specific phobia and 31.1% for obsession (Dunn et al., 2009). Similarly, in some studies epilepsy patients reported a higher burden of past trauma compared to people without chronic illness or psychiatric symptoms (78% vs 52%). More epilepsy patients (26%) scored above the diagnostic score for PTSD than the control group (7%). Patients had significantly more severe PTSD symptoms than the control group. As a group, 72% and 33% of patients reported anxiety and depression, respectively, which were significantly correlated with PTSD symptoms. Patients with high levels of PTSD severity reported higher levels of depressive symptoms than patients without PTSD (Soncin et al., 2021).

Investigating the relationship between PTSD as a result of past trauma and epilepsy is only one way to investigate this relationship. Some studies have been conducted to investigate PTSD resulting from the traumatic perspective of epilepsy (post-epileptic seizure PTSD). One study found that 51% met the diagnostic criteria for full PTSD, 30% for partial PTSD, and 19% for no PTSD. People with epilepsy reported higher levels of anxiety and depression than the healthy control group (Chung & Allen, 2013). PTSD following epileptic seizures and psychiatric comorbidity were associated with self-efficacy and alexithymia, specifically difficulty identifying feelings. Alexithymia mediated the impact that self-efficacy had on post-epileptic seizure PTSD and psychiatric comorbidity (Chung et al., 2013).

In a more recent study, the above findings were also confirmed: 36.2% of the patient group reported that seizures were triggered by certain thoughts, situations, or times of day; 24.4% reported avoidance symptoms to avoid situations, places, or thoughts that could trigger a seizure. In addition, 37.6% reported hypervigilant symptoms at the onset of seizures and 38.8% reported reliving traumatic memories or experiencing emotions over which they had no control during their seizure (ictal period). Patients who had PTSD due to previous trauma reported significantly more PTSD items during the interictal and peri-ictal periods after the epileptic seizure than patients without PTSD due to previous trauma (Soncin et al., 2021). The impact of prior trauma on post-epileptic seizure PTSD also reflects a previous study which found that some of their participants (22%) with epilepsy had also experienced prior trauma. The impact of previous trauma may attenuate the effects of emotional processing difficulties on distress outcomes (Chung et al., 2013).

However, the controversy continues. One study looked at PTSD following an epileptic seizure and found a low rate. While fifty of the 120 patients reported a seizure that met the criteria for a traumatic event, twenty-eight of them reported a seizure that did not meet the criteria. Only six patients met all the criteria for PTSD following an epileptic seizure, three of them also had regular PTSD, and in two other patients their PTSD-like symptoms could have been better explained by an adjustment disorder. Furthermore, the study was unable to distinguish specific features between traumatic and non-traumatic seizures. These findings have led to the conclusion that PTSD following epileptic seizures is a rare condition (Labudda, Illies, et al., 2018). Some sceptics might even argue in favour of the mental condition misattribution hypothesis. This is the argument that some patients might remember a past traumatic event during the seizure, which then leads to a PTSD diagnosis. In fact, this event never occurred, which means that PTSD occurs as a result of misattribution of mental states that accompany a seizure (Cohen et al., 2010).

Caregiver

Caring for one's own children with epilepsy can be very stressful and have an impact on the mental health of caregivers. One study looked at PTSD and depression in parents of children with epilepsy, finding that the prevalence rates for both PTSD and depression were the same (31.5%); 56% of people with PTSD also had a diagnosis of depression. They showed more symptoms of re-experiencing (88.8%) and arousal (80%) than symptoms of avoidance and numbing (32.5%) (Iseri et al., 2006). Another study showed that 43.5% met the diagnostic criteria for one or more disorders, namely PTSD, depression, and anxiety, and 11% showed symptoms of subclinical PTSD (Jakobsen et al., 2020).

Other studies have reported that 10.4% and 37.3% of parents of children with epilepsy met the diagnostic criteria for full and partial PTSD, respectively, in relation to the traumatic aspects of their children's epilepsy diagnosis. Mothers reported higher levels of PTSD symptom clusters other than avoidance than fathers, while an association between PTSD and mood spectrum symptoms was only found in the subgroup of fathers (Carmassi et al., 2018). A follow-up study found higher percentages: 25% of parents met criteria for PTSD, with higher prevalence rates among mothers (36% and 14%); 44% of parents had partial PTSD, with higher percentages among mothers (48% vs 40%). Gender differences were also evident on all cluster dimensions of the trauma and loss spectrum except avoidance. Mothers reported significantly higher scores on these dimensions (intrusion: 84% vs 58%; negative alterations in cognitions and mood: 64% vs 28%; changes in arousal and reactivity: 66% vs 44%). There were more mothers showing fear and sadness as well as somatic symptoms than fathers (Carmassi et al., 2020).

To focus on PTSD and depression, another study conducted by Carmassi et al. found that prevalence rates for PTSD were 19.5% for mothers and 8.1% for fathers, and rates for major depression were 10.2% for mothers and 1.8% for fathers. Being a mother, witnessing tonic–clonic seizures, and having experienced trauma or loss in the past were associated with depression (Carmassi et al., 2019). The changes in the above prevalence rates were partly due to the use of different diagnostic criteria: 9.1% and 12.1% for PTSD according to DSM-5 (American Psychiatric Association, 2013) and DSM-IV-TR (American Psychiatric Association, 2000) criteria, respectively, on one day. However, an overall consistency of 92.9% was found in the study (Carmassi et al., 2017).

Children's difficulties, perceived control over their own situation, and social support predicted perceived caregiver stress (Jakobsen et al., 2020). Children's difficulties also correlated with PTSD, depression, and anxiety in caregivers. Interestingly, the caregivers' own resources (social support and perceived control over their own circumstances) and children's behavioural difficulties had the strongest effect on their distress and psychiatric symptoms, in contrast to factors related to epilepsy (Jakobsen et al., 2020).

The above findings reflect the results of a meta-analysis that found 18.9% of parents of children and adolescents with chronic physical illness met criteria for PTSD. Parental PTSS was most common in parents of children with epilepsy, followed by diabetes. PTSS was associated with motherhood, child

PTSS severity, severity of illness, and duration/intensity of treatment. On the other hand, low levels of parental PTSS were associated with longer duration of illness, longer time since active treatment, and better social resources (Pinquart, 2019).

Of course, living with and caring for people who have epilepsy can be demanding, stressful, and potentially traumatising not only for patients' parents but also for their partners. One study found that 7.7% of partners of people with epilepsy met criteria for PTSD and that 43.9% reported subclinical levels of PTSD. Clinical and subclinical anxiety was also found in 9.3% of participants (Norup & Elklit, 2013).

PTSD and dementia

In addition to studying epilepsy as a neurological condition associated with PTSD, research has also focused on dementia. Dementia is not a specific disease. Rather, it is an umbrella term that describes symptoms that affect people's ability to cope with daily life because their memory, thinking, reasoning or judgement, attention, and speech and behaviour decline. There are different types or causes of dementia, including Lewy body dementia, frontotemporal dementia, vascular dementia, limbic-predominant age-related TDP-43 encephalopathy, Parkinson's disease dementia, Huntington's disease, and others.

There is evidence that PTSD due to past trauma is associated with risk of dementia. Some researchers even argue that there may be a genetic risk (e.g. the ε4 allele of the apolipoprotein E (APOE) gene) for cognitive decline and dementia in people with PTSD (Averill et al., 2019). People with dementia and comorbid PTSD may show difficult behavioural symptoms, although the level of aggression does not necessarily increase (Kramer et al., 2022). In addition to a case study showing that a middle-aged woman developed frontotemporal dementia after recalling an experience of childhood sexual abuse (Cohen & Brody, 2015), a nationwide longitudinal study showed that the association between PTSD due to past trauma and dementia risk is relevant not only for certain populations, such as survivors of war, but also for the general population. It showed that PTSD is a risk factor for dementia in later life (hazard ratio (HR): 4.37). A dose effect was also shown in that the frequency of attending a psychiatric clinic for PTSD problems was correlated with the risk of dementia later in life (<5: HR: 2.81; >10: HR: 18.13). Psychiatric and medical comorbidities also appeared to play a role, as patients with depression and medical conditions (e.g. cerebrovascular disease, diabetes) were more prone to developing dementia (Wang et al., 2016).

A subsequent large cohort study of nearly 5,000 veterans also concluded that PTSD and major depressive disorder were associated with nearly twice the risk of developing dementia or cognitive impairment in veterans aged >56 years. While gender had only a small moderating effect on the results, race—especially black veterans with depression—increased the risk almost twofold. In other words, PTSD and major depressive disorder were important risk factors for dementia and cognitive impairment, especially for black veterans with depression (Bhattarai et al., 2019). It has even been argued that the increased incidence of dementia in veterans with PTSD poses a challenge to the provision of long-term care that meets the needs of these individuals (Sorrell & Durham, 2011). These findings were based on individuals aged >56 years and reflect research on traumatised older people. Older people with PTSD had a smaller right parahippocampal gyrus compared to healthy controls who had been exposed to trauma. As PTSD patients get older, their brain structure could change quite significantly, although more research is needed to verify this claim (Basavaraju et al., 2021).

The above study examining veterans with PTSD and depression suggests that the focus may not only be on the unique impact of PTSD on dementia. This link also needs to be considered in the context of comorbidities. For example, depression has been shown to be a risk factor for organic diseases such as dementia and Alzheimer's disease, and the mechanisms underpinning this relationship involve chronic or acute stressors including PTSD (Bica et al., 2017). Comorbidities could include some psychosocial factors, such as low socioeconomic status, marital status, work stress, and vital exhaustion. These factors and trauma-related stress characterised by PTSD have been associated with increased levels of dementia in later life, although the robustness of these findings has been questioned (Bougea et al., 2022).

As mentioned earlier, dementia is an umbrella term for the symptoms of cognitive impairment in people. Alzheimer's disease, on the other hand, is the most common form of dementia. Since there is evidence of a link between PTSD and dementia, it is not surprising that some researchers have investigated the link between PTSD and Alzheimer's disease. One review study claims that traumatic life events in the past may act as a risk factor for Alzheimer's disease in later life, either directly or indirectly (or mediated by) PTSD or PTSD correlates. Alzheimer's-related experiential trauma is also associated with cognitive decline, either directly or indirectly (mediated) by PTSD or PTSD correlates (Burnes & Burnette, 2013). Notwithstanding this, the studies of PET have not linked PTSD to the specific pathology of Alzheimer's disease or neurodegenerative diseases underlying other dementia syndromes. In other words, although PTSD may be associated with an increased risk of dementia according to some studies, there is little evidence that PTSD causes or increases the likelihood of Alzheimer's disease, which in turn causes the most common forms of dementia (Elias et al., 2021).

Summary

It has been suggested that patients with SAH may develop PTSD and anxiety. The course of PTSD symptoms appears to be stable over time, although some differences are observed at the individual level, with some patients experiencing chronic symptoms, others recovering, and still others developing delayed symptoms. In addition to SAH, studies have also been conducted to investigate the posttraumatic effects of stroke. In some patients, post-stroke PTSD may be stable over time. In terms of risk factors, alexithymia (especially difficulty identifying feelings), cognitive appraisals, and negative cognitions about oneself and the world are associated with post-stroke PTSD.

Trauma can alter brain structure and affect neurological function. Although a link between PTSD and epilepsy has been advocated, it is controversial when comparing patients with ES with those who had NES or PNES. In addition to the association between PTSD due to past trauma and epilepsy, studies have also been conducted examining PTSD due to the traumatic event of epilepsy (post-epileptic seizure PTSD). Self-efficacy may influence post-epileptic seizure PTSD and other psychological symptoms through alexithymia.

Research has also studied caregivers of children with epilepsy. They too may suffer from PTSD symptoms and comorbid psychiatric symptoms. Although both parents show different PTSD symptoms, mothers seem to report more PTSD symptoms and comorbid psychiatric symptoms than fathers. Among parents of children and adolescents with chronic physical illnesses, parental PTSD was found to be most prevalent in parents of children with epilepsy.

Apart from epilepsy, an association between PTSD due to past trauma and risk of dementia has also been found in war survivors and in the general population. Depression may also play a role in the development of dementia, raising the question of the unique contribution of PTSD to this condition. Early trauma may also be a risk factor for Alzheimer's disease later in life. Despite the above evidence supporting the link between PTSD and vascular and neurological diseases, the evidence is much weaker in comparison when considering the link between PTSD and other diseases such as cardiovascular disease, cancer and HIV/AIDS. In other words, we need more research to better understand the link between trauma and vascular and neurological diseases, for which risk factors also need to be further explored.

References

Abubakr, A., Kablinger, A., & Caldito, G. (2003). Psychogenic seizures: Clinical features and psychological analysis. *Epilepsy & Behavior, 4*(3), 241–245. https://doi.org/10.1016/S1525-5050(03)00082-9

American Psychiatric Association. (2000). *Diagnostic and statistical manual of mental disorders* (4th ed., text rev.).

American Psychiatric Association. (2013). *Diagnostic and statistical manual of mental disorders* (5th ed.). https://doi.org/10.1176/appi.books.9780890425596

Averill, L. A., Abdallah, C. G., Levey, D. F., Han, S., Harpaz-Rotem, I., Kranzler, H. R., Southwick, S. M., Krystal, J. H., Gelernter, J., & Pietrzak, R. H. (2019). Apolipoprotein E gene polymorphism, posttraumatic stress disorder, and cognitive function in older US veterans: Results from the National Health and Resilience in Veterans Study. *Depression and Anxiety, 36*(9), 834–845. https://doi.org/10.1002/da.22912

Basavaraju, R., France, J., Maas, B., Brickman, A. M., Flory, J. D., Szeszko, P. R., Yehuda, R., Neria, Y., Rutherford, B. R., & Provenzano, F. A. (2021). Right parahippocampal volume deficit in an older population with posttraumatic stress disorder. *Journal of Psychiatric Research, 137*, 368–375. https://doi.org/10.1016/j.jpsychires.2021.03.015

Berry, E. (1998). Post-traumatic stress disorder after subarachnoid haemorrhage. *British Journal of Clinical Psychology, 37*(3), 365–367. https://doi.org/https://doi.org/10.1111/j.2044-8260.1998.tb01392.x

Bhattarai, J. J., Oehlert, M. E., Multon, K. D., & Sumerall, S. W. (2019). Dementia and cognitive impairment among US Veterans with a history of MDD or PTSD: A retrospective cohort study based on sex and race. *Journal of Aging and Health, 31*(8), 1398–1422. https://doi.org/10.1177/0898264318781131

Bica, T., Castello, R., Toussaint, L. L., & Monteso-Curto, P. (2017). Depression as a risk factor of organic diseases: An international integrative review. *Journal of Nursing Scholarship, 49*(4), 389–399.

Bougea, A., Anagnostouli, M., Angelopoulou, E., Spanou, I., & Chrousos, G. (2022). Psychosocial and trauma-related stress and risk of dementia: A meta-analytic systematic review of longitudinal studies. *Journal of Geriatric Psychiatry and Neurology, 35*(1), 24–37. https://doi.org/10.1177/0891988720973759

Brandt, C., Schoendienst, M., Trentowska, M., May, T. W., Pohlmann-Eden, B., Tuschen-Caffier, B., Schrecke, M., Fueratsch, N., Witte-Boelt, K., & Ebner, A. (2010). Prevalence of anxiety disorders in patients with refractory focal epilepsy—A prospective clinic based survey. *Epilepsy & Behavior, 17*(2), 259–263. https://doi.org/10.1016/j.yebeh.2009.12.009

Burnes, D. P. R., & Burnette, D. (2013). Broadening the etiological discourse on Alzheimer's disease to include trauma and posttraumatic stress disorder as psychosocial risk factors. *Journal of Aging Studies, 27*(3), 218–224. https://doi.org/10.1016/j.jaging.2013.03.002

Carek, V., Norman, P., & Barton, J. (2010). Cognitive appraisals and posttraumatic stress disorder symptoms in informal caregivers of stroke survivors. *Rehabilitation Psychology, 55*(1), 91–96. https://doi.org/10.1037/a0018417

Carmassi, C., Corsi, M., Bertelloni, C. A., Carpita, B., Gesi, C., Pedrinelli, V., Massimetti, G., Peroni, D. G., Bonuccelli, A., Orsini, A., & Dell'Osso, L. (2018). Mothers and fathers of children with epilepsy: Gender differences in post-traumatic stress symptoms and correlations with mood spectrum symptoms. *Neuropsychiatric Disease and Treatment, 14.* https://doi.org/10.2147/NDT.S158249

Carmassi, C., Corsi, M., Bertelloni, C. A., Pedrinelli, V., Massimetti, G., Peroni, D., Bonuccelli, A., Orsini, A., & Dell'Osso, L. (2020). Post-traumatic stress spectrum symptoms in parents of children affected by epilepsy: Gender differences. *Seizure, 80,* 169–174. https://doi.org/10.1016/j.seizure.2020.06.021

Carmassi, C., Corsi, M., Bertelloni, C. A., Pedrinelli, V., Massimetti, G., Peroni, D. G., Bonuccelli, A., Orsini, A., & Dell'Osso, L. (2019). Post-traumatic stress and major depressive disorders in parent caregivers of children with a chronic disorder. *Psychiatry Research, 279,* 195–200. https://doi.org/10.1016/j.psychres.2019.02.062

Carmassi, C., Corsi, M., Gesi, C., Bertelloni, C. A., Faggioni, F., Calderani, E., Massimetti, G., Saggese, G., Bonuccelli, A., Orsini, A., & Dell'Osso, L. (2017). DSM-5 criteria for PTSD in parents of pediatric patients with epilepsy: What are the changes with respect to DSM-IV-TR? *Epilepsy & Behavior, 70*(Part A), 97–103. https://doi.org/10.1016/j.yebeh.2017.02.025

Chardavoyne, J., & Frechette, V. E. (2006). Occult PTSD with panic attacks in a patient post-TIA: Case report. *International Journal of Psychiatry in Medicine, 36*(4), 427–434. https://doi.org/10.2190/8672-8623-8460-7K45

Chung, M. C., & Allen, R. D. (2013). Alexithymia and posttraumatic stress disorder following epileptic seizure. *Psychiatric Quarterly, 84*(3), 271–285.

Chung, M. C., Allen, R. D., & Dennis, I. (2013). The impact of self-efficacy, alexithymia and multiple traumas on posttraumatic stress disorder and psychiatric co-morbidity following epileptic seizures: A moderated mediation analysis. *Psychiatry Research, 210*(3), 1033–1041. https://doi.org/10.1016/j.psychres.2013.07.041

Cohen, L. J., & Brody, D. (2015). Frontotemporal dementia-like syndrome following recall of childhood sexual abuse. *Journal of Traumatic Stress, 28*(3), 240–246. https://doi.org/10.1002/jts.22016

Cohen, M. L., Rozensky, R. H., Zlatar, Z. Z., Averbuch, R. N., & Cibula, J. E. (2010). Posttraumatic stress disorder caused by the misattribution of seizure-related experiential responses. *Epilepsy & Behavior, 19*(4), 652–655. https://doi.org/10.1016/j.yebeh.2010.09.029

Cornelius, T., Birk, J. L., Derby, L., Ellis, J., & Edmondson, D. (2021). Effect of cohabiting partners on the development of posttraumatic stress symptoms after emergency department visits for stroke and transient ischemic attack. *Social Science & Medicine, 281,* 114088. https://doi.org/10.1016/j.socscimed.2021.114088

Cyr, S., Guo, D. X., Marcil, M.-J., Dupont, P., Jobidon, L., Benrimoh, D., Guertin, M.-C., & Brouillette, J. (2021). Posttraumatic stress disorder prevalence in medical populations: A systematic review and meta-analysis. *General Hospital Psychiatry, 69,* 81–93. https://doi.org/10.1016/j.genhosppsych.2021.01.010

D'Alessio, L., Giagante, B., Oddo, S., Silva, W., Solis, P., Consalvo, D., & Kochen, S. (2006). Psychiatric disorders in patients with psychogenic non-epileptic seizures, with and without comorbid epilepsy. *Seizure, 15*(5), 333–339. https://doi.org/10.1016/j.seizure.2006.04.003

Dikel, T. N., Fennell, E. B., & Gilmore, R. L. (2003). Posttraumatic stress disorder, dissociation, and sexual abuse history in epileptic and nonepileptic seizure patients. *Epilepsy & Behavior, 4*(6), 644–650. https://doi.org/10.1016/j.yebeh.2003.08.006

Dunn, D. W., Austin, J. K., & Perkins, S. M. (2009). Prevalence of psychopathology in childhood epilepsy: Categorical and dimensional measures. *Developmental Medicine & Child Neurology, 51*(5), 364–372. https://doi.org/10.1111/j.1469-8749.2008.03172.x

Edmondson, D., Richardson, S., Fausett, J. K., Falzon, L., Howard, V. J., & Kronish, I. M. (2013). Prevalence of PTSD in survivors of stroke and transient ischemic attack: A meta-analytic review. *PLoS ONE, 8*(6), ArtID e66435.

Elias, A., Rowe, C., & Hopwood, M. (2021). Risk of dementia in posttraumatic stress disorder. *Journal of Geriatric Psychiatry and Neurology, 34*(6), 555–564. https://doi.org/10.1177/08919 88720957088

Field, E. L., Norman, P., & Barton, J. (2008). Cross-sectional and prospective associations between cognitive appraisals and posttraumatic stress disorder symptoms following stroke. *Behaviour Research and Therapy, 46*(1), 62–70.

Gagny, M., Grenevald, L., El-Hage, W., Chrusciel, J., Sanchez, S., Schwan, R., Klemina, I., Biberon, J., de Toffol, B., Thiriaux, A., Visseaux, J. F., Martin, M. L., Meyer, M., Maillard, L., & Hingray, C. (2021). Explanatory factors of quality of life in psychogenic non-epileptic seizure. *Seizure, 84*, 6–13. https://doi.org/10.1016/j.seizure.2020.10.028

García-Bueno, B., Caso, J. R., & Leza, J. C. (2008). Stress as a neuroinflammatory condition in brain: Damaging and protective mechanisms. *Neuroscience and Biobehavioral Reviews, 32*(6), 1136–1151. https://doi.org/10.1016/j.neubiorev.2008.04.001

Guillen, A., Curot, J., Birmes, P. J., Denuelle, M., Garès, V., Taib, S., Valton, L., & Yrondi, A. (2019). Suicidal ideation and traumatic exposure should not be neglected in epileptic patients: A multidimensional comparison of the psychiatric profile of patients suffering from epilepsy and patients suffering from psychogenic nonepileptic seizures. *Frontiers in Psychiatry, 10*. https://doi.org/10.3389/fpsyt.2019.00303

Ho, R., Ocol, J., Lu, C., Dolim, S., Yang, M., Carrazana, E., & Liow, K. K. (2019). Presentation of psychogenic nonepileptic seizures in Hawaii's ethnoracially diverse population. *Epilepsy & Behavior, 96*, 150–154. https://doi.org/10.1016/j.yebeh.2019.04.024

Huenges Wajer, I. M. C., Smits, A. R., Rinkel, G. J. E., van Zandvoort, M. J. E., Wijngaards-de Meij, L., & Visser-Meily, J. M. A. (2018). Exploratory study of the course of posttraumatic stress disorder after aneurysmal subarachnoid hemorrhage. *General Hospital Psychiatry, 53*, 114–118. https://doi.org/10.1016/j.genhosppsych.2018.03.004

Iseri, P. K., Ozten, E., & Aker, A. T. (2006). Posttraumatic stress disorder and major depressive disorder is common in parents of children with epilepsy. *Epilepsy & Behavior, 8*(1), 250–255. https://doi.org/10.1016/j.yebeh.2005.10.003

Jakobsen, A. V., Møller, R. S., Nikanorova, M., & Elklit, A. (2020). The impact of severe pediatric epilepsy on experienced stress and psychopathology in parents. *Epilepsy & Behavior, 113*. https://doi.org/10.1016/j.yebeh.2020.107538

Jiang, C. (2020). Posttraumatic stress disorder after a first-ever intracerebral hemorrhage in the Chinese population: A pilot study. *Applied Neuropsychology: Adult, 27*(1), 1–8. https://doi.org/10.1080/23279095.2018.1451334

Kendall-Tackett, K. (Ed.) (2010). *The psychoneuroimmunology of chronic disease: Exploring the links between inflammation, stress, and illness.* American Psychological Association. https://doi.org/10.1037/12065-000

Kessler, R. C., Lane, M. C., Shahly, V., & Stang, P. E. (2012). Accounting for comorbidity in assessing the burden of epilepsy among US adults: Results from the National Comorbidity Survey Replication (NCS-R). *Molecular Psychiatry, 17*(7), 748–759. https://doi.org/10.1038/mp.2011.56

Koby, D. G., Zirakzadeh, A., Staab, J. P., Seime, R., Cha, S. S., Nelson, C. L., Sengem, S., Berge, R., Marshall, E. A., Varner, J. E., Vickers, K. S., Trenerry, M. R., & Worrell, G. A. (2010). Questioning the role of abuse in behavioral spells and epilepsy. *Epilepsy & Behavior, 19*(4), 584–590. https://doi.org/10.1016/j.yebeh.2010.09.014

Kramer, A., Kovach, S., & Wilkins, S. (2022). An integrative review of behavioral disturbances in veterans with dementia and PTSD. *Journal of Geriatric Psychiatry and Neurology, 35*(3), 262–270. https://doi.org/10.1177/0891988721993572

Kronenberg, G., Schoner, J., Nolte, C., Heinz, A., Endres, M., & Gertz, K. (2017). Charting the perfect storm: Emerging biological interfaces between stress and stroke. *European Archives of Psychiatry and Clinical Neuroscience, 267*(6), 487–494.

Kühn, S., & Gallinat, J. (2013). Gray matter correlates of posttraumatic stress disorder: A quantitative meta-analysis. *Biological Psychiatry, 73*(1), 70–74. https://doi.org/10.1016/j.biopsych.2012.06.029

Kutlubaev, M. A., Barugh, A. J., & Mead, G. E. (2012). Fatigue after subarachnoid haemorrhage: A systematic review. *Journal of Psychosomatic Research, 72*(4), 305–310. https://doi.org/10.1016/j.jpsychores.2011.12.008

Labudda, K., Frauenheim, M., Illies, D., Miller, I., Schrecke, M., Vietmeier, N., Brandt, C., & Bien, C. G. (2018). Psychiatric disorders and trauma history in patients with pure PNES and patients with PNES and coexisting epilepsy. *Epilepsy & Behavior, 88*, 41–48. https://doi.org/10.1016/j.yebeh.2018.08.027

Labudda, K., Illies, D., Bien, C. G., & Neuner, F. (2018). Postepileptic seizure PTSD: A very rare psychiatric condition in patients with epilepsy. *Epilepsy & Behavior, 78*, 219–225. https://doi.org/10.1016/j.yebeh.2017.08.043

Liu, C., Yi, X., Li, T., Xu, L., Hu, M., Zhang, S., & Jiang, R. (2019). Associations of depression, anxiety and PTSD with neurological disability and cognitive impairment in survivors of Moyamoya disease. *Psychology, Health & Medicine, 24*(1), 43–50. https://doi.org/10.1080/13548506.2018.1467024

Martin, R. C., Faught, E., Richman, J., Funkhouser, E., Kim, Y., Clements, K., & Pisu, M. (2014). Psychiatric and neurologic risk factors for incident cases of new-onset epilepsy in older adults: Data from U S Medicare beneficiaries. *Epilepsia, 55*(7), 1120–1127. https://doi.org/10.1111/epi.12649

McKenna, P., & Neil-Dwyer, G. (1993). Helping patients recover from subarachnoid haemorrhage. *Journal of Mental Health, 2*(4), 315–320. https://doi.org/10.3109/09638239309016966

Meyers, E. E., McCurley, J., Lester, E., Jacobo, M., Rosand, J., & Vranceanu, A.-M. (2020). Building resiliency in dyads of patients admitted to the neuroscience intensive care unit and their family caregivers: Lessons learned from William and Laura. *Cognitive and Behavioral Practice.* https://doi.org/10.1016/j.cbpra.2020.02.001

Myers, L., Trobliger, R., & Goszulak, S. (2021). Firefighter with co-morbid psychogenic non-epileptic seizures and post-traumatic stress disorder treated with prolonged exposure therapy: Long-term follow-up. *Clinical Case Studies, 20*(2), 95–114. https://doi.org/10.1177/1534650120963181

Noble, A. J., & Schenk, T. (2014). Psychological distress after subarachnoid hemorrhage: Patient support groups can help us better detect it. *Journal of the Neurological Sciences, 343*(1–2), 125–131. https://doi.org/10.1016/j.jns.2014.05.053

Norup, D. A., & Elklit, A. (2013). Post-traumatic stress disorder in partners of people with epilepsy. *Epilepsy & Behavior, 27*(1), 225–232. https://doi.org/10.1016/j.yebeh.2012.11.039

O'Carrol, R. E., Masterton, G., Gooday, R., Cossar, J. A., Couston, M. C., & Hayes, P. C. (1999). Variceal haemorrhage and post-traumatic stress disorder. *British Journal of Clinical Psychology, 38*(2), 203–208. https://doi.org/10.1348/014466599162755

Papavasiliou, A., Vassilaki, N., Paraskevoulakos, E., Kotsalis, C., Bazigou, H., & Bardani, I. (2004). Psychogenic status epilepticus in children. *Epilepsy & Behavior, 5*(4), 539–546. https://doi.org/10.1016/j.yebeh.2004.04.011

Partlow, B. H., & Birkley, E. L. (2022). Cognitive processing therapy for concurrent posttraumatic stress disorder (PTSD) and psychogenic nonepileptic seizures (PNES): A case study. *Cognitive and Behavioral Practice, 30*(2), 299–310. https://doi.org/10.1016/j.cbpra.2021.12.003

Pinquart, M. (2019). Posttraumatic stress symptoms and disorders in parents of children and adolescents with chronic physical illnesses: A meta-analysis. *Journal of Traumatic Stress,* *32*(1), 88–96. https://doi.org/10.1002/jts.22354

Sala, M., Perez, J., Soloff, P., di Nemi, S. U., Caverzasi, E., Soares, J. C., & Brambilla, P. (2004). Stress and hippocampal abnormalities in psychiatric disorders. *European Neuropsychopharmacology,* *14*(5), 393–405. https://doi.org/10.1016/j.eurone uro.2003.12.005

Salinsky, M., Evrard, C., Storzbach, D., & Pugh, M. J. (2012). Psychiatric comorbidity in veterans with psychogenic seizures. *Epilepsy & Behavior,* *25*(3), 345–349. https://doi.org/10.1016/j.yebeh.2012.07.013

Salinsky, M., Rutecki, P., Parko, K., Goy, E., Storzbach, D., Markwardt, S., Binder, L., & Joos, S. (2019). Health-related quality of life in Veterans with epileptic and psychogenic nonepileptic seizures. *Epilepsy & Behavior, 94*, 72–77. https://doi.org/10.1016/j.yebeh.2019.02.010

Say, G. N., Tasdemir, H. A., Akbas, S., Yüce, M., & Karabekiroglu, K. (2014). Self-esteem and psychiatric features of Turkish adolescents with psychogenic non-epileptic seizures: A comparative study with epilepsy and healthy control groups. *International Journal of Psychiatry in Medicine, 47*(1), 41–53. https://doi.org/10.2190/PM.47.1.d

Scévola, L., Teitelbaum, J., Oddo, S., Centurión, E., Loidl, C. F., Kochen, S., & D'Alessio, L. (2013). Psychiatric disorders in patients with psychogenic nonepileptic seizures and drug-resistant epilepsy: A study of an Argentine population. *Epilepsy & Behavior, 29*(1), 155–160. https://doi.org/10.1016/j.yebeh.2013.07.012

Soncin, L.-D., McGonigal, A., Kotwas, I., Belquaid, S., Giusiano, B., Faure, S., & Bartolomei, F. (2021). Post-traumatic stress disorder (PTSD) in patients with epilepsy. *Epilepsy & Behavior, 121*(Part A). https://doi.org/10.1016/j.yebeh.2021.108083

Sorrell, J. M., & Durham, S. (2011). Meeting the mental health needs of the aging veteran population: A challenge for the 21st century. *Journal of Psychosocial Nursing and Mental Health Services, 49*(1), 22–25. https://doi.org/10.3928/02793695-20101207-01

Taylor, J., Jonsson, G., Paruk, L., & Philippides, A. (2020). A South African review of routinely-collected health data of psychogenic nonepileptic seizure patients referred to psychiatrists in Johannesburg. *Epilepsy & Behavior, 114*, 107578. https://doi.org/10.1016/j.yebeh.2020.107578

Vilyte, G., & Pretorius, C. (2019). Personality traits, illness behaviors, and psychiatric comorbidity in individuals with psychogenic nonepileptic seizures (PNES), epilepsy, and other nonepileptic seizures (oNES): Differentiating between the conditions. *Epilepsy & Behavior, 98*(Part A), 210–219. https://doi.org/10.1016/j.yebeh.2019.05.043

Wang, T.-Y., Wei, H.-T., Liou, Y.-J., Su, T.-P., Bai, Y.-M., Tsai, S.-J., Yang, A. C., Chen, T.-J., Tsai, C.-F., & Chen, M.-H. (2016). Risk for developing dementia among patients with post-traumatic stress disorder: A nationwide longitudinal study. *Journal of Affective Disorders, 205*, 306–310. https://doi.org/10.1016/j.jad.2016.08.013

Wang, X., Chung, M. C., Hyland, M. E., & Bahkeit, M. (2011). Posttraumatic stress disorder and psychiatric co-morbidity following stroke: The role of alexithymia. *Psychiatry Research, 188*(1), 51–57. https://doi.org/http://dx.doi.org/10.1016/j.psychres.2010.10.002

Zeber, J. E., Copeland, L. A., Amuan, M., Cramer, J. A., & Pugh, M. J. V. (2007). The role of co-morbid psychiatric conditions in health status in epilepsy. *Epilepsy & Behavior, 10*(4), 539–546. https://doi.org/10.1016/j.yebeh.2007.02.008

Zijlmans, M., van Campen, J. S., & de Weerd, A. (2017). Post traumatic stress-sensitive epilepsy. *Seizure, 52*, 20–21. https://doi.org/10.1016/j.seizure.2017.09.010

8

Posttraumatic stress disorder and respiratory illnesses

Trauma exposure can lead to the onset of respiratory problems. At discharge of patients suffering from acute respiratory distress syndrome (ARDS), one study found that 43% met criteria for posttraumatic stress disorder (PTSD) and <1% for partial PTSD. These symptoms appeared to persist over time, with the median follow-up time being 8 years. Those with PTSD also reported somatic and anxiety symptoms, as well as impairments in health-related quality of life. Somewhat unexpectedly, there were no significant differences between the groups with PTSD, partial PTSD and no PTSD in terms of social support and cognitive impairment (Kapfhammer et al., 2004).

Similarly, in patients suffering from acute lung injury with ARDS, a systematic review suggested that between 21% and 35% of patients met clinically significant criteria for PTSD. In addition, depression was found to range from 17% to 43% and non-specific anxiety from 23% to 48%. These distresses were associated with poor quality of life. The prevalence rates for PTSD at the time of hospital discharge, and 5 and 8 years later were 44%, 25%, and 24%, respectively. Risk factors for PTSD and depression after acute lung injury/ARDS included intensive care unit (ICU) stay, sedation, and long duration of mechanical ventilation (Davydow et al., 2008). A small study also showed that PTSD symptoms occurred in patients who had to be ventilated after acute respiratory distress. The PTSD symptoms were related to the traumatic medical experiences. Patients with PTSD symptoms tended to use emotional words to describe their experiences. To cope with distress, denial can be useful as a coping strategy in the short term (Shaw et al., 2001).

PTSD and asthma

After the World Trade Center disaster, many victims reported lower and upper respiratory symptoms, largely due to breathing in the intense dust cloud from

Posttraumatic Stress in Physical Illness. Man Cheung Chung, Oxford University Press. © Oxford University Press 2024.
DOI: 10.1093/oso/9780198727323.003.0008

the collapse of the buildings (Mauer et al., 2007). As a result, they had significant physical health problems, including asthma. Exposure to this disaster increased the likelihood of moderate-to-severe asthma symptoms threefold and of seeking medical treatment and physician consultation (Fagan et al., 2003). One study showed that 10% of people who had no history of asthma before the disaster were diagnosed with asthma after exposure to the disaster. Professional and volunteer rescue and recovery workers also reported asthma and lower respiratory symptoms. Working long hours at the disaster site, acute and prolonged exposure to the disaster, and breathing in a heavy layer of dust at home or in the office were considered risk factors (Brackbill et al., 2009; Debchoudhury et al., 2011).

World Trade Center disaster victims with probable PTSD were one and a half times more likely to have asthma after the disaster than those without probable PTSD (Shiratori & Samuelson, 2012). In other words, the severity of asthma could also be influenced by whether or not they developed PTSD as a result of the disaster. PTSD could play the role of a mediator that mediates the impact of trauma characteristics on asthma severity. This is not surprising as PTSD is known to be associated with respiratory dysfunction (Blechert et al., 2007; Spitzer et al., 2011) and specific changes in the inflammatory response (O'Toole & Catts, 2008) and can coexist with respiratory conditions that affect the lives of many (Waszczuk et al., 2017), including asthma (Hayatbakhsh et al., 2010; Weiser, 2007). Community adults suffering from PTSD may be two-and-a-half to three times more likely to develop asthma, along with other problems such as bronchitis, liver disease, and peripheral artery disease (Spitzer et al., 2009). However, it was claimed that PTSD was associated with a lower likelihood of asthma compared to conditions such as myocardial infarction and emphysema (odds ratio (OR): 4.06) (Tsai & Shen, 2017).

However, it does not necessarily have to be trauma that has a clear direct cause, such as the World Trade Center disaster. One study examined the relationship between PTSD and asthma in survivors of Hurricane Katrina. Results showed that a 1-point increase in avoidance score was associated with twice the odds of experiencing an asthma attack or episode since the hurricane (Arcaya et al., 2014). A nationwide longitudinal study over 10 years was conducted to investigate the association between PTSD due to various traumatic events and asthma. It was found that patients with PTSD had an increased risk of asthma during the follow-up period of the study (hazard ratio (HR): 2.27), especially in the youngest age group (HR: 4.01). The study further supported the idea that the risk of developing asthma was consistently higher in patients with PTSD than in controls, although further research is needed to investigate the underlying mechanisms (Hung et al., 2019). It has been argued that there is a need to understand the neurobiology, mechanisms, and inflammatory mediators that may contribute to the association between asthma and PTSD (Allgire et al., 2021).

One study showed that 74% of children with severe asthma had experienced a traumatic event in the past, of which a quarter met diagnostic criteria for PTSD (Vanderbilt et al., 2008). Among adolescents in an inpatient behavioural health facility, asthma (32%) was the most common medical co-morbidity, while PTSD (63%) was the most common psychiatric comorbidity (Krass et al., 2020). Another study also showed that 20% of adolescents with life-threatening asthma met the criteria for PTSD due to past trauma. This was compared to 11% and 8% of the asthma and normal control groups, respectively. PTSD symptoms were positively associated with asthma severity (Kean et al., 2006). Parents of adolescents with life-threatening asthma may also be affected by the effects of PTSD in these adolescents; 29% of parents met criteria for PTSD compared with 14% and 2% of parents of asthma and normal controls, respectively (Kean et al., 2006). Parents who had experienced trauma in the past were more prone to be traumatised by the onset of their children's asthma and treatment than parents without previous trauma (Wamboldt et al., 1995).

These studies show that treating asthma is not just about giving patients medication. It should also include attempts to reduce the severity of PTSD symptoms. Treating PTSD symptoms could have an impact on the severity of respiratory symptoms. One study has shown that lower respiratory symptoms (LRS) can be reduced by treating PTSD symptoms using group-based weekly comprehensive trauma management and smoking cessation treatment in smokers exposed to the World Trade Center disaster. A 0.50 standard deviation reduction in LRS symptoms was achieved. The reduction in PTSD symptoms was correlated with the improvement in LRS. In other words, the PTSD symptoms maintained the chronicity of LRS and the treatment of the PTSD was able to alleviate LRS symptoms (Waszczuk et al., 2017).

Notwithstanding, it is also important not to focus only on the PTSD symptom. Compared to non-asthmatics, asthma patients were at least one-and-a-half times more likely to suffer from psychological disorders other than PTSD, such as depression, anxiety, and alcohol abuse (Scott et al., 2007). Increased anxiety and depressive symptoms have been associated with medical conditions such as asthma and other conditions such as cardiovascular disease, back problems, ulcers, migraines, and vision problems (Niles et al., 2015). All of these psychological symptoms, along with PTSD, can in turn interfere with asthma management. An approach to address a broader range of psychological disorders is needed, which in turn should impact asthma disease control (Weiser, 2007).

An interesting observation from the above studies is that most, if not all, do not address PTSD due to the traumatic impact of asthma. Do people develop post-asthma attack PTSD? This is a valid question because an asthma attack or exacerbation is a potentially life-threatening condition. After contact with allergens, the airways become sensitive, causing the muscles around the airways to tighten (i.e. bronchospasm). The lining of the airways swells or becomes inflamed, producing an abnormal amount of mucus, resulting in mucus plugs. As a result of the bronchospasm, inflammation, and mucus plugging, the airways narrow, making it difficult for air to enter or leave the lungs. This leads to symptoms such as shortness of breath, difficulty breathing and respiratory failure, which can lead to chest tightness, wheezing, chronic cough, itchy throat, difficulty speaking or even death. The increase in severity of symptoms is usually accompanied by increased wheezing and pulse rate, decreased peak expiratory rate, fatigue, chest pain, anxiety, drowsiness, and confusion.

Post-asthma attack PTSD with a low prevalence rate was found among university students. Only 3% met criteria for full PTSD, although 44% and 53% met criteria for partial and no PTSD, respectively. The severity of asthma was associated with PTSD symptoms and psychiatric comorbid symptoms (Chung et al., 2012). Another study showed that after an asthma attack, 2%, 42%, and 56% met diagnostic criteria for full PTSD, partial PTSD, or no PTSD, respectively. The asthma group reported significantly more somatic problems, social dysfunction, and depression than the control group and had five times the risk of developing a general psychiatric disorder (Chung & Wall, 2013). However, another study found a much higher percentage of PTSD following an asthma attack, with 20% as the prevalence rate for full PTSD; PTSD, asthma severity, and psychiatric comorbidity were highly correlated (Wagner et al., 2017).

In terms of risk factors, one study examined the role of alexithymia, which is characterised by difficulty identifying feelings and distinguishing between feelings and bodily sensations, difficulty describing and expressing feelings to others, and a tendency to focus on external events rather than internal experiences (Taylor & Bagby, 2012). Alexithymia essentially helps individuals prevent access to internal feelings and provides a way to avoid emotional distress (Declercq et al., 2010; Kupchik et al., 2007). One would therefore assume that alexithymia is related to PTSD symptoms, of which avoidance is one. Unexpectedly, alexithymia did not predict PTSD after controlling for age, marital status, asthma experience, and symptoms. However, difficulty identifying feelings predicted psychiatric comorbidity. Asthma symptoms partially mediated the association between difficulty identifying feelings and psychiatric comorbidity. In other words, people who have difficulty identifying feelings may have increased asthma symptoms, which affect psychiatric comorbidity (Chung & Wall, 2013).

Surprisingly, coping strategies did not appear to be related to distress outcomes, contradicting literature suggesting that emotion-focused coping is associated with poor well-being in asthma patients (González-Freire et al., 2010; Hesselink et al., 2004). This also contradicted the literature indicating an association between maladaptive coping (emotion-focused and avoidance-focused) and psychiatric comorbid symptoms in people who have experienced life-threatening illnesses (Alonzo & Reynolds, 1998; Chung et al., 2008; Hampton & Frombach, 2000). Similarly, locus of control beliefs were not associated with distress outcomes in asthma patients. Self-efficacy, on the other hand, was highly associated with all distress outcomes and was a significant mediator between asthma and both post-asthma attack PTSD and psychiatric comorbidity. In other words, for these asthma patients, the belief that they were in control of their own destiny did not seem to have a major impact on their distress. Rather, the belief in their ability to cope with the challenges in their lives contributes to reducing the severity of distress (Wagner et al., 2017).

PTSD and severe acute respiratory syndrome

The foregoing sections have provided us with examples of how PTSD might be related to respiratory diseases. In addition to these diseases, coronaviruses are a family of viruses that infect humans and animals, of which there are several types. These include the viruses responsible for severe acute respiratory syndrome (SARS), Middle Eastern respiratory syndrome, and Covid-19 epidemics. Among patients suffering from these diseases, the most common disorders were undifferentiated psychiatric morbidity (20–56%), PTSD (10–26%), and depression (9–27%). Infected or recovering adults (18–56%) reported the highest prevalence of each disorder, followed by medical personnel (11–28%) and adults in the community (11–20%). The impact that a coronavirus pandemic could have on various psychological disorders, including PTSD, in different populations cannot be overestimated (Boden et al., 2021; Kaseda & Levine, 2020).

Rather than focusing on all the different types of coronavirus-related illness, much of this chapter will focus on SARS and Covid-19, with an emphasis on the latter. Before we begin this review, it should be mentioned that the studies cited below have not always explicitly addressed the cause of PTSD. While some studies measured PTSD due to various traumatic aspects of SARS or Covid-19, others included trauma unrelated to SARS or Covid-19. For example, some researchers may be interested in investigating whether PTSD due to a previous trauma could be a triggering factor for the severity of Covid-19 and psychiatric comorbidities.

Following the outbreak of SARS, patients were found to have PTSD, with prevalence rates ranging from 9.4% to 55% (Fang et al., 2004; Hong et al., 2009; Kwek et al., 2006; Maunder, 2009; Sim et al., 2004; Wu et al., 2005; Xu et al., 2005). Their PTSD symptoms were significantly more severe than those of non-patients living in areas where the disease was prevalent (Xu et al., 2005). Among these uninfected residents, the prevalence rates for posttraumatic and psychiatric comorbidities were about 26% and 23%, respectively (Sim et al., 2010; Xu et al., 2005). Those with PTSD had more anxiety, depression, and global psychological and social dysfunction than those without PTSD (Hong et al., 2009). These distress symptoms persisted over a period of 3–46 months (Hong et al., 2009; Kwek et al., 2006; Lee et al., 2007; Maunder, 2009). In the acute and early recovery phase, people reported symptoms of psychosis, fear of survival, and fear of infecting others. In addition to these psychological reactions, they also had to endure the negative effects of stigma and reduced quality of life (Gardner & Moallef, 2015).

SARS has also produced secondary victims, namely health care workers and hospital staff working with SARS patients (Gardner & Moallef, 2015), through whom they could potentially become infected. However, both hospital staff and health care workers (SARS) were more concerned about infecting others (e.g. especially family members), although fear tended to be greater among healthcare workers. Hospital staff were also concerned about additional health problems and discrimination (Ho et al., 2005). They frequently reported posttraumatic stress symptoms (PTSS) and general psychiatric disorders. The estimated prevalence of PTSS in the acute phase was 23.4% and 11.9% at ≥12 months. For general psychiatric disorders, the estimated prevalence in the acute phase was 34.1%, followed by 17.9% at 6–12 months and 29.3% at ≥12 months. There appears to be a high prevalence of psychological disorders among health care workers, especially immediately after the outbreak of the pandemic (Allan et al., 2020).

When the outbreak began, high-risk health care workers did not differ from low-risk health care workers in terms of their stress levels. However, the former were more likely to report fatigue, difficulty sleeping, health-related anxiety, and fear of social contact, even though they were confident they had the infection under control. Towards the end of the outbreak, the stress levels of the high-risk group increased significantly more than those of the low-risk health care workers. Their stress levels were associated with increased levels of depression, anxiety, and SARS-related PTSD. In other words, SARS survivors who were health care workers suffered high levels of chronic psychological distress related to the infectious disease (Lee et al., 2007; McAlonan et al., 2007). However, these findings are not without controversy. One study showed that health care workers who worked in high-risk departments that treated and had close contact with SARS patients reported less distress than those who worked in low-risk areas (Styra et al., 2008). In addition, one would assume that cumulative exposure to patient care would be associated with increased distress (a dose effect). However, this assumption has been challenged as health care workers who cared for only one SARS patient showed more PTSD symptoms than those who cared for multiple patients (Styra et al., 2008).

Nevertheless, most of the above evidence suggests that the long-term impact of SARS on frontline health care workers should not be underestimated. One study looked at people infected with SARS who survived 1, 4, and 7 years after the outbreak. The results showed that clinically significant levels of PTSD, depression and anxiety among these workers did not decrease over the past 7 years. Rather, they reported persistent problems with pain, decreased vitality, and impaired physical, psychological, and social functioning (Moallef et al., 2021). These long-term effects of SARS were not only present in infected health workers. They also affected the uninfected health workers who cared for SARS patients. They continued to suffer significant psychological distress, if not psychological disorders, for 1–2 years after the outbreak (Maunder, 2009). Given the psychological distress that health workers might experience, it is not surprising that stress management has been recommended as part of preparing health workers for future outbreaks (McAlonan et al., 2007).

Risk factors

Several risk factors have been identified for predicting distress in SARS survivors. Starting with background variables, women and patients with low levels of education were more likely to report PTSD symptoms, especially avoidance behaviours. Younger age, being married and being in fever units were associated with PTSD and psychiatric comorbid symptoms, although direct contact with SARS patients or working in fever units was not always related to the occurrence of distress. Patients who personally knew someone who had contracted or died from SARS were more likely to be affected by depression. Patients' self-perception also seemed to be related to distress. For example, when patients perceived themselves to be at high risk of SARS or to be in life-threatening situations, they tended to have increased PTSD symptoms and psychiatric comorbidity (Fang et al., 2004; Sim et al., 2010; Sim et al., 2004; Styra et al., 2008; Wu et al., 2005; Xu et al., 2005). In addition, hospital staff who worked in high-risk locations (e.g. SARS wards) and had been quarantined or had friends or relatives infected with SARS were two to three times more likely to have higher severity of PTSS symptoms than those who had other experiences (Wu et al., 2009). In other words, the impact of working in a high-risk environment on distress symptoms may be exacerbated by one's own experience of quarantine or concern for the safety of loved ones.

Coping strategies such as denial, self-distraction, behavioural disengagement, religion, low levels of venting, use of humour, acceptance, and emotional support have been associated with PTSD and psychiatric comorbidity (Sim et al., 2004). When patients blame themselves for what happened to them, they tend to have increased psychiatric morbidity (Sim et al., 2010). In terms of personality traits, low self-efficacy tended to be associated with greater fear about SARS, which was positively correlated with PTSD symptoms. Some personality factors were protective in that high self-esteem could buffer distress for SARS patients. Altruism was seen as helpful in protecting medical staff. On the other hand, their depressive affect and feeling that SARS was affecting their work life and that they had to work in a high-risk unit were associated with distress (Ho et al., 2005; Sim et al., 2010; Sim et al., 2004; Styra et al., 2008; Wu et al., 2005; Wu et al., 2009; Xu et al., 2005).

PTSD and COVID-19

Covid-19 is a disease caused by a highly contagious coronavirus (severe acute respiratory syndrome coronavirus 2, SARS-CoV-2). It was first detected in Wuhan, China, in December 2019 and declared a pandemic in March 2020 (World Health Organization, 2019). This pandemic has affected the whole world and has led to increased unemployment, social isolation, psychosocial burden, existential threats, health fears, uncertainty, uncontrollability, and psychological distress (Estes & Thompson, 2020; Kesner & Horacek, 2020; Mucci et al., 2020; Rajkumar, 2020; Shakespeare-Finch et al., 2020; Wytrychiewicz et al., 2020).

In terms of psychological distress, there was evidence of mild (5.67%) and moderate (0.67%) anxiety and mild (14.33%), moderate (2.5%), and severe

(0.33%) depression in Chinese individuals (Wang et al., 2020). Another study also found higher overall scores for anxiety (mild: 10.1%; moderate: 6.0%; severe: 12.9%) and depression (mild: 10.2%; moderate: 17.8%; severe: 9.1%). In addition, 29.1%, 9.5%, and 1.6% reported an increase in hazardous drinking, harmful drinking, and alcohol dependence, respectively; 32.1% reported having low psychological well-being (Ahmed et al., 2020). More than 70% of Chinese citizens in different parts of China were found to have moderate and high levels of compulsive behaviour, interpersonal sensitivity, phobic anxiety, and psychoticism (Tian et al., 2020).

During the Covid-19 pandemic, Italy was found to have mild (19.4%) and moderate-to-severe (18.6%) levels of global psychological distress (Moccia et al., 2020). In Poland, 75% of adults recruited from the general public considered Covid-19, a highly stressful event, the strongest predictor of adjustment disorder; 49% who reported symptoms of adjustment disorder tended to be women and those without full-time employment. These adults also suffered from generalised anxiety (44%) and depression (26%). After adjusting for co-occurring symptoms, 14% were found to meet the diagnostic criteria for adjustment disorder (Dragan et al., 2021). Other psychiatric disorders include suicidal thoughts or attempts (Dutheil et al., 2020; Mucci et al., 2020) or substance abuse (Banducci & Weiss, 2020; Shakespeare-Finch et al., 2020).

PTSD in the general public

Apart from the psychiatric disorders mentioned above, Covid-19 is also associated with an increased risk of posttraumatic stress disorder (Covid-19 PTSD) (Boyraz & Legros, 2020; Coleman, 2020; Gallagher et al., 2021), which has been the subject of a large number of studies in different parts of the world since its onset. Although Covid-19 is a life-threatening disease, the question of whether Covid-19 should be considered a traumatic stressor remains controversial. The idea of a pandemic does not necessarily fit the existing diagnostic criteria for PTSD. To substantiate Covid-19 as a traumatic stressor, some researchers studied more than 1000 participants from five Western countries to determine whether Covid-19 would be a traumatic stressor leading to PTSD symptoms. The results showed that the participants had PTSD-like symptoms during events that had not occurred. These PTSD-like symptoms also occurred when participants had been exposed to Covid-19 directly (e.g. through contact with the virus) or indirectly (e.g. through the media). In addition, 13.2% likely met a probable PTSD diagnosis, although lockdown, a type of exposure characteristic of Covid-19, does not fit the DSM-5 (American Psychiatric Association, 2013) criteria. Participants reported that the emotional impact of the 'worst' expected events was most strongly associated with PTSD-like symptoms. These findings suggest that Covid-19 may potentially be a traumatic stressor that can trigger PTSD-like reactions and exacerbate psychiatric comorbid symptoms such as anxiety, depression, and psychosocial functioning (Bridgland et al., 2021).

Among adults living in Wuhan and surrounding cities in China, the prevalence rate of Covid-19 PTSD was 7% (Liu et al., 2020). One month after the outbreak, 4.6% met criteria for PTSD in another study of >2000 Chinese respondents, although the prevalence rate was higher (18.4%) among those with a suspected or confirmed Covid-19 diagnosis or those who had close contact with someone who had Covid-19 (Sun et al., 2020). However, the impact of PTSD can be far-reaching. For example, the network analysis revealed that the PTSD networks of students from Hubei Province and other provinces were similarly connected and shared some symptoms such as flashbacks, irritability and anger, although there were differences across networks. In the Hubei network, distorted cognition and no positive emotions had high network centrality, while in the non-Hubei network, physiological reactions and an exaggerated startle response had high centrality (Sun et al., 2021).

In another study, 36.6% Covid-19 exhibited PTSD symptoms, with avoidance being the most common symptom (Rodriguez-Rey et al., 2020; Taylor et al., 2020). In addition to avoidance behaviour, fear, anger, and hopelessness were also prevalent. Interestingly, fear was more about fear of the negative impact of Covid-19 on household income, and reduced access to health care and food supply, rather than threats to life (Trnka & Lorencova, 2020). Clearly, this fear was specifically related to the consequences of Covid-19 on one's life. However, there are people who tend to fear diseases and viruses in general. In one study, it was found that people from a non-clinical sample exposed to Covid-19 who had higher levels of such fears were more likely to have depression and PTSD symptoms at baseline. These higher levels of fears at baseline in turn predicted higher levels of Covid-19 PTSD one week later (Cottin et al., 2021).

A longitudinal study examined the impact 2 weeks after confinement began, 1 and 2 months after removal of lockdown, showing a downward trend in PTSD in the general population. There was a significant difference between the first and third assessments. Depressive symptoms increased significantly throughout the confinement; although symptoms decreased at the last assessment, they did not decrease to pre-crisis levels. For anxiety, there were no significant changes between the three assessments, although there was a downward trend over time (González-Sanguino et al., 2021).

Poor sleep quality is also related to Covid-19 PTSD (Geng et al., 2021; Sun et al., 2020). Sleep quality differed significantly between those with and without PTSD symptoms and between those with different frequencies of contact. Those with PTSD had poorer sleep quality overall. They also found that sleep quality mediated the effect of exposure level on PTSD (Yin et al., 2020). This is consistent with previous research suggesting that the impact of PTSD on patients' respiratory symptoms or lung function can be exacerbated by poor sleep and insomnia (Waszczuk et al., 2019). Other psychosomatic reactions besides sleep include fatigue and headaches, which have been associated with Covid-19 PTSD (Wytrychiewicz et al., 2020).

Covid-19 affects not only adults but also young people. A systematic review and meta-analysis was conducted to examine children and adolescents during the Covid-19 pandemic. It showed that the pooled prevalence of depression, anxiety, sleep disorders, and PTSD were 29%, 26%, 44%, and 48% respectively. Adolescents and women reported a higher prevalence of depression and anxiety than children and men, respectively (Ma et al., 2021).

In Covid-19, 14.4% of young people from China reported PTSD symptoms, and nearly 40.4% reported psychiatric comorbidity (Liang et al., 2020b). These traumatic effects can last a long period of time, partly due to unresolved traumatic distress in schools and families (Zhou, 2020). One study examined the mental health of some Chinese adolescents before school lockdown and after school resumption. They found that 10.4% met criteria for probable PTSD due to Covid-19. Perceived threat was positively correlated with PTSD symptoms, while positive youth development (PYD) qualities were negatively correlated with these symptoms at baseline. There was also a moderating effect in that the negative impact of perceived threat on PTSD symptoms depended on the level of PYD qualities. These findings seem to suggest that PYD may protect adolescents from the negative impact of Covid-19 on adolescent mental health (Shek et al., 2021).

Compared to healthy controls, adolescents with major depressive disorder (MDD) had higher levels of PTSD symptoms. Male and female adolescents with MDD did not differ significantly in total PTSD symptoms or subscales. However, junior high school students had higher avoidance rates than senior high school students. The totality of PTSD symptoms was associated with MDD. 'Flashbacks' or avoidance of traumatic memories were prominent among Covid-19 PTSD symptoms (Hang Zhang et al., 2021). Adolescents were more likely than adults to report moderate-to-severe depression (55%

vs 29%), anxiety (48% vs 29%), PTSD (45% vs 33%), suicidal thoughts or behaviours (38% vs 16%), and sleep disturbances (69% vs 57%). Fifty-five per cent of the adolescents who had lost someone to Covid-19 suffered intense grief reactions. Loneliness was the most common predictor of all distress outcomes in adolescents (Murata et al., 2021). This has also been confirmed elsewhere (González-Sanguino et al., 2021). Increased time spent on social media and exposure to media related to Covid-19 have been associated with depression and suicidal thoughts or behaviour in adolescents (Murata et al., 2021).

One study examined adolescents exposed to Covid-19 and Typhoon Lekima, finding that PTSD–depression networks were similar for both Covid-19 and Lekima PTSD–depression. However, comorbid PTSD–depression symptoms were more complicated in the Covid-19 network but appeared to be more consistent in the Lekima network. Distinct bridge symptoms contributed to the heterogeneity of comorbid PTSD–depression symptoms in the two networks. The PTSD–depression comorbidity network appeared to overlap across trauma types. However, specific symptom-level associations and some bridging symptoms appeared to differ across trauma types (Qi et al., 2021).

PTSD in inpatients from COVID-19

Among patients hospitalised for Covid-19 in China, 13.2% reported Covid-19 PTSD, 21% reported depression, and 16.4% reported anxiety (Chen et al., 2021). Prior to their discharge from temporary quarantine hospitals in Wuhan, 96.2% of Covid-19 inpatients met diagnostic criteria for PTSD, even among those with clinically stable Covid-19 (Bo et al., 2021). In other words, it is of utmost importance that psychological interventions and follow-up are provided to these patients in the long term (Bo et al., 2020). The fact that almost all patients in the Bo et al. study met the PTSD criteria contradicts the literature, which states that even in the most devastating disasters, the prevalence of PTSD rarely exceeds 50% (McFarlane, 1990). This unusually high prevalence could be due to the fact that although these patients had been treated and were awaiting discharge, they were still constantly reminded of the trauma—of the threat that could strike them again soon after discharge to the community. This constant reminder may have exacerbated the severity of the PTSD symptoms. There is even an argument that just thinking about Covid-19 associated health problems or social isolation could reduce self-efficacy and impair psychological well-being, especially in people with high levels of PTSS or Covid-related functional impairment (Lockett et al., 2021). On the other hand, a study compared Covid-19 patients admitted to a hospital in China with mild symptoms with patients without Covid-19 (matched controls). They found that while the former reported higher levels of PTSD, depression, and anxiety overall than the latter, only one Covid-19 patient (1%) met criteria for probable PTSD, who nevertheless reported helplessness, fear, guilt, and worry about the course of the illness (Guo et al., 2020).

Among patients who had recovered from acute Covid-19 infection, one study showed that 1 month after discharge 36% still met the cut-off for a probable PTSD diagnosis attributable to distressing aspects of Covid-19 (Ju et al., 2021). Another study showed that, on average, 34.5% reported clinically significant PTSD, anxiety and/or depression 50 days after diagnosis, with PTSD being the most common (25.4%). In addition, 44.3% reported one or more protracted symptoms (e.g. fatigue, muscle pain, headache), which predicted the severity of PTSD according to Covid-19 (Poyraz et al., 2021). PTSD correlated with increased anxiety (OR: 1.34) and lack of emotional support during hospitalisation (OR: 0.41) in these recovered individuals (Ju et al., 2021).

PTSD in health care workers caring for patients with COVID-19

A review and meta-analysis based on an outbreak of an emerging virus states that health care workers exposed to a high-risk situation (direct contact) working with infected patients tended to have an almost twofold increase (OR: 1.71) in acute and PTSD compared to those exposed to a low risk situation, along with an almost equal increase in other psychological symptoms (OR: 1.74) (Kisely et al., 2020). It is therefore not surprising that several studies have found prevalence rates for PTSD or PTSS resulting from Covid-19 among health care workers ranging from 3.8% to 31.6% (Chew et al., 2020; Geng et al., 2021; Hou et al., 2022; Kang et al., 2020; Lai et al., 2020; Yin et al., 2020; Zakeri et al., 2021). In one study, 34.4%, 22.4%, and 6.2% of medical personnel in Wuhan were found to have mild, moderate, and severe levels of Covid-19 PTSD, respectively (Kang et al., 2020). Those who lived in Wuhan reported a higher prevalence rate (12.6%) of severe PTSD symptoms than those who worked outside Wuhan (7.2%) (Lai et al., 2020). Compared to medical staff working outside Wuhan, those working in Wuhan reported higher levels of feelings of danger, worry about their own and their family infection, poor sleep quality, feeling they needed psychological help, and a higher likelihood of contracting the disease. At the same time, they felt less confident about fighting the pandemic than their counterparts (Wu et al., 2020).

In addition to Covid-19 PTSD, health care workers also reported general psychological disorders (45.5%), generalised anxiety disorder (25.3%) (Zakeri et al., 2021), and depression (50.4%) (Lai et al., 2020). In another study, 5.3%, 8.7%, and 2.2% of health care workers tested positive for moderate-to-very-severe depression, moderate-to-extremely-severe anxiety, and moderate-to-extremely-severe stress, respectively. They also suffered from headaches (31.9%), sore throat (33.6%), lethargy (26.6%), and insomnia (21.0%); more than half (54%) reported multiple symptoms. Covid-19 PTSD, anxiety, depression, and stress were all associated with physical symptoms (Chew et al., 2020). Among another group of health care workers in Wuhan, 34.4%, 22.4%, and 6.2% reported mild, moderate, and severe disorders, respectively, characterised by Covid-19 PTSD, depression, anxiety, and insomnia symptoms (Kang et al., 2020).

A longitudinal study also reported that, during the pandemic, the rates for health care workers reporting probable anxiety, depression, and/or Covid-19 PTSD were 72% at baseline, 62% at 30 days, and 64% at 90 days (Amsalem et al., 2021). Although psychological distress decreases over time among health workers working with patients infected with coronaviruses, they may still be suffering from insomnia, burnout, and PTSS 3 years after the pandemic outbreak. In the mean time, there are few interventions to help these people and their effectiveness has not yet been evaluated (Magill et al., 2020).

A large-scale national survey examined the psychological well-being and quality of life of health care workers during Covid-19. It found that of 1,685 people, 14% reported Covid-19 PTSD, along with 31% mild anxiety, 33% clinically significant anxiety, 29% mild depression, 17% moderate-to-severe depressive symptoms, and 5% suicidal ideation. Health workers' psychiatric history increased the risk of anxiety disorders (OR: 2.78) and depression (OR: 3.49). Similarly, barriers to working were also associated with moderate-to-severe anxiety (OR: 2.50) and moderate depressive symptoms (OR: 2.15) (Young et al., 2021). Nurses and physicians may develop acute stress disorder leading to chronic PTSD, partly due to the fearful impact of inadequate human and technical resources when working with infected patients (Dutheil et al., 2020).

Another large-scale survey of nearly 4000 health care workers found that 50.2% reported moderate/severe Covid-19 PTSD symptoms, 24.6% anxiety, and 31.5% depression. Interestingly, those who had worked during the 2003 SARS outbreak had lower scores for PTSD, anxiety, and depression than those who had not worked during the SARS outbreak. This is probably unexpected since, as we will see later in the section on risk factors, studies suggest that people who have experienced previous trauma (in this case SARS) tend to report higher levels of distress during the pandemic. On the contrary, previous traumatic experiences related to the current trauma and clinical experiences seemed to be protective factors. Non-clinical health workers had a higher risk of anxiety (OR: 1.68) and depressive symptoms (OR: 2.03) during this pandemic. Health workers who took sedatives (OR: 2.55), who cared for only two to five patients with Covid-19 (OR: 1.59), and who were isolated due to Covid-19 (OR: 1.36) were more likely to report moderate/severe symptoms of PTSD. Sleep difficulties were also associated with PTSD symptoms (OR: 4.68), anxiety (OR: 3.09), and depression (OR: 5.07) (Styra et al., 2021).

Furthermore, 57% of health care workers in New York reported acute stress, and 48% and 33% reported depressive and anxiety symptoms, respectively. Despite this, 61% reported an increased sense of meaning or purpose in life since the outbreak (Shechter et al., 2020). This suggests that a sense of posttraumatic growth is developing in these workers. This is not surprising given that their work is characterised by a double-edged sword. It is extremely dangerous, traumatic and yet extremely important, meaningful, and rewarding. They risk their lives to defeat the virus and save the lives of others, for which they are praised and morally supported by the entire country. Yet, working with Covid-19 patients can cause health care workers such as psychiatrists, psychologists, and psychotherapists to experience emotional exhaustion, a common symptom of vicarious trauma or burnout (Blackman, 2020; Shortland et al., 2020). One study showed that 15% experienced high levels of vicarious trauma, while the rest reported moderate levels (Aafjes-van Doorn et al., 2022).

Social workers can also be affected by Covid-19 PTSD. One study shows that 26.2% of social workers met the diagnostic criteria for PTSD and 16.2% reported severe grief symptoms. Yet, almost all (99.1%) reported average-to-high levels of compassion satisfaction, while 63.7% and 49.5% reported burnout and secondary trauma, respectively. Support was clearly needed for the psychological well-being of these professionals (Holmes et al., 2021).

Health workers were compared with the general population and it was found that in the overall group 14.9% suffered from PTSS due to Covid-19, along with 16% depression and 11.7% anxiety. More people from the general population (28.6%) reported these symptoms than health workers (17.9%). The triad model of fear of Covid-19, anxiety, and stress was supported in this sample. This model is about short- or medium-term fear, anxiety, and a stressful situation (in this case Covid-19). Fear refers to a concrete and clearly defined stressor or situation (the possibility of contracting Covid-19). Anxiety, on the other hand, is not necessarily related to a concrete or defined situation such as the pandemic. It can be understood as a kind of non-specific and diffuse emotion. Fear, anxiety, and Covid-19 (the stressful situation) are linked in such a way that they trigger acute stress or PTSD symptoms. Specifically, this model explains depressive symptoms in >70% of the general population and health care workers combined. In the general population, the Covid-19 PTSD mediated the effects of anxiety on depression. In other words, anxiety may have triggered PTSD symptoms, which then affected depression. However, this indirect relationship was not found in health care workers (Villarreal-Zegarra et al., 2021).

PTSD in specific populations

Some studies have focused on the experiences of women who had gynaecological experiences during Covid-19. Among pregnant women who had given birth during the Covid-19 pandemic, concern for the foetus or baby correlated with social support, anxiety, and depression. Compared to a control group of new mothers who had given birth outside the lockdown period, participants in the study also had higher levels of anxiety, but no postpartum PTSD (Gonzalez-Garcia et al., 2021). Women who had given birth during the pandemic also tended to report more acute stress reactions related to childbirth than the control group (i.e. women who had given birth before the pandemic). Specifically, higher levels of acute stress related to childbirth were associated with increased birth-related PTSD symptoms, which affected postpartum adjustment and lower levels of bonding with the infant (Mayopoulos et al., 2021). In another study, 36.5% of puerperal women met criteria for PTSD related to their birth experience, 8.9% had a probable PTSD diagnosis, 28.8% had some symptoms related to PTSD, and 25.6% had no symptoms. The avoidance dimension of PTSD was prominent (Vitale, 2021). It appears that the experience during the pandemic may have exacerbated their distress symptoms related to their birth.

Regarding other populations, a national survey found that the prevalence of generalised anxiety disorder increased from pre- to peri-pandemic (from 7.1% to 9.4%, especially among veterans aged 45–64 years (from 8.2% to 13.5%)). In contrast, the prevalence of major depressive disorder and PTSD remained stable. Veterans with a larger social network and a secure attachment style before the pandemic tended not to experience an increase in distress, whereas veterans who experienced more loneliness before the pandemic tended to experience an increase in distress. Concerns about Covid-19 social losses, Covid-19 impact on psychological well-being, and about residential stability during the pandemic were associated with increased distress, over and above pre-pandemic factors (Hill et al., 2021). Among psychiatric patients, >45% reported PTSD-like symptoms related to Covid-19. They also had high levels of pandemic-related depressive symptoms. Rumination or worries about the Covid-19 outbreak and feelings of social isolation were associated with high levels of PTSD-like symptoms and hypervigilance to pandemic-related stimuli (Ting et al., 2021).

Having presented all these different rates of PTSD, it is worth noting that the differences in prevalence of PTSD, as highlighted in previous chapters, could result from the different PTSD measures used (e.g. Impact of Event Scale—Revised, PTSD Checklist for DSM-5) with different cut-off scores. It is also worth pointing out some recent arguments that simply responding to population prevalence estimates for psychological disorders or focusing on changes in mean scores over time may not be the best way to examine heterogeneity in mental health in response to the Covid-19 pandemic. People's response to the pandemic is heterogeneous, not homogeneous. For example, a longitudinal study with three waves in about 5 months was conducted to show the heterogeneity of these responses. Rather than looking at changes in mean scores over time, a latent class growth analysis was used to show that while Covid-19 PTSD declined between waves 2 and 3, the overall prevalence of anxiety and depression remained stable. Three classes reflecting heterogeneity in mental health responses were identified: (i) stability, (ii) improvement, and (iii) deterioration in mental health. It is likely that different psychological mechanisms underlie these classes of individuals. For example, in the stability group there were individuals with a low stability profile (i.e. they were resilient individuals with little to no psychological distress). Their psychological mechanisms would be quite different from those of the other groups (Shevlin et al., 2021).

In another study, a latent class analysis was used to show that there are three classes of health and social care workers who respond to distress: high-exposure (19.5%), betrayal-only (31.3%), and minimal exposure (49.4%). Individuals who had high levels of perceived stress were more likely to be in the high-exposure and betrayal-only classes. Individuals in these classes also reported higher levels of depressive, anxiety, and posttraumatic symptoms, as well as more symptoms of moral injury, lower levels of self-compassion, but higher levels of self-criticism than the minimal exposure class (Zerach & Levi-Belz, 2021). Moral injury is a psychological phenomenon whereby they feel that their values and beliefs have been betrayed. They may have witnessed the most devastating effects of the acute Covid-19 situation and feel helpless to respond. Increased moral injury has been linked to a range of psychological symptoms, including suicidal ideation (Amsalem et al., 2021).

While the above literature is primarily concerned with Covid-19 PTSD, awareness has been raised of Covid-19 peritraumatic distress (CPD), which includes immediate physiological arousal, and emotional and cognitive responses to the threat of Covid-19. One study found that 35.5% and 17.2% of individuals met clinical diagnostic criteria for CPD at baseline and follow-up (3–4 months later), respectively. Baseline CPD explained between 14 and 20% of the variance in Covid-19 PTSS, depression, and anxiety symptoms. Further analysis revealed that chronic CPD and PTSS were most common in individuals who were worried about the Covid-19 crisis. Depression and anxiety, on the other hand, were more common among people who were single and who had pre-existing mental health problems (Megalakaki et al., 2021).

Risk factors

In terms of risk factors, a number of 'victim variables' have been identified as risk factors, in line with the literature reviewed in previous chapters.

Demographic variables

Younger age is thought to be associated with distress, including depression and Covid-19 PTSD (Aafjes-van Doorn et al., 2020; Boyraz & Legros, 2020; González-Sanguino et al., 2021; Kisely et al., 2020; Mukherjee & Maity, 2021; Rodriguez-Rey et al., 2020). On the other hand, older people are less likely than younger people to experience pandemic-related stressors such as losing their job or the fear of losing it, having to go to work, worrying about being infected by or infecting family members, as many of them no longer live with their families. They should therefore be more resilient (Boyraz & Legros, 2020). However, a word of caution for Chinese families: due to their collectivist culture, many older people live with their family members. This could have an impact on their resilience. Nevertheless, age was negatively correlated with negative affect (sadness, depression, anxiety) in responding to distress during quarantine. In other words, older people seemed to be less prone to negative affect (Pérez-Fuentes et al., 2021). Similarly, older health care workers (aged 51–60 years) reported lower levels of Covid-19 PTSS than younger (aged 31–40 years) or those in a lower (job) position (Hou et al., 2022; Kisely et al., 2020). One should not conclude from the above findings that older adults are therefore not vulnerable groups. In fact, they have their own unique stressors that should not be ignored. For example, in the context of Covid-19 vaccine-related stressors, older adults struggled with depressive symptoms, ageism, vaccine hesitancy, and severity of side-effects associated with their clinical level of current PTSD from before Covid-19 trauma (Palgi et al., 2021).

People with a junior high school or lower level of education reported higher levels of Covid-19 PTSD and psychiatric comorbidity than those who had a high school or university education (Liang et al., 2020a). This association between a low level of education (high school or below) and the occurrence of distress was also found in another study examining people who recovered from Covid-19 (Ju et al., 2021). In addition, people with low incomes also tended to have higher levels of Covid-19 PTSD than their counterparts (Mukherjee & Maity, 2021). Other social inequalities include poor housing, financial or occupational loss (Boyraz & Legros, 2020), and living with a disability (e.g. spinal cord injury) (Boyraz & Legros, 2020). These disparities or inequalities could increase infections and deaths from Covid-19, which in turn could further increase disparities or inequalities (Kira et al., 2021).

As mentioned earlier, social inequalities such as inadequate housing, financial loss, or job loss are examples of resource losses that people may experience during Covid-19. These losses can affect the relationship between partners. A three-wave study over a 67-month period examined the impact of loss and gain on partner strain, finding that increased Covid-19 PTSS at baseline was correlated with both loss and gain in the second wave within and between partners. However, loss in wave 2 was correlated with PTSS in wave 3 with partners. In other words, increased loss was a consistent factor associated with increased PTSD within and between partners over time. Loss is an important clinical factor to consider when treating PTSD in a dyadic relationship, although this does not mean that gains should be ignored (Banford Witting et al., 2022).

Gender differences

Several studies have looked at women's psychological responses to PTSD associated with Covid-19. One month after the outbreak, Covid-19 PTSD was associated with gender (Sun et al., 2020). Female gender is a consistent factor predicting distress, including severity of PTSD (Boyraz & Legros, 2020; Poyraz et al., 2021; Rodriguez-Rey et al., 2020; Sun et al., 2020; Yin et al., 2020). Women have been shown to report higher levels of anxiety and PTSD (González-Sanguino et al., 2021; Ju et al., 2021). Women reported significantly higher PTSS symptoms in terms of re-experiencing, negative alterations in cognition or mood, and hyperarousal symptoms than men (Liu et al., 2020). Women had more sadness–depression, anxiety, and negative affect than men; whereas men showed more happiness and positive affect than women. Women appeared to be at greater risk of negative affective balance during quarantine (Pérez-Fuentes et al., 2021). It was also estimated that female workers had twice the risk (HR: 2.13) of Covid-19 PTSD than male workers (Yin et al., 2020).

Also, when comparing the burden of the Covid-19 pandemic and the mental health of female and male caregivers of 5–18-year-old children, female caregivers reported higher levels of distress or disruption related to Covid, higher levels of anxiety, and higher levels of PTSD related to other traumas than Covid-19. They also reported more adverse childhood experiences (ACEs) than male caregivers. It appears that women are disproportionately burdened or disturbed by the pandemic. Among female caregivers, increased Covid stress/disruption and ACEs independently predicted all distress outcomes. For male caregivers, however, there was an interaction effect, i.e. the impact of Covid stress/disruption on mental health was stronger for those with elevated ACEs. There appear to be differences between the sexes in terms of pre-existing vulnerability to adaptation to the current situation (Wade et al., 2021) and the psychological mechanisms underlying these distress responses.

Minority groups

People belonging to ethnic minorities may have to cope with stressors related to Covid-19 and racial prejudice and discrimination, which could increase the risk of PTSD and psychiatric comorbid symptoms (Lund, 2021). The impact of Covid-19 discrimination on mental health was examined in a study of Asian and Asian American young adults during the first three months of the pandemic. Eighty-six per cent of these young adults reported that they or their family experienced Covid-19 discrimination, and some of them (15%) also experienced verbal or physical assault. Increased PTSD was not only associated with Covid-19 discrimination, but also with lifelong discrimination and pre-existing mental health diagnoses. However, anxiety and depression were not correlated with these variables (Hahm et al., 2021).

Parenthood

Parents who have dependent children also appear to be a vulnerable population. This is not surprising, as parents' concerns about who would care for their children if they were infected would increase their psychological distress or exacerbate their Covid-19 PTSD symptoms and psychiatric comorbidity (Kisely et al., 2020). Healthcare workers who have at least one child were also more likely to develop PTSS as a result of Covid-19 (Hou et al., 2022). Parents of children aged <18 years have been found to face additional Covid-19 parenting-related stressors and may therefore suffer from increased psychological distress. In a national sample of >2,000 parents, 38.3% met or exceeded the clinical cut-off for parents with PTSS. Younger parents reported higher levels of stress, Covid-19 PTSS, and adjustment disorder. Younger parents and parents of colour reported higher levels of distress related to the pandemic. These findings seem to indicate that parents are at higher risk for pandemic stress, Covid-19 PTSS, and adjustment disorder (Wamser-Nanney et al., 2021). During the pandemic, parents and children reported poor well-being and psychological distress. Their well-being was lower than before the pandemic. For children, the perception of social support from family members and friends can buffer the severity of distress. Social support is a protective factor that can mitigate the distress caused by the pandemic (Mactavish et al., 2021).

Pre-existing mental health problems

People who have pre-existing mental health problems could also have an impact on the distress associated with Covid-19. For example, health care workers with a history of psychiatric problems tended to manifest their perceived stress and PTSD in relation to the impact of Covid-19 on symptoms. They felt that the impact of the pandemic had exacerbated and worsened their psychiatric symptoms and that their perceived stress had increased as a result of avoiding physical contact with others (MacKenzie et al., 2021). Another study also claimed that pre-existing psychological problems such as previous anxiety about one's health, hypersensitivity to anxiety, intolerance of uncertainty, disgust tendencies, worries about germs, and obsessive–compulsive contamination and checking rituals were more vulnerable to Covid stress (Taylor et al., 2020). People with a history of psychological disorders, especially those who are sexual minorities (e.g. lesbian, gay, bisexual, trans-gender), also tended to have higher levels of distress symptoms, anxiety, de-pression, PTSD related to the pandemic, and physical complaints. They also tended to use maladaptive coping strategies. People with these two conditions had the highest severity on these symptoms (Fallahi et al., 2021).

Past trauma

Past trauma can often contribute significantly to pre-existing mental health problems and has been shown to play a role in influencing Covid-19 PTSD (Poyraz et al., 2021). One study looked at Syrian refugees, who had been trau-matised by fleeing their own country, to see whether their cumulative trau-matic stress had an impact on Covid-19 distress. Torture (75%) was a strong predictor of hospitalisation for Covid-19. The sample had high scores for PTSD, depression, and anxiety, especially among those who had been hospi-talised for Covid-19 and those who had been tortured in the past. Covid-19 PTSS was directly related to increased PTSD due to past trauma, depression, and comorbid anxiety symptoms, and indirectly via existential death and status anxiety as mediators. In other words, the relationship between PTSD due to previous trauma and psychiatric comorbid symptoms (anxiety and de-pression) and current Covid-19 PTSS could be influenced by existential death and status anxiety (Alpay et al., 2021).

Among the descendants of Holocaust survivors (OHS), their heightened sensitivity to life-threatening challenges may have played a role in influencing distress during the pandemic. Older OHS during Covid-19 with two parents who suffered from PTSD reported the highest levels of PTSD as a result of past trauma and had higher levels of loneliness than OHS whose parents did not suffer from PTSD. However, both groups did not differ in concerns about Covid-19 and social support. On the whole, although OHS received good so-cial support, some felt lonely, which could be due to the particular interper-sonal difficulties that some OHS families are prone to. In other words, these ageing OHS with parental PTSD appeared to suffer more from, or be more vulnerable to, the negative psychological effects of the pandemic than their counterparts (Shrira & Felsen, 2021).

Whereas the above studies suggest that past trauma may influence current distress related to Covid-19, the severity of symptoms related to past trauma may also increase during the pandemic. One study looked at people with PTSD due to past trauma, depression, and somatic symptoms and compared them to healthy controls. The group was found to have an increase in general psychological distress and severity of PTSD symptoms (ω^2: 0.07–0.08) during Covid-19. In particular, childhood trauma was associated with increased PTSD symptom severity. However, this association was mediated by a lack of perceived social support (indirect effect: 0.101), not by fear of Covid-19. In other words, during the pandemic, people's childhood trauma experiences may have influenced their perceptions of social support received, which in turn influenced PTSD symptoms. This also means that, during the pandemic, it is important to promote social inclusion or improve perceptions of social inclusion to alleviate the psychological distress of people with childhood trauma experiences (Seitz et al., 2021).

One study explored the claim that traumatised sexual minority women (SMW) may be at higher risk of PTSD than traumatised heterosexual women due to past trauma and risky alcohol use. SMW reported higher severity of PTSD symptoms due to past trauma, probable PTSD, and indicators of risky alcohol use (i.e. alcohol use disorder and heavy episodic drinking) than general samples of SMW. Living in or near the initial epicentres of Covid-19 contributed to their psychological and behavioural distress. In other words, it is important to integrate PTSD and alcohol use prevention for traumatised SMW during Covid-19 (Helminen et al., 2021).

Covid-19-related factors

There are also specific Covid-19-related factors that are thought to be associated with increased Covid-19 PTSD and psychiatric comorbidity (Boyraz & Legros, 2020). Hospitalised patients who reported higher levels of Covid-19 PTSD, depression, and anxiety tended to be those who had been more exposed to traumatic experiences related to Covid-19 while perceiving low levels of social support (Chen et al., 2021). Those with high exposure reported significantly more hyperarousal symptoms (HR: 4.02) than those with low exposure (Yin et al., 2020). Various indicators were used to measure trauma exposure in the context of Covid-19. For example, people who lived in the epicentre of Wuhan tended to report higher levels of PTSD than those who lived in surrounding areas (Liu et al., 2020; Sun et al., 2020). Having contracted the virus themselves was another feature of high trauma exposure Covid-19. While university lecturers during the Covid-19 outbreak reported that the overall incidence rate of PTSD was 24.5%, compared to those without confirmed Covid-19, among university lecturers for whom Covid-19 was confirmed, the ratio of PTSD (Covid-19 PTSD) increased up to 2.81 (i.e. an 181% increase)

(C. Fan et al., 2021). Subsequent stigmatisation (Samantha K. Brooks et al., 2020; Guo et al., 2020; Kisely et al., 2020; Poyraz et al., 2021), contact with an infected family member (Kisely et al., 2020; Wytrychiewicz et al., 2020), being friends or family members of a Covid-19 health care worker, and having friends or family members who have recently visited Wuhan could also represent high trauma exposure to Covid-19. This trauma exposure has been associated with moderate or severe PTSD symptomatology (Jiang et al., 2020).

The experience of hospitalisation for Covid-19 (Boyraz & Legros, 2020) is another risk factor for Covid-19 PTSD. Some family members would have been separated from their loved ones who were admitted to the ICU. This would exacerbate the intrinsically high level of ICU-related stress on PTSD and other trauma-related symptoms (Montauk & Kuhl, 2020). In addition, patients suffering from Covid-19 may develop some medical complications, which may be exacerbated by some psychological complications resulting from the illness or other factors such as hospitalisation and quarantine. After discharge from Covid treatment in the ICU, patients may experience medical trauma, acute stress and Covid-19 PTSD, cognitive dysfunction, fatigue and depression, social stress and adjustment problems, and illness anxiety, for which psychological treatments should be provided (Guck et al., 2021).

Another Covid-19-related factor associated with increased distress is the loss of a loved one (Boyraz & Legros, 2020; Kokou-Kpolou et al., 2020). Compared to those who had no deaths of family members or relatives due to Covid-19, the ratio increased to 5.59 (a 459% increase) for university teachers (C. Fan et al., 2021). For many surviving family members, this experience of loss due to Covid-19 can lead to Covid-19 PTSD symptoms and psychiatric comorbid symptoms, fear, a sense of uncertainty, and delayed grief responses (Blackman, 2020; Dutheil et al., 2020). Other symptoms may include feelings of guilt, somatisation, regret, and anger. This highlights the importance of allowing the bereaved to engage in meaning-making practices which are an important part of the grieving process (Kokou-Kpolou et al., 2020).

Whereas lockdown, staying at home, social isolation, and quarantine can be useful as physical forms of prevention to slow the spread of the virus, they can also have negative effects on people's distress (Banducci & Weiss, 2020; Boyraz & Legros, 2020; Kisely et al., 2020; Taylor et al., 2020) and feelings of uncertainty, fear, despair (Mucci et al., 2020), health anxiety (Tull et al., 2020), frustration, boredom (Samantha K. Brooks et al., 2020), loneliness, lack of social support (Tull et al., 2020), confusion, anger (Samantha K. Brooks et al., 2020; Wytrychiewicz et al., 2020), financial worries (Tull et al., 2020), and even Covid-19 PTSD (S. K. Brooks et al., 2020; Wytrychiewicz et al., 2020). Lockdown or quarantine also means that families spend more time together, which could lead to an increased likelihood of domestic violence, which is associated with Covid-19 PTSD symptoms (Blackman, 2020; Dutheil et al., 2020). Among people living in domestic quarantine for ≥4 weeks, one study showed that the prevalence rate for PTSD was 28.2%; 36.3%, 26.9%, 9.4%, and 4.7% had minimal, mild, moderate, and severe depression, respectively. The number of household members, occupation and PTSD were correlated with depression (Singh & Khokhar, 2021).

The media may also influence PTSD symptoms associated with the outbreak Covid-19. High levels of media exposure were associated with increased Covid-19 PTSD (Mukherjee & Maity, 2021). Hospital patients who reported higher levels of Covid-19 PTSD, depression, and anxiety tended to be those affected by negative news reports (Chen et al., 2021). Watching news about Covid-19 could affect the severity of past traumatic experiences. In one study, Israeli ex-prisoners of war (ex-POWs) from the 1973 Yom Kippur War were compared with veterans of the same war (the control group). They were followed up longitudinally (1991, 2003, 2008, 2015, and 2020 during the outbreak of Covid-19). The former POWs were more likely to watch news on Covid-19, which in turn contributed to the severity of PTSD during the time of the pandemic. Furthermore, the delayed course of PTSD (i.e. participants who did not meet the PTSD criteria in the first two assessment periods but did in subsequent periods) was associated with an increased frequency of watching the television news on Covid-19, which in turn contributed to increased severity of PTSD during the pandemic. In other words, watching the television news on Covid-19 appeared to have negative effects for viewers and may potentially exacerbate previous PTSD in trauma survivors (Solomon et al., 2021). It is likely that this exposure to the media or experiencing the above Covid-19 events could increase people's fear of infection or danger of Covid-19 (Samantha K. Brooks et al., 2020; Taylor et al., 2020) and risk perception of Covid-19. Risk or negative perception was positively correlated with the severity of Covid-19 PTSD (Geng et al., 2021; Poyraz et al., 2021).

In addition to the above Covid-19-related factors, according to the COVID stress syndrome hypothesis, other factors should also be considered, including viral anxiety, lower socioeconomic status anxiety, and vicarious PTSD (Brooks et al., 2020; Taylor et al., 2020). In addition, this syndrome also includes fear of foreign visitors entering and spreading the virus (xenophobia) and compulsive checking behaviour. One study found that 38% of those affected suffered from this stress syndrome to some degree, while 16% were distressed to the point of needing psychiatric help (Taylor et al., 2020). These additional factors represent a 'parallel pandemic' triggered by the devastating and long-term effects of Covid (Mucci et al., 2020).

As mentioned previously, working in a Covid-19 health care environment can be stressful. Healthcare workers employed in Covid-19 and non-Covid-19 wards were found to have different distress outcomes. Witnessing the death of patients on the Covid-19 wards was associated with a fourfold higher likelihood of developing PTSS (OR: 3.97) compared to those not on Covid-19 wards (OR: 0.91). In other words, witnessing the death of patients appeared to be a unique risk factor for PTSS for health care workers who directly dealt with and treated Covid-19 patients. Helping these workers cope with Covid-19 deaths could reduce their risk for PTSS (Mosheva et al., 2021). Risk factors for psychological distress included mental exhaustion, fear of contracting the virus, and of infecting family members (Mosheva et al., 2021). Less experience in their profession as a health professional (Aafjes-van Doorn et al., 2020; Kisely et al., 2020) and negative experiences in providing online treatment (Aafjes-van Doorn et al., 2020) were also associated with distress.

Coping

Since dealing with the effects of Covid-19 is not an option for us, it is not surprising that coping strategies are central to the discussion when risk factors are identified. The use of negative coping strategies such as avoidance coping has been associated with psychological distress, including Covid-19 PTSD, in young people (Liang et al., 2020b). Other negative coping strategies such as withdrawal thinking, distraction, and blaming others were correlated with all three Covid-19 PTSD clusters. In addition, fatigue mediated the impact that negative coping had on PTSS (Hou et al., 2022).

Some people might take the approach that this outbreak is something over which one has no control. In other words, fatalism is an approach someone might have taken to cope with this stressful event. One study showed that 48.8% of respondents reported moderate-to-severe Covid-19 PTSS and that 79% had to change their daily routine because of the pandemic. Fatalism was associated with PTSS and with a lack of behavioural change in response to Covid-19 (i.e. people felt unable to adopt health-protective behaviours) (Bogolyubova et al., 2021).

Rather than focusing on negative coping strategies as risk factors, some researchers have taken a positive psychology approach. For example, spiritual fortitude, i.e. the ability to draw on spiritual resources to transcend negative emotions in the face of stressors (Van Tongeren et al., 2019), could be considered as a way of coping with Covid-19. It has been shown to have positive psychological effects, including higher levels of meaning in life, spiritual well-being, adoption of positive religious coping, and perceptions of posttraumatic growth (Hansong Zhang et al., 2021). This reflects the assertion that spiritual well-being is the greatest protector against Covid-19 depression, anxiety, and PTSD (González-Sanguino et al., 2021).

Practices of acceptance, mindfulness, and loving-kindness are also considered useful in reducing stress, improving resilience and recovery, empowering people to make sense of their current situation, tolerating distress, improving social support and interpersonal relationships, and taking purposeful action (Polizzi et al., 2020). However, for some people, such as health care workers, it is more important to advocate some practically oriented types of coping strategies. One study showed that physical activity or exercise was the most common coping behaviour (59%), although a third (33%) of them also received individual therapy with some kind of online self-help counselling (Shechter et al., 2020). Another study showed that more than one-third (36.3%) of medical staff used mental health education materials, half (50.4%) used online psychological self-help resources, and 17.5% used counselling or psychotherapy (Kang et al., 2020). Otherwise, clear communication, adequate personal protection, rest, and practical and psychological support are important coping or protective factors for them (Kisely et al., 2020). Other practical protective factors include government plans to reduce the risk of infection and the availability of food (Wytrychiewicz et al., 2020).

To look at coping from a defence mechanism perspective, psychoanalysts would argue that Covid-19 can trigger unconscious defence mechanisms, including the use of humour, denial, and obsessional cleaning behaviour. This compulsive cleaning behaviour is a form of defence aimed at alleviating the fear of contracting the virus in oneself or family members. This type of anxiety is arguably a real-angst. However, for some people, the constant fear causes insomnia, so they use the cleansing behaviour to ward off other types of fears triggered by the virus. For example, a mother might compulsively clean herself to protect her husband or son, i.e. to ward off her fear for their safety. In reality, however, she may be doing it to defend against her feelings of guilt for not wanting to marry or have a son. Unresolved attachment or childhood issues may also come to the fore (Blackman, 2020). However, defence alone may not be the most effective way to protect oneself. The combination of defence and mindfulness has been suggested as a potential adaptive defence strategy to buffer the experience of Covid-19 (Di Giuseppe et al., 2020).

Personality trait

There is evidence that a personality trait, particularly narcissism, can be a risk factor. This is a trait characterised by grandiose self-perception and preoccupation with self-interest. People with high levels of narcissism tend to have high levels of 'narcissistic vulnerability', i.e. they have difficulty regulating their emotions, especially when their grandiosity is challenged. One might therefore suspect that these individuals also have difficulty regulating distressing Covid-19 PTSD-related symptoms (Coleman, 2020). Notwithstanding, narcissism can also be understood as a defence mechanism, in line with the above. Psychoanalysts would argue that grandiosity is an attempt to hide deep-seated feelings of inferiority, a negative self-schema characterised by negative self-worth or insecurity. This is the basis for the 'mask model of narcissism', which asserts the relationship between grandiosity and negative self-schema, where people interpret past and present experiences negatively (Thomas et al., 2013). It could therefore be hypothesised that individuals with high levels of narcissism would exacerbate the threat of Covid-19 and the distress associated with Covid-19 through a distorted schema.

Anxiety sensitivity, a stable personality trait (Hovenkamp-Hermelink et al., 2019), is thought to influence the association between PTSD due to past trauma and respiratory symptoms. Specifically, the somatic concerns of anxiety sensitivity significantly contributed to the overlap between PTSD and respiratory symptoms in individuals with PTSD symptoms due to past trauma (Mahaffey et al., 2017). This paves the way for further studies on whether this trait may also similarly influence Covid-19 PTSD.

Other factors

While the above are mainly person-related factors, there are some state factors that should also be considered. These could include population density, the proportion of certain ethnic groups, gross domestic product per capita, and the number of Covid-19 cases. For example, states with higher populations and Covid-19 cases were associated with higher levels of Covid-19 PTSS. People's perceived community resilience may have an impact on PTSD, but this outcome varies by ethnic group (e.g. African Americans) (Shigemoto, 2021). In other words, while it is important to examine the psychological mechanisms underlying Covid-19 in individuals, the ways in which the pandemic may affect the occurrence of PTSD and depression and how professionals should respond should also be considered. Evidence gained at the individual level should be complemented by population-level modelling, which will allow us to estimate long-term psychiatric morbidity as a result of the pandemic (Waters et al., 2021). Given the traumatic impact and societal consequences of Covid-19 around the world, what has been presented so far will only be expanded by future research aimed at understanding the traumatic aspect of Covid-19 (Horesh & Brown, 2020).

Intervention

In addition to disease and death, this virus has also caused great fear of contamination, helplessness, hopelessness, economic hardship, physical distancing, forced isolation, and a broken social network, all of which can lead to high levels of mental health problems. Psychotherapy, crisis intervention, or counselling are at the forefront, which could increase the demand for psychological services related to PTSD. These interventions can be integrated into primary care (Kanzler & Ogbeide, 2020).

The effects of narrative exposure therapy—a typical cognitive behavioural therapy targeting trauma-related psychological disorders—on Covid-19 patients just prior to discharge were examined. Patients who received this therapy and a personalised psychological intervention reduced their PTSD significantly more than the control group who received only a personalised psychological intervention. Although there was evidence of improvement in sleep quality, anxiety, and depression after the intervention, the two groups did not differ in these variables (Y. Fan et al., 2021).

A randomised controlled trial examined changes in mental health, health behaviours, executive functioning, emotion regulation, and mindfulness in adolescents who participated in a service-learning mentoring programme during the Covid-19 pandemic. The aim of this programme was to empower adolescents to build positive relationships, achieve academic success and develop pro-social interests. Mindfulness training was integrated into this programme. The follow-up period is about 6 months. However, it was found that their health did not improve. Instead, they improved on average in the areas of sleep, emotion regulation, executive functions and mindfulness over time (about 6 months). Those who participated in mentoring and mindfulness reported significantly less PTSD and emotional impulsivity at follow-up compared to those who participated in the mentoring-as-usual condition. It appears that mentoring combined with mindfulness may be effective in protecting adolescent mental health during the pandemic period (Miller et al., 2021).

The pandemic may trigger existential questions, including the question of the meaning of life, for which existential–humanistic and relational psychotherapy may be relevant. This approach advocates the importance of self-awareness, meaning making, taking responsibility for one's life, and choosing and realising ways of living in the world that are consistent with one's values. It empowers people to focus on their own values, assumptions, and priorities in life, their actions, self-efficacy, agency, and commitment to their lives, and the relationship between self and others (Gordon et al., 2021). Other interventions include art therapy, which has been suggested to promote expression, hope, and inspiration, to combat stigma, to foster family and personal relationships, to combat distress, and to develop coping and resilience skills (Potash et al., 2020). Due to restricted access to human contact, pet therapy can also provide social support (Nieforth & O'Haire, 2020).

However, access to physically normal mental health services or interventions has become increasingly difficult due to social distancing rules, lockdown, and the like. One innovative way to provide these interventions is through telepsychotherapy (Inchausti et al., 2020). Several studies have argued that telepsychotherapy may be a new way to offer psychotherapeutic treatments in the community. Telepsychotherapy is a framework that can be combined with various forms of therapy such as cognitive behavioural therapy or cognitive processing therapy, a trauma-focused, evidence-based treatment for posttraumatic stress disorder (Moring et al., 2020). It has been argued that the strength-based philosophy should form the basis for telepsychotherapy. It is a preventative measure for individuals who may have experienced a life threat, loss, and PTSD symptoms (Anton et al., 2020; Polizzi et al., 2020; Rosen et al., 2020). It aims to enable families to strengthen attachment relationships (Ronen-Setter & Cohen, 2020), learn online family problem solving and provide parenting skills training alongside traditional treatments (Wade et al., 2020). It aims to empower victims to manage distressing emotions during the Covid-19 pandemic, increase resilience (Lissoni et al., 2020) and posttraumatic growth (Shakespeare-Finch et al., 2020). The extent of the increase would depend on a number of factors, including the severity of exposure, individual differences (e.g. optimism), family context (e.g. family cohesion, good communication between family members, financial management), and community characteristics (e.g. access to health care, socioeconomic status) (Chen & Bonanno, 2020).

Some preliminary findings have also suggested that telepsychotherapy is a trustworthy alternative to traditional interventions that can be used for anxiety, depression, and PTSD, for example. However, clients' technological knowledge and ability to communicate effectively over the Internet may influence the effectiveness of telepsychotherapy (Poletti et al., 2020). The effectiveness of telepsychotherapy has been demonstrated in a non-Covid-19 situation. For example, a pilot study examined the feasibility and potential effectiveness of trauma-focused cognitive behavioural therapy delivered via telepsychotherapy for youths who have experienced trauma. There was a reduction in PTSD symptoms at follow-up with large effect sizes for both the youths and the caregivers (Stewart et al., 2020). A case study was also reported in which a veteran receiving prolonged PTSD treatment for military sexual trauma became infected with Covid-19 halfway through treatment. The treatment modality therefore had to be changed, including a switch to telehealth. Despite technological, environmental, and pandemic difficulties, the patient persevered through a course of prolonged exposure treatment, reduced his PTSD symptoms, and achieved a good level of functional recovery (Banducci, 2021).

COVID Coach, a public mental health app that provides tools and resources for coping with Covid-19 stress, was studied. Users of this app tended to have problems with anxiety, depression, and PTSD. People with higher levels of distress tended to use this app more often. App users with moderate-to-severe anxiety or depression tended to reuse the app more often than those with minimal symptoms. Similarly, those with significant PTSD symptoms tended to continue using the app more often than those with fewer symptoms (Jaworski et al., 2021). Similarly, it has been suggested that clinical virtual reality (VR) can be used to address the psychological distress associated with Covid-19. Clinical programmes based on the delivery of trauma-focused VR exposure therapy (VRET) have been developed to address PTSD. This type of programme can now be extended to a range of other traumas, including those serving on the frontlines of the Covid-19 pandemic (Rizzo et al., 2021).

PTSD and other respiratory disorders

To conclude this chapter, it is worth briefly discussing the relationship between PTSD and other, less well- known respiratory illnesses. It has been postulated that there is a link between trauma and environmental sensitivity in the form of allergies. This is in line with the trauma/hypersensitivity hypothesis that patients with PTSD tend to be more sensitive or less tolerant to certain environmental substances (Sansone et al., 2009). War-related trauma, childhood abuse and PTSD due to other traumas have been associated with allergies, urticaria and/or angioedema. These allergy symptoms could be triggered by exposure to certain trauma-related stimuli (Gupta, 2010). Several studies have also found an association between allergies such as chronic idiopathic urticaria (CIU) and PTSD. CIU patients were almost twice as likely to have a diagnosis of PTSD due to previous trauma than non-CIU patients. In addition, CIU patients were almost one and a half times more likely to meet the threshold for psychiatric comorbidity than healthy controls (Chung et al., 2010a, 2010b; Hunkin & Chung, 2012).

Although CIU is not life-threatening as an allergic reaction, some allergic reactions such as anaphylaxis can be a severe, life-threatening, generalised or systemic hypersensitivity reaction, according to the European Academy of Allergology and Clinical Immunology Nomenclature Committee. In anaphylaxis, there are sudden and rapidly developing life-threatening airway and/or breathing difficulties and/or circulatory problems (i.e. a drop in blood pressure that may lead to collapse and loss of consciousness), as well as skin and/or mucosal changes, i.e. flushing, a nettle rash or hives (urticaria) and/or swelling of the face (angioedema). In severe cases, either the breathing difficulties or the drop in blood pressure can lead to death. Anaphylaxis can be triggered by food (e.g. peanuts or shellfish), poison, bee or wasp stings, or drugs (e.g. antibiotics, aspirin).

Because of the potentially life-threatening nature of anaphylaxis, some researchers have investigated whether patients can develop PTSD symptoms after anaphylactic shock (i.e. post-anaphylactic shock–PTSD). One study showed that 12% of people with anaphylactic shock experiences met the diagnostic criteria for full PTSD. They also reported significantly more traumatic past experiences and psychiatric comorbidity than the control group. In other words, there may be a cumulative stress phenomenon in which the effects of previous trauma may have exacerbated the PTSD following anaphylactic shock, although this hypothesis has not yet been confirmed. Trauma exposure characteristics (i.e. anaphylactic shock symptoms) influenced PTSD symptoms and psychiatric comorbidity following anaphylactic shock, which in turn influenced coping strategies (Chung et al., 2011).

PTSD is also associated with an increased risk of chronic obstructive pulmonary disease (COPD) (adjusted odds: 1.22) (Taylor-Clift et al., 2016). One study found that 74% of patients with COPD had experienced trauma in the past, with half identifying lung disease as the traumatic event. However, only 8% met the diagnostic criteria for PTSD and reported worse health than patients without PTSD. The severity of their PTSD symptoms persisted after pulmonary rehabilitation, although exercise capacity and quality of life improved after rehabilitation (Jones et al., 2009). In a study focusing on older patients, it was found that 6% of patients met criteria for full PTSD and 39% met criteria for partial PTSD. PTSD correlated with the severity of COPD, which in turn correlated with health-related quality of life and psychiatric co-morbidity. Specifically, the emotional dimension of COPD mediated the impact of PTSD on mental health functioning of health-related quality of life and the impact of PTSD on depression (Chung et al., 2016).

Summary

Patients suffering from respiratory distress syndrome and acute lung injury have been found to have PTSD. People with PTSD who were victims of the World Trade Centre disaster were more likely to suffer from asthma symptoms than were victims without PTSD. PTSD symptoms were also associated with asthma severity in children and adolescents. Treating PTSD symptoms could reduce the severity of respiratory disease. In addition to the association between PTSD due to past trauma and asthma severity, some studies have also looked at PTSD due to the traumatic effects of asthma (i.e. PTSD following an asthma attack). Self-efficacy plays a role in influencing PTSD following an asthma attack and psychiatric comorbidity.

Studies have also examined PTSD associated with SARS. People with PTSD, health care workers and hospital staff working with SARS patients may report a range of psychological and physical symptoms as well as fear of infecting others, and social contact and discrimination. Several risk factors play a role in the distress experienced by SARS patients. These include being female, having a low level of education, being younger, being married, being seen in fever stations, knowing someone who has SARS, feeling exposed to the risk of SARS, working in high-risk places, and being under quarantine. Maladaptive coping strategies and low levels of self-efficacy are also risk factors, while high levels of self-esteem and altruism can be protective factors.

Covid-19 is associated with a whole range of general psychological disorders. Different prevalence rates for PTSD have been reported. Covid-19 affects adults, children, and adolescents. Adolescents are more likely than adults to report moderate-to-severe levels of mental health difficulties. Those who have lost someone to Covid-19 suffer intense grief reactions. Loneliness is the most common predictor of all distress conditions in adolescents. When examining PTSD in Covid-19 inpatients, different proportions of Covid-19 patients reported PTSD, depression, and anxiety. Healthcare workers who care for patients with Covid-19 may also develop PTSD. However, more people from the general population report Covid-19 PTSS, depression, and anxiety than health workers. Research has informed us about the psychological responses during Covid-19 in specific populations such as pregnant women who have given birth during the Covid-19 pandemic, military veterans, and psychiatric patients. It is worth noting that people's reactions to the pandemic are heterogeneous. For some, responses are stable; for some, mental health has improved, whereas for others, it has deteriorated.

Risk factors for Covid-19 PTSD include younger age, low educational attainment, low income and other social inequalities, loss of resources and disability, and gender differences, with women being a consistent predictor of PTSD severity and other distress outcomes. People belonging to ethnic minorities not only have to cope with stressors related to Covid-19, but also with racial prejudice and discrimination, which can increase the risk of PTSD and comorbid psychiatric symptoms. Parents and parents of colour who have dependent children are also vulnerable to Covid-19 PTSD. People who have a history of mental health problems are also vulnerable to PTSD related to the effects of Covid-19 and other distress outcomes. Past trauma may contribute to pre-existing mental health problems and influence the severity of Covid-19 PTSD.

Covid-19-related factors may also be associated with increased Covid-19 PTSD and comorbid psychiatric symptoms. These include greater exposure to traumatic Covid-19-related experiences, living in the Wuhan epicentre, infection with the virus and subsequent stigma, contact with infected family members, and experience of hospitalisation for Covid-19. Loss of a loved one is another factor associated with Covid-19. Other factors include lockdown, staying at home, social isolation, quarantine, domestic violence, and media exposure. Witnessing the death of patients due to Covid-19 may also be associated with PTSS.

Coping strategies are also associated with Covid-19 PTSD. These include negative coping strategies and fatalistic beliefs. On the other hand, spiritual fortitude can be an effective approach to produce posttraumatic growth traits. Other positive psychology coping strategies include acceptance, mindfulness, and loving kindness. Some people benefit from more practical types of coping strategies, and individual therapy with online self-help counselling. In addition to coping strategies, narcissism is also mentioned as a risk factor. Anxiety sensitivity is also a personality trait thought to influence respiratory symptoms in people with PTSD.

Research is also focusing on intervention strategies for people with Covid-19. Narrative exposure therapy appears to be effective in reducing PTSS. A service-learning mentoring programme has been shown to improve sleep, emotion regulation, executive functioning and mindfulness in adolescents during Covid-19. Those who received mentoring and mindfulness reported less PTSD and emotional impulsivity. Telepsychotherapy based on a strengths-based philosophy was suggested as another psychotherapeutic treatment for the community. Another suggested intervention tool is COVID coach, a public mental health app. Clinical programmes could also include trauma-focused virtual reality exposure therapy to help those on the front lines of the Covid-19 pandemic. Other interventions have also been suggested, including existential–humanistic and relational psychotherapy as well as art therapy.

References

Aafjes-van Doorn, K., Békés, V., Luo, X., Prout, T. A., & Hoffman, L. (2022). Therapists' resilience and posttraumatic growth during the COVID-19 pandemic. *Psychological Trauma*, *14*(S1), S165–S173. https://doi.org/10.1037/tra000109710.1037/tra0001097

Aafjes-van Doorn, K., Békés, V., Prout, T. A., & Hoffman, L. (2020). Psychotherapists' vicarious traumatization during the COVID-19 pandemic. *Psychological Trauma*, 12(S1), S148–S150. https://doi.org/10.1037/tra0000868

Ahmed, M. Z., Ahmed, O., Aibao, Z., Hanbin, S., Siyu, L., & Ahmad, A. (2020). Epidemic of COVID-19 in China and associated psychological problems. *Asian Journal of Psychiatry*, *51*, 102092. https://doi.org/https://doi.org/10.1016/j.ajp.2020.102092

Allan, S. M., Bealey, R., Birch, J., Cushing, T., Parke, S., Sergi, G., Bloomfield, M., & Meiser-Stedman, R. (2020). The prevalence of common and stress-related mental health disorders in healthcare workers based in pandemic-affected hospitals: a rapid systematic review and meta-analysis. *European Journal of Psychotraumatology*, *11*(1), 1810903. https://doi.org/10.1080/20008198.2020.1810903

Allgire, E., McAlees, J. W., Lewkowich, I. P., & Sah, R. (2021). Asthma and posttraumatic stress disorder (PTSD): Emerging links, potential models and mechanisms. *Brain, Behavior, and Immunity*, *97*, 275–285. https://doi.org/10.1016/j.bbi.2021.06.001

Alonzo, A., & Reynolds, N. (1998). The structure of emotions during acute myocardial infarction: a model of coping. *Social Science & Medicine*, *46*, 1099–1110.

Alpay, E. H., Kira, I. A., Shuwiekh, H. A. M., Ashby, J. S., Turkeli, A., & Alhuwailah, A. (2021). The effects of COVID-19 continuous traumatic stress on mental health: The case of Syrian refugees in Turkey. *Traumatology*, *27*, 375–387. https://doi.org/10.1037/trm0000347

American Psychiatric Association. (2013). *Diagnostic and statistical manual of mental disorders* (5th ed.). https://doi.org/10.1176/appi.books.9780890425596

Amsalem, D., Lazarov, A., Markowitz, J. C., Naiman, A., Smith, T. E., Dixon, L. B., & Neria, Y. (2021). Psychiatric symptoms and moral injury among us healthcare workers in the COVID-19 era. *BMC Psychiatry*, *21*. https://doi.org/10.1186/s12888-021-03565-9

Anton, M. T., Ridings, L. E., Gavrilova, Y., Bravoco, O., Ruggiero, K. J., & Davidson, T. M. (2020). Transitioning a technology-assisted stepped-care model for traumatic injury patients to a fully remote model in the age of Covid-19. *Counselling Psychology Quarterly*, *34*(11), 1–12. https://doi.org/10.1080/09515070.2020.1785393

Arcaya, M. C., Lowe, S. R., Rhodes, J. E., Waters, M. C., & Subramanian, S. V. (2014). Association of PTSD symptoms with asthma attacks among hurricane Katrina survivors. *Journal of Traumatic Stress*, *27*(6), 725–729. https://doi.org/10.1002/jts.21976

Banducci, A. N. (2021). Prolonged exposure therapy in the time of COVID-19: Modifying PTSD treatment for a military sexual trauma survivor who contracted COVID-19 mid-treatment. *Clinical Case Studies, 20*(4), 331–348. https://doi.org/10.1177/1534650121993547

Banducci, A. N., & Weiss, N. H. (2020). Caring for patients with posttraumatic stress and substance use disorders during the COVID-19 pandemic. *Psychological Trauma, 12*(S1), S113–S114. https://doi.org/10.1037/tra0000824

Banford Witting, A., Tambling, R., & Hobfoll, S. (2022). Resource loss, gain, and traumatic stress in couples during COVID-19. *Psychological Trauma, 15*(3), 502–510. https://doi.org/10.1037/tra0001276

Blackman, J. S. (2020). A psychoanalytic view of reactions to the coronavirus pandemic in China. *American Journal of Psychoanalysis, 80*(2), 119–132. https://doi.org/10.1057/s11231-020-09248-w

Blechert, J., Michael, T., Grossman, P., Lajtman, M., & Wilhelm, F. H. (2007). Autonomic and respiratory characteristics of posttraumatic stress disorder and panic disorder. *Psychosomatic Medicine, 69*(9), 935–943.

Bo, H.-X., Li, W., Yang, Y., Wang, Y., Zhang, Q., Cheung, T., Wu, X., & Xiang, Y.-T. (2021). Posttraumatic stress symptoms and attitude toward crisis mental health services among clinically stable patients with COVID-19 in China. *Psychological Medicine, 51*(6), 1052–1053. https://doi.org/10.1017/S0033291720000999

Boden, M., Cohen, N., Froelich, J. M., Hoggatt, K. J., Abdel Magid, H. S., & Mushiana, S. S. (2021). Mental disorder prevalence among populations impacted by Coronavirus pandemics: A multilevel meta-analytic study of COVID-19, MERS & SARS. *General Hospital Psychiatry, 70*, 124–133. https://doi.org/10.1016/j.genhosppsych.2021.03.006

Bogolyubova, O., Fernandez, A. S.-M., Lopez, B. T., & Portelli, P. (2021). Traumatic impact of the COVID-19 pandemic in an international sample: Contribution of fatalism to psychological distress and behavior change. *European Journal of Trauma & Dissociation, 5*(2), 100219. https://doi.org/https://doi.org/10.1016/j.ejtd.2021.100219

Boyraz, G., & Legros, D. N. (2020). Coronavirus disease (Covid-19) and traumatic stress: Probable risk factors and correlates of posttraumatic stress disorder. *Journal of Loss and Trauma, 25*(6–7), 503–522. https://doi.org/10.1080/15325024.2020.1763556

Brackbill, R. M., Hadler, J. L., DiGrande, L., Ekenga, C. C., Farfel, M. R., Friedman, S., Perlman, S. E., Stellman, S. D., Walker, D. J., Wu, D., Yu, S., & Thorpe, L. E. (2009). Asthma and posttraumatic stress symptoms 5 to 6 years following exposure to the World Trade Center terrorist attack. *JAMA, 302*(5), 502–516. https://doi.org/10.1001/jama.2009.1121

Bridgland, V. M. E., Moeck, E. K., Green, D. M., Swain, T. L., Nayda, D. M., Matson, L. A., Hutchison, N. P., & Takarangi, M. K. T. (2021). Why the COVID-19 pandemic is a traumatic stressor. *PLoS ONE, 16*(1), e0240146. https://doi.org/10.1371/journal.pone.0240146

Brooks, S. K., Webster, R. K., Smith, L. E., Woodland, L., Wessely, S., Greenberg, N., & Rubin, G. J. (2020). The psychological impact of quarantine and how to reduce it: rapid review of the evidence. *Lancet, 395*(10227), 912–920. https://doi.org/10.1016/s0140-6736(20)30460-8

Chen, S., & Bonanno, G. A. (2020). Psychological adjustment during the global outbreak of COVID-19: A resilience perspective. *Psychological Trauma, 12*(S1), S51–S54. https://doi.org/10.1037/tra0000685

Chen, Y., Huang, X., Zhang, C., An, Y., Liang, Y., Yang, Y., & Liu, Z. (2021). Prevalence and predictors of posttraumatic stress disorder, depression and anxiety among hospitalized patients with coronavirus disease 2019 in China. *BMC Psychiatry, 21*(1), 80. https://doi.org/10.1186/s12888-021-03076-7

Chew, N. W. S., Lee, G. K. H., Tan, B. Y. Q., Jing, M., Goh, Y., Ngiam, N. J. H., Yeo, L. L. L., Ahmad, A., Ahmed Khan, F., Napolean Shanmugam, G., Sharma, A. K., Komalkumar, R. N., Meenakshi, P. V., Shah, K., Patel, B., Chan, B. P. L., Sunny, S., Chandra, B., Ong, J. J. Y.,

… Sharma, V. K. (2020). A multinational, multicentre study on the psychological outcomes and associated physical symptoms amongst healthcare workers during COVID-19 outbreak. *Brain, Behavior, and Immunity, 88*, 559–565. https://doi.org/https://doi.org/10.1016/j.bbi.2020.04.049

Chung, M. C., & Wall, N. (2013). Alexithymia and posttraumatic stress disorder following asthma attack. *Psychiatric Quarterly, 84*, 287–302.

Chung, M. C., Berger, Z., & Rudd, H. (2008). Coping with posttraumatic stress disorder and co-morbidity after myocardial infarction. *Comprehensive Psychiatry, 49*(1), 55–64. https://doi.org/http://dx.doi.org/10.1016/j.comppsych.2007.08.003

Chung, M. C., Jones, R. C. M., Harding, S. A., & Campbell, J. (2016). Posttraumatic stress disorder among older patients with chronic obstructive pulmonary disease. *Psychiatric Quarterly, 87*(4), 605–618. https://doi.org/10.1007/s11126-015-9413-z

Chung, M. C., Rudd, H., & Wall, N. (2012). Posttraumatic stress disorder following asthma attack (post-asthma attack PTSD) and psychiatric co-morbidity: The impact of alexithymia and coping. *Psychiatry Research, 197*(3), 246–252.

Chung, M. C., Symons, C., Gilliam, J., & Kaminski, E. R. (2010a). The relationship between posttraumatic stress disorder, psychiatric comorbidity, and personality traits among patients with chronic idiopathic urticaria. *Comprehensive Psychiatry, 51*(1), 55–63.

Chung, M. C., Symons, C., Gilliam, J., & Kaminski, E. R. (2010b). Stress, psychiatric co-morbidity and coping in patients with chronic idiopathic urticaria. *Psychology & Health, 25*(4), 477–490.

Chung, M. C., Walsh, A., & Dennis, I. (2011). Trauma exposure characteristics, past traumatic life events, coping strategies, posttraumatic stress disorder and psychiatric co-morbidity among people with anaphylactic shock experience. *Comprehensive Psychiatry, 52*, 394–404.

Coleman, S. R. M. (2020). A commentary on potential associations between narcissism and trauma-related outcomes during the coronavirus pandemic. *Psychological Trauma, 12*(S1), S41–S42. https://doi.org/10.1037/tra0000768

Cottin, M., Hernández, C., Núñez, C., Labbé, N., Quevedo, Y., Davanzo, A., & Behn, A. (2021). "What if we get sick?": Spanish adaptation and validation of the fear of illness and virus evaluation scale in a non-clinical sample exposed to the COVID-19 pandemic. *Frontiers in Psychology, 12*, 590283. https://doi.org/10.3389/fpsyg.2021.590283

Davydow, D. S., Desai, S. V., Needham, D. M., & Bienvenu, O. J. (2008). Psychiatric morbidity in survivors of the acute respiratory distress syndrome: a systematic review. *Psychosomatic Medicine, 70*(4), 512–519. https://doi.org/10.1097/PSY.0b013e31816aa0dd

Debchoudhury, I., Welch, A. E., Fairclough, M. A., Cone, J. E., Brackbill, R. M., Stellman, S. D., & Farfel, M. R. (2011). Comparison of health outcomes among affiliated and lay disaster volunteers enrolled in the World Trade Center Health Registry. *Preventive Medicine, 53*(6), 359–363. https://doi.org/10.1016/j.ypmed.2011.08.034

Declercq, F., Vanheule, S., & Deheegher, J. (2010). Alexithymia and posttraumatic stress: subscales and symptom cluster. *Journal of Clinical Psychology, 66*, 1076–1089.

Di Giuseppe, M., Gemignani, A., & Conversano, C. (2020). Psychological resources against the traumatic experience of COVID-19. *Clinical Neuropsychiatry, 17*(2), 85–87.

Dragan, M., Grajewski, P., & Shevlin, M. (2021). Adjustment disorder, traumatic stress, depression and anxiety in Poland during an early phase of the COVID-19 pandemic. *European Journal of Psychotraumatology, 12*(1), 1860356. https://doi.org/10.1080/20008198.2020.1860356

Dutheil, F., Mondillon, L., & Navel, V. (2021). PTSD as the second tsunami of the SARS-CoV-2 pandemic. *Psychological Medicine, 51*(10), 1773–1774. https://doi.org/10.1017/S0033291720001336

Estes, K. D., & Thompson, R. R. (2020). Preparing for the aftermath of COVID-19: Shifting risk and downstream health consequences. *Psychological Trauma, 12*(S1), S31–S32. https://doi.org/10.1037/tra0000853

Fagan, J., Galea, S., Ahern, J., Bonner, S., & Vlahov, D. (2003). Relationship of self-reported asthma severity and urgent health care utilization to psychological sequelae of the September 11, 2001 terrorist attacks on the World Trade Center among New York City area residents. *Psychosomatic Medicine, 65*(6), 993–996. https://doi.org/10.1097/01.psy.0000097334.48556.5f

Fallahi, C. R., Blau, J. J. C., Mitchell, M. T., Rodrigues, H. A., Daigle, C. D., Heinze, A. M., LaChance, A., & DeLeo, L. (2021). Understanding the pandemic experience for people with a preexisting mental health disorder. *Traumatology, 27*(4), 471–478. https://doi.org/10.1037/trm0000344

Fan, C., Fu, P., Li, X., Li, M., & Zhu, M. (2021). Trauma exposure and the PTSD symptoms of college teachers during the peak of the Covid-19 outbreak. *Stress and Health, 37*(5), 914–927. https://doi.org/10.1002/smi.3049

Fan, Y., Shi, Y., Zhang, J., Sun, D., Wang, X., Fu, G., Mo, D., Wen, J., Xiao, X., & Kong, L. (2021). The effects of narrative exposure therapy on COVID-19 patients with post-traumatic stress symptoms: A randomized controlled trial. *Journal of Affective Disorders, 293*, 141–147. https://doi.org/10.1016/j.jad.2021.06.019

Fang, Y., Zhe, D., & Shuran, L. (2004). Survey on mental status of subjects recovered from SARS. [In Chinese.] *Chinese Mental Health Journal, 18*(10), 675–677.

Gallagher, M. W., Smith, L. J., Richardson, A. L., & Long, L. J. (2021). Examining associations between Covid-19 experiences and posttraumatic stress. *Journal of Loss and Trauma, 26*(8), 752–766. https://doi.org/10.1080/15325024.2021.1886799

Gardner, P. J., & Moallef, P. (2015). Psychological impact on SARS survivors: Critical review of the English language literature. *Canadian Psychology/Psychologie canadienne, 56*(1), 123–135. https://doi.org/10.1037/a0037973

Geng, S., Zhou, Y., Zhang, W., Lou, A., Cai, Y., Xie, J., Sun, J., Zhou, W., Liu, W., & Li, X. (2021). The influence of risk perception for COVID-19 pandemic on posttraumatic stress disorder in healthcare workers: A survey from four designated hospitals. *Clinical Psychology & Psychotherapy, 28*(5), 1146–1159. https://doi.org/https://doi.org/10.1002/cpp.2564

González-Freire, B., Vázquez-Rodríguez, I., Marcos-Velázquez, P., & de la Cuesta, C. G. (2010). Repression and coping styles in asthmatic patients. *Journal of Clinical Psychology in Medical Settings, 17*(3), 220–229. https://doi.org/10.1007/s10880-010-9198-z

Gonzalez-Garcia, V., Exertier, M., & Denis, A. (2021). Anxiety, post-traumatic stress symptoms, and emotion regulation: A longitudinal study of pregnant women having given birth during the COVID-19 pandemic. *European Journal of Trauma & Dissociation, 5*(2), 100225. https://doi.org/10.1016/j.ejtd.2021.100225

González-Sanguino, C., Ausín, B., Castellanos, M. A., Saiz, J., & Muñoz, M. (2021). Mental health consequences of the Covid-19 outbreak in Spain A longitudinal study of the alarm situation and return to the new normality. *Progress in Neuro-Psychopharmacology & Biological Psychiatry, 107*, 110219. https://doi.org/10.1016/j.pnpbp.2020.110219

Gordon, R. M., Dahan, J. F., Wolfson, J. B., Fults, E., Lee, Y. S. C., Smith-Wexler, L., Liberta, T. A., & McGiffin, J. N. (2021). Existential–humanistic and relational psychotherapy during COVID-19 with patients with preexisting medical conditions. *Journal of Humanistic Psychology, 61*(4), 470–492. https://doi.org/10.1177/0022167820973890

Guck, A. J., Buck, K., & Lehockey, K. (2021). Psychological complications of COVID-19 following hospitalization and ICU discharge: Recommendations for treatment. *Professional Psychology: Research and Practice, 52*(4), 318–327. https://doi.org/10.1037/pro0000402

Guo, Q., Zheng, Y., Shi, J., Wang, J., Li, G., Li, C., Fromson, J. A., Xu, Y., Liu, X., Xu, H., Zhang, T., Lu, Y., Chen, X., Hu, H., Tang, Y., Yang, S., Zhou, H., Wang, X., Chen, H., ... Yang, Z. (2020). Immediate psychological distress in quarantined patients with COVID-19 and its association with peripheral inflammation: A mixed-method study. *Brain, Behavior, and Immunity, 88*, 17–27. https://doi.org/https://doi.org/10.1016/j.bbi.2020.05.038

Gupta, M. (2010). Dermatological conditions. In Fink, G. (Ed.), *Stress consequences: Mental, neuropsychological and socioeconomic* (pp. 420–424). Elsevier/Academic Press.

Hahm, H. C., Ha, Y., Scott, J. C., Wongchai, V., Chen, J. A., & Liu, C. H. (2021). Perceived COVID-19-related anti-Asian discrimination predicts post traumatic stress disorder symptoms among Asian and Asian American young adults. *Psychiatry Research, 303*, 114084. https://doi.org/10.1016/j.psychres.2021.114084

Hampton, M. R., & Frombach, I. (2000). Women's experience of traumatic stress in cancer treatment. *Health Care for Women International, 21*(1), 67–76. https://doi.org/10.1080/0739 93300245410

Hayatbakhsh, M. R., Najman, J. M., Clavarino, A., Bor, W., Williams, G. M., & O'Callaghan, M. J. (2010). Association of psychiatric disorders, asthma and lung function in early adulthood. *Journal of Asthma, 47*(7), 786–791. https://doi.org/10.3109/02770903.2010.489141

Helminen, E. C., Scheer, J. R., Jackson, S. D., Brisbin, C. D., Batchelder, A. W., Cascalheira, C. J., & Sullivan, T. P. (2021). PTSD symptoms and hazardous drinking indicators among trauma-exposed sexual minority women during heightened societal stress. *Behavioral Medicine, 49*(2), 183–194. https://doi.org/10.1080/08964289.2021.2006132

Hesselink, A. E., Penninx, B. W., Schlösser, M. A., Wijnhoven, H. A., van der Windt, D. A., Kriegsman, D. M., & van Eijk, J. T. (2004). The role of coping resources and coping style in quality of life of patients with asthma or COPD. *Quality of Life Research, 13*(2), 509–518. https://doi.org/10.1023/B:QURE.0000018474.14094.2f

Hill, M. L., Nichter, B., Na, P. J., Norman, S. B., Morland, L. A., Krystal, J. H., & Pietrzak, R. H. (2021). Mental health impact of the Covid-19 pandemic in US Military veterans: A population-based, prospective cohort study. *Psychological Medicine, 53*(3), 945–956. https://doi.org/10.1017/S0033291721002361

Ho, S. M., Kwong-Lo, R. S., Mak, C. W., & Wong, J. S. (2005). Fear of severe acute respiratory syndrome (SARS) among health care workers. *Journal of Consulting and Clinical Psychology, 73*(2), 344–349.

Holmes, M. R., Rentrope, C. R., Korsch-Williams, A., & King, J. A. (2021). Impact of COVID-19 pandemic on posttraumatic stress, grief, burnout, and secondary trauma of social workers in the United States. *Clinical Social Work Journal, 49*(4), 495–504. https://doi.org/10.1007/s10 615-021-00795-y

Hong, X., Currier, G. W., Zhao, X., Jiang, Y., Zhou, W., & Wei, J. (2009). Posttraumatic stress disorder in convalescent severe acute respiratory syndrome patients: A 4-year follow-up study. *General Hospital Psychiatry, 31*(6), 546–554. https://doi.org/10.1016/j.genhospps ych.2009.06.008

Horesh, D., & Brown, A. D. (2020). Traumatic stress in the age of COVID-19: A call to close critical gaps and adapt to new realities. *Psychological Trauma, 12*(4), 331–335. https://doi. org/10.1037/tra0000592

Hou, T., Yin, Q., Cai, W., Song, X., Deng, W., Zhang, J., & Deng, G. (2022). Posttraumatic stress symptoms among health care workers during the COVID-19 epidemic: The roles of negative coping and fatigue. *Psychology, Health & Medicine, 27*(2), 367–378. https://doi.org/10.1080/ 13548506.2021.1921228

Hovenkamp-Hermelink, J. H. M., van der Veen, D. C., Oude Voshaar, R. C., Batelaan, N. M., Penninx, B. W. J. H., Jeronimus, B. F., Schoevers, R. A., & Riese, H. (2019). Anxiety sensitivity, its stability and longitudinal association with severity of anxiety symptoms. *Scientific Reports,* *9*(1), 4314. https://doi.org/10.1038/s41598-019-39931-7

Hung, Y. H., Cheng, C. M., Lin, W. C., Bai, Y. M., Su, T. P., Li, C. T., Tsai, S. J., Pan, T. L., Chen, T. J., & Chen, M. H. (2019). Post-traumatic stress disorder and asthma risk: A nationwide longitudinal study. *Psychiatry Research, 276,* 25–30. https://doi.org/10.1016/j.psychres.2019.04.014

Hunkin, V., & Chung, M. C. (2012). Chronic idiopathic urticaria, psychological co-morbidity and posttraumatic stress: The impact of alexithymia and repression. *Psychiatric Quarterly,* *83*(4), 431–447. https://doi.org/10.1007/s11126-012-9213-7

Inchausti, F., MacBeth, A., Hasson-Ohayon, I., & Dimaggio, G. (2020). *Telepsychotherapy in the age of COVID-19: A commentary. Journal of Psychotherapy Integration, 30*(2), 394–405.

Jaworski, B. K., Taylor, K., Ramsey, K. M., Heinz, A., Steinmetz, S., Pagano, I., Moraja, G., & Owen, J. E. (2021). Exploring usage of COVID Coach, a public mental health app designed for the COVID-19 pandemic: Evaluation of analytics data. *Journal of Medical Internet Research, 23*(3), e26559. https://doi.org/10.2196/26559

Jiang, F., Deng, L., Zhang, L., Cai, Y., Cheung, C. W., & Xia, Z. (2020). Review of the clinical characteristics of coronavirus disease 2019 (COVID-19). *Journal of General Internal Medicine, 35*(5), 1545–1549. https://doi.org/10.1007/s11606-020-05762-w

Jones, R. C., Harding, S. A., Chung, M. C., & Campbell, J. (2009). The prevalence of posttraumatic stress disorder in patients undergoing pulmonary rehabilitation and changes in PTSD symptoms following rehabilitation. *Journal of Cardiopulmonary Rehabilitation and Prevention, 29*(1), 49–56. https://doi.org/10.1097/HCR.0b013e318192787e

Ju, Y., Liu, J., Ng, R. M. K., Liu, B., Wang, M., Chen, W., Huang, M., Yang, A., Shu, K., Zhou, Y., Zhang, L., Liao, M., Liu, J., & Zhang, Y. (2021). Prevalence and predictors of post-traumatic stress disorder in patients with cured coronavirus disease 2019 (COVID-19) one month post-discharge. *European Journal of Psychotraumatology, 12*(1). https://doi.org/10.1080/20008198.2021.1915576

Kang, L., Ma, S., Chen, M., Yang, J., Wang, Y., Li, R., Yao, L., Bai, H., Cai, Z., Xiang Yang, B., Hu, S., Zhang, K., Wang, G., Ma, C., & Liu, Z. (2020). Impact on mental health and perceptions of psychological care among medical and nursing staff in Wuhan during the 2019 novel coronavirus disease outbreak: A cross-sectional study. *Brain, Behavior, and Immunity, 87,* 11–17. https://doi.org/https://doi.org/10.1016/j.bbi.2020.03.028

Kanzler, K. E., & Ogbeide, S. (2020). Addressing trauma and stress in the COVID-19 pandemic: Challenges and the promise of integrated primary care. *Psychological Trauma, 12*(S1), S177–S179. https://doi.org/10.1037/tra0000761

Kapfhammer, H. P., Rothenhäusler, H. B., Krauseneck, T., Stoll, C., & Schelling, G. (2004). Posttraumatic stress disorder and health-related quality of life in long-term survivors of acute respiratory distress syndrome. *American Journal of Psychiatry, 161*(1), 45–52. https://doi.org/10.1176/appi.ajp.161.1.45

Kaseda, E. T., & Levine, A. J. (2020). Post-traumatic stress disorder: A differential diagnostic consideration for COVID-19 survivors. *Clinical Neuropsychology, 34*(7–8), 1498–1514. https://doi.org/10.1080/13854046.2020.1811894

Kean, E. M., Kelsay, K., Wamboldt, F., & Wamboldt, M. Z. (2006). Posttraumatic stress in adolescents with asthma and their parents. *Journal of the American Academy of Child & Adolescent Psychiatry, 45*(1), 78–86. https://doi.org/10.1097/01.chi.0000186400.67346.02

Kesner, L., & Horáček, J. (2020). Three challenges that the Covid-19 pandemic represents for psychiatry. *British Journal of Psychiatry, 217*(3), 475–476. https://doi.org/10.1192/bjp.2020.106

Kira, I. A., Shuwiekh, H. A. M., Alhuwailah, A., Ashby, J. S., Sous Fahmy Sous, M., Baali, S. B. A., Azdaou, C., Oliemat, E. M., & Jamil, H. J. (2021). The effects of COVID-19 and collective identity trauma (intersectional discrimination) on social status and well-being. *Traumatology*, *27*, 29–39. https://doi.org/10.1037/trm0000289

Kisely, S., Warren, N., McMahon, L., Dalais, C., Henry, I., & Siskind, D. (2020). Occurrence, prevention, and management of the psychological effects of emerging virus outbreaks on healthcare workers: Rapid review and meta-analysis. *BMJ*, *369*, ArtID m1642.

Kokou-Kpolou, C. K., Fernandez-Alcantara, M., & Cenat, J. M. (2020). Prolonged grief related to COVID-19 deaths: Do we have to fear a steep rise in traumatic and disenfranchised griefs? *Psychological Trauma*, *12*(S1), S94–S95. https://doi.org/10.1037/tra0000798

Krass, P., Zimbrick-Rogers, C., Iheagwara, C., Ford, C. A., & Calderoni, M. (2020). COVID-19 outbreak among adolescents at an inpatient behavioral health hospital. *Journal of Adolescent Health*, *67*(4), 612–614. https://doi.org/10.1016/j.jadohealth.2020.07.009

Kupchik, M., Strous, R. D., Erez, R., Gonen, N., Weizman, A., & Spivak, B. (2007). Demographic and clinical characteristics of motor vehicle accident victims in the community general health outpatient clinic: a comparison of PTSD and non-PTSD subjects. *Depression and Anxiety*, *24*, 244–250. https://doi.org/10.1002/da.20189

Kwek, S.-K., Chew, W.-M., Ong, K.-C., Ng, A. W.-K., Lee, L. S.-U., Kaw, G., & Leow, M. K.-S. (2006). Quality of life and psychological status in survivors of severe acute respiratory syndrome at 3 months postdischarge. *Journal of Psychosomatic Research*, *60*(5), 513–519. https://doi.org/10.1016/j.jpsychores.2005.08.020

Lai, J., Ma, S., Wang, Y., Cai, Z., Hu, J., Wei, N., Wu, J., Du, H., Chen, T., Li, R., Tan, H., Kang, L., Yao, L., Huang, M., Wang, H., Wang, G., Liu, Z., & Hu, S. (2020). Factors associated with mental health outcomes among health care workers exposed to coronavirus disease 2019. *JAMA Network Open*, *3*(3), e203976–e203976. https://doi.org/10.1001/jamanetworko pen.2020.3976

Lee, A. M., Wong, J. G., McAlonan, G. M., Cheung, V., Cheung, C., Sham, P. C., Chu, C. M., Wong, P. C., Tsang, K. W., & Chua, S. E. (2007). Stress and psychological distress among SARS survivors 1 year after the outbreak. *Canadian Journal of Psychiatry*, *52*(4), 233–240. https://doi.org/10.1177/070674370705200405

Liang, L., Ren, H., Cao, R., Hu, Y., Qin, Z., Li, C., & Mei, S. (2020a). The effect of COVID-19 on youth mental health. *Psychiatric Quarterly*, *91*(3), 841–852. https://doi.org/10.1007/s11 126-020-09744-3

Lissoni, B., Del Negro, S., Brioschi, P., Casella, G., Fontana, I., Bruni, C., & Lamiani, G. (2020). Promoting resilience in the acute phase of the COVID-19 pandemic: Psychological interventions for intensive care unit (ICU) clinicians and family members. *Psychological Trauma*, *12*(S1), S105–S107. https://doi.org/10.1037/tra0000802

Liu, N., Zhang, F., Wei, C., Jia, Y., Shang, Z., Sun, L., Wu, L., Sun, Z., Zhou, Y., Wang, Y., & Liu, W. (2020). Prevalence and predictors of PTSS during COVID-19 outbreak in China hardest-hit areas: Gender differences matter. *Psychiatry Research*, *287*, 112921. https://doi.org/https://doi.org/10.1016/j.psychres.2020.112921

Lockett, M., Pyszczynski, T., & Koole, S. L. (2021). Pandemic reminders as psychological threat: Thinking about Covid-19 lowers coping self-efficacy among trauma-exposed adults. *Cognition and Emotion*, *36*(1), 23–30. https://doi.org/10.1080/02699931.2021.2020731

Lund, E. M. (2021). Even more to handle: Additional sources of stress and trauma for clients from marginalized racial and ethnic groups in the united states during the Covid-19 pandemic. *Counselling Psychology Quarterly*, *34*(3–4), 321–330. https://doi.org/10.1080/09515 070.2020.1766420

Ma, L., Mazidi, M., Li, K., Li, Y., Chen, S., Kirwan, R., Zhou, H., Yan, N., Rahman, A., Wang, W., & Wang, Y. (2021). Prevalence of mental health problems among children and adolescents during the COVID-19 pandemic: A systematic review and meta-analysis. *Journal of Affective Disorders*, *293*, 78–89. https://doi.org/10.1016/j.jad.2021.06.021

MacKenzie, M., Daviskiba, S., Dow, M., Johnston, P., Balon, R., Javanbakht, A., & Arfken, C. L. (2021). The impact of the coronavirus disease 2019 (COVID-19) pandemic on healthcare workers with pre-existing psychiatric conditions. *Psychiatric Quarterly*, *92*(3), 1011–1020. https://doi.org/10.1007/s11126-020-09870-y

Mactavish, A., Mastronardi, C., Menna, R., Babb, K. A., Battaglia, M., Amstadter, A. B., & Rappaport, L. M. (2021). Children's mental health in Southwestern Ontario during summer 2020 of the COVID-19 pandemic. *Journal of the Canadian Academy of Child and Adolescent Psychiatry/Journal de l'Académie canadienne de psychiatrie de l'enfant et de l'adolescent*, *30*(3), 177–190.

Magill, E., Siegel, Z., & Pike, K. M. (2020). The mental health of frontline health care providers during pandemics: A rapid review of the literature. *Psychiatric Services*, *71*(12), 1260–1269. https://doi.org/10.1176/appi.ps.202000274

Mahaffey, B. L., Gonzalez, A., Farris, S. G., Zvolensky, M. J., Bromet, E. J., Luft, B. J., & Kotov, R. (2017). Understanding the connection between posttraumatic stress symptoms and respiratory problems: Contributions of anxiety sensitivity. *Journal of Traumatic Stress*, *30*(1), 71–79. https://doi.org/10.1002/jts.22159

Mauer, M. P., Cummings, K. R., & Carlson, G. A. (2007). Health effects in New York State personnel who responded to the World Trade Center disaster. *Journal of Occupational and Environmental Medicine*, *49*(11), 1197–1205. https://doi.org/10.1097/JOM.0b013e318 157d31d

Maunder, R. G. (2009). Was SARS a mental health catastrophe? *General Hospital Psychiatry*, *31*(4), 316–317. https://doi.org/10.1016/j.genhosppsych.2009.04.004

Mayopoulos, G. A., Ein-Dor, T., Dishy, G. A., Nandru, R., Chan, S. J., Hanley, L. E., Kaimal, A. J., & Dekel, S. (2021). COVID-19 is associated with traumatic childbirth and subsequent mother–infant bonding problems. *Journal of Affective Disorders*, *282*, 122–125. https://doi.org/10.1016/j.jad.2020.12.101

McAlonan, G. M., Lee, A. M., Cheung, V., Cheung, C., Tsang, K. W. T., Sham, P. C., Chua, S. E., & Wong, J. G. W. S. (2007). Immediate and sustained psychological impact of an emerging infectious disease outbreak on health care workers. *The Canadian Journal of Psychiatry/La Revue canadienne de psychiatrie*, *52*(4), 241–247. https://doi.org/10.1177/07067437070 5200406

McFarlane, A. C. (1990). Vulnerability to posttraumatic stress disorder. In M. E. Wolf & A. D. Mosnaim (Eds.), *Posttraumatic stress disorder: Etiology, phenomenology and treatment* (pp. 3–20). American Psychiatric Association.

Megalakaki, O., Kokou-Kpolou, C. K., Vaudé, J., Park, S., Iorfa, S. K., Cénat, J. M., & Derivois, D. (2021). Does peritraumatic distress predict PTSD, depression and anxiety symptoms during and after COVID-19 lockdown in France? A prospective longitudinal study. *Journal of Psychiatric Research*, *137*, 81–88. https://doi.org/10.1016/j.jpsychires.2021.02.035

Miller, R. L., Moran, M., Shomaker, L. B., Seiter, N., Sanchez, N., Verros, M., Rayburn, S., Johnson, S., & Lucas-Thompson, R. (2021). Health effects of COVID-19 for vulnerable adolescents in a randomized controlled trial. *School Psychology*, *36*(5), 293–302. https://doi.org/10.1037/spq0000458

Moallef, P., Lueke, N. A., Gardner, P. J., & Patcai, J. (2021). Chronic PTSD and other psychological sequelae in a group of frontline healthcare workers who contracted and survived SARS. *Canadian Journal of Behavioural Science/Revue canadienne des sciences du comportement*, *53*(3), 342–352. https://doi.org/10.1037/cbs0000252

Moccia, L., Janiri, D., Pepe, M., Dattoli, L., Molinaro, M., De Martin, V., Chieffo, D., Janiri, L., Fiorillo, A., Sani, G., & Di Nicola, M. (2020). Affective temperament, attachment style, and the psychological impact of the COVID-19 outbreak: an early report on the Italian general population. *Brain, Behavior, and Immunity*, *87*, 75–79. https://doi.org/https://doi.org/10.1016/j.bbi.2020.04.048

Montauk, T. R., & Kuhl, E. A. (2020). COVID-related family separation and trauma in the intensive care unit. *Psychological Trauma*, *12*(S1), S96–S97. https://doi.org.10.1037/tra0000839

Moring, J. C., Dondanville, K. A., Fina, B. A., Hassija, C., Chard, K., Monson, C., LoSavio, S. T., Wells, S. Y., Morland, L. A., Kaysen, D., Galovski, T. E., & Resick, P. A. (2020). Cognitive processing therapy for posttraumatic stress disorder via telehealth: Practical considerations during the Covid-19 pandemic. *Journal of Traumatic Stress*, *33*(4), 371–379.

Mosheva, M., Gross, R., Hertz-Palmor, N., Hasson-Ohayon, I., Kaplan, R., Cleper, R., Kreiss, Y., Gothelf, D., & Pessach, I. M. (2021). The association between witnessing patient death and mental health outcomes in frontline COVID-19 healthcare workers. *Depression and Anxiety*, *38*(4), 468–479. https://doi.org/10.1002/da.23140

Mucci, F., Mucci, N., & Diolaiuti, F. (2020). Lockdown and isolation: Psychological aspects of COVID-19 pandemic in the general population. *Clinical Neuropsychiatry*, *17*(2), 63–64. https://doi.org/10.36131/CN20200205

Mukherjee, M., & Maity, C. (2021). Influence of media engagement on the post traumatic stress disorder in context of the COVID-19 pandemic: An empirical reflection from India. *Journal of Human Behavior in the Social Environment*, *31*(1–4), 409–424. https://doi.org/10.1080/10911359.2020.1833806

Murata, S., Rezeppa, T., Thoma, B., Marengo, L., Krancevich, K., Chiyka, E., Hayes, B., Goodfriend, E., Deal, M., Zhong, Y., Brummit, B., Coury, T., Riston, S., Brent, D. A., & Melhem, N. M. (2021). The psychiatric sequelae of the COVID-19 pandemic in adolescents, adults, and health care workers. *Depression and Anxiety*, *38*(2), 233–246. https://doi.org/10.1002/da.23120

Nieforth, L. O., & O'Haire, M. E. (2020). The role of pets in managing uncertainty from COVID-19. *Psychological Trauma*, *12*(S1), S245–S246. https://doi.org/10.1037/tra0000678

Niles, A. N., Dour, H. J., Stanton, A. L., Roy-Byrne, P. P., Stein, M. B., Sullivan, G., Sherbourne, C. D., Rose, R. D., & Craske, M. G. (2015). Anxiety and depressive symptoms and medical illness among adults with anxiety disorders. *Journal of Psychosomatic Research*, *78*(2), 109–115. https://doi.org/10.1016/j.jpsychores.2014.11.018

O'Toole, B. I., & Catts, S. V. (2008). Trauma, PTSD, and physical health: an epidemiological study of Australian Vietnam veterans. *Journal of Psychosomatic Research*, *64*(1), 33–40. https://doi.org/10.1016/j.jpsychores.2007.07.006

Palgi, Y., Greenblatt-Kimron, L., Hoffman, Y., Goodwin, R., & Ben-Ezra, M. (2021). Factors associated with current posttraumatic stress disorder among COVID-19 vaccinated older adults in Israel. *Journal of Psychiatric Research*, *142*, 272–274. https://doi.org/10.1016/j.jpsychores.2021.08.005

Pérez-Fuentes, M. d. C., Molero Jurado, M. d. M., Martos Martínez, Á., Simón Márquez, M. d. M., & Gázquez Linares, J. J. (2021). Mood and affective balance of Spaniards confined by COVID-19: A cross-sectional study. *International Journal of Psychological Research*, *14*(1), 55–65. https://doi.org/10.21500/20112084.4765

Poletti, B., Tagini, S., Brugnera, A., Parolin, L., Pievani, L., Ferrucci, R., Compare, A., & Silani, V. (2020). Telepsychotherapy: A leaflet for psychotherapists in the age of Covid-19. A review of the evidence. *Counselling Psychology Quarterly*, *34*(3–4), 352–367. https://doi.org/10.1080/09515070.2020.1769557

Polizzi, C., Lynn, S. J., & Perry, A. (2020). Stress and coping in the time of COVID-19: Pathways to resilience and recovery. *Clinical Neuropsychiatry*, *17*(2), 59–62. https://doi.org/10.36131/CN20200204

Potash, J. S., Kalmanowitz, D., Fung, I., Anand, S. A., & Miller, G. M. (2020). Art therapy in pandemics: Lessons for Covid-19. *Art Therapy*, *37*(2), 105–107. https://doi.org/10.1080/07421656.2020.1754047

Poyraz, B. Ç., Poyraz, C. A., Olgun, Y., Gürel, Ö., Alkan, S., Özdemir, Y. E., Balkan, İ. İ., & Karaali, R. (2021). Psychiatric morbidity and protracted symptoms after COVID-19. *Psychiatry Research*, *295*, 113604. https://doi.org/https://doi.org/10.1016/j.psychres.2020.113604

Qi, J., Sun, R., & Zhou, X. (2021). Network analysis of comorbid posttraumatic stress disorder and depression in adolescents across COVID-19 epidemic and Typhoon Lekima. *Journal of Affective Disorders*, *295*, 594–603. https://doi.org/10.1016/j.jad.2021.08.080

Rajkumar, R. P. (2020). COVID-19 and mental health: A review of the existing literature. *Asian Journal of Psychiatry*, *52*, 102066. https://doi.org/10.1016/j.ajp.2020.102066

Rizzo, A. S., Hartholt, A., & Mozgai, S. (2021). From combat to COVID-19—Managing the impact of trauma using virtual reality. *Journal of Technology in Human Services*, *39*(3), 314–347. https://doi.org/10.1080/15228835.2021.1915931

Rodriguez-Rey, R., Garrido-Hernansaiz, H., & Collado, S. (2020). Psychological impact of COVID-19 in Spain: Early data report. *Psychological Trauma*, *12*(5), 550–552. https://doi.org/10.1037/tra0000943

Ronen-Setter, I. H., & Cohen, E. (2020). Becoming "teletherapeutic": Harnessing accelerated experiential dynamic psychotherapy (AEDP) for challenges of the Covid-19 era. *Journal of Contemporary Psychotherapy*, *50*, 265–273. https://doi.org/10.1007/s10879-020-09462-8

Rosen, C. S., Glassman, L. H., & Morland, L. A. (2020). Telepsychotherapy during a pandemic: A traumatic stress perspective. *Journal of Psychotherapy Integration*, *30*(2), 174–187.

Sansone, R. A., Sinclair, J. D., & Wiederman, M. W. (2009). Drug allergies and childhood trauma among chronic pain patients. *Psychiatry*, *6*, 17–18.

Scott, K. M., Von Korff, M., Ormel, J., Zhang, M. Y., Bruffaerts, R., Alonso, J., Kessler, R. C., Tachimori, H., Karam, E., Levinson, D., Bromet, E. J., Posada-Villa, J., Gasquet, I., Angermeyer, M. C., Borges, G., de Girolamo, G., Herman, A., & Haro, J. M. (2007). Mental disorders among adults with asthma: results from the World Mental Health Survey. *General Hospital Psychiatry*, *29*(2), 123–133. https://doi.org/10.1016/j.genhosppsych.2006.12.006

Seitz, K. I., Bertsch, K., & Herpertz, S. C. (2021). A prospective study of mental health during the Covid-19 pandemic in childhood trauma-exposed individuals: Social support matters. *Journal of Traumatic Stress*, *34*(3), 477–486. https://doi.org/10.1002/jts.22660

Shakespeare-Finch, J., Bowen-Salter, H., Cashin, M., Badawi, A., Wells, R., Rosenbaum, S., & Steel, Z. (2020). Covid-19: An Australian perspective. *Journal of Loss and Trauma*, *25*(8), 662–672. https://doi.org/10.1080/15325024.2020.1780748

Shaw, R. J., Harvey, J. E., Nelson, K. L., Gunary, R., Kruk, H., & Steiner, H. (2001). Linguistic analysis to assess medically related posttraumatic stress symptoms. *Psychosomatics*, *42*(1), 35–40. https://doi.org/10.1176/appi.psy.42.1.35

Shechter, A., Diaz, F., Moise, N., Anstey, D. E., Ye, S., Agarwal, S., Birk, J. L., Brodie, D., Cannone, D. E., Chang, B., Claassen, J., Cornelius, T., Derby, L., Dong, M., Givens, R. C., Hochman, B., Homma, S., Kronish, I. M., Lee, S. A. J., . . . Abdalla, M. (2020). Psychological distress, coping behaviors, and preferences for support among New York healthcare workers during the COVID-19 pandemic. *General Hospital Psychiatry*, *66*, 1–8. https://doi.org/10.1016/j.genhosppsych.2020.06.007

Shek, D. T. L., Zhao, L., Dou, D., Zhu, X., & Xiao, C. (2021). The impact of positive youth development attributes on posttraumatic stress disorder symptoms among Chinese adolescents under COVID-19. *Journal of Adolescent Health*, *68*(4), 676–682. https://doi.org/10.1016/j.jadohealth.2021.01.011

Shevlin, M., Butter, S., McBride, O., Murphy, J., Gibson-Miller, J., Hartman, T. K., Levita, L., Mason, L., Martinez, A. P., McKay, R., Stocks, T. V. A., Bennett, K., Hyland, P., & Bentall, R.

P. (2021). Refuting the myth of a 'tsunami' of mental ill-health in populations affected by COVID-19: evidence that response to the pandemic is heterogeneous, not homogeneous. *Psychological Medicine*, *53*(2), 1–9. https://doi.org/10.1017/s0033291721001665

Shigemoto, Y. (2021). Exploring state-level variabilities between perceived community resilience and posttraumatic stress symptoms during the COVID-19 pandemic: Multilevel modeling approach. *Traumatology*, *27*(1), 98–106. https://doi.org/10.1037/trm0000303

Shiratori, Y., & Samuelson, K. W. (2012). Relationship between posttraumatic stress disorder and asthma among New York area residents exposed to the World Trade Center disaster. *Journal of Psychosomatic Research*, *73*(2), 122–125. https://doi.org/10.1016/j.jpsychores.2012.05.003

Shortland, N., McGarry, P., & Merizalde, J. (2020). Moral medical decision-making: Colliding sacred values in response to COVID-19 pandemic. *Psychological Trauma*.

Shrira, A., & Felsen, I. (2021). Parental PTSD and psychological reactions during the COVID-19 pandemic among offspring of Holocaust survivors. *Psychological Trauma*, *13*(4), 438–445. https://doi.org/10.1037/tra0001014

Sim, K., Chan, Y. H., Chong, P. N., Chua, H. C., & Soon, S. W. (2010). Psychosocial and coping responses within the community health care setting towards a national outbreak of an infectious disease. *Journal of Psychosomatic Research*, *68*(2), 195–202. https://doi.org/10.1016/j.jpsychores.2009.04.004

Sim, K., Chong, P. N., Chan, Y. H., & Soon, W. S. (2004). Severe acute respiratory syndrome-related psychiatric and posttraumatic morbidities and coping responses in medical staff within a primary health care setting in Singapore. *Journal of Clinical Psychiatry*, *65*(8), 1120–1127. https://doi.org/10.4088/jcp.v65n0815

Singh, S. P., & Khokhar, A. (2021). Prevalence of posttraumatic stress disorder and depression in general population in India during COVID-19 pandemic home quarantine. *Asia–Pacific Journal of Public Health*, *33*(1), 154–156. https://doi.org/10.1177/1010539520968455

Solomon, Z., Ginzburg, K., Ohry, A., & Mikulincer, M. (2021). Overwhelmed by the news: A longitudinal study of prior trauma, posttraumatic stress disorder trajectories, and news watching during the COVID-19 pandemic. *Social Science & Medicine*, *278*, 113956. https://doi.org/10.1016/j.socscimed.2021.113956

Spitzer, C., Barnow, S., Volzke, H., John, U., Freyberger, H. J., & Grabe, H. J. (2009). Trauma, posttraumatic stress disorder, and physical illness: Findings from the general population. *Psychosomatic Medicine*, *71*(9), 1012–1017.

Spitzer, C., Koch, B., Grabe, H. J., Ewert, R., Barnow, S., Felix, S. B., Ittermann, T., Obst, A., Völzke, H., Gläser, S., & Schäper, C. (2011). Association of airflow limitation with trauma exposure and post-traumatic stress disorder. *European Respiratory Journal*, *37*(5), 1068–1075. https://doi.org/10.1183/09031936.00028010

Stewart, R. W., Orengo-Aguayo, R., Young, J., Wallace, M. M., Cohen, J. A., Mannarino, A. P., & de Arellano, M. A. (2020). Feasibility and effectiveness of a telehealth service delivery model for treating childhood posttraumatic stress: A community-based, open pilot trial of trauma-focused cognitive-behavioral therapy. *Journal of Psychotherapy Integration*, *30*(2), 274–289.

Styra, R., Hawryluck, L., McGeer, A., Dimas, M., Sheen, J., Giacobbe, P., Dattani, N., Lorello, G., Rac, V. E., Francis, T., Wu, P. E., Luk, W.-S., Ng, E., Nadarajah, J., Wingrove, K., & Gold, W. L. (2021). Surviving SARS and living through COVID-19: Healthcare worker mental health outcomes and insights for coping. *PLoS ONE*, *16*(11), e0258893. https://doi.org/10.1371/journal.pone.0258893

Styra, R., Hawryluck, L., Robinson, S., Kasapinovic, S., Fones, C., & Gold, W. L. (2008). Impact on health care workers employed in high-risk areas during the Toronto SARS outbreak. *Journal of Psychosomatic Research*, *64*(2), 177–183. https://doi.org/10.1016/j.jpsychores.2007.07.015

Sun, L., Sun, Z., Wu, L., Zhu, Z., Zhang, F., Shang, Z., Jia, Y., Gu, J., Zhou, Y., Wang, Y., Liu, N., & Liu, W. (2020). Prevalence and risk factors of acute posttraumatic stress symptoms during the COVID-19 outbreak in Wuhan, China. *medRxiv*, 2020.2003.2006.20032425. https://doi. org/10.1101/2020.03.06.20032425

Sun, R., Qi, J., Huang, J., & Zhou, X. (2021). Network analysis of PTSD in college students across different areas after the COVID-19 epidemic. *European Journal of Psychotraumatology*, *12*(1), 1920203. https://doi.org/10.1080/20008198.2021.1920203

Taylor-Clift, A., Holmgreen, L., Hobfoll, S. E., Gerhart, J. I., Richardson, D., Calvin, J. E., & Powell, L. H. (2016). Traumatic stress and cardiopulmonary disease burden among low-income, urban heart failure patients. *Journal of Affective Disorders*, *190*, 227–234. https://doi. org/10.1016/j.jad.2015.09.023

Taylor, G. J., & Bagby, R. M. (2012). The alexithymia personality dimension. In T. A. Widiger (Ed.), *The Oxford handbook of personality disorders* (pp. 648–673). Oxford University Press.

Taylor, S., Landry, C. A., Paluszek, M. M., Fergus, T. A., McKay, D., & Asmundson, G. J. G. (2020). Covid stress syndrome: Concept, structure, and correlates. *Depression and Anxiety*, *37*(8), 706–714. https://doi.org/doi: 10.1002/da.23071

Thomas, J., Hashmi, A. A., Chung, M. C., Morgan, K., & Lyons, M. (2013). The narcissistic mask: An exploration of 'the defensive grandiosity hypothesis'. *Personality and Mental Health*, *7*(2), 160–167.

Tian, F., Li, H., Tian, S., Yang, J., Shao, J., & Tian, C. (2020). Psychological symptoms of ordinary Chinese citizens based on SCL-90 during the level I emergency response to COVID-19. *Psychiatry Research*, *288*, 112992. https://doi.org/10.1016/j.psychres.2020.112992

Ting, T. C. M., Wong, A. W. S., Liu, W. S., Leung, F. L. T., & Ng, M. T. (2021). Impact of COVID-19 outbreak on posttraumatic stress in patients with psychiatric illness. *Psychiatry Research*, *303*, 114065. https://doi.org/10.1016/j.psychres.2021.114065

Trnka, R., & Lorencova, R. (2020). Fear, anger, and media-induced trauma during the outbreak of COVID-19 in the Czech Republic. *Psychological Trauma*, *12*(5), 546–549. https://doi.org/ 10.1037/tra0000675

Tsai, J., & Shen, J. (2017). Exploring the link between posttraumatic stress disorder and inflammation-related medical conditions: An epidemiological examination. *Psychiatric Quarterly*, *88*(4), 909–916. https://doi.org/10.1007/s11126-017-9508-9

Tull, M. T., Edmonds, K. A., Scamaldo, K. M., Richmond, J. R., Rose, J. P., & Gratz, K. L. (2020). Psychological outcomes associated with stay-at-home orders and the perceived impact of COVID-19 on daily life. *Psychiatry Research*, *289*, 113098. https://doi.org/https://doi.org/ 10.1016/j.psychres.2020.113098

Van Tongeren, D. R., Aten, J. D., McElroy, S., Davis, D. E., Shannonhouse, L., Davis, E. B., & Hook, J. N. (2019). Development and validation of a measure of spiritual fortitude. *Psychological Trauma*, *11*, 588–596. https://doi.org/10.1037/tra0000449

Vanderbilt, D., Young, R., MacDonald, H. Z., Grant-Knight, W., Saxe, G., & Zuckerman, B. (2008). Asthma severity and PTSD symptoms among inner city children: a pilot study. *Journal of Trauma Dissociation*, *9*(2), 191–207. https://doi.org/10.1080/15299730802046136

Villarreal-Zegarra, D., Copez-Lonzoy, A., Vilela-Estrada, A. L., & Huarcaya-Victoria, J. (2021). Depression, post-traumatic stress, anxiety, and fear of COVID-19 in the general population and health-care workers: Prevalence, relationship, and explicative model in Peru. *BMC Psychiatry*, *21*, Art. 455. https://doi.org/10.1186/s12888-021-03456-z

Vitale, E. (2021). How the Italian women perceived distress from their puerperal conditions during the COVID-19 outbreak. *Journal of Psychopathology*, *27*(3), 135–139.

Wade, M., Prime, H., Johnson, D., May, S. S., Jenkins, J. M., & Browne, D. T. (2021). The disparate impact of COVID-19 on the mental health of female and male caregivers. *Social Science & Medicine*, *275*, 113801. https://doi.org/10.1016/j.socscimed.2021.113801

Wade, S. L., Gies, L. M., Fisher, A. P., Moscato, E. L., Adlam, A. R., Bardoni, A., Corti, C., Limond, J., Modi, A. C., & Williams, T. (2020). Telepsychotherapy with children and families: Lessons gleaned from two decades of translational research. *Journal of Psychotherapy Integration*, 30(2), 332–347.

Wagner, E. H., Hoelterhoff, M., & Chung, M. C. (2017). Posttraumatic stress disorder following asthma attack: the role of agency beliefs in mediating psychiatric morbidity. *Journal of Mental Health*, 26(4), 342–350. https://doi.org/10.1080/09638237.2017.1340628

Wamboldt, M. Z., Weintraub, P., Krafchick, D., Berce, N., & Wamboldt, F. S. (1995). Links between past parental trauma and the medical and psychological outcome of asthmatic children: A theoretical model. *Families, Systems, & Health*, 13, 129–149. https://doi.org/10.1037/h0089303

Wamser-Nanney, R., Nguyen-Feng, V., Lotzin, A., & Zhou, X. (2021). Parenting amidst COVID-19: Pandemic-related stressors, inequities, and treatment utilization and perceptions. *Couple and Family Psychology: Research and Practice*, 12(2), 55–65. https://doi.org/10.1037/cfp0000189

Wang, Y., Di, Y., Ye, J., & Wei, W. (2021). Study on the public psychological states and its related factors during the outbreak of coronavirus disease 2019 (COVID-19) in some regions of China. *Psychology, Health & Medicine*, 26(1), 13–22. https://doi.org/10.1080/13548506.2020.1746817

Waszczuk, M. A., Li, X., Bromet, E. J., Gonzalez, A., Zvolensky, M. J., Ruggero, C., Luft, B. J., & Kotov, R. (2017). Pathway from PTSD to respiratory health: Longitudinal evidence from a psychosocial intervention. *Health Psychology*, 36(5), 429–437. https://doi.org/10.1037/hea0000472 10.1037/hea0000472

Waszczuk, M. A., Ruggero, C., Li, K., Luft, B. J., & Kotov, R. (2019). The role of modifiable health-related behaviors in the association between PTSD and respiratory illness. *Behaviour Research and Therapy*, 115, 64–72. https://doi.org/10.1016/j.brat.2018.10.018

Waters, E. K., Pellen, D., & Buus, N. (2021). Psychiatry research in the COVID-19 era and beyond: A role for mathematical models. *Australian & New Zealand Journal of Psychiatry*, 55(2), 221–222. https://doi.org/10.1177/0004867420978460

Weiser, E. B. (2007). The prevalence of anxiety disorders among adults with asthma: A meta-analytic review. *Journal of Clinical Psychology in Medical Settings*, 14(4), 297–307. https://doi.org/10.1007/s10880-007-9087-2

World Health Organization. (2019). Coronavirus disease (COVID-19) pandemic. https://www.who.int/emergencies/diseases/novel-coronavirus-2019

Wu, K. K., Chan, S. K., & Ma, T. M. (2005). Posttraumatic stress, anxiety, and depression in survivors of severe acute respiratory syndrome (SARS). *Journal of Traumatic Stress*, 18(1), 39–42. https://doi.org/10.1002/jts.20004

Wu, P., Fang, Y., Guan, Z., Fan, B., Kong, J., Yao, Z., Liu, X., Fuller, C. J., Susser, E., Lu, J., & Hoven, C. W. (2009). The psychological impact of the SARS epidemic on hospital employees in China: exposure, risk perception, and altruistic acceptance of risk. *Canadian Journal of Psychiatry*, 54(5), 302–311. https://doi.org/10.1177/070674370905400504

Wu, W., Zhang, Y., Wang, P., Zhang, L., Wang, G., Lei, G., Xiao, Q., Cao, X., Bian, Y., Xie, S., Huang, F., Luo, N., Zhang, J., & Luo, M. (2020). Psychological stress of medical staffs during outbreak of COVID-19 and adjustment strategy. *Journal of Medical Virology*, 92(10), 1962–1970. https://doi.org/10.1002/jmv.25914

Wytrychiewicz, K., Pankowski, D., Jasinski, M., & Fal, A. M. (2020). Commentary on COVID-19 situation in Poland: Practical and empirical evaluation of current state. *Psychological Trauma*, 12(5), 542–545. https://doi.org/10.1037/tra0000676

Xu, Y., Zhang, K., & Liu, Z. (2005). Control study on posttraumatic stress response in SARS patients and the public in SARS prevalent area. *Chinese Journal of Clinical Psychology, 13*(2), 210–212.

Yin, Q., Sun, Z., Liu, T., Ni, X., Deng, X., Jia, Y., Shang, Z., Zhou, Y., & Liu, W. (2020). Posttraumatic stress symptoms of health care workers during the corona virus disease 2019. *Clinical Psychology & Psychotherapy, 27*(3), 384–395. https://doi.org/10.1002/cpp.2477

Young, K. P., Kolcz, D. L., O'Sullivan, D. M., Ferrand, J., Fried, J., & Robinson, K. (2021). Health care workers' mental health and quality of life during COVID-19: Results from a mid-pandemic, national survey. *Psychiatric Services, 72*(2), 122–128. https://doi.org/10.1176/appi.ps.202000424

Zakeri, M. A., Dehghan, M., Ghaedi Heidari, F., Pakdaman, H., Mehdizadeh, M., Ganjeh, H., Sanji Rafsanjani, M., & Hossini Rafsanjanipoor, S. M. (2021). Mental health outcomes among health-care workers during the COVID-19 outbreak in Iran. *Mental Health Review Journal, 26*(2), 152–160. https://doi.org/10.1108/MHRJ-10-2020-0075

Zerach, G., & Levi-Belz, Y. (2021). Moral injury and mental health outcomes among Israeli health and social care workers during the COVID-19 pandemic: A latent class analysis approach. *European Journal of Psychotraumatology, 12*(1), 1945749. https://doi.org/10.1080/20008198.2021.1945749

Zhang, H., Hook, J. N., Van Tongeren, D. R., Davis, E. B., Aten, J. D., McElroy-Heltzel, S., Davis, D. E., Shannonhouse, L., Hodge, A. S., & Captari, L. E. (2021). Spiritual fortitude: A systematic review of the literature and implications for COVID-19 coping. *Spirituality in Clinical Practice, 8*, 229–244. https://doi.org/10.1037/scp0000267

Zhang, H., Xu, H., Huang, L., Wang, Y., Deng, F., Wang, X., Tang, X., Wang, W., Fu, X., Tao, Y., & Yin, L. (2021). Increased occurrence of PTSD symptoms in adolescents with major depressive disorder soon after the start of the COVID-19 outbreak in China: A cross-sectional survey. *BMC Psychiatry, 21*, Art 395. https://doi.org/10.1186/s12888-021-03400-1

Zhou, X. (2020). Managing psychological distress in children and adolescents following the COVID-19 epidemic: A cooperative approach. *Psychological Trauma, 12*(S1), S76–S78. https://doi.org/10.1037/tra0000754

9

Posttraumatic stress disorder and autoimmune diseases

The relationship between posttraumatic stress disorder (PTSD) and autoimmune diseases, including arthritis, type 1 diabetes, and multiple sclerosis, has been documented. Previous studies have focused on the relationship between PTSD and autoimmune diseases in general, while some studies have combined autoimmune diseases with non-autoimmune diseases. One large study looked at more than 120,000 military personnel and found that the risk of any of the selected autoimmune diseases (rheumatoid arthritis, systemic lupus erythematosus, inflammatory bowel disease, and multiple sclerosis) was 58% (hazard ratio: 1.58) higher in those with PTSD due to prior trauma than in those without PTSD. These results did not change significantly even after accounting for body mass index, smoking habits, alcohol consumption, combat experience, and past physical or sexual assault (Bookwalter et al., 2020). These findings seemed to mirror the results of a previous study of 666,269 veterans in which 30.6% met criteria for PTSD and 19.5% developed psychiatric disorders other than PTSD. Those with PTSD had a higher risk of any of the autoimmune disorders (thyroiditis, inflammatory bowel disease, rheumatoid arthritis, multiple sclerosis, lupus) alone or in combination than veterans without psychiatric disorders (adjusted relative risk (aRR): 2.00) and those with non-PTSD-related psychiatric disorders (aRR: 1.51). Military sexual trauma was associated with an increased risk of autoimmune disorders in both genders (O'Donovan et al., 2015).

Turning to patients in primary care, of 502 patients with at least one anxiety disorder, approximately 46% met diagnostic criteria for PTSD. Patients with PTSD reported significantly more current and lifetime illnesses than patients with other, non-PTSD anxiety disorders. Those with PTSD tended to have a range of medical problems, including arthritis, diabetes, as well as anaemia, asthma, back pain, eczema, kidney or lung disease, and ulcers. PTSD was the strongest predictor of these medical problems along with other predictors such as trauma history, physical injury, lifestyle characteristics, or depression

Posttraumatic Stress in Physical Illness. Man Cheung Chung, Oxford University Press. © Oxford University Press 2024.
DOI: 10.1093/oso/9780198727323.003.0009

(Weisberg et al., 2002). In another study on patients in primary care, a gender effect was observed. In female primary care patients, early trauma was not associated with arthritis, but with digestive disease and cancer. In male patients, however, prior trauma was associated with arthritis and diabetes. PTSD carried the impact of prior trauma on arthritis but not on diabetes (Norman et al., 2006).

Gulf War veterans were also thought to have developed PTSD, depression and chronic disease. After controlling for demographic variables, combat exposure, and nuclear, biological, and chemical warfare agents, veterans with experiential avoidance coping tended to have a higher likelihood of PTSD, arthritis, as well as gastrointestinal problems, irritable bowel syndrome, fibromyalgia, and chronic fatigue syndrome (odds ratio (OR) ranging from 1.25 to 2.89) (Blakey et al., 2021). In a large-scale study based on a nationally representative sample of veterans, a gender effect was observed in that female veterans reported higher prevalence rates of lifetime PTSD (OR: 3.33), lifetime (OR: 2.10) and current depression (OR: 2.79), and lifetime arthritis along with migraine and osteoporosis (OR: 2.14–9.74) compared to male veterans (Ziobrowski et al., 2017). Refugees also tended to have poorer psychological and physical health, and more chronic diseases (e.g. type 2 diabetes mellitus) than the population they were resettled in. They seemed to lack knowledge about their disease, symptoms, and self-management, resulting in a lower ability to control their chronic diseases (Shahin et al., 2018).

A population survey also showed that, after controlling for sociodemographic variables and psychiatric disorders, participants with potentially traumatic events had an increased likelihood of all physical illnesses (e.g. arthritis, chronic pain, cardiovascular disease, respiratory disease) compared to adults who were not exposed to traumatic events, with an OR of 1.48 for the autoimmune disease arthritis. Traumatic events included sexual and physical violence and the unexpected death of a loved one. There was evidence of a dose–response phenomenon in that as the number of traumatic events in the past increased, so did the likelihood of all physical illnesses. Traumatic life events appeared to increase the risk of chronic physical illness, independent of psychiatric disorders (Atwoli et al., 2016).

Another epidemiological study also showed that, after controlling for sociodemographic variables and psychological disorders, psychological trauma (e.g. neglect) was associated with arthritis and diabetes along with cardiovascular and gastrointestinal diseases. Natural disasters or terrorism were associated with arthritis, cardiovascular disease, and gastrointestinal disease, while surprisingly, combat-related trauma and other trauma were not associated with any physical disease. A dose–response effect was also observed in the relationship between the number of traumatic events and physical illness. It appears that certain types and number of traumas can influence physical health problems differently and independently of PTSD (Husarewycz et al., 2014). This is in contrast to a previous study suggesting that specific trauma (i.e. childhood trauma) influences autoimmune diseases such as rheumatoid arthritis and other autoimmune diseases through the effects of PTSD, rather than independently (Mulvihill, 2005).

As mentioned in previous chapters, PTSD is not a discrete clinical syndrome, but is often comorbid with other psychological disorders. These coexisting conditions may play a role in influencing physical illness. The physical illnesses appear to vary depending on whether individuals have PTSD alone or a comorbidity of PTSD and major depressive disorder (MDD). After controlling for demographic factors and substance use, veterans with comorbid PTSD and MDD were more likely to suffer from rheumatoid arthritis as well as cardiovascular disease, migraine, and fibromyalgia than those with MDD alone. The former were about three times more likely to report disability than the latter. Veterans with concurrent PTSD and MDD, as well as with PTSD alone, reported more physical dysfunction than those with MDD alone. Veterans with concurrent PTSD and MDD appeared to be at high risk for physical health problems (Nichter et al., 2019). Similarly, the percentage of PTSD and/or depression was higher in people with diabetes (PTSD: 5.9%; depression: 24.4%), along with other chronic conditions such as anaemia, angina, cataract, dyslipidaemia, chronic bronchitis, heart failure, stroke, kidney disease, and tuberculosis in a group of middle-aged people (Pengpid & Peltzer, 2020).

PTSD and arthritis

PTSD is a stronger predictor of common medical complaints than trauma history, physical injury, lifestyle factors, or comorbid depression in primary care patients. Compared to patients without PTSD, patients with PTSD were more than four times as likely to report arthritis. In comparison, people with PTSD were more than twice as likely to have anaemia, lung disease, or an ulcer. They were also more than three times as likely to develop kidney disease (Weisberg et al., 2002). Their trauma-related stress responses can be characterised by arousal and passive cognitive–affective avoidance responses as well as re-experiencing and active avoidance responses (Livneh & Martz, 2006).

Some researchers focusing on arthritis with pain as a dominant clinical feature found that in patients with chronic pain due to arthritis and low back pain, trauma symptoms predicted pain intensity. Emotional reactivity as a temperament trait was associated with increased global trauma symptoms, which in turn were associated with increased pain intensity (Rzeszutek et al., 2015). There appear to be gender differences in response to chronic pain. Trauma symptoms and body image were associated with pain intensity in men, while trauma symptoms and age were associated with pain intensity in women (Rzeszutek et al., 2016). Age may also play a role in that older adults with these painful conditions (e.g. arthritis, back pain, and migraine) tend to have increased anxiety disorder symptoms, including PTSD. Those who had anxiety and physical problems such as arthritis and others (allergies, cataracts and lung disease) tended to report worse physical and/or mental health problems after adjusting for confounding variables (El-Gabalawy et al., 2011).

Painful conditions, including arthritis/rheumatism, appear to be related not only to PTSD and other psychiatric comorbid symptoms (e.g. depression and bipolar disorder), but also to certain types of trauma. People who had negative experiences in childhood tended to report increased painful medical complaints. Childhood trauma was associated with increased anxiety and mood disorders, which in turn were associated with increased painful medical conditions (Sachs-Ericsson et al., 2017).

Cannabis has been prescribed for possible relief of PTSD symptoms and pain intensity, but this may increase the likelihood of cannabis use disorder (CUD) in people with musculoskeletal pain such as arthritis. Compared to people without PTSD, people with PTSD reported higher rates of CUD (9.4% vs 2.2%). People with PTSD and digestive pain, PTSD and nerve pain, and PTSD and any chronic pain had higher odds of CUD, ranging from 1.88 to 2.32, than people who had neither PTSD nor chronic pain (Bilevicius et al., 2019). Similarly, opioids are often prescribed as a treatment strategy for patients with chronic pain. Chronic pain and PTSD may coexist, which is associated with opioid use disorder (OUD). Patients with PTSD have been found to have a higher prevalence rate of OUD than those without PTSD (4.3% vs 0.7%). Musculoskeletal pain and nerve pain were significantly associated with OUD in both chronic pain condition alone and comorbid PTSD and chronic pain condition, with the largest effect size in the group with comorbid PTSD and chronic pain condition (musculoskeletal pain + PTSD: aOR1: 4.2; nerve pain + PTSD: aOR1: 3.1) (Bilevicius et al., 2018).

PTSD and type 1 diabetes

An international integrative review argued that PTSD, alterations in the hypothalamic–pituitary axis, an unhealthy lifestyle, and elevated C-reactive protein may play a role in the link between depression and physical illness, including type 1 diabetes (Bica et al., 2017). The association between diabetes and PTSD in adults in the community has been established. Diabetes was associated with an increased likelihood of PTSD (OR: 2.3), even after controlling for differences in sociodemographic characteristics. Interestingly, diabetes was not associated with an increased likelihood of other psychological disorders (Goodwin & Davidson, 2005).

A national comorbidity survey looking at comorbidity and burden of disease also showed that PTSD was among the most burdensome psychological disorders at the individual level, along with panic/agoraphobia, bipolar disorder, and major depression, while diabetes was also among them, along with neurological disorders and chronic pain conditions (Gadermann et al., 2012). In addition, patients with diabetes (28% overall) reported symptoms of depression and coexisting PTSD (58%) and generalised anxiety (77%) (Vanderlip et al., 2014). Compared to people without diabetes, people with diabetes have been shown to have higher prevalence rates for anxiety disorders and PTSD, mood disorders, major depressive disorder, and specific phobias, but lower prevalence rates for substance use disorders, alcohol and tobacco use, and cannabis use. Those with diabetes and comorbid psychological disorders reported lower levels of physical and mental functioning. Psychological disorders were associated with gender, age, race, and ethnicity in people with diabetes (Boden, 2018). Similarly, people with type 1 diabetes tended to report higher levels of depression than healthy controls and greater fear about disease progression than childhood cancer survivors. Young people with diabetes were more vulnerable to these distress outcomes (Kremer et al., 2017).

Similarly, people who had survived a major disaster such as the 9/11 attack showed a significant association between PTSD and diabetes (aOR: 1.28) (Miller-Archie et al., 2014). After wars, veterans with PTSD tend to suffer from diabetes in addition to osteoarthritis, heart disease, depression, obesity, and elevated lipid levels and are more likely to use medical services (David et al., 2004). Primary care patients with PTSD due to past trauma reported a higher number of current and lifetime medical conditions, including diabetes, than patients with other, non-PTSD-related anxiety disorders.

Notwithstanding this, an epidemiological study examining the association between PTSD and inflammation-related illnesses found that PTSD was strongly associated with an increased likelihood of insulin resistance, but with the lowest likelihood of type 1 diabetes (OR: 0.43) (Tsai & Shen, 2017). Also, a national survey of veterans found that overall, 6.1% of the sample met diagnostic criteria for full PTSD and 9.0% for subthreshold PTSD. However, only subthreshold PTSD was associated with an increased likelihood of diabetes (aOR: 1.42). Dysphoric arousal symptoms, characterised by difficulty sleeping, anger/irritability, and difficulty concentrating appeared to play a role in influencing these outcomes (El-Gabalawy et al., 2018).

Rather than looking at diabetes as a whole, one study examined hypoglycaemia fear and hypoglycaemia-specific posttraumatic stress in people with type 1 diabetes, >25% of whom met diagnostic criteria for current PTSD. Perceived threat of death related to hypoglycaemia and hypoglycaemia fear was significantly associated with PTSD. The number of recent hypoglycaemic episodes did not predict posttraumatic stress symptoms (PTSS)/PTSD (Myers et al., 2007). Another study also confirmed PTSS associated with hyperglycaemia in adults with type 1 diabetes. It found that >30% of respondents reported PTSD symptoms associated with hyperglycaemia, using standard scoring. PTSD was associated with diabetes self-management behaviours and perceived helplessness to hyperglycaemia. Perceived helplessness, severity of hypoglycaemia, perceived threat of death, HbA1c (glycated haemoglobin) level, and self-management behaviour were associated with severity of PTSS. The combination of fear, helplessness, and perceived death threat was the strongest predictor of PTSD and PTSS (Renna et al., 2016). Another study confirmed this finding: it showed that individuals with PTSD and depression in the past month reported the highest hyperglycaemia and hospitalisations in the past year, but had low health status (Aronson et al., 2016).

The relationship between PTSD and diabetes appears to be influenced by several factors. Adverse childhood experiences may lead to coexisting psychological and somatic disorders such as PTSD and diabetes, in addition to other disorders such as depression, borderline personality disorder, and obesity (Herzog & Schmahl, 2018). The impact of childhood trauma on the development of psychological disorders and physical illness is perhaps no surprise. Adverse childhood circumstances are considered a factor in the occurrence of psychobiological maladjustments, which can be explained by changes in physiological systems (e.g. low cortisol levels, elevated inflammatory markers) in children and in their developmental stages of childhood and adolescence (Ehlert, 2013). Childhood trauma may be associated with PTSD, other psychological disorders (e.g. anxiety, depression, bipolar disorder) and physical diseases such as diabetes and cardiovascular disease, but the heritability of phenotypes associated with adverse childhood experiences, such as PTSD, depression, and resilience, is low to moderate and may vary for a given phenotype, suggesting that there may be an interaction between genes and environment in the development of these phenotypes (Jiang et al., 2019).

There appears to be a gender effect influencing the relationship between PTSD and diabetes. In male primary care patients, past trauma was associated with both diabetes and arthritis, although PTSD did not mediate the association between trauma and diabetes. In female primary care patients, trauma was not associated with diabetes but with other diseases such as digestive disorders and cancer (Norman et al., 2006). Also, a large-scale study looking at veterans found that female veterans had a higher prevalence of lifetime PTSS (OR: 3.33) and lifetime (OR: 2.10) and current (OR: 2.76) major depressive disorder compared to male veterans, but lower prevalence estimates for diabetes, myocardial infarction, and high blood pressure (OR ranging from 0.05 to 0.49) (Ziobrowski et al., 2017). However, a systematic review shows that there is a significant association between PTSD and diabetes in female veterans, although other psychological disorders (e.g. depression and substance use disorders) and physical illnesses (e.g. cardiovascular disease, gastrointestinal disease, hypertension, obesity, pain, and urinary symptoms) were also found. These associations may impact health behaviours, such as preventive care and treatment adherence (Creech et al., 2021). Self-management of diabetes mellitus, which is characterised by adherence to medication, exercise, healthy diet, and blood glucose testing, was also found to be influenced by other health problems. For example, early stage cancer survivors with cancer-related PTSS symptoms could affect adherence to some diabetes mellitus self-management behaviours. One study found that 33% of these cancer survivors with cancer-related PTSS symptoms had problems with an unhealthy diet (James et al., 2018).

Ethnicity also appears to play a role, as according to a population-based national survey, the association between lifetime PTSD and diabetes was stronger among non-Latino blacks than whites. Prior PTSD was associated with a significantly higher risk of diabetes in blacks than in whites (Nobles et al., 2016). Another study also examined the association between PTSD and chronic disease in Latino and non-Latino whites. Significant interactions were found between Latino ethnicity and PTSD for the likelihood of diabetes (OR Latino: 2.18 vs 0.81 non-Latino white) and cardiovascular disease (OR Latino: 3.23 vs 1.28 non-Latino white) and hypertension (OR Latino: 1.61 vs 0.98 non-Latino white). Among US-born Latinos, a significant interaction between ethnicity and PTSD was found for the odds of cardiovascular disease (OR Latino: 4.18 vs 1.28 non-Latino white) and diabetes (OR Latino: 2.27 vs 0.81 non-Latino white) (Valentine et al., 2017). One study looked at different countries in Europe, the Middle East, Africa, and Asia, finding that the risk of mood and anxiety disorders was higher in people with diabetes than in people without diabetes, with ORs for anxiety disorders including PTSD and depression of 1.20 and 1.38, respectively, after adjusting for age and gender. The OR estimates did not differ significantly between countries (Lin & Von Korff, 2008).

It has been suggested that helping people with anxiety and a comorbid condition such as diabetes or MI is one of the most costly and demanding interventions (Marciniak et al., 2005). A preliminary study shows that a weekly telephone-based intervention to promote self-care behaviour or diabetes management appears to be effective for veterans with diabetes and PTSS. Veterans were satisfied with and benefited from the intervention, reduced their psychological distress, exercised more, and ate healthier (Collins et al., 2014).

Secondary victims of diabetes

According to a systematic review, parents of children hospitalised for conditions such as type 1 diabetes, cancer, meningococcal disease, severe injury, and other serious conditions requiring intensive care reported acute stress disorder at rates ranging from 12% to 63%; the prevalence rate for PTSD ranged from 8% to 68% (Woolf et al., 2016). A meta-analysis also showed that parents of children and adolescents with paediatric chronic physical illness may have high levels of PTSS and PTSD. The reason for using two outcome indicators is that although some chronic conditions no longer meet the exposure criteria for a PTSD diagnosis according to the DSM-5 (American Psychiatric Association, 2013), parents of children with these conditions may still experience PTSS; 18.9% of parents met the criteria for PTSD related to their children's chronic illness (e.g. effects associated with the illness, treatment complications, painful medical interventions, emergency hospitalisation, etc.). These parents were significantly more likely to meet PTSD criteria (OR: 7.12) than parents in the other normative samples. PTSS was most frequent in parents of children with diabetes ($g = 1.16$) and epilepsy ($g = 1.25$). PTSS was also positively associated with maternity, severity of illness, duration/intensity of treatment, and child PTSS. Parents who have experienced traumatic events related to their child's chronic illnesses could thus develop

PTSS and PTSD. Psychological interventions might be warranted for these parents (Pinquart, 2019).

To distinguish psychological responses between parents of children with type 1 diabetes mellitus or cancer, 16% of fathers and 23.9% of mothers met the full DSM-IV (American Psychiatric Association, 1994) criteria for current PTSD related to their children's illness (Landolt et al., 2003). Among fathers of children who had either cancer, type 1 diabetes mellitus, or who had suffered an unintentional injury, the former fathers reported higher rates of PTSD (26% at Time 1 and 21% at Time 2, respectively) than did the fathers of children with unintentional injuries (12% at Time 1 and 6% at Time 2, respectively). The severity of PTSS decreased over time (six months after the child's diagnosis or accident) in both groups (Ribi et al., 2007). Compared to mothers of children with cancer, mothers of children with type 1 diabetes reported higher cortisol levels. In other words, mothers of children with type 1 diabetes mellitus may be vulnerable to stress, which is characterised by the biological marker cortisol (Greening et al., 2017). Two groups of mothers with type 1 diabetes or cancer may not differ in the frequency of PTSD related to their children's illnesses. Overall, 7% of mothers met criteria for PTSD using the structured clinical interview, while 17% met criteria using self-report. Mothers with elevated depressive and anxiety symptoms and stressful life events tended to report significantly more PTSD symptoms (Stoppelbein & Greening, 2007).

To distinguish stress reactions between parents of children with type 1 diabetes, 24% of mothers and 22% of fathers met the full diagnosis for full PTSD related to their children's illness, while 51% of mothers and 41% of fathers met criteria for partial or subclinical PTSD. PTSD was not related to children's age and gender, socioeconomic status, family structure, or length of hospital stay (Landolt et al., 2002). Among mothers of youth with type 1 diabetes, PTSS was most severe at the onset of the disease and symptoms often persisted for 1–5 years after diagnosis. The level of stress and PTSS of the mothers in turn affected the health of the children. In other words, improving mothers' stress responses can lead to improved behavioural and metabolic outcomes in children (Rechenberg et al., 2017). Another study also showed that 10% of mothers of children with diabetes met criteria for full PTSD, while 15% met criteria for partial PTSD. More than half (55%) reported that the news of their child's diagnosis was the most traumatic stressor. Forty per cent and 17% also reported moderate-to-severe anxiety and depression, respectively (Horsch et al., 2007). Negative cognitive appraisals and dysfunctional cognitive appraisals were positively associated with PTSD symptoms related to diabetes trauma. On the other hand, social support was negatively associated with PTSD symptoms (Horsch et al., 2012). In addition, children of mothers with PTSD related to their children's diagnosis of type 1 diabetes reported more problems with adherence to the treatment regime than those without PTSD. However, this result depended on the mothers who had younger children (aged ≤8 years) and who were more actively involved in their children's treatment (Horsch & McManus, 2014).

PTSD and type 2 diabetes

Whether type 2 diabetes is an autoimmune disease is controversial. Nevertheless, studies have been conducted looking at the relationship between PTSD and type 2 diabetes, which deserves some attention. A large-scale population study found that 1.7% of people met the diagnosis of full PTSD, 8.8% met partial PTSD, and 11.2% met type 2 diabetes and 16.8% met prediabetes. After controlling for sociodemographic characteristics and metabolic risk factors, full PTSD was significantly associated with type 2 diabetes (OR: 3.90) compared to those who did not have a traumatic event. The same results persisted after controlling for psychopathological conditions (OR: 3.56). Meanwhile, no significant associations were found in those with pre-diabetes. In other words, PTSD could influence chronic stress symptoms and physiological mechanisms leading to type 2 diabetes (Lukaschek et al., 2013).

After controlling for age, the cumulative incidence of diabetes was significantly higher in twins with PTSD (18.9%) than in twins without PTSD (14.4%) (OR: 1.4) and in twins with subthreshold PTSD (16.4%) (OR: 1.2). PTSD was associated with a 40% increased risk of new-onset type 2 diabetes, which could be partly explained by metabolic and behavioural risk factors such as overweight and hypertension. These factors are known to influence insulin resistance. PTSD appears to be a marker of neuroendocrine and metabolic dysregulation that could lead to the development of type 2 diabetes (Vaccarino et al., 2014).

PTSD and other autoimmune diseases

Some studies have investigated PTSD and multiple sclerosis (MS), another form of autoimmune disease. Of patients with MS, 16% met symptom criteria for PTSD, with 75% reporting intrusions related to their worries about their prognosis (Chalfant et al., 2004). Higher MS-related disability and comorbid health conditions were both significantly associated with PTSD symptoms (Counsell et al., 2013). A case study has raised awareness of the link between PTSD and Guillain–Barré syndrome. This patient was successfully treated with interventions for PTSD (Chemtob & Herriott, 1994).

Summary

The association between PTSD and autoimmune diseases has been established in a variety of samples, including primary care patients, veterans, and the general population. People with PTSD are more than four times more likely to develop arthritis. Trauma and emotional reactivity are associated with arthritis pain intensity. The link between diabetes and PTSD in community adults has also been established. In addition to PTSD, diabetics also suffer from depression and anxiety. People with diabetes have been shown to have higher prevalence rates for a range of psychiatric disorders, compared to people without diabetes. Victims of terrorist attacks, war veterans, and primary care patients have been shown to have diabetes among other conditions, although this link is not always consistent. Research has also examined hypoglycaemic fear and hypoglycaemia-specific posttraumatic stress in people with type 1 diabetes.

The relationship between PTSD and diabetes is influenced by several factors. These include adverse childhood experiences and gender differences, with trauma being associated with diabetes and arthritis in more men than women. However, a systematic review has also found a significant association between PTSD and diabetes in female veterans. Ethnicity is another factor that suggests that the association between PTSD and diabetes appears to be stronger in black people than in white people.

The literature also looks at PTSD and PTSS in parents of children with diabetes and other conditions. Both parents appear to respond differently to their children with diabetes or other illnesses, with mothers more likely to encounter PTSD related to their children's illness than fathers. Looking at the stress reactions of parents of children who only have type 1 diabetes, more mothers than fathers tend to have a diagnosis of full, partial or subclinical PTSD in relation to their children's illness.

Research has also been conducted on PTSD associated with other autoimmune diseases, including type 2 diabetes, although whether or not it is an autoimmune disease is still controversial. It has been postulated that PTSD may influence chronic stress and physiological mechanisms leading to type

2 diabetes. In addition, PTSD may serve as a marker for neuroendocrine and metabolic dysregulation that could lead to the development of type 2 diabetes. Limited research has looked at PTSD in people suffering from multiple sclerosis and Guillain–Barré syndrome.

References

American Psychiatric Association. (1994). *Diagnostic and statistical manual of mental disorders* (4th ed.).

American Psychiatric Association. (2013). *Diagnostic and statistical manual of mental disorders* (5th ed.). https://doi.org/10.1176/appi.books.9780890425596

Aronson, B. D., Palombi, L. C., & Walls, M. L. (2016). Rates and consequences of posttraumatic distress among American Indian adults with type 2 diabetes. *Journal of Behavioral Medicine, 39*(4), 694–703. https://doi.org/10.1007/s10865-016-9733-y

Atwoli, L., Platt, J. M., Basu, A., Williams, D. R., Stein, D. J., & Koenen, K. C. (2016). Associations between lifetime potentially traumatic events and chronic physical conditions in the South African Stress and Health Survey: A cross-sectional study. *BMC Psychiatry 16*, Art. 214.

Bica, T., Castello, R., Toussaint, L. L., & Monteso-Curto, P. (2017). Depression as a risk factor of organic diseases: An international integrative review. *Journal of Nursing Scholarship, 49*(4), 389–399.

Bilevicius, E., Sommer, J. L., Asmundson, G. J. G., & El-Gabalawy, R. (2018). Posttraumatic stress disorder and chronic pain are associated with opioid use disorder: Results from a 2012–2013 American nationally representative survey. *Drug and Alcohol Dependence, 188*, 119–125. https://doi.org/10.1016/j.drugalcdep.2018.04.005

Bilevicius, E., Sommer, J. L., Asmundson, G. J. G., & El-Gabalawy, R. (2019). Associations of PTSD, chronic pain, and their comorbidity on cannabis use disorder: Results from an American nationally representative study. *Depression and Anxiety, 36*(11), 1036–1046. https://doi.org/10.1002/da.22947

Blakey, S. M., Halverson, T. F., Evans, M. K., Patel, T. A., Hair, L. P., Meyer, E. C., DeBeer, B. B., Beckham, J. C., Pugh, M. J., Calhoun, P. S., & Kimbrel, N. A. (2021). Experiential avoidance is associated with medical and mental health diagnoses in a national sample of deployed Gulf War veterans. *Journal of Psychiatric Research, 142*, 17–24. https://doi.org/10.1016/j.jpsychires.2021.07.033

Boden, M. T. (2018). Prevalence of mental disorders and related functioning and treatment engagement among people with diabetes. *Journal of Psychosomatic Research, 106*, 62–69. https://doi.org/10.1016/j.jpsychores.2018.01.001

Bookwalter, D. B., Roenfeldt, K. A., LeardMann, C. A., Kong, S. Y., Riddle, M. S., & Rull, R. P. (2020). Posttraumatic stress disorder and risk of selected autoimmune diseases among US military personnel. *BMC Psychiatry, 20*(1), 23. https://doi.org/10.1186/s12888-020-2432-9

Chalfant, A. M., Bryant, R. A., & Fulcher, G. (2004). Posttraumatic stress disorder following diagnosis of multiple sclerosis. *Journal of Traumatic Stress, 17*(5), 423–428. https://doi.org/10.1023/B:JOTS.0000048955.65891.4c

Chemtob, C. M., & Herriott, M. G. (1994). Post-traumatic stress disorder as a sequela of Guillain–Barré syndrome. *Journal of Traumatic Stress, 7*(4), 705–711. https://doi.org/10.1002/jts.2490070415

Collins, A. E., Niles, B. L., Mori, D. L., Silberbogen, A. K., & Seligowski, A. V. (2014). A telephone-based intervention to promote diabetes management in veterans with posttraumatic stress symptoms. *Professional Psychology: Research and Practice*, 45(1), 20–26. https://doi.org/ 10.1037/a0032604

Counsell, A., Hadjistavropoulos, H. D., Kehler, M. D., & Asmundson, G. J. G. (2013). Posttraumatic stress disorder symptoms in individuals with multiple sclerosis. *Psychological Trauma*, 5(5), 448–452. https://doi.org/10.1037/a0029338

Creech, S. K., Pulverman, C. S., Crawford, J. N., Holliday, R., Monteith, L. L., Lehavot, K., Olson-Madden, J., & Kelly, U. A. (2021). Clinical complexity in women veterans: A systematic review of the recent evidence on mental health and physical health comorbidities. *Behavioral Medicine*, 47(1), 69–87. https://doi.org/10.1080/08964289.2019.1644283

David, D., Woodward, C., Esquenazi, J., & Mellman, T. A. (2004). Comparison of comorbid physical illnesses among veterans with PTSD and veterans with alcohol dependence. *Psychiatric Services*, 55(1), 82–85. https://doi.org/10.1176/appi.ps.55.1.82

Ehlert, U. (2013). Enduring psychobiological effects of childhood adversity. *Psychoneuroendocrinology*, 38(9), 1850–1857. https://doi.org/10.1016/j.psyne uen.2013.06.007

El-Gabalawy, R., Blaney, C., Tsai, J., Sumner, J. A., & Pietrzak, R. H. (2018). Physical health conditions associated with full and subthreshold PTSD in US military veterans: Results from the National Health and Resilience in Veterans Study. *Journal of Affective Disorders*, 227, 849–853. https://doi.org/10.1016/j.jad.2017.11.058

El-Gabalawy, R., Mackenzie, C. S., Shooshtari, S., & Sareen, J. (2011). Comorbid physical health conditions and anxiety disorders: A population-based exploration of prevalence and health outcomes among older adults. *General Hospital Psychiatry*, 33(6), 556–564. https://doi.org/ 10.1016/j.genhosppsych.2011.07.005

Gadermann, A. M., Alonso, J., Vilagut, G., Zaslavsky, A. M., & Kessler, R. C. (2012). Comorbidity and disease burden in the National Comorbidity Survey Replication (NCS-R). *Depression and Anxiety*, 29(9), 797-806.

Goodwin, R. D., & Davidson, J. R. (2005). Self-reported diabetes and posttraumatic stress disorder among adults in the community. *Preventive Medicine*, 40(5), 570–574. https://doi.org/ 10.1016/j.ypmed.2004.07.013

Greening, L., Stoppelbein, L., & Cheek, K. (2017). Racial/ethnic disparities in the risk of posttraumatic stress disorder symptoms among mothers of children diagnosed with cancer and Type-1 diabetes mellitus. *Psychological Trauma*, 9(3), 325–333. https://doi.org/10.1037/tra 0000230

Herzog, J. I., & Schmahl, C. (2018). Adverse childhood experiences and the consequences on neurobiological, psychosocial, and somatic conditions across the lifespan. *Frontiers in Psychiatry*, 9. https://doi.org/10.3389/fpsyt.2018.00420

Horsch, A., & McManus, F. (2014). Brief report: Maternal posttraumatic stress symptoms are related to adherence to their child's diabetes treatment regimen. *Journal of Health Psychology*, 19(8), 987–992. https://doi.org/10.1177/1359105313482169

Horsch, A., McManus, F., & Kennedy, P. (2012). Cognitive and non-cognitive factors associated with posttraumatic stress symptoms in mothers of children with type 1 diabetes. *Behavioural and Cognitive Psychotherapy*, 40(4), 400–411. https://doi.org/10.1017/S1352465812000112

Horsch, A., McManus, F., Kennedy, P., & Edge, J. (2007). Anxiety, depressive, and posttraumatic stress symptoms in mothers of children with type 1 diabetes. *Journal of Traumatic Stress*, 20(5), 881–891. https://doi.org/10.1002/jts.20247

Husarewycz, M., El-Gabalawy, R., Logsetty, S., & Sareen, J. (2014). The association between number and type of traumatic life experiences and physical conditions in a nationally representative sample. *General Hospital Psychiatry*, 36(1), 26–32.

James, J., Harris, Y. T., Kronish, I. M., Wisnivesky, J. P., & Lin, J. J. (2018). Exploratory study of impact of cancer-related posttraumatic stress symptoms on diabetes self-management among cancer survivors. *Psycho-Oncology*, *27*(2), 648–653. https://doi.org/10.1002/pon.4568

Jiang, S., Postovit, L., Cattaneo, A., Binder, E. B., & Aitchison, K. J. (2019). Epigenetic modifications in stress response genes associated with childhood trauma. *Frontiers in Psychiatry*, *10*, 808. https://doi.org/10.3389/fpsyt.2019.00808

Kremer, A.-L., Schieber, K., Metzler, M., Schuster, S., & Erim, Y. (2017). Long-term positive and negative psychosocial outcomes in young childhood cancer survivors, type 1 diabetics and their healthy peers. *International Journal of Adolescent Medicine and Health*, *29*(6), 1–8.

Landolt, M. A., Ribi, K., Laimbacher, J., Vollrath, M., Gnehm, H. E., & Sennhauser, F. H. (2002). Posttraumatic stress disorder in parents of children with newly diagnosed Type 1 diabetes. *Journal of Pediatric Psychology*, *27*(7), 647–652. https://doi.org/10.1093/jpepsy/27.7.647

Landolt, M. A., Vollrath, M., Ribi, K., Gnehm, H. E., & Sennhauser, F. H. (2003). Incidence and associations of parental and child posttraumatic stress symptoms in pediatric patients. *Journal of Child Psychology & Psychiatry*, *44*(8), 1199–1207. https://doi.org/10.1111/1469-7610.00201

Lin, E. H. B., & Von Korff, M. (2008). Mental disorders among persons with diabetes—Results from the world mental health surveys. *Journal of Psychosomatic Research*, *65*(6), 571–580. https://doi.org/10.1016/j.jpsychores.2008.06.007

Livneh, H., & Martz, E. (2006). On structure of trauma-related stress reactions among people with diabetes mellitus. *Psychological Reports*, *99*(1), 209–212. https://doi.org/10.2466/PR0.99.5.209-212

Lukaschek, K., Baumert, J., Kruse, J., Emeny, R. T., Lacruz, M. E., Huth, C., Thorand, B., Holle, R., Rathmann, W., Meisinger, C., & Ladwig, K.-H. (2013). Relationship between posttraumatic stress disorder and type 2 diabetes in a population-based cross-sectional study with 2970 participants. *Journal of Psychosomatic Research*, *74*(4), 340–345. https://doi.org/10.1016/j.jpsychores.2012.12.011

Marciniak, M. D., Lage, M. J., Dunayevich, E., Russell, J. M., Bowman, L., Landbloom, R. P., & Levine, L. R. (2005). The cost of treating anxiety: the medical and demographic correlates that impact total medical costs. *Depression and Anxiety*, *21*(4), 178–184. https://doi.org/10.1002/da.20074

Miller-Archie, S. A., Jordan, H. T., Ruff, R. R., Chamany, S., Cone, J. E., Brackbill, R. M., Kong, J., Ortega, F., & Stellman, S. D. (2014). Posttraumatic stress disorder and new-onset diabetes among adult survivors of the World Trade Center disaster. *Preventive Medicine*, *66*, 34–38. https://doi.org/10.1016/j.ypmed.2014.05.016

Mulvihill, D. (2005). The health impact of childhood trauma: an interdisciplinary review, 1997–2003. *Issues in Comprehensive Pediatric Nursing*, *28*(2), 115–136. https://doi.org/10.1080/01460860590950890

Myers, V. H., Boyer, B. A., Herbert, J. D., Barakat, L. P., & Scheiner, G. (2007). Fear of hypoglycemia and self reported posttraumatic stress in adults with Type I diabetes treated by intensive regimens. *Journal of Clinical Psychology in Medical Settings*, *14*(1), 11–21. https://doi.org/10.1007/s10880-007-9051-1

Nichter, B., Norman, S., Haller, M., & Pietrzak, R. H. (2019). Physical health burden of PTSD, depression, and their comorbidity in the US veteran population: Morbidity, functioning, and disability. *Journal of Psychosomatic Research*, *124*, 109744. https://doi.org/10.1016/j.jpsychores.2019.109744

Nobles, C. J., Valentine, S. E., Borba, C. P. C., Gerber, M. W., Shtasel, D. L., & Marques, L. (2016). Black–white disparities in the association between posttraumatic stress disorder and chronic illness. *Journal of Psychosomatic Research*, *85*, 19–25. https://doi.org/10.1016/j.jpsychores.2016.03.126

Norman, S. B., Means-Christensen, A. J., Craske, M. G., Sherbourne, C. D., Roy-Byrne, P. P., & Stein, M. B. (2006). Associations between psychological trauma and physical illness in primary care. *Journal of Traumatic Stress, 19*(4), 461–470. https://doi.org/10.1002/jts.20129

O'Donovan, A., Cohen, B. E., Seal, K. H., Bertenthal, D., Margaretten, M., Nishimi, K., & Neylan, T. C. (2015). Elevated risk for autoimmune disorders in Iraq and Afghanistan veterans with posttraumatic stress disorder. *Biological Psychiatry, 77*(4), 365–374. https://doi.org/10.1016/j.biopsych.2014.06.015

Pengpid, S., & Peltzer, K. (2020). Mental morbidity and its associations with socio-behavioural factors and chronic conditions in rural middle- and older-aged adults in South Africa. *Journal of Psychology in Africa, 30*(3), 257–263. https://doi.org/10.1080/14330237.2020.1767956

Pinquart, M. (2019). Posttraumatic stress symptoms and disorders in parents of children and adolescents with chronic physical illnesses: A meta-analysis. *Journal of Traumatic Stress, 32*(1), 88–96. https://doi.org/10.1002/jts.22354

Rechenberg, K., Grey, M., & Sadler, L. (2017). Stress and posttraumatic stress in mothers of children with type 1 diabetes. *Journal of Family Nursing, 23*(2), 201–225. https://doi.org/10.1177/1074840716687543

Renna, C. P., Boyer, B. A., Prout, M. F., & Scheiner, G. (2016). Posttraumatic stress related to hyperglycemia: Prevalence in adults with type I diabetes. *Journal of Clinical Psychology in Medical Settings, 23*(3), 269–284. https://doi.org/10.1007/s10880-016-9463-x

Ribi, K., Vollrath, M. E., Sennhauser, F. H., Gnehm, H. E., & Landolt, M. A. (2007). Prediction of posttraumatic stress in fathers of children with chronic diseases or unintentional injuries: A six-months follow-up study. *Child and Adolescent Psychiatry and Mental Health, 1*(1), 16 https://doi.org/10.1186/1753-2000-1-16

Rzeszutek, M., Oniszczenko, W., Schier, K., Biernat-Kałuża, E., & Gasik, R. (2015). Trauma symptoms, temperament traits, social support and the intensity of pain in a Polish sample of patients suffering from chronic pain. *Personality and Individual Differences, 83*, 13–17. https://doi.org/10.1016/j.paid.2015.03.036

Rzeszutek, M., Oniszczenko, W., Schier, K., Biernat-Kałuża, E., & Gasik, R. (2016). Sex differences in trauma symptoms, body image and intensity of pain in a Polish sample of patients suffering from chronic pain. *Psychology, Health & Medicine, 21*(7), 827–835. https://doi.org/10.1080/13548506.2015.1111393

Sachs-Ericsson, N. J., Sheffler, J. L., Stanley, I. H., Piazza, J. R., & Preacher, K. J. (2017). When emotional pain becomes physical: Adverse childhood experiences, pain, and the role of mood and anxiety disorders. *Journal of Clinical Psychology, 73*(10), 1403–1428. https://doi.org/10.1002/jclp.22444

Shahin, W., Stupans, I., & Kennedy, G. (2018). Health beliefs and chronic illnesses of refugees: A systematic review. *Ethnicity & Health, 26*(5), 756–768. https://doi.org/10.1080/13557858.2018.1557118

Stoppelbein, L., & Greening, L. (2007). Brief report: the risk of posttraumatic stress disorder in mothers of children diagnosed with pediatric cancer and type I diabetes. *Journal of Pediatric Psychology, 32*(2), 223–229. https://doi.org/10.1093/jpepsy/jsj120

Tsai, J., & Shen, J. (2017). Exploring the link between posttraumatic stress disorder and inflammation-related medical conditions: An epidemiological examination. *Psychiatric Quarterly, 88*(4), 909–916. https://doi.org/10.1007/s11126-017-9508-9

Vaccarino, V., Goldberg, J., Magruder, K. M., Forsberg, C. W., Friedman, M. J., Litz, B. T., Heagerty, P. J., Huang, G. D., Gleason, T. C., & Smith, N. L. (2014). Posttraumatic stress disorder and incidence of type-2 diabetes: A prospective twin study. *Journal of Psychiatric Research, 56*, 158–164. https://doi.org/10.1016/j.jpsychires.2014.05.019

Valentine, S. E., Nobles, C. J., Gerber, M. W., Vaewsorn, A. S., Shtasel, D. L., & Marques, L. (2017). The association of posttraumatic stress disorder and chronic medical conditions by ethnicity. *Journal of Latina/o Psychology, 5*(3), 227–241.

Vanderlip, E. R., Katon, W., Russo, J., Lessler, D., & Ciechanowski, P. (2014). Depression among patients with diabetes attending a safety-net primary care clinic: Relationship with disease control. *Psychosomatics, 55*(6), 548–554. https://doi.org/10.1016/j.psym.2014.01.008

Weisberg, R. B., Bruce, S. E., Machan, J. T., Kessler, R. C., Culpepper, L., & Keller, M. B. (2002). Nonpsychiatric illness among primary care patients with trauma histories and posttraumatic stress disorder. *Psychiatric Services, 53*(7), 848–854. https://doi.org/10.1176/appi.ps.53.7.848

Woolf, C., Muscara, F., Anderson, V. A., & McCarthy, M. C. (2016). Early traumatic stress responses in parents following a serious illness in their child: A systematic review. *Journal of Clinical Psychology in Medical Settings, 23*(1), 53–66. https://doi.org/10.1007/s10880-015-9430-y

Ziobrowski, H., Sartor, C. E., Tsai, J., & Pietrzak, R. H. (2017). Gender differences in mental and physical health conditions in U.S. veterans: Results from the National Health and Resilience in Veterans Study. *Journal of Psychosomatic Research, 101*, 110–113. https://doi.org/10.1016/j.jpsychores.2017.08.011

10

A hypothesised model and theoretical issues related to posttraumatic stress disorder in physical illnesses

In reviewing the literature in the previous chapters on posttraumatic stress disorder (PTSD) in physical illness, several observations are noteworthy. The reason for mentioning and discussing these observations is (1) to raise awareness of knowledge gaps and develop overarching research questions for future research and (2) to tentatively outline a hypothesised model as a springboard for future debates.

PTSD subtypes in patients with chronic illnesses

The diseases examined in the previous chapters have been argued to potentially trigger PTSD symptoms and comorbid psychiatric symptoms that are closely linked. This is consistent with claims in the literature that PTSD is not a discrete clinical entity, but is expressed through psychiatric comorbid symptoms (Miller et al., 2003, 2004). This raises the question of whether there may be subtypes of PTSD in patients suffering from PTSD associated with physical illness. PTSD is a complex disorder that has been divided into different subtypes depending on the manifestation of symptoms. For example, people may 'internalise' PTSD symptoms by directing them inward through avoidance and numbing (López & Guarnaccia, 2000; Miller et al., 2004), whereas others 'externalise' PTSD symptoms, for example through anger or hostility (hyperarousal symptoms) towards others. In other words, there are internalising and externalising subtypes of posttraumatic symptoms (Miller et al., 2003).

Following trauma survivors with non-physical illnesses, among female survivors of sexual assault, externalisers are classified as those who exhibit symptoms of disinhibition, substance dependence, and personality disorder traits, while internalisers are classified as those with low levels of positive

Posttraumatic Stress in Physical Illness. Man Cheung Chung, Oxford University Press. © Oxford University Press 2024.
DOI: 10.1093/oso/9780198727323.003.0010

temperament, high rates of major depressive disorder, and elevated levels of schizoid and avoidant personality disorders (Miller & Resick, 2007). Three PTSD subtypes have been distinguished in Vietnam veterans: externalisers, internalisers, and low pathology. Veterans with externalising and internalising subtypes had higher mortality rates and were more likely to die from cardiovascular disease than those without PTSD (Flood et al., 2010). Another study also focused on veterans and identified three classes of individuals: average, severe, and highly severe symptom groups. The severe and/or highly severe symptom classes consisted of veterans who had higher levels of traumatic experiences, used more avoidant and problem-focused coping strategies, and exhibited more dysfunctional personality traits (e.g. neuroticism) (Jongedijk et al., 2019). A recent study also showed that there are subtypes of PTSD in veterans. It identified a three-cluster solution (veterans with low, most serious symptoms, and moderate symptoms of anxiety, depression, and neurobehavioural symptoms) (Palmer & Palmer, 2021). Limited research has investigated whether patients with physical illnesses would exhibit PTSD subtypes. This is a knowledge gap that needs to be addressed.

The effects of cumulative trauma

The studies discussed in the previous chapters have shown that whereas PTSD can be triggered by the illness itself, previous trauma can also influence the severity of the illness and other distress outcomes. In other words, there is a possible impact of cumulative trauma on the health outcomes of people suffering from physical illness. Cumulative trauma is the total number of traumas that a person has experienced in their lifetime, including the traumatic impact before and after the onset of the disease. Cumulative trauma can be a form of cumulative risk, causing people to develop more symptoms than those who have been exposed to less trauma (Appleyard et al., 2005; Follette et al., 1996). Exposure to different traumas can have an additive effect on the degree of psychological and physical health problems. These effects go beyond the effect resulting from exposure to a single traumatic event (Pat-Horenczyk et al., 2013).

The concept of cumulative trauma needs further investigation. According to the enduring somatic threat (EST) of PTSD (Edmondson, 2014), life-threatening illness related PTSD may have clinical features that differ from the features of PTSD symptoms that result from past discrete or external traumatic events. In patients with a life-threatening illness that is chronic or somatic (e.g. a heart attack), symptoms of PTSD often focus on the ongoing threat of disease recurrence and loss of function rather than the past traumatic event that no longer poses a threat to the patient's current life. For these patients with chronic illnesses, factors associated with intrusion symptoms could include fear of disease progression, physical symptoms, and doctor's appointments. Notably, a strong positive association was found between PTSD triggered by heart disease and fear of disease progression, even after controlling for anxiety and depression (Fait et al., 2018). Similarly, patients' avoidance, negative alterations in cognition or mood, and hyperarousal symptoms may manifest differently and have different psychological, behavioural, and health consequences than symptoms of PTSD resulting from discrete or external traumatic events. In patients with chronic illnesses, avoidance behaviours may be associated with non-adherence to preventive medications. Hyperarousal symptoms may be associated with inflammation for cardiovascular events in people with myocardial infarction (MI). The EST model states that fear of mortality maintains PTSD for both types of discrete/external and persistent/somatic events (Edmondson, 2014). It thus seems necessary to distinguish PTSD from a life-threatening illness and from past discrete or external traumatic events, the combination of which constitutes the phenomenology of cumulative trauma.

People may experience cumulative physical and psychological changes or distress resulting from having to survive exposure to repeated threats that are detrimental to their mental and physical health. Exposure to various traumas can lead to a phenomenon of 'allostatic load' (McEwen & Stellar, 1993), in which our bodies are worn down by such repeated and chronic distress over time. Our physiological systems are constantly fluctuating as we respond to and recover from stress (a state of allostasis). Over time, recovery becomes less and less complete. Our bodies are increasingly depleted and more likely to become ill when allostatic load is high. A meta-analysis shows that high allostatic load was associated with an increased risk of death of 22% for all-cause mortality and 31% for cardiovascular disease mortality (Parker et al., 2022). In addition, trauma can cause prolonged distress (allostatic load) to psychobiological systems characterised by affect dysregulation, hyperarousal, personality changes, failure to adapt to stress in the sensory nervous system, and 'wear and tear' of coping (McEwen, 1998, 2002). Furthermore, according to the conservation of resources model (Hobfoll, 1989), PTSD can deplete personal resources, including those (e.g. psychological resources) that are important for maintaining one's survival and well-being. In addition to personal resources, the chronic illnesses examined in previous chapters may also involve the loss of resources in the form of income, employment, and a sense of personal efficacy, which can influence responses to extreme stress (Hobfoll et al., 1996).

It is not known to what extent cumulative trauma resulting from PTSD due to previous trauma and chronic illness might play a role in affecting patients with chronic illness. This is another knowledge gap that needs to be addressed. One can treat physical illness not only with physical treatments, but also with psychological ones, including treating the traumatic aspects of the illness or the past trauma. Integrating these two approaches might be the best way to understand and help patients with chronic diseases.

The risk factors for PTSD in physical illness

The risk factors examined in studies of PTSD in physical illness can be broadly categorised according to demographic characteristics, specific illness-related variables, personality traits and coping strategies. In some ways, the study of these broad categories as risk factors is not surprising, as they are considered in some theoretical frameworks to be the important components to consider in understanding people's health and well-being. Moreover, a good understanding of the relationship between these risk factors is likely to have important implications for the design and implementation of psychotherapeutic interventions for patients with chronic illness.

To elaborate on this, the integrative conceptual framework of the health psychology literature (Moos & Holahan, 2007; Moos & Schaefer, 1993), which describes the process of coping with a critical illness, highlights the role of the above risk factors. To begin conceptualising this coping process, two systems are distinguished. The environmental system consists of persistent life stressors and social coping resources. The personal system refers to the socio-demographic characteristics of patients and their personal coping resources. These relatively stable environmental and personal factors influence the way patients cope with life crises and transitions that often involve significant changes in their circumstances. These combined influences in turn affect health and well-being directly and indirectly through cognitive appraisal and coping responses. In other words, cognitive and coping responses are seen as mediators in the stress process.

The risk factors for PTSD in physical illness reflect some of the processes in this framework. For example, the environmental system can be conceptualised in terms of ongoing life stressors such as past trauma. The personal system is composed of socio-demographic variables such as gender, age, ethnicity, and social deprivation, and personal coping resources in the form of hostile personality, neuroticism, Type D or Big Five traits, and self-efficacy. These are victim variables that have been shown to influence distress outcomes (Vogt et al., 2007). These factors might then interact to influence how patients cope with the changes in their lives and the outcomes of distress, whether it be severity of illness and psychiatric comorbidity or PTSD resulting from the traumatic illness, directly and indirectly through cognitive appraisal (e.g. awareness during the illness, experience of pain, helplessness, perception of illness, fear of progression of the illness, uncertainty about the impact of the illness), and coping (e.g. repression, avoidance-focused, emotion-focused, or problem-focused coping).

The risk factors for PTSD in physical illness also reflect the positive health-belief model, which states that humans are not defined by a reactive and passive response to stresses from some biological changes, as described in the classic General Adaptation Syndrome (Selye, 1950). We are not simply the product of physical resistance to stress, waiting to return to homeostasis as long as the body is not exhausted or depleted by chronic stress, causing illness. Rather, the way we think (i.e. cognitive appraisal) can influence our emotions and distress. According to the two-stage appraisal of stress model (Lazarus, 1993; Lazarus & Folkman, 1984), we confront the stressor (e.g. a chronic illness) and actively engage in psychological processes in which we appraise (primary appraisal) whether the stressor is potentially or actually harmful to our psychological well-being. If it is harmful, we cope with the resulting distress by choosing to act in a certain way (secondary appraisal). This action, roughly speaking, leads to two types of coping responses: emotion-focused and problem-focused. In emotion-focused coping, we make an effort to reduce the discomfort associated with the stressful situation without changing the situation itself. Problem-focused coping involves planned action to change the stressful situation by acting on the environment or ourselves. It has been postulated that people tend to respond to stress in a consistent way with a coping style even when the situation changes (Endler, 1983; Endler & Edwards, 1986).

Notwithstanding, the way people cope with stress can be influenced by personality traits (Costa Jr et al., 1996) which play an important role in influencing distress outcomes. This postulate is reflected in the literature reviewed in the previous chapters. Personality traits and coping strategies are not independent of each other. The differential choice-effectiveness model also points to the fact that personality traits can influence the choice of coping strategy (Bolger & Zuckerman, 1995). Take some of the Big Five factors—for example, people with high levels of neuroticism tend to reduce distress or negative affect by resorting to emotion-focused coping or disengagement (Carver & Connor-Smith, 2010). They may also seek social support to vent their emotions (Vollrath, Alnæs, & Torgersen, 1998; Vollrath, Torgersen, & Alnæs, 1998). On the other hand, people with high levels of conscientiousness tend to engage in cognitive restructuring, where they evaluate their negative thoughts and shift them from negative to positive thoughts or activities (Connor-Smith & Flachsbart, 2007; Vollrath & Torgersen, 2000).

Personality and coping can be linked in different ways and influence the outcome of stress. Personality factors may determine certain coping strategies, which then lead to maladjustment or distress (a mediation model). Alternatively, personality and coping may contribute independently to psychological outcomes. In other words, personality factors and coping strategies contribute independently or are uniquely related to outcomes (an additive model). Furthermore, personality factors may interact with coping strategies and lead to outcomes (an interaction model) (Chung et al., 2005; Hewitt & Flett, 1996).

The deviation amplification model also assumes that the way people respond to trauma is regulated by either processes of deviation countering or deviation amplification. The former process is similar to the homeostatic process, that is, when people are confronted with trauma and experience high levels of distress, they want to find a way to reduce the distress and return to homeostatic levels. In the latter process, however, when confronted with the trauma, they experience positive or negative effects depending on whether they magnify the small changes in adaptive or maladaptive coping responses. Pre-trauma psychological resources, including personality traits, can influence these responses. Before the trauma, victims with high self-esteem or high levels of personal mastery are likely to use adaptive coping strategies that lead to positive outcomes. On the other hand, victims with low levels of these traits are likely to use maladaptive coping strategies that lead to negative outcomes (Aldwin & Brustrom, 1997; Aldwin et al., 1996; Updegraff & Taylor, 2000).

An overarching research question

Given the broad risk factors of personality traits, coping strategies demographic characteristics, and specific disease-related variables, and considering the two gaps in knowledge mentioned above—namely cumulative trauma (PTSD due to a life-threatening illness and due to previous discrete or external traumatic events) and PTSD subtypes in patients with physical illnesses—a research question might be: To what extent would cumulative trauma affect distress (including PTSD subtypes) and whether this relationship is moderated by the interaction between personality and coping strategies, after controlling for demographic variables and specific disease-related variables? To the best of my knowledge, this research has not yet been attempted in patients with physical illness.

What is missing in the research question?

However, the above question misses a larger context, as it does not take into account the distorted self-structure that underlies the complex interaction between cumulative trauma and risk factors, especially personality and coping. The concept of the self is a complex issue that has been discussed and debated in different ways in philosophy for decades. It is beyond the scope of this chapter to try to capture this complexity. One definition is that of a reflexive process of self-awareness (Mischel & Morf, 2003), in which people focus on themselves, gather information about themselves, and are aware of their internal states and reactions as well as their external behaviours. This information forms the basis for the development of the self-concept, which continues to develop and change as people expand their information and ideas about who they are (Baumeister, 1987). This view is similar to William James' idea that the self is defined by the person who is able to introspectively assess how they are doing, or who is the source of agency, that is, their body or mind can regulate their perception, thoughts and behaviour (James, 1890). According to Kohut (1971), the self is a coherent, stable and yet dynamic experience of our individuality, continuity in time and space, autonomy, and efficacy.

However, trauma researchers have highlighted the fact that trauma can distort the concept of self by distorting the process of self-awareness or agency in regulating one's perception, thoughts and behaviour. After trauma, people can 'reconfigure' and develop a traumatised schema that is incompatible with the existing schema and causes great psychological distress (Janoff-Bulman, 1992). The word 'reconfiguration' means a permanent adaptation to the trauma or a change as a result of the trauma. People may experience changes to accommodate the demands of the traumatic situation and they may change the way they respond to future events (Morland et al., 2008). People may shatter their assumptions about their invulnerability or safety, about the benevolence, meaningfulness, and predictability of the world, and the goodness of people (Janoff-Bulman, 1992). These assumptions have been replaced by feelings of negativity, difficulties in trusting the world and others, and perceptions of the world and others as threatening, challenging, and dangerous. These are some of the examples of cognitive changes that manifest in different ways in different people with different trauma experiences, whether experiences from the traumatic impact of the illness or previous traumas that may not be illness-related.

To further explain the distortion of the self in terms of cognitive changes following trauma, the cognitive model of PTSD (Ehlers & Clark, 2000) explains the interrelationship between cognitive changes and the regulation or management of distressing emotions. Put simply, trauma can distort cognitions and cause victims to develop an overly negative appraisal of the trauma and/ or its aftermath, disrupting autobiographical memory related to the trauma, which in turn can create a sense of current external or internal threat. They may thereby overgeneralise the trauma and, for example, see the world as a dangerous place (external threat) or see themselves as unacceptable, helpless, hopeless, and unable to achieve important goals in life (internal threat). Problematic behaviours and cognitive strategies would only prevent these negative appraisals and memories of the trauma from changing. This would in turn perpetuate PTSD and create distressing emotions such as anxiety and depression (e.g. Cieslak et al., 2008; Mayou et al., 2002; Owens et al., 2008; Wenninger & Ehlers, 1998). Distorted cognitions about oneself and external reality can lead to self-blame, self-criticism, feelings of helplessness or hopelessness, and hypervigilance about dangers in the world (Briere & Spinazzola, 2005). These dysfunctional thoughts influence the subjective inner state and psychological distress later in life (Briere, 1996; Briere, 2002).

Trauma centrality is another perspective to look at the cognitive changes of the distorted self (Berntsen & Rubin, 2006a, 2007). Past trauma or the chronic illness itself may constantly remind patients of the trauma or traumatic aspect of the illness, keeping traumatic memories alive and accessible, which can serve as reference points from which patients ascribe meaning to existing beliefs, feelings, experiences, and future expectations (Berntsen, 2001; Porter & Birt, 2001; Reviere & Bakeman, 2001; Rubin et al., 2004). These traumatic memories can shatter assumptions about the world (Janoff-Bulman, 1992), leading to oversimplification of the life situation (i.e. different aspects of life are explained in terms of traumatic experiences) and rejection of contradictory experiences (Berntsen & Rubin, 2006a, 2006b; Linde, 1993; Robinson, 1996). These accessible trauma memories can also lead people to overestimate the frequency of traumatic events, increasing the likelihood of re-traumatisation as well as hypervigilance and avoidance behaviour. The link between memories and traumatisation further echoes the dual representation model, which states that psychological and physiological states can be influenced by accessing trauma material in different memory systems (Brewin et al., 1996). Consequently, one's outlook on life changes, the course of one's life is redirected, and turning points become a causal agent in one's life story (Pillemer, 1998; Pillemer, 2003). Since life histories define who we are and how we understand ourselves (Fitzgerald, 1988), traumatic memories, when they become turning points, also affect the way we define ourselves and become central components of personal identity and an integral feature of our self concept, resulting in a traumatised self in different situations (Berntsen & Rubin, 2007; Wilson, 2006). Trauma centrality is associated with increased PTSD and psychiatric comorbidity (Bernard et al., 2015; Berntsen & Rubin, 2006a; Boals & Schuettler, 2011; Brown et al., 2010; Lancaster et al., 2011; Ogle et al., 2014, 2016; Schuettler & Boals, 2011).

As mentioned earlier, the development of a traumatic schema that is incompatible with the existing schema can be a major psychological burden. According to the 'completion principle' advocated in Stress Response Syndrome (Horowitz, 1976), victims would attempt to prevent distress by making the internal psychological trauma model coherent with existing mental schemas and by revising, accommodating, and assimilating the trauma information with the existing schema. This process could further exacerbate the extent of psychiatric comorbid symptoms. In order to resist, tolerate, and control the aforementioned experiences or to prevent emotional exhaustion, victims might use defence mechanisms to inhibit the flow of traumatic information to a tolerable level (Ihilevich & Gleser, 1993; McDougall, 1985; Thome, 1990).

However, as part of the distorted self, people's self-capacities, such as emotion regulation and resilience, are distorted by trauma (Briere & Runtz, 2002; Briere, 1992; Wilson, 2006), resulting in maladaptive defence mechanisms or coping strategies that increase the level of psychological distress. However, these defence mechanisms are maladaptive and include tension reduction and avoidance activities (e.g. illicit drug use and/or self-harm). They are inhibitory mechanisms aimed at preventing emotional exhaustion, keeping distressing emotions in check (Horowitz, 1986), inhibiting intense and negative emotions, and avoiding frightening or intolerable feelings (Busch, 2014). Alexithymia can also be considered as another inhibitory or avoidance mechanism or a defensive response (Fang & Chung, 2019; Fang et al., 2020; Kooiman et al., 1998). Alexithymia is defined as a degree of difficulty in identifying and describing feelings but relies on external oriented thinking (Nemiah & Sifneos, 1970; Taylor et al., 1997). These difficulties would help in coping with overwhelming emotional distress by limiting access to internal feelings but focusing on external facts. Alexithymia has been associated with anxiety, depression (Honkalampi et al., 2007), and poor physical health and somatisation (Sayar et al., 2003; Taylor et al., 1997).

Similarly, according to psychoanalytic literature, suppression is a conscious defence mechanism (Myers et al., 2004) in which victims, when they recognise the distressing emotions associated with the trauma, deliberately avoid thinking about it and inhibit their emotional expressive behaviour (Gross, 1998). A study showed that increased emotional suppression was associated with lower psychological distress (such as depression) in cancer patients (Cohen, 2013). Emotional suppression was also found to reduce sadness in the short term, although it was not effective for moderate and higher levels of anxiety (Liverant et al., 2008). However, it is controversial whether suppression can actually protect psychological well-being (Vaillant, 2000). One consequence of these avoidance, inhibition, and suppression mechanisms is that distressing emotions become pent up in the body unprocessed and unresolved, causing disturbances in the physiological and neurological systems that lead to health or psychological impairment (Pennebaker, 1995; Pennebaker & Traue, 1993; Temoshok et al., 2008), anxiety and depression (Amstadter & Vernon, 2008; Ho et al., 2004; Iwamitsu et al., 2005), negative affect (Gross & John, 2003), and increased severity of PTSD symptoms (Amir et al., 1997; Clohessy & Ehlers, 1999).

So far, it has been outlined how the concept of the self can be distorted on a cognitive level. It is also argued that the self can be divided by trauma. According to the model of the posttraumatic self, there is an internal psychological structure or essential structural part of the personality that forms the basis for self-esteem, self-worth, well-being, and uniqueness of individual identity. It is a central processing unit of the personality that organises our experiences with others, the validation of our own individuality by others, our existence, and our adaptation. There are different dimensions of self-structure described by the terms coherence, connection, continuity, energy, autonomy, and vitality, all of which are integrated and interconnected with their own functions and reflective capacities. Trauma can disrupt coherence, leading to a fragmentation of oneself and a sense of disconnection, thereby affecting one's sense of stability or order in daily life. As a result, people may experience a loss of continuity, self-sameness, and connectedness. They may lose their physical and mental energy, motivation, and purposeful behaviour, but also experience fatigue. They may also lose their self-esteem and reduce their ability to regulate themselves freely. Their health is also affected and they lose an essential personal vitality (Wilson, 2006). This traumatised self can be considered a loss of self. The lack of a coherent but unstable sense of self contributes to the inability of victims to reflect on themselves and their feelings, make sense of their trauma, and to cope with PTSD symptoms later in life (Janoff-Bulman, 1992). This loss of self can be accompanied by feelings of despair, depression, PTSD and inability to concentrate, mood swings, and harmful behaviours (Nevid & Rathus, 2007).

Several posttraumatic personality typologies have been proposed: the insert self, the empty self, the fragmented self, the imbalanced self, the over-controlled self, the anomic self, the conventional self, the grandiose self, the cohesive self, the accelerated self, and the integrated–transcendent self (Wilson, 2006). Without going into detail, take some of these typologies as examples. People with the insert self tend to display characteristics such as blunt and blank feelings, withdrawal, helplessness, inexpressiveness, and alexithymia. People with an empty self tend to exhibit characteristics such as passivity, depressiveness, and lack of energy. They lose interest in activities and relationships and tend to isolate themselves and withdraw from others. They also tend to be self-centred, insecure, dependent safety-seeking, and lack joy and positive affect. They are often depressed and despairing. They are chronically worried and fearful, so they try to hide. They also have doubts and lose confidence in the world. People with a fragmented self experience themselves as someone who is not whole, who is broken, who is falling apart and falling to pieces. They suffer from chronic anxiety and when confronted with suffering they tend to dissociate (Wilson, 2006). People with an over-controlled self, on the other hand, tend to be emotionally constricted and are afraid of losing control. They tend to behave compulsively and lead rigid lives in order to cope with anxiety. They are afraid of 'letting go', which would lead to overwhelming anxiety. Therefore, they tend to overorganise their lives and their interactions with others. Their rigidity and compulsive behaviour are aimed at protecting themselves and gaining a sense of control over their inner fears. To cope with the effects of the trauma, they tend to use denial, overwork and maintain routines, living a disciplined and rigid pattern of daily life (Wilson, 2006).

A revised overarching research question

In view of the distorted self presented in relation to the cognitive changes and the 'divided' self, a further revision of the above research question is required. One might ask: To what extent would this distorted self affect how personality and coping strategies interact to moderate the impact of cumulative trauma on distress, including PTSD subtypes, after controlling for demographic variables and specific disease-related variables?

Imagine that Ms Johnson is a victim of child abuse that led her to develop some characteristics of an empty self (e.g. passivity, withdrawal, insecurity, seeking safety, despair) and a fragmented self (e.g. feeling disjointed and falling apart, chronic anxiety, dissociation). She describes herself as an anxious person and worrier and scored high on the neuroticism subscale. To cope with her distress, she avoids talking and thinking about her fears, but she smokes and drinks. Two months ago, she suffered a life-threatening heart attack, which led to her meeting the diagnostic criteria for PTSD, displaying anxiety and depressive symptoms.

With this case as an example in the background, to return to and unpack the research question above, the component questions are: (1) controlling for patient demographic variables (e.g. age, gender, socioeconomic status) and specific disease-related variables (e.g. awareness of having the MI, feelings of pain and helplessness during the MI), whether the patient's past experiences of trauma (e.g. child abuse) are related to a combination of MI PTSD and depressive symptoms; (2) whether the effect of this relationship is exacerbated by the interaction effects between their empty and fragmented self-characteristics and neuroticism and avoidance coping strategies. Again, to my knowledge, this research question has not been studied in patients who have undergone life-threatening illnesses.

Some conceptual issues of the self

Philosophers have been debating the concept of the self for decades. It is beyond the scope of this chapter to summarise all the debates. Given the experience of the distorted self, one might ask how we can know ourselves, that is, the problem of self-knowledge. We believe that we have privileged access (Heil, 1992, 1998), immediate and direct self-knowledge, and that we enjoy a privileged epistemic position, since our access to our mental states is infallible and incorrigible, as Descartes (1641/1960) said. Similarly, when we are in a mental state, undergoing a mental process, or experiencing something, we cannot help but know at that time that we are in such a mental state (omniscience) (Audi, 2010). Considering how patients' self-perception may be distorted after trauma, as described above, they can still claim that their access to their own mental states is infallible and incorrigible, but what it is that they have access to is unclear. Can they say that it is this or that to which they have access? What they have access to is a bundle of distressing experiences and disrupting experiences that interfere with their daily functioning. In other words, patients may claim that they know they are in certain mental states, but the nature of these states is opaque.

This is similar to Hume's (1739/1974) argument that we never grasp the self directly. For him, there is no substantial self. If we proceed introspectively, we find that the self is merely a 'bundle' of perceptions, for example, heat or cold, light or darkness, love or anger, pain or pleasure. We can never observe anything and catch our 'self' without a perception at any time. The so-called self or person is simply a bundle or collection of different perceptions that follow each other in an uninterrupted flow and movement. It would not be surprising if patients, when introspecting and looking inwards, experienced a bundle of negative perceptions of experiences previously described in terms of PTSD symptoms, trauma centrality, posttraumatic self typologies, and others.

Some patients have difficulty defining their self. It has been postulated that the self is a unified, persistent, conscious subject that owns its own experiences, thinks its own thoughts, and is responsible for its own actions (Albahari, 2006). This definition of the self is difficult to maintain for these patients with a distorted self. For example, people who have a fragmented self feel disjointed, falling apart, broken, and anxious, and use dissociation to cope with distress, contradicting what was described above as a unified, conscious, and agentive self. Some traumatised patients would rather subscribe to some philosophers who argue that there is no such thing as conscious mental agency, which is interpreted as conscious mental causation (i.e. our own unique mental properties are causally responsible for bringing about our behaviour) and is in fact neither a unique nor a common form of human agency. Instead, patients may experience an action as theirs without experiencing it as caused by conscious mental states for specific reasons, even if they interpret it that way (Pacherie, 2011). In other words, these patients with a fragmented self might behave in this or that way without really experiencing it as caused by conscious mental states or conscious reasons.

Arguably, what has been presented contradicts the philosophical argument that there is a holistic conception of the self (Mele, 2011). This concept states that someone does not have to be merely some mental states or brain states, but rather a concerned individual who is motivated to exercise self-control and cares about how they conduct themselves practically. Concern about how they live their lives is what defines the concept of personhood. However, in the case of a patient with a distorted self, there seem to be times when the patient is confused about how to conduct themselves practically and manage their life, and may even say, 'I do not experience being the agent performing the I-action'.

This problematic notion of the self could lead to the problem of identity. Philosophers like Parfit (1986) radically argue that we could describe reality without claiming that persons exist. He even believes that we should eliminate references to persons, such as the word 'I'. Instead, we should speak with reference to the series of experiences that are causally dependent on their own bodies. Of course, it is difficult to say how to put this claim into practise. However, one interesting point in his argument might reflect the experiences of patients with PTSD. Who am I?, or who is the 'I' after a life-threatening experience with some distorted aspects of oneself? The 'I' is interwoven with the negative experiences of PTSD symptoms, the distorted self-characteristics that are different from the 'I' before the trauma. They may even be more inclined to focus on the perception that they are involved in a series of traumatic experiences that are causally dependent on their own body.

These philosophical arguments are perhaps helpful in illuminating the subjective experience of patients with a distorted self. Whether these arguments can serve as the basis for some hypotheses that can be systematically investigated remains to be seen.

How posttraumatic growth occurs in people with physical illnesses

In reviewing the literature on PTSD in physical illness in the previous chapters, it has become clear that we also need to consider posttraumatic growth (PTG) in order to understand the experiences of people with PTSD symptoms in relation to their chronic illnesses. While the traumas mentioned in the literature suggest that they can have a negative impact on the distress outcomes of people who have experienced PTSD in a physical illness, the studies on PTG also suggest that they can have both positive and negative effects. Positive psychologists consider psychological disorders to be those that differ only in degree, not in kind, from normal life problems. That is, these disorders lie on a continuum of human functioning. Psychological disorders result not only from people's internal problems, but also from the way they interact with their environment, including other people and culture. Positive psychologists aim to identify human strengths and promote mental health (Joseph & Linley, 2008). They focus on positive changes triggered within oneself that go beyond previous levels of functioning and well-being and vice versa.

The inoculation hypothesis (Eysenck, 1983) states that exposure to stress or past crises could increase one's defences or resistance to later stress and allow people to develop coping strategies that would help them adapt to traumatic events. People who have successfully adapted to earlier trauma tend to cope better with later stresses in life (e.g. Gibbs, 1989; Norris & Murrell, 1988). Similarly, stress inoculation and resilience theory argues that past success in coping with stressful events can be an important resource for strengthening resilience and coping skills that act as a buffer against future distress, functional impairment, and posttraumatic stress symptoms (PTSS). On the other hand, people who have had little experience of coping with adversity in the past may find current or future adversity extremely challenging. The idea is that what did not kill us in the past may make us stronger in the future (Joseph, 2011; Meichenbaum & Novaco, 1985; Seery, 2011; Updegraff & Taylor, 2000).

Although the topic of PTG is not the main concern of this book, the information reviewed suggests that it is an important topic for PTSD in physical illness. PTG involves the co-existence of trauma and resilience. According to the psychosocial framework integrating PTSD and PTG, personality (traumatic schema) may influence trauma appraisal, emotional states, and coping (e.g. avoidance strategies), which in turn may paradoxically influence positive changes in personality or psychological well-being, that is, understanding their place and significance in the world and coping with existential challenges in life including trauma (Joseph & Linley, 2008). Among university students who experienced various traumas in the past, cumulative adversity was positively correlated with PTG, and coping with trauma adversity could facilitate the development of PTG (Jirek & Saunders, 2018). Another study examined multicultural individuals and found that people's struggle with cumulative adversity was related to the development of the psychological well-being outcomes of personal growth and positive relationships with others. These findings highlight the importance of incorporating cumulative adversity into the PTG process. Valuing diversity and positive framing could also be important mechanisms for growth following adversity (Sadaghiyani et al., 2022). Similarly, in non-clinical adolescents, experiencing more events was associated with greater PTSS and some forms of PTG, including changing priorities, increasing self-reliance, and finding a new path in life, although the majority of adolescents attributed their PTG to one specific event rather than multiple events. Trauma severity and PTSS were also linearly correlated with PTG (Fraus et al., 2023).

It has also been argued that PTG is a useful coping resource for cumulative trauma. Research has shown that PTG was associated with attenuating the impact of trauma on subjective well-being in helping professionals with experience of cumulative trauma (Veronese et al., 2017). In other words, whether the impact of cumulative trauma affects the severity of people's distress could depend on the level of PTG. However, previous studies have not always confirmed this link between cumulative trauma and PTG. One study found that women with breast cancer had higher levels of PTG (new possibilities, personal strengths, and spiritual changes) than healthy women with a severe non-cancer-related stressful life event and allostatic load. In other words, chronic stress could hinder growth after adversity (Ruini et al., 2015).

People have the ability to understand and meaningfully integrate traumatic experiences while optimising their psychological well-being and rebuilding their lives. Their traumatic experience has motivated them to think about how to develop adaptive beliefs that help them cope better with future difficulties. As a result, they develop new characteristics and strengths. In other words, the event has changed them in a positive way. They can integrate these positive changes into their lives, which in turn promotes growth and meaning in life (Calhoun et al., 2010; Janoff-Bulman, 2006; Tedeschi & Calhoun, 2004).

PTG involves positive changes in personality schema and adopted assumptive worlds that are related to psychological well-being. This well-being is characterised by changes in life philosophy (purpose in life, autonomy), self-perception (mastery of the environment, personal growth and self-acceptance) and relationships with others (building positive relationships with others) (Joseph & Linley, 2008). As mentioned in Chapter 2, 'organismic valuing theory' explains the cognitive processes involved. To reiterate, after trauma, people may integrate the trauma experience into their pre-trauma belief systems or worldviews (the assimilation process), while they may also change their pre-trauma beliefs in light of their trauma experience (the accommodation process). Assimilators can accept the fact that unfortunate events happen in life and that they can recover from the trauma and restore their pre-trauma psychological well-being. In other words, they have not 'grown' from their trauma, but have regained their level of wellbeing before the trauma. They are vulnerable to future stressful events. However, some accommodators may change their pre-trauma beliefs in a negative way. For example, they may believe that unfortunate events happen in life and that there is absolutely nothing they can do to prevent them. As a result, they tend to experience increased hopelessness, PTSD symptoms, and other psychiatric symptoms. Other accommodators may appropriately or positively change their beliefs before the trauma; for example, that unfortunate events happen in life, which means that life is unpredictable, and therefore we should cherish our lives and live life to the fullest. These people tend to 'grow' from the trauma and experience higher levels of well-being or lower levels of psychiatric symptoms (Joseph, 2011; Joseph & Linley, 2005).

Rather than growing by adopting the above lines of thought, it has been argued that some people can grow by living in a kind of illusion. For example, comparing our own situation with that of others can also be a motivating factor for growth, although such a comparison may not correspond to reality. This is called a 'positive illusion', which reflects the degree of divergence between personal belief and reality. According to cognitive adaptation theory, while trauma may affect victims' self-concept, they can still take an active role in preventing this attack on the self by adopting a particular belief. Whether this belief accurately reflects reality is another matter. Nevertheless, it can help them to protect their self. For example, they might compare themselves to other people's situation and believe that there are people who are much worse off than they are. As a result, they feel better—their self-esteem is strengthened and they are more optimistic about the future. Such a perception is a kind of illusion, but a positive one. What is important here is that people adapt to the stressor by being able to develop and maintain such an illusion. This is particularly useful to protect yourself in the early stages of the trauma, which can later strengthen your ability to accept the predicament. It is worth noting that the departure between positive illusions and reality should not be too great. Otherwise, one wonders whether it is actually a form of dissociation, self-deception, or delusion (Taylor, 1989; Taylor & Armor, 1996).

Comparing oneself to others in relation to one's situation is only one positive illusory example. According to the Janus-face model of self-perceived growth, some may enhance this illusory or self-deceptive aspect of PTG by exaggerating their sense of control and developing unrealistic optimism about the future. This type of illusion can coexist with PTG and affect distress outcomes. This is almost comparable to the placebo effect in the sense that my belief (e.g. that I have taken a newly developed medicine, but in fact I have not) can influence outcomes. Similarly, if they have a belief that they have a sense of control, that their future is optimistic and that other people are worse off than they are, this will make them stronger and encourage their growth, which in turn should provide a buffer against distress. Now that patients have become stronger and have adapted to the trauma, the self-deceptive aspect of PTG will diminish, while the non-self-deceptive or constructive aspect of growth will increase. This is the point at which concrete actions take place that lead to real positive change (Maercker & Zoellner, 2004; Zoellner & Maercker, 2006).

Two unexplored issues related to posttraumatic growth

In light of what has been said, two issues are worth mentioning. First, PTG is not independent of the distorted self-structure described above. So the question is how people with a physical illness can experience growth when they experience distorted self-structure. This question has not been addressed in the literature for people with PTSD in physical illness. In order to say that someone has developed PTG, they must experience changes in their personality or their assumed world that occur as part of their process of adjustment in relation to new appraisals. These changes must involve a positive reconfiguration of the schema. How would people with a distorted self trigger these positive changes in themselves or develop a positive schema if their schema has been changed or reconfigured into a traumatised schema?

The process by which people with certain functioning personality traits from before the trauma—who see their trauma as a reference point in their lives, explain various aspects of their lives in terms of the trauma, have changed their outlook on life, and may feel empty, fragmented, overcontrolled, and unbalanced—can transform into someone who has the psychological well-being described by PTG researchers has yet to be explored. For example, when people with some of the posttraumatic typologies have problems that are opposite to the characteristics of psychological well-being (e.g. feeling despair, depressed vs feeling meaning in life; passivity, helplessness vs autonomy; being self-absorbed, insecure, dependent vs self-accepting; withdrawing from others, isolating, distrusting others and the world vs having positive relationships with others), we might investigate how their notion of psychological well-being can be developed. In respect of the organismic valuing theory, there is a need for a better understanding of the process by which people with these posttraumatic typologies and traumatic physical illness experiences can become positive accommodators who accept life as unpredictable, value their lives to the fullest, and thereby grow.

The second issue concerns illusory growth. This illusory or self-deceptive approach reminds us of a similar, though not identical, debate in philosophy about the nature of self-deception. That debate is about how self-deceivers deliberately trick themselves into believing something while knowing or believing full well that that something is not true. In other words, self-deceivers must (1) hold contradictory beliefs and (2) intentionally trick themselves into having a belief that they know or believe is false (Mele, 2001). The question of the possibility of self-deception has given rise to many philosophical debates.

In the case of illusory growth, the self-deceivers (the patients themselves) must (1) hold contradictory beliefs and (2) deliberately trick themselves into having a belief (e.g. they have a sense of control and have an optimistic future) that they know or believe may be false. Interestingly, positive psychologists seem to believe that some people develop PTG under this kind of paradox.

Some philosophers have argued that there is a temporal or psychological partitioning. Put simply, the former means that when self-deception occurs, the deceiver may, over time, forget the deception due to normal degradation of memory that can interrupt awareness of one's intention. It could be argued that self-deception is in some sense subintentional (Johnston, 1988). The latter refers to the fact that there is a strong division in the self, where the deceiving part is a relatively autonomous subagency capable of belief, desire, and intention (Rorty, 1988). In self-deception, however, this deceiving sub-system is hidden from the conscious self that is being deceived. This seems to correspond to the idea of dissociation, where patients with a fragmented self experience themselves not as a whole person but as broken into pieces, are chronically anxious, and engage in dissociation. Does this mean that dissociation partly facilitates the growth process? The question remains: How can this kind of self-deceptive process help patients suffering from PTSD related to their illness to initiate a growth process? To take the question even further: How can patients with physical illness and a distorted self use this self-deception process to trigger growth? These conceptual questions need to be explored further.

Family relationships in PTSD in connection with physical illnesses

The literature reviewed in Chapters 4, 6, and 9 has shown that chronic illnesses can affect both the patients themselves and their family members. One cannot ignore the importance of family or intimate relationships when examining PTSD in physical illness. The secondary victims are mostly family members as secondary or vicarious trauma victims of cancer (Figley, 1998; Figley & Kleber, 1995). These studies describe how children's distress (cancer or PTSD) can affect parents' distress, how parents' distress can affect their children's distress, how children's distress can affect their siblings' distress, and how patients' distress can affect their partners' distress. However, one should remember that the impact of family member A on family member B is not independent of the impact of family member A or B on family member C. All family members—parents, children, siblings, and partners—are connected in some way. The studies reviewed in this book do not examine how the chronic illness and PTSD of all family members interact to affect distress outcomes, although studies of this kind can be very labour intensive.

Nonetheless, PTSD is found in physical illness in patients and their secondary trauma victims in the context of a family relationship. Much emphasis has been placed on how families adapt to stressors such as a physical illness. For example, the Family Adjustment and Adaptation Response Model (Patterson, 1988) assumes that an important function of the family is to maintain a homeostatic state or equilibrium (balanced functioning) by using its capabilities, characterised by resources and coping behaviours, to meet demands (i.e. stressors). Successful coping with demands would mean that families have achieved family adjustment or adaptation.

To explain this model a little further, all families are confronted with a stressor at some point and have to face its demands. A stressor is defined as a life event that occurs at a particular time, amplifies the demands, disrupts the homeostatic state and thereby causes change and ongoing stress in the family's social system. If families can use their existing capacities to meet these demands and cause only minor changes within the family, they can be considered to be living in a relatively stable period and going through a period of adjustment. The way in which family members interact with each other is predictable and stable. However, when families are faced with different demands at the same time, which may accumulate over time, they are in an adaptation phase in which they try to reduce the demands, change their perception of the current situation, and finally restore homeostasis by acquiring new adaptive resources and relying on new coping behaviours. However, demands may accumulate to such an extent that the demand load may exceed the families' existing capacities to cope. A major stressor such as cancer within the family can also push the burden beyond their capacity. Families would find themselves in a state of instability, imbalance, or disequilibrium. They therefore fail to cope, leading to tension, stress and strain, and possibly exhaustion. In other words, stress does not arise from the occurrence of demands, but from an imbalance between demands and capacities.

We should say a few words about capacities, which can be defined in terms of resources (i.e. what families have) and coping behaviours (i.e. what families do). Personal resources include, for example, personality traits, self-esteem, physical and emotional health of family members, and the feeling of being able to cope with difficulties. Family resources include the degree of cohesion (e.g. unity, trust, appreciation, support, and integration between family members), adaptability (how the family can overcome challenges together), and communication within the family system. Other resources include community-based resources that families can rely on, including services from health facilities, schools, religious organisations, or some government agencies. These resources ultimately provide families with a range of social support, whether emotional, informational, or instrumental.

As for coping behaviour, it is defined in terms of the efforts family members make to cope with a demand or to reduce its impact. This coping behaviour aims to maintain family integration and cooperation in order to care for a sick child, for example. In this way, balance or homeostatic status is maintained and restored. Some examples of these coping strategies are spending time together as a family, mutual emotional and informal support, expression of emotions, cognitive reappraisal of demands, maintaining an optimistic outlook, and an accepting attitude.

In light of this model, one can ask how a family of patients with PTSD-related illnesses and family members with secondary traumatic effects would interact to maintain a homeostatic state by acquiring new adaptive resources and adopting new coping behaviours to manage cumulative stress demands, change their appraisal of the current situation, and restore homeostasis. These cumulative effects can lead to a kind of overwhelming demand that exceeds the families' existing capacity to cope with the stress. It is important to understand the implications of the family being in a state of instability or imbalance. The resources of personality (e.g. personality traits), family (e.g. integration between family members), adaptability (how the family cohere together), communication between family members and family coping behaviours (emotional and informal support for each other, emotional expressiveness) mentioned earlier can also be distorted by the trauma, as mentioned in the previous section on the concept of self. The distortion of these components inevitably affects their ability to meet the demands mentioned above.

The above speaks to the study of a suffering family unit, as opposed to suffering between family members A and B, or family member A, or B and C. The transmissible traumatic effect between family members is likely to be exacerbated because, according to Bowen family systems theory (Bowen, 1978), the family is an interdependent and emotional unit in which family members are emotionally connected. Family members influence each other's thoughts, feelings, and behaviours, seek each other's attention, approval, and support, and respond to each other's needs, expectations, and emotions as if they shared the same 'emotional skin'. Some changes in the psychological or social functioning of one family member (e.g. PTSD in the children with cancer) result in reciprocal changes in other family members. Increased anxiety in one member (the sick children) can often exacerbate the anxiety of the other members, cause a lot of stress, leading them to feel overwhelmed and to begin to isolate themselves. These members, whether the parents or the siblings, are usually the ones who try to adapt to the stressful situation, absorb the anxiety within the family and risk developing psychological problems such as depression, PTSD, or some physical illnesses.

In addition, trauma can also affect interpersonal relationships, leading to interpersonal conflict, and chaotic and emotionally upsetting relationships. They might even experience idealisation–disillusionment, drastically changing their opinion about important people and shifting from a positive to a negative view. They may also feel that they have been abandoned by others. Trauma victims may have difficulty maintaining a coherent sense of identity and self-awareness in different contexts. Consequently, they may have problems understanding themselves and experience identity diffusion as they tend to confuse their feelings, thoughts, or perspectives with those of others (Briere & Runtz, 2002). The point is that these changes in self would likely increase communication problems, problems with trust, support, cooperation and integration between family members to cope with the challenges and care of the ill person. Thus, they are likely to spend less time together as a family, sharing emotions and supporting each other. What remains is suffering in silence between family members.

To the complex relationships that exist between the family members of this suffering family, another level is added. Namely, while the illness itself plays a major role in creating the stress within the family, according to family stress theory (Boss & Greenberg, 1984), the distress can also result from an ambiguous loss. Loss and separation due to events such as divorce, death, or children moving out of the parental home are common or even inevitable in some cases. However, the term 'missing family members' is not limited to physical disappearance, but also to psychological disappearance. For example, a family member (e.g. a parent) suffering from a chronic illness (e.g. cancer) may be physically present but at the same time psychologically absent. This type of loss can be a major stressor for the family as a whole (Boss, 1999, 2007).

Following this loss, family members may feel uncertain about who is and who is not in the family, and who performs what roles and tasks within the family. As a result, immobilisation occurs within the family, where family decisions are postponed, certain tasks are taken over by family members who do not have the capacity to do so, and some members take on more tasks than before. The psychological absence of a family member, together with the sense of loss, could increase the likelihood of other family members experiencing psychological distress and disrupt family dynamics and cohesion. At the same time, family members might try to cope with the changes within the family and protect the affected family member (in this case, the cancer patient), for example, by avoiding issues that might upset the patient or by encouraging the patient to detach behaviourally or emotionally from their current situation. However, one consequence of this is reduced emotional expressiveness, self-disclosure, or trauma-related disclosure, which in turn impairs emotional processing of trauma memories and recovery, but perpetuates traumatic distress (Monson et al., 2012).

Another level of complexity concerns the attachment experiences between children and parents. Attachment (Bowlby, 1969, 2005) is a relevant concept in current discussions because attachment experiences and emotional regulation play a crucial role in coping and regulating distress, maintaining resilience, and sustaining psychological well-being (Mikulincer & Shaver, 2007, 2012; Mikulincer et al., 2003). The ways in which we learned to acknowledge and express emotions, restore emotional balance, understand emotions and communicate feelings in socially acceptable ways, and use emotion regulation strategies were largely based on a secure foundation in terms of relationships with others and were influenced by whether, at the time we faced distress or some obstacles or difficulties and felt we needed help, caregivers (e.g. parents) were available, responsive, emotionally accessible, approachable, and supportive. The experience of such security and the resulting feelings of relief and comfort that come from being close to caregivers would help us face difficulties with confidence and move on to other activities (Cassidy, 1994; Waters & Waters, 2006). In other words, when this secure attachment is activated, the feeling of safety would guide behaviour, alleviate distress, promote positive emotions, and enhance adaptive or effective coping strategies (Mikulincer et al., 2009).

On the contrary, when care is poor or insecure, the development of effective or adaptive coping strategies or emotional regulation strategies is interrupted, so that people feel physically and emotionally insecure. This kind of insecurity and the lack of observing a role model for constructive or non-threatening expression of emotions would lead to discomfort or ambivalence in expressing one's emotions. Instead, the emotions of their thoughts and actions create a sense of extreme discomfort or extreme fear, which they resist or try to block. In this way, however, distressing emotions are suppressed, unprocessed, and thus remain unresolved, which in turn means that they are unable to cope with difficulties in life (Berenbaum & James, 1994). They therefore increase the risk of developing psychological symptoms, psychosomatic problems, or negative affect due to accumulated, unresolved, and unprocessed distressing feelings in the physiological and neurological system (Amstadter & Vernon, 2008; Gross & John, 2003; Pennebaker, 1995; Rachman, 1980).

When examining how a family of patients with PTSD-related illnesses and family members with secondary traumatic effects would work together to cope with cumulative stressful demands by using certain resources and adopting certain coping strategies, interpersonal functioning between family members, ambiguous loss in the family, and attachment experiences are some of the other factors that also need to be considered.

A hypothesised model

Taken together with what has been discussed so far, a hypothesised model (see Figure 10.1) can now be created to illustrate the relationship between the psychological constructs mentioned in the overarching research question, PTG, and family functioning. It is important to note that the main intention behind the diagram is to conceptualise the relationship between the constructs. Thus, although the diagram seems to advocate a structural equation model, which is an acceptable way of looking at it, this does not mean that it must be interpreted in this way. In considering this model, one might wonder whether a distorted self interacts with coping or defence to mitigate the effects of cumulative trauma (i.e. PTSD due to previous trauma plus illness-related PTSD subtypes) on people with physical illnesses, or whether growth also has a similar mitigating effect. Whether distorted self, coping or defence, and growth should be considered mediators or moderators depends on individual interpretation.

Alternatively, this model could focus on the coexisting relationship between facets of the distorted self and coping or defence and how this relationship might influence cumulative trauma. A person-centred latent class analysis approach can be used for this purpose. Discrete subgroups (classes) of people with physical illnesses who exhibit similar patterns of response would be identified. Whereas homogeneity is found between persons within each subgroup, heterogeneity is found between persons in different subgroups (Lubke & Muthen, 2007).

The family construct is a broad one that includes an indicator of the wellbeing of family members. In this sense, the model is concerned with how people with chronic illnesses who have specific profiles of a distorted self and coping or defence strategies, or who have developed different types of growth, influence the psychological or physical well-being of family members, be they parents, siblings, or partners. At the same time, the family construct also

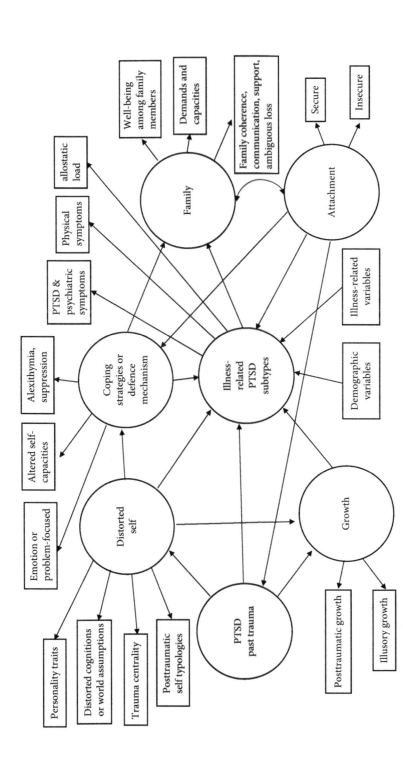

Figure 10.1 The hypothesised model.

PTSD, posttraumatic stress disorder.

includes indicators that measure family functioning, family dynamics, or family cohesion as seen by different family members, rather than the well-being of family members *per se*.

As far as attachment is concerned, it could be argued that it should be treated as one of the indicators of the family construct and not as a construct in its own right. Nevertheless, there is a wealth of studies that have examined the impact of attachment on PTSD as a coping process rather than in a family psychology context (Mikulincer et al., 2015). This is the reason for treating it as a separate construct in this model.

Summary

This chapter has aimed to outline some gaps in knowledge from existing research, to formulate an overarching research question, and to build a hypothesised model. As PTSD often co-occurs with other and psychiatric symptoms, one research gap is whether PTSD subtypes are a possible area of investigation for patients with chronic illnesses. It is clear from the existing literature that PTSD symptoms can be triggered by traumatic events in the past prior to the onset of chronic illness or by the illness itself, both of which manifest their clinical features differently. Such cumulative trauma could affect the outcome of distress. The risk factors examined in the previous chapters can be broadly categorised according to demographic characteristics, specific disease-related variables, personality traits, and coping strategies. Another research gap is whether the relationship between cumulative trauma and distress outcomes, including PTSD subtypes, would be moderated by the interaction between personality and coping strategies after controlling for demographic variables and specific disease-related variables.

However, a distorted self may underpin the complex interaction between cumulative trauma and risk factors. The notion of a distorted self has been taken up in literature addressing cognitive changes in trauma survivors, including the shattered assumption hypothesis, the cognitive model of PTSD, and the trauma centrality hypothesis. The literature also addresses the disjointedness of the self. Trauma can affect the coherence, connection, continuity, and integration of the self, leading to fragmentation and splitting of the self, characterised by different types of posttraumatic personality typologies. Another research gap then concerns how the distorted self may affect the complex interaction between cumulative trauma and personality and coping risk factors in people who have experienced PTSD in the context of their physical illness.

This phenomenon of the distorted self is also relevant to PTG, which forms another research gap, namely how people with physical illness can experience growth when they experience a distorted self-structure. It is a puzzling phenomenon how people with a distorted self can develop a positive schema that has been reconfigured into a traumatised schema. More research is needed to understand the process by which people with certain personality traits that were functioning before the trauma—who see their trauma as a reference point in their lives, life histories, and new outlook on life, and who experience emptiness, fragmentation and other posttraumatic self characteristics—can transform into someone who has the kind of psychological well-being described in the literature from PTG. Another research gap is how illusory growth, as a kind of self-deception process, can help trigger growth in patients with PTSD who suffer from their illnesses and a distorted self.

The chronic illness of one family member can affect the psychological well-being of other family members. The role of PTSD in family and intimate relationships cannot be ignored. It is not clear how a family with patients with PTSD-related illnesses and family members with secondary traumatic effects would work together to manage cumulative stress demands. To extend this even further, it is not clear how a family can manage or reduce the demands resulting from the cumulative effects of PTSD and secondary traumatic effects of different family members, change their appraisal of the current situation, and restore homeostasis within a family. A family's ability to cope needs to be examined in the context of the distorted self mentioned earlier, other problems related to interpersonal conflict, ambiguous losses within a family, and attachment experiences between caregivers and children.

References

Albahari, M. (2006). *Analytical Buddhism: The two-tiered illusion of self.* Palgrave-Macmillan.

Aldwin, C. M., & Brustrom, J. (1997). Theories of coping with chronic stress: Illustrations from the health psychology and aging literatures. In B. H. Gottlieb (Ed.), *Coping with chronic stress* (pp. 75–103). Plenum Press. https://doi.org/10.1007/978-1-4757-9862-3_3

Aldwin, C. M., Sutton, K. J., & Lachman, M. (1996). The development of coping resources in adulthood. *Journal of Personality, 64,* 837–2871.

Amir, M., Kaplan, Z., Efroni, R., Levine, Y., Benjamin, J., & Kotler, M. (1997). Coping styles in post-traumatic stress disorder (PTSD) patients. *Personality and Individual Differences, 23,* 399–2405.

Amstadter, A. B., & Vernon, L. L. (2008). A preliminary examination of thought suppression, emotion regulation, and coping in a trauma-exposed sample. *Journal of Aggression, Maltreatment & Trauma, 17*(3), 279–295.https://doi.org/10.1080/10926770802403236

Appleyard, K., Egeland, B., van Dulmen, M. H., & Sroufe, L. A. (2005). When more is not better: The role of cumulative risk in child behavior outcomes. *Journal of Child Psychology & Psychiatry, 46*(3), 235–245. https://doi.org/10.1111/j.1469-7610.2004.00351.x

Audi, R. (2010). *Epistemology: A contemporary introduction to the theory of knowledge.* Routledge.

Baumeister, R. F. (1987). How the self became a problem: A psychological review of historical research. *Journal of Personality and Social Psychology, 52,* 163–176. https://doi.org/10.1037/0022-3514.52.1.163

Berenbaum, H., & James, T. (1994). Correlates and retrospectively reported antecedents of alexithymia. *Psychosomatic Medicine, 56*(4), 353–359. https://doi.org/10.1097/00006842-199407000-00011

Bernard, J. D., Whittles, R. L., Kertz, S. J., & Burke, P. A. (2015). Trauma and event centrality: Valence and incorporation into identity influence well-being more than exposure. *Psychological Trauma, 7*(1), 11–17.

Berntsen, D. (2001). Involuntary memories of emotional events: Do memories of traumas and extremely happy events differ? *Applied Cognitive Psychology, 15,* S135–S158. https://doi.org/10.1002/acp.838

Berntsen, D., & Rubin, D. C. (2006a). The centrality of event scale: A measure of integrating a trauma into one's identity and its relation to post-traumatic stress disorder symptoms. *Behaviour Research and Therapy, 44*(2), 219–231.

Berntsen, D., & Rubin, D. C. (2006b). Flashbulb memories and posttraumatic stress reactions across the life span: Age-related effects of the German occupation of Denmark during World War II. *Psychology and Aging, 21*(1), 127–139.

Berntsen, D., & Rubin, D. C. (2007). When a trauma becomes a key to identity: Enhanced integration of trauma memories predicts posttraumatic stress disorder symptoms. *Applied Cognitive Psychology, 21*(4), 417–431.

Boals, A., & Schuettler, D. (2011). A double-edged sword: Event centrality, PTSD and post-traumatic growth. *Applied Cognitive Psychology, 25*(5), 817–822.

Bolger, N., & Zuckerman, A. (1995). A framework for studying personality in the stress process. *Journal of Personality & Social Psychology, 69,* 890–902.

Boss, P. (1999). *Ambiguous loss.* Harvard University Press.

Boss, P. (2007). Ambiguous loss theory: Challenges for scholars and practitioners. *Family Relations, 56*(2), 105–110. http://www.jstor.org/stable/4541653

Boss, P., & Greenberg, J. (1984). Family boundary ambiguity: A new variable in family stress theory. *Family Process, 23,* 535–546. https://doi.org/10.1111/j.1545-5300.1984.00535.x

Bowen, M. (1978). *Family therapy in clinical practice.* Jason Aronson.

Bowlby, J. (1969). *Attachment and loss.* Basic Books.

Bowlby, J. (2005). *A secure base.* Routledge.

Brewin, C. R., Dalgleish, T., & Joseph, S. (1996). A dual representation theory of posttraumatic stress disorder. *Psychological Review, 103*(4), 670–686.

Briere, J. (1996). A self-trauma model for treating adult survivors of severe child abuse. In J. Briere, L. Berliner, J. A. Bulkley, C. Jenny, & T. Reid (Eds.), *The APSAC handbook on child maltreatment* (pp. 140–157). Sage Publications.

Briere, J. (2002). Treating adult survivors of severe childhood abuse and neglect: future development of an integrative model. In J. Briere, L. Berliner, J. A. Bulkley, C. Jenny, & T. Reid (Eds.), *The APSAC handbook on child maltreatment* (pp. 175–204.). Sage Publications.

Briere, J., & Runtz, M. (2002). The Inventory of Altered Self-Capacities (IASC): A standardized measure of identity, affect regulation, and relationship disturbance. *Assessment, 9,* 230–239.

Briere, J., & Spinazzola, J. (2005). Phenomenology and psychological assessment of complex posttraumatic states. *Journal of Traumatic Stress, 18,* 401–412.

Briere, J. N. (1992). *Child abuse trauma: Theory and treatment of the lasting effects.* Sage Publications.

Brown, A. D., Antonius, D., Kramer, M., Root, J. C., & Hirst, W. (2010). Trauma centrality and PTSD in veterans returning from Iraq and Afghanistan. *Journal of Traumatic Stress, 23*(4), 496–499.

Busch, F. N. (2014). Clinical approaches to somatization. *Journal of Clinical Psychology, 70*(5), 419–427.

Calhoun, L. G., Cann, A., & Tedeschi, R. G. (2010). The posttraumatic growth model: Sociocultural considerations. In Weiss, T., & Berger, R. (Eds.), *Posttraumatic growth and culturally competent practice: Lessons learned from around the globe* (pp. 1–14). John Wiley & Sons.

Carver, C. S., & Connor-Smith, J. (2010). Personality and coping. *Annual Review of Psychology, 61*, 679–704.

Cassidy, J. (1994). Emotion regulation: Influences of attachment relationships. *Monographs of the Society for Research in Child Development, 59*(2–3), 228–283.

Chung, M. C., Dennis, I., Easthope, Y., Werrett, J., & Farmer, S. (2005). A multiple-indicator multiple-cause model for posttraumatic stress reactions: Personality, coping and maladjustment. *Psychosomatic Medicine, 67*, 251–259.

Cieslak, R., Benight, C. C., & Lehman, V. C. (2008). Coping self-efficacy mediates the effects of negative cognitions on posttraumatic distress. *Behaviour Research and Therapy, 46*, 788–798.

Clohessy, S., & Ehlers, A. (1999). PTSD symptoms, response to intrusive memories and coping in ambulance service workers. *British Journal of Clinical Psychology, 38*(3), 251–265.

Cohen, M. (2013). The association of cancer patients' emotional suppression and their self-rating of psychological distress on short screening tools. *Behavioral Medicine, 39*, 29–35.

Connor-Smith, J. K., & Flachsbart, C. (2007). Relations between personality and coping: A meta-analysis. *Journal of Personality and Social Psychology, 93*, 1080–1107. https://doi.org/10.1037/0022-3514.93.6.1080

Costa Jr, P. T., Somerfield, M. R., & McCrae, R. R. (1996). Personality and coping: A reconceptualization. In M. Zeidner & Endler, N. S. (Eds.), *Handbook of coping: Theory, research, applications* (pp. 44–61). John Wiley & Sons.

Descartes, R. (1641/1960). *Meditations on first philosophy.* The Liberal Arts Press.

Edmondson, D. (2014). An enduring somatic threat model of posttraumatic stress disorder due to acute life-threatening medical events. *Social and Personality Psychology Compass, 8*(3), 118–134. https://doi.org/10.1111/spc3.12089

Ehlers, A., & Clark, D. M. (2000). A cognitive model of posttraumatic stress disorder. *Behaviour Research Therapy, 38*, 319–345.

Endler, N. S. (1983). Interactionism: A personality model, but not yet a theory. In M. M. Page (Ed.), *Nebraska Symposium on Motivation, 1982: Personality-Current theory and research* (pp. 155–200). Lincoln: University of Nebraska Press.

Endler, N. S., & Edwards, J. M. (1986). Interactionism in personality in the twentieth century. *Personality and Individual Differences, 7*(3), 379–384. https://doi.org/https://doi.org/10.1016/0191-8869(86)90013-9

Eysenck, H. J. (1983). Stress, disease and personality: The "inoculation effect." In C. L. Cooper (Ed.), *Stress and research* (pp. 121–146). John Wiley & Sons.

Fait, K., Vilchinsky, N., Dekel, R., Levi, N., Hod, H., & Matetzky, S. (2018). Cardiac-disease-induced PTSD and fear of illness progression: Capturing the unique nature of disease-related PTSD. *General Hospital Psychiatry, 53*, 131–138. https://doi.org/10.1016/j.genhosppsych.2018.02.011

Fang, S., & Chung, M. C. (2019). The impact of past trauma on psychological distress among Chinese students: The roles of cognitive distortion and alexithymia. *Psychiatry Research, 271,* 136–143.

Fang, S., Chung, M. C., & Wang, Y. (2020). The impact of past trauma on psychological distress: The roles of defense mechanisms and alexithymia. *Frontiers in Psychology, 11*(992). https://doi.org/10.3389/fpsyg.2020.00992

Figley, C. R. (1998). Burnout as systemic traumatic stress: A model for helping traumatized family members. In C. R. Figley (Ed.), *Burnout in families: The systemic costs of caring* (pp. 15–28). CRC Press.

Figley, C. R., & Kleber, R. J. (1995). Beyond the "victim": Secondary traumatic stress. In R. J. Kleber, C. R. Figley, & B. P. R. Gersons (Eds.), *Beyond trauma: Cultural and societal dynamics* (pp. 75–98). Plenum Press. https://doi.org/10.1007/978-1-4757-9421-2_5

Fitzgerald, J. M. (1988). Vivid memories and the reminiscence phenomenon: The role of a self narrative. *Human Development, 31,* 261–273.

Flood, A. M., Boyle, S. H., Calhoun, P. S., Dennis, M. F., Barefoot, J. C., Moore, S. D., & Beckham, J. C. (2010). Prospective study of externalizing and internalizing subtypes of posttraumatic stress disorder and their relationship to mortality among Vietnam veterans. *Comprehensive Psychiatry, 51*(3), 236–242.

Follette, V. M., Polusny, M. A., Bechtle, A. E., & Naugle, A. E. (1996). Cumulative trauma: The impact of child sexual abuse, adult sexual assault, and spouse abuse. *Journal of Traumatic Stress, 9,* 25–35. https://doi.org/10.1002/jts.2490090104

Fraus, K., Dominick, W., Walenski, A., & Taku, K. (2023). The impact of multiple stressful life events on posttraumatic growth in adolescence. *Psychological Trauma, 15*(1), 10–17. https://doi.org/10.1037/tra0001181

Gibbs, M. S. (1989). Factors in the victim that mediate between disaster and psychopathology: A review. *Journal of Traumatic Stress, 2*(4), 489–514. https://doi.org/https://doi.org/10.1002/jts.2490020411

Gross, J. J. (1998). The emerging field of emotion regulation: An integrative review. *Review of General Psychology, 2,* 271–299.

Gross, J. J., & John, O. P. (2003). Individual differences in two emotion regulation processes: Implications for affect, relationships, and well-being. *Journal of Personality and Social Psychology, 85,* 348–362.

Heil, J. (1992). *The nature of true minds.* Cambridge University Press. https://doi.org/DOI: 10.1017/CBO9780511625367

Heil, J. (1998). Privileged access. In P. Ludlow & N. Martin (Eds.), *Externalism and self-knowledge* (p. 264). University of Chicago Press.

Hewitt, P. L., & Flett, G. L. (1996). Personality traits and the coping process. In M. Zeidner, & N. S. Endler (Eds.), *Handbook of coping: Theory, research, applications* (pp. 410–433). John Wiley & Sons.

Ho, R. T. H., Chan, C. L. W., & Ho, S. M. Y. (2004). Emotional control in Chinese female cancer survivors. *Psycho-Oncology, 13,* 808–817.

Hobfoll, S. E. (1989). Conservation of resources: A new attempt at conceptualizing stress. *The American Psychologist, 44,* 513–524.

Hobfoll, S. E., Freedy, J. R., Green, B. L., & Solomon, S. D. (1996). Coping in reaction to extreme stress: The roles of resource loss and resource availability. In M. Zeidner & Endler, N. S. (Eds.), In *Handbook of coping: Theory, research, applications.* (pp. 322–349). John Wiley & Sons.

Honkalampi, K., Hintikka, J., Koivumaa-Honkanen, H., Antikainen, R., Haatainen, K., & Viinamaki, H. (2007). Long-term alexithymic features indicate poor recovery from depression and psychopathology: A six-year follow-up. *Psychotherapy and Psychosomatics,* *76*(5), 312–314.

Horowitz, M. J. (1976). *Stress response syndromes.* Aronson.

Horowitz, M. J. (1986). Stress-response syndromes: A review of posttraumatic and adjustment disorders. *Hospital & Community Psychiatry, 37,* 241–249.

Hume, D. (1739/1974). *Treatise of human nature.* Clarendon.

Ihilevich, D., & Gleser, G. C. (1993). *Defense mechanisms: Their classification, correlates, and measurement with the Defence Mechanisms Inventory.* Psychological Assessment Resources.

Iwamitsu, Y., Shimoda, K., Abe, H., & Tani, T. (2005). Anxiety, emotional suppression, and psychological distress before and after breast cancer diagnosis. *Psychosomatics, 46,* 19–24.

James, W. (1890). *The principles of psychology.* H. Holt & Company.

Janoff-Bulman, R. (1992). *Shattered assumptions: Towards a new psychology of trauma.* Free Press.

Janoff-Bulman, R. (2006). Schema-change perspectives on posttraumatic growth. In L. G. Calhoun & R. G. Tedeschi (Eds.), *Handbook of posttraumatic growth: Research & practice* (pp. 81–99). Lawrence Erlbaum Associates.

Jirek, S. L., & Saunders, D. G. (2018). Cumulative adversity as a correlate of posttraumatic growth: The effects of multiple traumas, discrimination, and sexual harassment. *Journal of Aggression, Maltreatment & Trauma, 27*(6), 612–630. https://doi.org/10.1080/10926 771.2017.1420720

Johnston, M. (1988). Self-deception and the nature of mind. In B. McLaughlin & A. O. Rorty (Eds.), *Perspectives on self-deception* (pp. 63–91). University of California Press.

Jongedijk, R. A., van der Aa, N., Haagen, J. F. G., Boelen, P. A., & Kleber, R. J. (2019). Symptom severity in PTSD and comorbid psychopathology: A latent profile analysis among traumatized veterans. *Journal of Anxiety Disorders, 62,* 35–44. https://doi.org/10.1016/j.janx dis.2018.11.004

Joseph, S. (2011). *What doesn't kill us.* Piatkus.

Joseph, S., & Linley, P. A. (2005). Positive adjustment to threatening events: An organismic valuing theory of growth through adversity. *Review of General Psychology, 9*(3), 262–280. https://doi.org/10.1037/1089-2680.9.3.262

Joseph, S., & Linley, P. A. (Eds.). (2008). *Trauma, recovery, and growth: Positive psychological perspectives on posttraumatic stress.* John Wiley & Sons.

Kohut, H. (1971). *The analysis of the self.* International Universities Press.

Kooiman, C., Spinhoven, P., Trijsburg, R., & Rooijmans, H. (1998). Perceived parental attitude, alexithymia and defense style in psychiatric outpatients. *Psychotherapy and Psychosomatics, 67*(2), 81–87.

Lancaster, S. L., Rodriguez, B. F., & Weston, R. (2011). Path analytic examination of a cognitive model of PTSD. *Behaviour Research and Therapy, 49*(3), 194–201.

Lazarus, R. S. (1993). From psychological stress to the emotions: A history of changing outlooks. *Annual Review of Psychology, 44,* 1–21.

Lazarus, R. S., & Folkman, S. (1984). *Stress, appraisal and coping.* Springer.

Linde, C. (1993). *Life stories. The creation of coherence.* Oxford University Press.

Liverant, G. I., Brown, T. A., Barlow, D. H., & Roemer, L. (2008). Emotion regulation in unipolar depression: The effects of acceptance and suppression of subjective emotional experience on the intensity and duration of sadness and negative affect. *Behaviour Research and Therapy, 46,* 1201–1209.

López, S. R., & Guarnaccia, P. J. (2000). Cultural psychopathology: uncovering the social world of mental illness. *Annual Review of Psychology, 51,* 571–598. https://doi.org/10.1146/annu rev.psych.51.1.571

Lubke, G., & Muthen, B. O. (2007). Performance of factor mixture models as a function of model size, covariate effects, and class-specific parameters. *Structural Equation Modeling*, *14*(1), 26–47.

Maercker, A., & Zoellner, T. (2004). The Janus face of self-perceived growth: toward a two-component model of posttraumatic growth. *Psychological Inquiry*, *15*, 41–48.

Mayou, R., Ehlers, A., & Bryant, B. (2002). Posttraumatic stress disorder after motor vehicle accidents: 3-year follow-up of a prospective longitudinal study. *Behaviour Research and Therapy*, *40*(6), 665–675.

McDougall, J. (1985). *Theatres of the mind. Illusion and truth on the psychoanalytic stage*. Free Association Books.

McEwen, B. S. (1998). Stress, adaptation, and disease. Allostasis and allostatic load. *Annals of the New York Academy of Science*, *840*, 33–44. https://doi.org/10.1111/j.1749-6632.1998.tb09546.x

McEwen, B. S. (2002). Sex, stress and the hippocampus: allostasis, allostatic load and the aging process. *Neurobiology of Aging*, *23*(5), 921–939. https://doi.org/10.1016/s0197-4580(02)00027-1

McEwen, B. S., & Stellar, E. (1993). Stress and the individual. Mechanisms leading to disease. *Archives of Internal Medicine*, *153*(18), 2093–2101.

Meichenbaum, D., & Novaco, R. (1985). Stress inoculation: A preventative approach. *Issues in Mental Health Nursing*, *7*, 419–435. https://doi.org/10.3109/01612848509009464

Mele, A. (2011). Self-control in action. In S. Gallagher (Ed.), *Oxford handbook of the self* (pp. 465–486). Oxford University Press.

Mele, A. R. (2001). *Self-deception unmasked*. Princeton University Press. http://www.jstor.org/stable/j.ctt7s4tg

Mikulincer, M., & Shaver, P. R. (2007). *Attachment in adulthood: Structure, dynamics, and change*. Guilford Press.

Mikulincer, M., & Shaver, P. R. (2012). Attachment theory expanded: A behavioral systems approach. In K. Deaux, & M. Snyder (Eds.), *The Oxford handbook of personality and social psychology* (pp. 467–492). Oxford University Press.

Mikulincer, M., Shaver, P. R., & Pereg, D. (2003). Attachment theory and affect regulation: The dynamics, development, and cognitive consequences of attachment-related strategies. *Motivation and Emotion*, *27*(2), 77–102.

Mikulincer, M., Shaver, P. R., Sapir-Lavid, Y., & Avihou-Kanza, N. (2009). What's inside the minds of securely and insecurely attached people? The secure-base script and its associations with attachment-style dimensions. *Journal of Personality and Social Psychology*, *97*(4), 615–633.

Mikulincer, M., Shaver, P., & Solomon, Z. (2015). An attachment perspective on traumatic and posttraumatic reactions. In M. Safir, H. Wallach, & A. Rizzo (Eds.), *Future directions in posttraumatic stress disorder* (pp. 79–96). Springer Science + Business Media. https://doi.org/10.1007/978-1-4899-7522-5_4

Miller, M. W., & Resick, P. A. (2007). Internalizing and externalizing subtypes in female sexual assault survivors: Implications for the understanding of complex PTSD. *Behavior Therapy*, *38*(1), 58–71. https://doi.org/10.1016/j.beth.2006.04.003

Miller, M. W., Greif, J. L., & Smith, A. A. (2003). Multidimensional personality questionnaire profiles of veterans with traumatic combat exposure: Internalizing and externalizing subtypes. *Psychological Assessment*, *15*, 205–215.

Miller, M. W., Kaloupek, D. G., Dillon, A. L., & Keane, T. M. (2004). Externalizing and internalizing subtypes of combat related PTSD: A replication and extension using the PSY-5 scales. *Journal of Abnormal Psychology*, *112*, 636–645.

Mischel, W., & Morf, C. C. (2003). The self as a psycho-social dynamic processing system: A meta-perspective on a century of the self in psychology. In *Handbook of self and identity*. (pp. 15–43). The Guilford Press.

Monson, C., Fredman, S., Dekel, R., & Macdonald, A. (2012). Family models of posttraumatic stress disorder. In J. G. Beck, & D. M. Sloan (Eds.), *The Oxford handbook of traumatic stress disorders* (pp. 219–232). Oxford Adademic. https://doi.org/10.1093/oxfordhb/9780195399 066.013.0015

Moos, R., & Holahan, C. (2007). Adaptive tasks and methods of coping with illness and disability. *Coping with Chronic Illness and Disability*, *107*, 107–126. https://doi.org/10.1007/978-0-387-48670-3_6

Moos, R. H., & Schaefer, J. A. (1993). Coping resources and processes: Current concepts and measures. In L. Goldberger & S. Breznitz (Eds.), *Handbook of stress: Theoretical and clinical aspects* (pp. 234–257). Free Press.

Morland, L. A., Butler, L. D., & Leskin, G. A. (2008). Resilience and thriving in a time of terrorism. In S. Joseph, & P. A. Linley (Eds.), *Trauma, recovery, and growth: Positive psychological perspectives on posttraumatic stress* (pp. 39–61). John Wiley & Sons.

Myers, L. B., Vetere, A., & Derakshan, N. (2004). Are suppression and repressive coping related? *Personality and Individual Differences*, *36*, 1009–1013.

Nemiah, J. C., & Sifneos, P. E. (1970). Psychosomatic illness: A problem in communication. *Psychotherapy and Psychosomatics*, *18*, 154–160. https://doi.org/10.1159/000286074

Nevid, J. S., & Rathus, S. A. (2007). *Psychology and the challenges of life: Adjustment in the new millennium* (10th ed.). John Wiley & Sons.

Norris, F. H., & Murrell, S. A. (1988). Prior experience as a moderator of disaster impact on anxiety symptoms in older adults. *American Journal of Community Psychology*, *16*, 665–683. https://doi.org/10.1007/BF00930020

Ogle, C. M., Rubin, D. C., & Siegler, I. C. (2014). Cumulative exposure to traumatic events in older adults. *Aging & Mental Health*, *18*(3), 316–325.

Ogle, C. M., Rubin, D. C., & Siegler, I. C. (2016). Maladaptive trauma appraisals mediate the relation between attachment anxiety and PTSD symptom severity. *Psychological Trauma*, *8*(3), 301–309.

Owens, G. P., Chard, K. M., & Cox, T. A. (2008). The relationship between maladaptive cognitions, anger expression, and posttraumatic stress disorder among veterans in residential treatment. *Journal of Aggression, Maltreatment & Trauma*, *17*(4), 439–452.

Pacherie, E. (2011). Self-agency. In S. Gallagher (Ed.), *The Oxford handbook of the self* (pp. 442–464). Oxford University Press.

Palmer, G. A., & Palmer, D. G. (2021). Subtypes in PTSD for veterans: Do similar profiles exist in polytrauma patients? *Journal of Loss and Trauma*, *26*(5), 409–420. https://doi.org/10.1080/15325024.2020.1833550

Parfit, D. (1986). Reasons and persons. Oxford University Press. https://doi.org/10.1093/019 824908x.001.0001

Parker, H., Abreu, A., Sullivan, M., & Vadiveloo, M. (2022). Allostatic load and mortality: A systematic review and meta-analysis. *American Journal of Preventive Medicine*, *63*(1), 131–140. https://doi.org/10.1016/j.amepre.2022.02.003

Pat-Horenczyk, R., Ziv, Y., Asulin-Peretz, L., Achituv, M., Cohen, S., & Brom, D. (2013). Relational trauma in times of political violence: Continuous versus past traumatic stress. *Peace and Conflict*, *19*, 125. https://doi.org/10.1037/a0032488

Patterson, J. M. (1988). Families experiencing stress: I. The Family Adjustment and Adaptation Response Model: II. Applying the FAAR Model to health-related issues for intervention and research. *Family Systems Medicine*, *6*, 202–237. https://doi.org/10.1037/h0089739

Pennebaker, J. W. (1995). *Emotion, disclosure & health*. American Psychological Association.

Pennebaker, J. W., & Traue, H. C. (1993). Inhibition and psychosomatic processes. In H. C. Traue & J. W. Pennebaker (Eds.), *Emotion, Inhibition and Health* (pp. 146–163). Hogrefe & Huber Publishers.

Pillemer, D. B. (1998). *Momentous events, vivid memories.* Harvard University Press.

Pillemer, D. B. (2003). Directive functions or autobiographical memory: The guiding power of the specific episode. *Memory, 11*, 193–202.

Porter, S., & Birt, A. R. (2001). Is traumatic memory special? A comparison of traumatic memory characteristics with memories for other life experiences. *Applied Cognitive Psychology, 15*, 101–117.

Rachman, S. (1980). Emotional processing. *Behaviour Research and Therapy, 18*, 51–60.

Reviere, S. L., & Bakeman, R. (2001). The effects of early trauma on autobiographical memory and schematic self-representation. *Applied Cognitive Psychology, 15*, 89–100.

Robinson, J. A. (1996). Perspective, meaning and remembering. In D. C. Rubin (Ed.), *Remembering our past: Studies in autobiographical memory* (pp. 199–217). Cambridge University Press.

Rorty, A. O. (1988). *The deceptive self: Liars, layers, and lairs.* University of California Press.

Rubin, D. C., Feldman, M. E., & Beckham, J. C. (2004). Reliving, emotions and fragmentation in the autobiographical memories of veterans diagnosed with PTSD. *Applied Cognitive Psychology, 18*, 17–35.

Ruini, C., Offidani, E., & Vescovelli, F. (2015). Life stressors, allostatic overload, and their impact on posttraumatic growth. *Journal of Loss and Trauma, 20*(2), 109–122. https://doi.org/10.1080/15325024.2013.830530

Sadaghiyani, S., Belgrade, A., Kira, M., & Lee, F. (2022). Finding strength in adversity: Exploring the process of posttraumatic growth among multicultural individuals. *Cultural Diversity and Ethnic Minority Psychology, 29*(3), 316–331. https://doi.org/10.1037/cdp0000517

Sayar, K., Kirmayer, L. J., & Taillefer, S. S. (2003). Predictors of somatic symptoms in depressive disorder. *General Hospital Psychiatry, 25*(2), 108–114. https://doi.org/10.1016/s0163-8343(02)00277-3

Schuettler, D., & Boals, A. (2011). The path to posttraumatic growth versus posttraumatic stress disorder: Contributions of event centrality and coping. *Journal of Loss and Trauma, 16*(2), 180–194.

Seery, M. D. (2011). Resilience: A silver lining to experiencing adverse life events? *Current Directions in Psychological Science, 20*(6), 390–394. https://doi.org/10.1177/0963721411424740

Selye, H. (1950). Stress and the general adaptation syndrome. *British Medical Journal, 1*(4667), 1383–1392. https://doi.org/10.1136/bmj.1.4667.1383

Taylor, G. J., Bagby, R. M., & Parker, J. D. A. (1997). *Disorders of affect regulation: Alexithymia in medical and psychiatric illness.* Cambridge University Press. https://doi.org/10.1017/CBO9780511526831

Taylor, S. E. (1989). *Positive illusions: Creative self-deception and the healthy mind.* Basic Books.

Taylor, S. E., & Armor, D. A. (1996). Positive illusions and coping with adversity. *Journal of Personality, 64*, 873–898. https://doi.org/10.1111/j.1467-6494.1996.tb00947.x

Tedeschi, R. G., & Calhoun, L. G. (2004). Target Article: "Posttraumatic growth: Conceptual foundations and empirical evidence". *Psychological Inquiry, 15*, 1–18. https://doi.org/10.1207/s15327965pli1501_01

Temoshok, L. R., Waldstein, S. R., Wald, R. L., Garzino-Demo, A., Synowski, S. J., Sun, L., & Wiley, J. A. (2008). Type C coping, alexithymia, and heart rate reactivity are associated independently and differentially with specific immune mechanisms linked to HIV progression. *Brain, Behaviour and Immunity, 22*, 781–792.

Thome, A. (1990). Alexithymia and acquired immune deficiency syndrome. *Psychotherapy and Psychosomatics, 54*, 40–43.

Updegraff, J. A., & Taylor, S. E. (2000). From vulnerability to growth: Positive and negative effects of stressful life events. In J. H. Harvey, & E. D. Miller (Eds.), *Loss and trauma: General and close relationship perspectives* (pp. 3–28). Brunner–Routledge.

Vaillant, G. E. (2000). Adaptive mental mechanisms. Their role in a positive psychology. *American Psychologist, 55*(1), 89–98. https://doi.org/10.1037//0003-066x.55.1.89

Veronese, G., Pepe, A., Massaiu, I., De Mol, A.-S., & Robbins, I. (2017). Posttraumatic growth is related to subjective well-being of aid workers exposed to cumulative trauma in Palestine. *Transcultural Psychiatry, 54*(3), 332–356. https://doi.org/10.1177/1363461517706288

Vogt, D., King, D., & King, L. (2007). Risk pathways in PTSD: Making sense of the literature. In M. Friedman, T. Kean, & P. Resick (Eds.), *Handbook of PTSD: Science and practice* (pp. 99–116). Guildford.

Vollrath, M., & Torgersen, S. (2000). Personality types and coping. *Personality and Individual Differences, 29*, 367–378. https://doi.org/10.1016/S0191-8869(99)00199-3

Vollrath, M., Alnæs, R., & Torgersen, S. (1998). Coping styles predict change in personality disorders. *Journal of Personality Disorders, 12*(3), 198–209. https://doi.org/10.1521/pedi.1998.12.3.198

Vollrath, M., Torgersen, S., & Alnæs, R. (1998). Neuroticism, coping and change in MCMI-II clinical syndromes: Test of a mediator model. *Scandinavian Journal of Psychology, 39*(1), 15–24. https://doi.org/10.1111/1467-9450.00051

Waters, H. S., & Waters, E. (2006). The attachment working models concept: Among other things, we build script-like representations of secure base experiences. *Attachment & Human Development, 8*(3), 185–197.

Wenninger, K., & Ehlers, A. (1998). Dysfunctional cognitions and adult psychological functioning in child sexual abuse survivors. *Journal of Traumatic Stress, 11*, 281–300. https://doi.org/10.1023/A:1024451103931

Wilson, J. P. (2006). The posttraumatic self. In J. P. Wilson (Ed.), *The posttraumatic self: restoring meaning and wholeness to personality* (pp. 9–68). Routledge.

Zoellner, T., & Maercker, A. (2006). Posttraumatic growth in clinical psychology—A critical review and introduction of a two component model. *Clinical Psychology Review, 26*, 626–653. https://doi.org/10.1016/j.cpr.2006.01.008

Index

For the benefit of digital users, indexed terms that span two pages (e.g., 52–53) may, on occasion, appear on only one of those pages.

Tables are indicated by an italic *t* following the page/paragraph number.